THE MYSTERY OF GLAUCOMA

Edited by **Tomas Kubena**
and **Martina Kofronova**

The Mystery of Glaucoma
Edited by Tomas Kubena and Martina Kofronova

Published by InTech
Janeza Trdine 9, 51000 Rijeka, Croatia

Publishing Process Manager Mirna Cvijic

Technical Editor Teodora Smiljanic

Cover Designer InTech Design Team

Additional hard copies can be obtained from orders@intechopen.com

The Mystery of Glaucoma, Edited by Tomas Kubena and Martina Kofronova
p. cm.
ISBN 978-953-307-567-9

For EU product safety concerns:
IN TECH d.o.o., Prolaz Marije Krucifikse Kozulić 3, 51000 Rijeka, Croatia,
info@intechopen.com or visit our website at intechopen.com.

Meet the editors

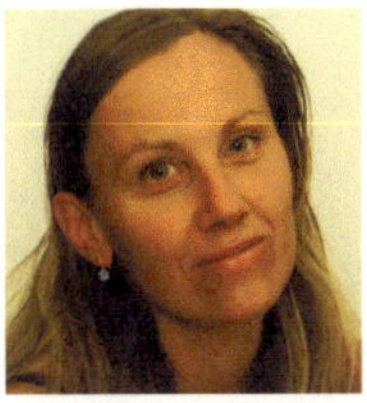

Martina Kofronova M.D., works currently in Glaucoma Service in Zlín, Czech Republic. She is the graduate of the Medical College at Masaryk University in Brno (2003). Since this year, she has been engaged in glaucoma and diabetic retinopathy. She enlarged her education also in the Eye Clinic of the Medical College at Palacky University in Olomouc (2006-2009). She is interested in diagnosis and treatment of patients with vascular dysregulation and also in biomechanical properties of cornea and lamina cribrosa. She presented her findings at international congress in Athens (Greece).

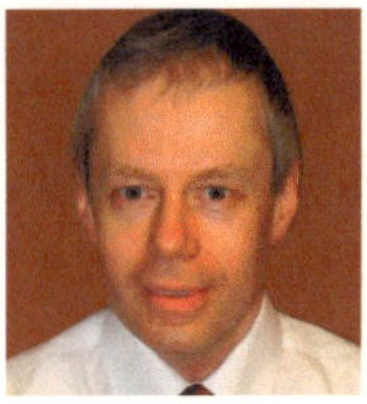

Tomas Kubena, M.D., works currently as head of the Glaucoma Service in Zlin, Czech Republic. He is the graduate of the Medical College at Masaryk University in Brno (1987). Since 1990 he has been engaged in glaucoma and myopia research. He studied glaucoma with Professor G.L.Spaeth at Wills Eye Hospital in Philadelphia (USA) and he is a fellow of Prof. Spaeth. He enlarged his education also in the department of Professor Airaxinen in Oulu (Finland), Professor Kriegelstein in Koln (Germany), and Professor Kessing in Copenhagen (Denmark). He improved the digital planimetry technology of the optic nerve head evaluation and the technology of imaging of retinal nerve fiber layer in a healthy eye and that of glaucoma eye. He presented his findings at the some international congresses: Athens (Greece), Boston (USA), Hong Kong, Taipei (Taiwan) and Hakone (Japan). One of his major concerns- other than medicine- is music- he is an active organ-builder and a local organist as well.

Contents

Preface XI

Part 1 Molecular Biology 1

Chapter 1 **Evidence of Oxidative Stress Damage in Glaucoma 3**
Sandra M Ferreira, Claudia G Reides, Fabián S Lerner and Susana F Llesuy

Chapter 2 **Differential Effects of Elevated Hydrostatic Pressure on Gene Expression and Protein Phosphorylation in Optic Nerve Head Astrocytes 19**
Thomas J. Lukas, Pan Du, Haixi Miao and Simon Lin

Chapter 3 **Homocysteine in the Pathogenesis of Chronic Glaucoma 41**
Mustafa R Kadhim and Colin I Clement

Chapter 4 **Expression of Metabolic Coupling and Adhesion Proteins in the Porcine Optic-Nerve Head: Relevance to a Flow Model of Glaucoma 61**
Francisco-Javier Carreras, David Porcel, Francisco Rodriguez-Hurtado, Antonio Zarzuelo, Ignacio Carreras and Milagros Galisteo

Chapter 5 **Anatomical and Molecular Responses Triggered in the Retina by Axonal Injury 91**
Marta Agudo-Barriuso, Francisco M. Nadal-Nicolás, Guillermo Parrilla-Reverter, María Paz Villegas-Pérez and Manuel Vidal-Sanz

Chapter 6 **Neuroprotective Agents in Glaucoma 115**
Eleni Bagli and George Kitsos

Part 2 Optic Nerve Head and Nerve Fiber Layer 145

Chapter 7 **The Optic Nerve in Glaucoma 147**
Ivan Marjanovic

Chapter 8 **The use of Confocal Scanning Laser Tomography in the Evaluation of Progression in Glaucoma 171**
Liamet Fernández Argones, Ibraín Piloto Díaz, Marerneda Domínguez Randulfe, Germán A. Álvarez Cisneros and Marcelino Río Torres

Chapter 9 **Nerve Fiber Layer Defects Imaging in Glaucoma 187**
Kubena T., Kofronova M. And Cernosek P.

Chapter 10 **Optic Neuropathy Mimicking Normal Tension Glaucoma Associated with Internal Carotid Artery Hypoplasia 199**
Kyoko Shidara and Masato Wakakura

Chapter 11 **Optic Nerve Head Blood Flow in Glaucoma 209**
Tetsuya Sugiyama, Maho Shibata, Shota Kojima and Tsunehiko Ikeda

Part 3 New Possibilities and Genetics 219

Chapter 12 **Measurement of Anterior Chamber Angle with Optical Coherence Tomography 221**
De Orta-Arellano F, Muñoz-Rodriguez P and Salinas-Gallegos JL

Chapter 13 **Association of TNF-α and TNF-β Gene Polymorphisms with Primary Open Angle and Primary Angle Closure Glaucoma 229**
Najwa Mohammed Al- Dabbagh, Nourah Al-Dohayan, Abdulrahman Al-Asmari, Misbahul Arfin and Mohammad Tariq

Chapter 14 **Immune Modulation in Glaucoma – Can Manipulation of Microglial Activation Help? 257**
Kin Chiu, Kwok-Fai So and Raymond Chuen-Chung Chang

Chapter 15 **Stem Cell Based Therapies for Glaucoma 269**
Hari Jayaram, Silke Becker and G. Astrid Limb

Chapter 16 **Functional and Structural Evaluation of Retrobulbar Glaucomateus Damage 293**
Kaya N Engin

Chapter 17 **Central Changes in Glaucoma: Neuroscientific Study Using Animal Models 307**
Kazuyuki Imamura, Masamitsu Shimazawa, Hirotaka Onoe, Yasuyoshi Watanabe, Kiyoshi Ishii, Chihiro Mayama, Takafumi Akasaki, Satoshi Shimegi, Hiromichi Sato, Kazuhiko Nakadate, Hideaki Hara and Makoto Araie

Chapter 18 **Using Artificial Neural Networks to Identify Glaucoma Stages 331**
Gustavo Santos-García and Emiliano Hernández Galilea

Preface

Since long ago scientists have been trying hard to show up the core of glaucoma. To its understanding we needed to penetrate gradually to its molecular level. The newest pieces of knowledge about the molecular biology of glaucoma are presented in the first section.

The second section deals with the clinical problems of glaucoma. Ophthalmologists and other medical staff may find here more important understandings for doing their work. What would our investigation be for, if not owing to the people's benefit?

The third section is full of new perspectives on glaucoma. After all, everybody believes and relies – more or less – on bits of hopes of a better future. Just let us engage in the mystery of glaucoma, to learn how to cure it even to prevent suffering from it.

Each information in this book is an item of great importance as a precious stone behind which genuine, through and honest piece of work should be observed.

It is a point of honour to edit such a book.

Tomas Kubena, M.D.
Head of the Glaucoma service, Zlin, Czech Republic

Martina Kofronova, M.D.
Glaucoma service, Zlin, Czech Republic

Part 1

Molecular Biology

1

Evidence of Oxidative Stress Damage in Glaucoma

Sandra M Ferreira, Claudia G Reides, Fabián S Lerner and Susana F Llesuy
Laboratory of Free Radical Biology (PRALIB, CONICET),
School of Pharmacy and Biochemistry,
University of Buenos Aires, Buenos Aires,
Argentine

1. Introduction

Oxidative stress has been implicated as a risk factor at several levels in the pathophysiology of glaucoma (Ferreira et al., 2004, 2009, 2010) as well as neurodegenerative diseases (Famulari et al., 1996); growing evidence supports the role of oxidative stress in glaucomatous neurodegeneration (Tezel, 2006). Reactive oxygen species are involved in signalling pathways during retinal ganglion cells death by acting as second messengers and/or modulating protein functions (Neufeld et al., 1999). Evidence of oxidative and nitrative processes was found in glaucoma in terms of activity of antioxidant enzymes, levels of low-molecular weight antioxidants and markers of lipid peroxidation (Aslan et al., 2008). Moreover it has been reported that nitric oxide may be an important mediator in retinal ganglion cells death in glaucoma (Neufeld et al., 1997). In the glaucoma eye, an altered oxidant/antioxidant balance may result in a number of molecular changes that contribute to the development of this ocular disease.

Glaucoma is a disease characterized by a specific pattern of optic nerve head and visual field damage in which if it is not controlled may lead to blindness. Although it has been traditionally associated with high intraocular pressure (IOP), glaucoma is now considered as a multifactorial disease. In this context, IOP is the most important known risk factor for the development of glaucomatous optic nerve damage. Even in normal-pressure glaucoma, reducing IOP can be beneficial in terms of halting visual field damage progression. However, lowering IOP may not be enough in every case, since different mechanisms that may or may not depend on the IOP level could contribute to this damage. Proposed mechanisms include ischemia (Lander, 1982), obstruction of axoplasmic flow (Anderson & Hendrickson 1974) and deprivation of one or more trophic factors (Quigley et al., 1995), excitoxicity (Vorwerk et al., 1997) and oxidative stress damage (Ferreira et al., 2004, 2009, 2010).

IOP is not elevated in all the eyes that exhibit characteristics of glaucomatous neurodegeneration but experimental elevation of IOP induces oxidative stress in the retina.

Aqueous humor is known to contain several active oxidative agents such as hydrogen peroxide and superoxide anion. Low molecular weight antioxidants, such as glutathione (GSH), and ascorbate, together with molecules with free radicals scavenging properties like cysteine and tyrosine, have been identified in the aqueous. Ascorbate is present at high concentrations in it (1-2 mM) (Richer & Rose, 1998) and antioxidant enzymes such as superoxide dismutase (SOD), catalase and glutathione peroxidase have been reported in aqueous humor (Garland, 1991; Varma, 1987).

It has been suggested that a chronic oxidative stress insult induced by this agents can compromise the trabecular meshwork function, the major route for aqueous outflow from the anterior chamber. The trabecular meshwork (TM) is exposed to chronic oxidative stress over the course of lifetime and therefore it has a sophisticated defense mechanism against ROS. Previous studies estimated that the rate of loss of cells of the TM is linear and approximately 0.58 % per year from birth through 81 years old (De la Paz & Epstein, 1996).

Exfoliation syndrome (XFS) is a clinically significant systemic disorder, involving abnormal production or turnover of extracellular matrix material or a combination of both processes (Ritch & Schlötzer-Schrehardt, 2001). The exact etiology of this syndrome remains unknown; the most accepted theory postulates that it is an age-related process of buildup of an abnormal elastotic material (Schlötzer-Schrehardt & Naumann, 2006). XFS is the most common cause of secondary open-angle glaucoma (Ritch, 1994). It is a generalized age-related disorder of the extracellular matrix with abnormalities in the basal membranes. Exfoliation syndrome: The clinical diagnosis is made by the presence of exfoliative material on the surface of the anterior capsule of the lens. Exfoliative material may also be present in the corneal endothelium and the trabecular meshwork. Other clinical features include atrophy of the pupillary border and iris transillumination defects (Naumann et al., 1998).

XFS may be associated with ocular problems such as high intraocular pressure (IOP), and glaucomatous optic neuropathy. It may be also associated with poor mydriasis, zonular instability, corneal endotheliopathy, central retinal vein occlusion and cataract (Ritch & Schlötzer-Schrehardt, 2001). Systemic associations found in XFS include angina pectoris, hypertension, myocardial infarction, and stroke. An active involvement of the trabecular meshwork in this abnormal matrix process that leads to a progressive accumulation of XFS material in the juxtacanalicular tissue is considered as the possible cause of chronic high pressure in XFS eyes (Schöltzer-Schrehardt et al., 1992; Koliakos et al., 2001). The principal ocular cells implicated in the production XFS material are those closely associated with the aqueous humor circulation and are influenced by the substances that are present in it. Increasing evidence suggests that ascorbic acid plays an important role in the defense mechanisms of the ocular tissues against free radical damage (Varma, 1987, 2001). A decrease in ascorbic acid and an increase of 8-isoprostaglandin F2a have been reported in the aqueous humor of patients with XFS (Koliakos et al., 2003). The principal ocular cells implicated in the production of exfoliative material are those closely associated with the aqueous humor circulation and are influenced by the substances present in it. Investigation of qualitative and quantitative alterations of the aqueous humor composition might, therefore, provide an important insight into the factors involved in this disorder. Recent studies reported differences in the concentration of matrix metalloproteinases (Schöltzer-Schrehardt et al., 2003) and growth factors (Koliakos et al., 2000, 2001) in the aqueous humor of XFS patients. It is well known that growth factors and proteases can be activated by free radicals, so the occurrence of oxidative stress and therefore the antioxidant status of the aqueous humor may play a role in the oxidative metabolism of the cells implicated in the production of exfoliative material.

The antioxidant status was evaluated in order to assess the occurrence of oxidative stress in the aqueous humor of glaucoma patients. It was meassured through the determination of Total Reactive Antioxidant Potential (TRAP) levels and antioxidant enzymes activities. Antioxidant status of biological samples is regarded as an indicator of oxidative stress (Evelson et al., 2001). A decrease in the antioxidant capacity of tissues and body fluids may

be the consequence of increased oxidative processes. The activities of superoxide dismutase, glutathione peroxidase and catalase were determined in the aqueous humor of both types of glaucoma patients and compared with those measured in control group.
An experimental glaucoma model in rats was performed by our group in order to evaluate the time course changes in oxidative stress markers. This model induced high intraocular pressure and optic nerve head damage. It appears to mimic features of primary open angle glaucoma; therefore, it may be useful to understand the time-course of this ocular disease (Ferreira et al., 2010).
The relationship between the development of glaucoma and oxidative stress was evaluated. The occurrence of oxidative stress was evaluated by the following markers: in vivo chemiluminescence of the eye surface, the total antioxidant capacity in the aqueous and vitreous humor, nitrite concentration and markers of lipid peroxidation in the optic nerve head.
Among oxidative stress markers, organ chemiluminiscence seems to afford a non-invasive assay that integratively measures the rate of formation of excited species, mostly singlet oxygen, through the measurement of light emission (Boveris et al., 1985).
Chemiluminiscence from in situ organs is related to the in vivo steady state concentration of reactive oxygen species. An increased chemiluminescence level reflects an increased intracellular concentration of excited states, singlet oxygen, excited carbonyls and peroxyl radicals. Increased levels of chemiluminescence indicated the occurrence of oxidative stress. Therefore chemiluminescence can be considered a non-invasive, nondestructive assay that can be useful in monitoring cellular damage in glaucomatous eyes (Ferreira et al., 2010).

2. Materials and methods

2.1 Aqueous humor sampling

Aqueous humor (0.1 mL to 0.2 mL) was rapidly and carefully collected at the beginning of the surgery through a paracentesis, using a 27 gauge needle connected to a tuberculin syringe under an operating microscope. Aqueous humor was immediately cooled at -70° C and transported to the laboratory to run all the assays. All the samples were protected from light. Samples were evaluated as soon as possible during the first 24 hours after the surgery.

2.2 Patients

Glaucoma patients included in the study had a diagnosis of Primary open angle glaucoma (POAG) or XFG. Structural definition: Vertical C/D of 0.7 or more, asymmetry in the C/D of 0.2 or more and/or thinning of the neuroretinal rim to disc ratio of less than 0.1 with corresponding perimetric damage. The Disc Damage Likelihood Scale system was used to evaluate the rim to disc ratio. Functional definition: Glaucoma hemifield test outside normal limits, and 3 adjacent points in the 5% level on the pattern deviation plot, using the 24-2 strategy of the Humphrey perimeter. Visual fields were considered reliable if false negative and false positive responses were below 33%. Unreliable visual fields were repeated on the same day. If the second visual field was also unreliable, inclusion was made only on the basis of structural damage (Foster et al., 2002; Quigley et al., 2001).
All individuals had advanced glaucoma and elevated IOP despite the use of maximum tolerated medical therapy, and were scheduled for trabeculectomy. Patients with glaucoma (XFG and POAG) were using a variety of topical anti-glaucoma medications. Maximal tolerated medical therapy usually included a combination of timolol-dorzolamide (or timolol and brimonidine), although we have eliminated patients on prostaglandin analogues. Anti-glaucoma medications were not stopped before the procedures. Patients

enrolled in the cataract group had senile cataract. Cataract patients received topical phenylephrine and tropicamide as dilating drops before surgery. Non-steroidal anti-inflammatory agents were not administered before the procedure. All patients in this group, did not have glaucoma. In all cases, this was the first intraocular surgical procedure.
All subjects underwent a complete ophthalmic examination. This included an anamnesis, best corrected visual acuity, slit-lamp examination, Goldmann applanation tonometry, and fundus examination with a dilated pupil. Gonioscopy was performed in all cases with a 4-mirror goniolens. All subjects (POAG and XFG) had an open-angle (grade 3 or 4 of the Shaffer classification). The optic nerve was evaluated with a 78 diopter lens, and the vertical and horizontal cup to disc ratio (C/D) was recorded, as well as the presence of any notch or hemorrhage, and the appearance of the neuroretinal rim. Computerized perimetry was performed with the Humphrey 750, threshold strategy 24-2, or similar program with the Octopus. In all glaucoma patients, no other explanation for the optic nerve damage and the visual field loss should be found apart from the glaucoma.
XFS was defined by the presence of exfoliation material on the anterior surface of the lens. Exfoliation material was also investigated in the pupillary border, corneal endothelium, anterior hyaloid, and angle. However, for the diagnosis of XFS only the presence of material in the anterior surface of the lens was considered. This surface, with the pupil dilated, was carefully examined for the presence of the exfoliative material, using the high magnification of the slit-lamp and adequate illumination. Patients with previous intraocular surgeries, laser treatment, uveitis, any posterior segment pathologies, diabetes mellitus or any other systemic disease that may have influenced the measurements were excluded. Patients with other ophthalmic conditions such as angle-closure, low-tension, congenital glaucoma, trauma, or pigment dispersion syndrome were excluded. None of the subjects smoked, had special diets, or were taking antioxidant vitamins, such as α-tocopherol, ascorbic acid, nonsteroidal anti-inflammatory agents, or on prostaglandin analogues treatment. The only systemic medications allowed were those for blood hypertension.
The patients were divided into three groups: patients with XFG, POAG and cataract. Each group consisted of 25 patients. All subjects were Caucasians and matched for age and sex. There were no statistically significant differences between the groups in terms of age and sex. Age was 73 ± 2 years old for the XFG group, 70 ± 10 years old for the POAG group, and 73 ± 2 years old for the cataract group.
Preoperative intraocular pressure (IOP) was 25 ± 5 mmHg for the XFG patients, 26 ± 4 mmHg for the POAG group and 14 ± 6 mmHg for the cataract group.
Vertical cup/disc ratio was 0.89 ± 0.01 for XFG patients and 0.89 ± 0.01 for the POAG group. A total of 75 aqueous humor samples were analysed, 25 for each of the following groups: patients with XFG, POAG and cataract. Aqueous humor samples were compared regarding the alterations in the levels of non-enzymatic antioxidants with two parameters: ascorbic acid concentration and the total reactive antioxidant potential. The activities of the antioxidant enzymes: glutathione peroxidase, catalase and superoxide dismutase were also measured. This study was approved by the Human Subjects Commitee of the University of Buenos Aires, and adhered to the Declaration of Helsinki. A written informed consent was obtained from all participants.

2.3 Experimental glaucoma model

The chronic ocular hypertension model following episcleral venous occlusion in rats was used (Shareef et al., 1995). Female Wistar rats (n= 18) weighting 250-300 g were operated under a microscope with a coaxial light. Animals were anesthetized with ketamine hydrochloride (50 mg/ kg) and xylazine hydrochloride (0.5 mg/ kg) administrated intraperitoneally. A specially designed small lid speculum was used to retract the eyelids. One drop of 0.5% proparacaine hydrochloride (Alcon Laboratorios Argentina) was instilled. Vannas scissors and a conjunctiva forceps were used to open the conjunctiva and expose the limbal veins. A cyclodyalisis spatula was used to gently lift the vein from the underlying sclera, and an ophthalmic cautery was used to cauterize the vein. Care was taken in order not to damage the sclera. Two of the large veins of the left eye were cauterized using this method for the glaucoma group (n=9). Retraction without bleeding was noted after cauterization. Only one eye per animal was used for the experiment.

A sham operation without cauterizing the vessels was performed in the left eye of the control group (n= 9). The right eye was only controlled in both groups.

Rats were housed in standard animal room in a 12 hours light/ dark cycle and were fed with food and water ad libitum under controlled conditions of temperature (21 ± 2° C) and humidity. After different periods of time (0, 7, 15, 30, 45, 60 days), eyes were enucleated under dim light immediately after anesthesia, and aqueous humor, vitreous humor and retinas were carefully removed. Vitreous and aqueous humor were collected in a syringe under a surgical microscope and the retinas were detached by blunt dissection. Immediately after dissecting, the optic nerves heads were homogenized.

To assess the occurrence of oxidative stress the following markers were evaluated: in vivo chemiluminescence of the eye surface, the total antioxidant capacity in the aqueous and vitreous humor, nitrite concentration and markers of lipid peroxidation (TBARS) in the optic nerve head.

All animals used procedures were in accordance with ARVO Statement for the Use of Animals in Ophthalmic and Vision Research.

3. Results

3.1 Glaucoma patients

The ascorbic acid concentration in the aqueous humor was 230 ± 20 μM for the XFG group, which represents a 45 % decrease when compared to the POAG group. The mean value of the POAG group was 415 ± 17 μM ($p < 0.001$). Ascorbic acid levels of both types of glaucoma were lower than in the cataract group (720 ± 30 μM; $p< 0.001$)

Ascorbic acid was significantly lower (67 %) in the exfoliation group in accordance with previously published values. Significantly reduced levels of ascorbic acid, an important free radical scavenger in the eye, have been reported in the aqueous humor of exfoliation patients, suggesting a faulty antioxidant defense system (Packer et al., 1979). Ascorbic acid is secreted into the aqueous by the ciliary epithelium and is essential in cells for its antioxidant capacity and its role in regenerating vitamin E and glutathione (Koliakos et al., 2003; Zhou et al., 1998). Beside its protective role against free radical damage, ascorbic acid modulates the synthesis of various extracellular matrix molecules such as collagen, elastin, laminin and glycosaminoglycans (Yimaz et al., 2005). The ascorbic acid levels in XFG patients were decreased 45 % compared to POAG patients. These findings seem to be significant because ascorbic acid is essential in cells for its antioxidant capacity and its role in regenerating vitamin E and glutathione (Parker et al., 1979). In addition to the protective role of ascorbic acid against free radical damage, it also modulates the synthesis of various extracellular matrix molecules such as collagen, elastin, laminin and glycosaminoglycans (Zhou et al.,

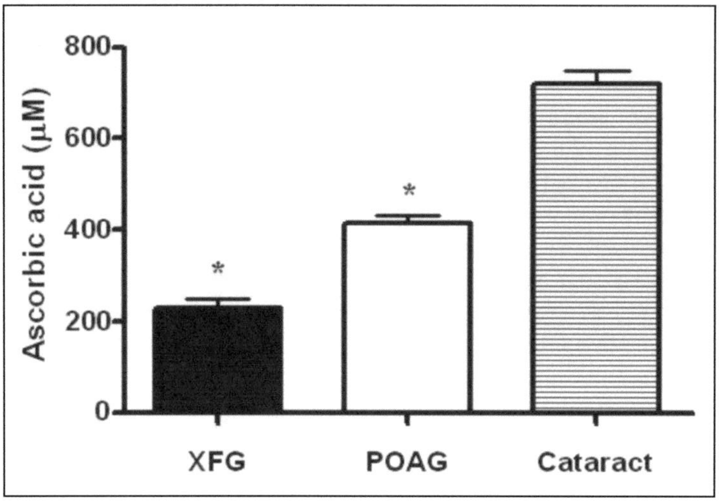

Fig. 1. Ascorbic acid concentration from the aqueous humor in patients with glaucoma associated with exfoliation syndrome (XFG), compared to primary open angle glaucoma (POAG) and cataract patients. The values are represented as mean ± SEM for 25 XFG patients, 25 POAG patients and 25 cataract patients. * $p < 0.001$.

1998). Thus, alterations in ascorbic acid concentrations may produce an increase in the fibrillar material deposits that affect the normal aqueous flow through the trabecular meshwork. Significantly reduced levels of ascorbic acid have been reported in the aqueous humor of exfoliation patients with cataract, suggesting a faulty antioxidant defense system (Koliakos et al., 2002).

The induction time for the aqueous humor from a glaucoma patient was 9.6 minutes, while the same volume of aqueous humor from a control patient rendered an induction time of 39.4 minutes. These results indicate that the concentration of antioxidants in the aqueous humor of glaucoma patients was lower than in control patients. The average TRAP values from glaucoma patients was significantly lower, by 64 %, than that obtained from control patients (124 ± 5 µM; $p < 0.001$). On the other hand, the mean values of the total reactive antioxidant potential were found to be 55 ± 8 µM Trolox in the aqueous humor of POAG group and 28 ± 2 µM Trolox in aqueous humor of the XFG group. In other words, the levels of TRAP were significantly decreased (49 %) in the XFG aqueous humor when compared to the POAG group ($p < 0.001$). TRAP values of both types of glaucoma were lower than the cataract value (124 ± 5 µM Trolox; $p < 0.001$) (Figure 2).

In addition to the decrease in ascorbic acid levels, a significant decay in the aqueous humor total reactive antioxidant potential level of XFG group was found when compared to the POAG group. These results indicate a significant reduction in the concentrations of water-soluble antioxidants in the aqueous humor, such as glutathione, ascorbic acid, tyrosine and cysteine. Homocysteine is a non-essential sulphur aminoacid produced as an intermediate in the metabolism of cysteine. In recent studies, the role of homocysteine in the development of exfoliation glaucoma was investigated (Bleich et al., 2004). The toxicity mechanism of homocysteine may be due to its oxidation in the presence of transition metals, generating superoxide anion, hydrogen peroxide, hydroxyl radical, and sulphurated radicals (Halliwell & Gutteridge , 1989). Homocysteine was found to be elevated in the aqueous humor and

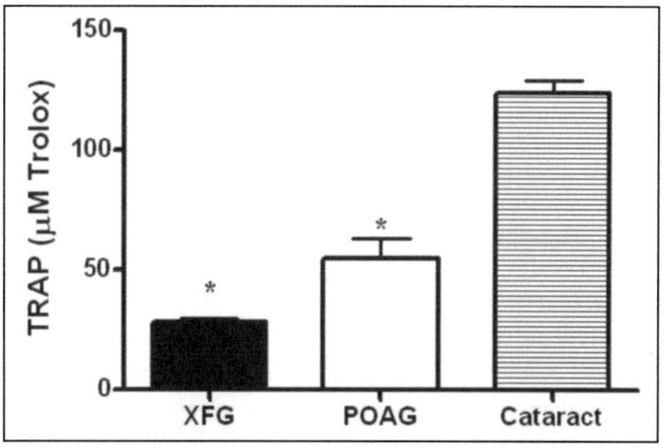

Fig. 2. Total reactive antioxidant potential from the aqueous humor in patients with glaucoma associated with exfoliation syndrome (XFG), compared to primary open angle glaucoma (POAG) and cataract patients. The values are represented as mean ± SEM for 25 XFG patients and 25 POAG patients and 25 cataract patients. * $p < 0.001$.

the plasma of patients with exfoliation syndrome coexistent with cataract and normal IOP (Bleich et al., 2002; Vessani et al., 2003). Moreover, low levels of glutathione were found in the aqueous humor of patients with exfoliation syndrome coexisting with cataract and normal IOP (Gartaganis et al., 2005).

These results indicate a significant reduction in the level of water-soluble antioxidants in the aqueous humor (that includes glutathione, ascorbic acid and tyrosine). These results indicate a significant reduction in the level of water-soluble antioxidants in the aqueous humor, mainly represented by glutathione and ascorbate. This decrease may be due to the occurrence of oxidative stress in a glaucomatous eye that make the organ more susceptible to damage associated with ROS production.

The activity of glutathione peroxidase (GPx), catalase (CAT) levels and superoxide dismutase (SOD) activity, were determined in the aqueous humor of XFG group and compared to those measured in the POAG and cataract groups. A significant increase in GPx activity was found in the aqueous humor of the XFG group, when compared to the POAG group, whereas no significant changes were found in CAT levels and SOD activity. Glutathione peroxidase activity in the aqueous humor of XFG patients showed a 87 % of increase when compared to the POAG group. The mean value of GPx in aqueous humor from the XFG group was 30 ± 2 U/ mL, and for the POAG group was 16 ± 3 U/ mL ($p < 0.001$). GPx of both glaucomas showed an increase when compared to the cataract group (6 ± 2 U/ mL, $p< 0.001$). On the other hand, no significant changes were found in catalase activity. Catalase levels in the aqueous humor from the XFG and POAG groups showed a mean value of 40 ± 5 fmol/ mL, and 42 ± 4 fmol/ mL respectively, while in the cataract patients it was 38 ± 7 fmol/mL. The mean value of SOD in aqueous humor of the XFG group was 44 ± 7 U SOD/ mL versus 42 ± 5 U SOD/ mL in the POAG group. A significant increase of 67% in the superoxide dismutase activity was observed in both glaucoma groups versus the cataract group (27 ± 3 U/ mL, $p< 0.001$), but no changes were found between both glaucomas. A significant increase in SOD and glutathione peroxidase activities was found in the aqueous humor of glaucoma patients, whereas catalase activity was not affected. These results imply a 57 % increase in SOD activity. Glutathione peroxidase activity in the aqueous humor of glaucoma patients showed a threefold increase when compared with value obtained in the control group. The changes observed in the antioxidant enzymes in glaucoma patients are consistent with the presence of oxidative stress.

SOD is an antioxidant key enzyme in the metabolism of oxygen free radicals, as it removes superoxide radical and prevents formation of other reactive radical species, such as peroxynitrite (Aslan et al., 2008). Superoxide anion is the first species in the cascade of univalent reductions of molecular oxygen and therefore the first indicator of an increased production of ROS. Steady state concentrations of superoxide anion are directly proportional to its rate of production and inversely proportional to the concentration of scavenging enzymes, such as SOD. Thus alterations in SOD activity will have important consequences on the steady state concentrations of superoxide in the aqueous humor.

Nitric oxide reacts extremely rapidly with superoxide to form peroxynitrite. The deleterious effects of peroxynitrite may be prevented by limiting its formation, lowering the concentration of superoxide radicals by increasing SOD levels (Enghild et al., 1999). When peroxynitrite is added to a biological fluid, rapid losses of important antioxidant defenses, like ascorbic acid, uric acid, and -SH groups present in small molecules and proteins are observed (Giuseppe et al., 1998). If there is an increase of SOD activity, there will be a decrease in superoxide anion and an increase in hydrogen peroxide production.

H_2O_2 is removed by two enzymes: catalase and glutathione peroxidase. Catalase directly catalizes the decomposition of H_2O_2 to ground state oxygen and water. Glutathione peroxidase removes H_2O_2 using glutathione as a cofactor. Hydrogen peroxide is an essential component of several signal transduction pathways (Evelson et al., 2000).

In this pathological condition in the eye, there is an increase rate of superoxide production, which leads to a depletion of low weight molecules antioxidants and an increase in H_2O_2 levels. According to this, glutathione peroxidase activity in the aqueous humor of glaucoma patients was found three fold higher than control group. Glutathione peroxidase activity was found increased and acts as a compensatory mechanism to ameliorate the oxidative stress in the aqueous humor of XFG and POAG patients (Ferreira et al., 2009). No significant changes were found in catalase levels, and this may be due to the nitric oxide (NO) inhibition of the catalase because of the union of NO to the heme group of the enzyme. NO competes with hydrogen peroxide for the union to the complex I of the catalase (Brown, 1995); if catalase is inhibited, hydrogen peroxide has to be metabolized by glutathione peroxidase. Nevertheless, in the present study we did not find any statistically significant differences in superoxide dismutase activity between XFG and POAG groups. Our results indicate that in both glaucoma groups, the activity of superoxide dismutase is increased compared to cataract group. Ischemia produced by changes in IOP and the resultant decrease of oxygen flow into the tissue may lead to an increase in intracellular calcium ions concentration, which may activate proteolysis and lead to conversion of xanthine reductase into xanthine oxidase which produces superoxide anion and a compensatory increase in superoxide dismutase activity (Tezel & Yang, 2004).

3.2 Experimental glaucoma model

Elevated IOP is the most important risk factor in the progression of glaucomatous damage. All animals, without any exception, responded with an increase in IOP after the development of the experimental glaucoma surgery. No differences in the IOP of control eyes were detected during the experimental period. A significantly increase in IOP compared to control eyes was observed at 7 days after the surgery.

Chemiluminescence is the emission of radiation resulting from a chemical reaction. The organ chemiluminescence is a method to evaluate signals of oxidative metabolism. This assay is specific and non-invasive for the organ and provides a time course evaluation of peroxidative breakdown of lipids. The termination reaction of peroxyl radicals and singlet oxygen yield excited states and chemiluminescence in parallel with malondialdehyde production and conjugated lipid dienes.

An analysis of spontaneous eye surface luminescence at 0, 7, 15, 30, 60 days was showed in Figure 3. During the first days the luminescence showed a decreased in the eye photoemission by 22 %, 35 % and 27 %, respectively at 7, 15 and 30 days after the surgery. An increase of 22 % in light emission was observed at 60 days. Chemiluminescence at 0 days was considered as 100 % of light emission and results were relative to this value. At the first 30 days we observed a decrease in the relative chemiluminescence; this situation may be due in part because of the consumption of non-enzymatic antioxidants. Up to 30 days the marked increase in the spontaneous chemiluminescence of the eye appears to indicate an increase in the steady state levels of oxidant species, suggesting the occurrence of oxidative stress. Increased eye chemiluminescence was associated with the development of cell injury after oxidative stress that could not be compensated by the antioxidant defenses.

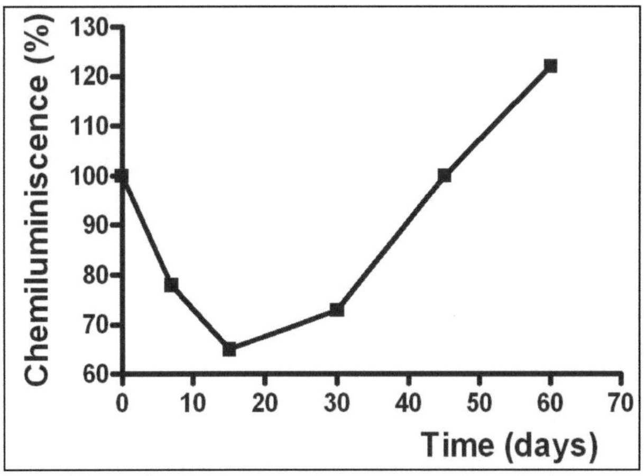

Fig. 3. Analysis of spontaneous chemiluminescence percentage at different times in the eye. surface. Experimental glaucoma model was performed at time 0.

Aqueous humor samples were compared regarding the alterations in the levels of non-enzymatic antioxidants measuring the total reactive antioxidant potential. A significant decrease in levels of non-enzymatic antioxidants was found in the aqueous humor of hypertensive eyes since 15 days after surgery. A significant decrease in TRAP values was observed at 30 days compared to 15 days; on the other hand the levels of this parameter did not change compared to 45 days. At 60 days TRAP levels were significantly higher than at 30 or 45 days, whereas, these levels were significantly lower than at 7 days of treatment (Figure 4).

Figure 5 shows the average of TRAP values in the vitreous humor of rats at 0, 7, 15, 30, 45, and 60 days after surgery. A significant decrease in levels of non-enzymatic antioxidants was found in the vitreous humor of hypertensive eyes since 7 days after surgery. No significant changes were observed in the levels of TRAP at 7 days compared to 15 days.

Since 15 until 60 days there was a significant and progressive decrease in levels of non-enzymatic antioxidants at all over the experimental period. The percent of decrease was 42 % for 15 days, and 78% for 60 days compared to control eyes.

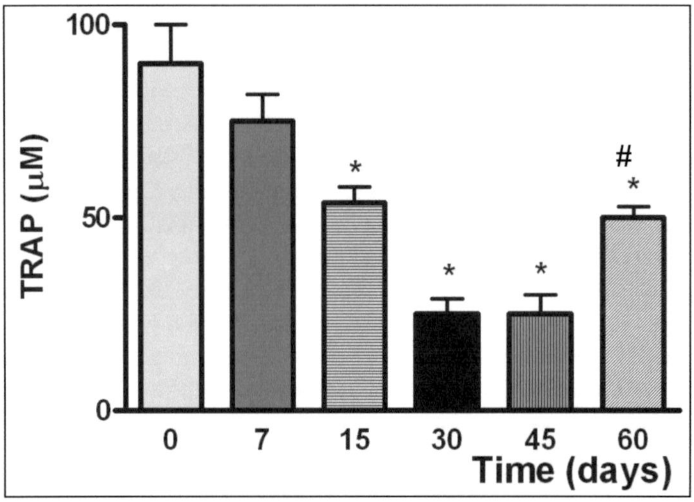

Fig. 4. TRAP in the aqueus humor at different times. Data are mean ± SEM. *$p< 0.05$ versus time 0, # $p<0.05$ versus time 30 and 45 days. Experimental glaucoma model was performed at time 0.

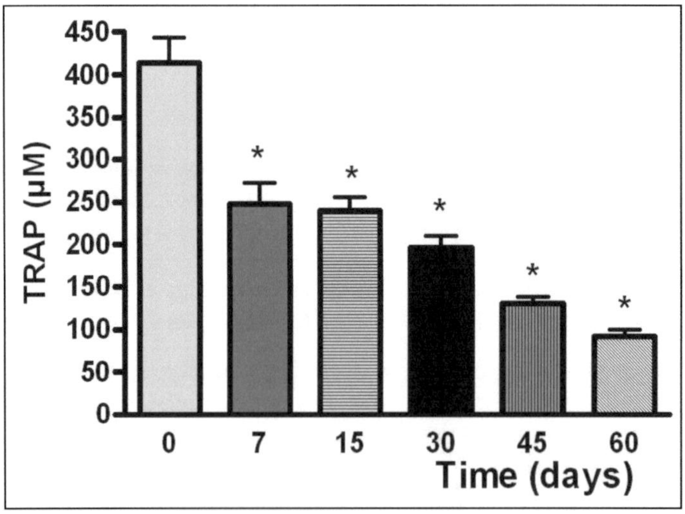

Fig. 5. TRAP in the vitreus humor at different times. Data are mean ± SEM. *$p<0.001$. Experimental glaucoma model was performed at time 0

TBARS levels as an index of lipid peroxidation were assessed in the optic nerve head from the hypertensive rats or from sham rats for the same periods (Figure 6). At 30 days of surgery, TBARS levels were significantly higher (200 %) in hypertensive rats than in sham ones (6.24 ± 0.42 nmol/ mg protein). A further significant increase was observed at 45 and

60 days (300 and 600%). No significant changes were observed at 7 and 15 days compared to control value (6.24 ± 0.42 nmol/ mg protein).
The retina exhibits a distinct susceptibility to oxidative stress due to its enhanced metabolic rate with high levels of oxygen demand, and higher lipid content in its membranes. The TBARS levels support this situation; the increase in them was time-dependent and correlated with high IOP. Figure 6 shown, a significant increase of lipid peroxidation occurred through 15 days after IOP elevation.

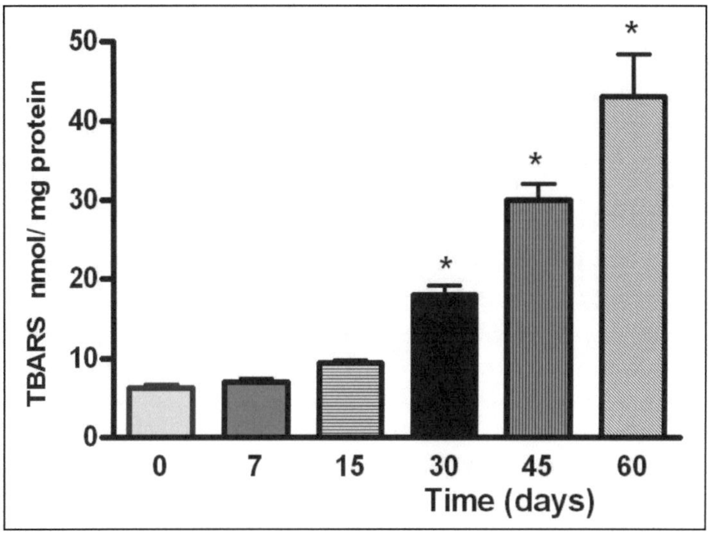

Fig. 6. Optic nerve head TBARS levels at different times. Data are mean ± SEM. *$p<0.001$.
Experimental glaucoma model was performed at time 0.

Negative correlation between TRAP and TBARS levels was found (Ferreira et al., 2010). The levels of lipid peroxidation products are increased meanwhile the levels of non- enzymatic antioxidants are decreased in the optic nerve head of rats with glaucoma. The oxidation of endogenous antioxidants reflects an increase in tissue oxidants that is assessed by the decrease in the total level of antioxidants. These molecules prevent or reduce the extent of the oxidative destruction of biomolecules.
The nitrite levels in the optic nerve head were represented at different times of surgery in Figure 7. A significant increase of nitrite concentration in the optic nerve head was found since 7 days of surgery and this increase was kept up until 60 days of treatment. There was no significant difference between nitrite levels at 7, 15, 30 and 45 days. Nanning et al have demonstrated the release of nitric oxide (NO) by superoxide. This would result in the formation of peroxynitrite that leads to cytotoxic effects in the surrounding cells (Manning et al., 2001). Therefore, NO may be a mediator in ganglion cells death. Different studies showed that NO levels were increased in retinas after IOP elevation (Siu et al., 2002), and increased levels of NOS isoforms in the optic nerve head were reported (Neufeld et al., 1997). NOS inhibitor provided protection for retinal ganglion cells neurodegeneration (Neufeld et al., 1999). Oral administration of an inducible nitric oxide synthase (iNOS) inhibitor did not protect the optic nerve in a rat model (Kasmala et al., 2004), on the other hand another report documented iNOS activity is not elevated in an experimental glaucoma

model (Morrison et al., 2003). The capacity of NO to induce apoptosis have been documented in astrocytes (Hu et al., 1996) and neuronal cells (Heneka et al., 1998). Further detailed studies are required to elucidate and clarify the role of NO in glaucoma.

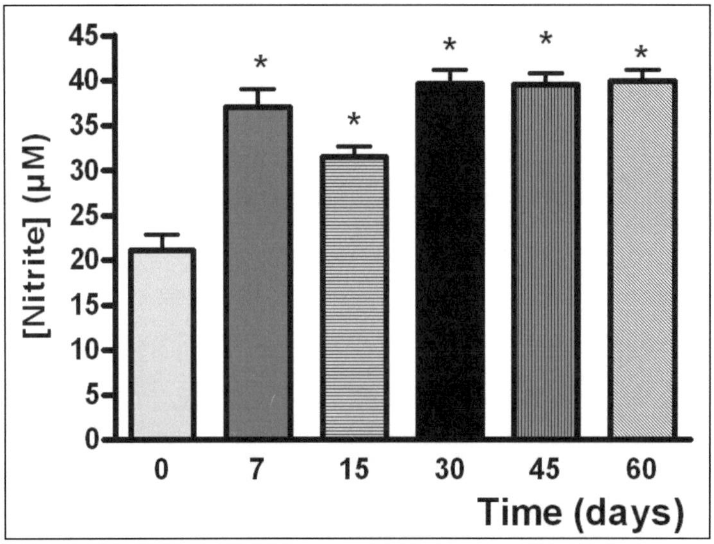

Fig. 7. Nitrite concentration in the optic nerve head at different times. Data are mean ± SEM. *$p<0.001$. Experimental glaucoma model was performed at time 0

4. Conclusion

The defense against the harmful effects of free radicals is achieved by endogenous antioxidant compounds and antioxidant enzymes present in the aqueous humor. The antioxidant status of aqueous humor might therefore provide an important insight into the factors involved in the development of glaucoma. If oxygen active species are implicated in trabecular meshwork cell damage, an associated antioxidant mechanism should be present to repair the oxidative injury.

The changes observed in the antioxidant defenses in the aqueous humor suggest a possible role of the active oxygen species in the tissue damage and the pathogenesis of XFG. Our findings suggest that free radicals action with a depleted endogenous non-enzymatic defense system play a role in the worse damage observed in XFG than in POAG eyes. At any level of IOP, damage in XFG is worse than in POAG, prognosis is also worse, progression is more rapid, response to medical therapy is worse, needs surgery more often and blinds more people. Our results would suggest that further research regarding the use of antioxidants as an adjunct therapy in glaucoma may be indicated. An important goal of future research in glaucoma is therefore to understand the mechanisms of retinal ganglion cell (RGC) death and to develop new ways to treat them. Progressive loss of retinal ganglion cells leads to optic nerve atrophy and visual fields defects in glaucoma patients. Oxidative stress caused by increased generation of reactive oxygen and nitrogen species has been implicated RCG death. Recent in vitro studies using primary culture of RGC have also provided evidence that different glaucomatous stimuli involves increased of reactive oxygen species generation and antioxidant treatment provides additional protection. However, although the involvement of free radicals in the pathophysiology of pseudoexfoliation glaucoma has not been confirmed yet, we suggest their likely role in this disease.

Oxidative stress is thought to contribute to the pathophysiology of many neurodegenerative diseases. The retina contains large amounts of polyunsaturated fatty acids and thus could be susceptible to oxidation by free radicals. Furthermore elevated intraocular pressure or vascular diseases altered blood flow. The consequence decrease in perfusion of the retina and optic nerve head can cause ischemia and this affects retinal ganglion cells survival. Reactive oxygen species are involved in signalling retinal ganglion cells death by acting as a second messenger and/ or modulating protein function. Oxidative stress induces dysfunction of retinal ganglion cells and may contribute to spreading neuronal damage. Chronic elevation of IOP demonstrated significant loss of retinal ganglion cells and has a measurable effect on the redox status.

Spontaneous organ chemiluminescence evaluates the redox status of the tissues in real time in several pathologies, including glaucoma. Spontaneous chemiluminescence of the eye in rats with experimental glaucoma and in control ones was measured for the first time in order to be a useful tool for studying the time course change of oxidative stress.

Reactive oxygen and nitrogen species were increased in glaucoma; this could be evidenced by the increase in chemiluminescence, nitrite levels and the increase in lipid peroxidation.

The glaucoma model was used to elucidate the role of oxidative stress and allows demonstrating the changes found in previous studies using human subjects with glaucoma.

The increased chemiluminescence observed at a later stage could be due to a decrease in the antioxidant defenses, evidenced by TRAP decrease in aqueous and vitreous humor. The levels of lipid peroxidation products and nitric oxide levels increased during the development of glaucomatous optic neuropathy.

According to several investigation lines, there is increase evidence that oxidative stress may be involved in the development and/ or progression of glaucomatous damage

Cells usually tolerate mild oxidative stress that results in up regulation of antioxidant defense system, in order to restore the antioxidant- oxidant balance.

It seems possible that the decrease in non-enzymatic antioxidant may overcome the ability of cells to resist oxidative damage. The increased levels of lipid peroxidation products and in vivo chemiluminescence demonstrate this damage.

The relationship between oxidative stress and neurodegeneration is not completely clear. Free radicals can act directly as neurotoxic, or may also function as secondary messengers to spread the damage. Our results would suggest that further research regarding the use of antioxidants as an adjunct therapy in glaucoma may be indicated. Treatment interventions to reduce in vivo oxidative stress may be important in patients with this disease. Future studies will improve our knowledge on the mechanisms of damage in glaucoma and thus devise more effective treatments, in addition to IOP reduction.

5. Acknowledgment

This work was supported by a grant (B 024) from the University of Buenos Aires, Argentina.

6. References

Anderson, D.R. & Hendrickson, A. (1974). Effect of intraocular pressure on rapid axoplasmic transport in monkey optic nerve. *Investative Ophthalmology Vision & Science*,Vol. 13, pp 771-783, ISSN 0146-0404.

Aslan, M.; Cort, A. & Yucel I . (2008). Oxidative and nitrative stress markers in glaucoma. *Free Radical Biology & Medicine* , Vol.45, pp.367- 376, ISSN 0891-5849.

Bleich, S.; Junemann, A.; Von Ahsen, N.; Lausen, B.; Ritter, K.; Beck, G.; Nauman, G.O. & Kornhuber, J. (2002) Homocysteine and risk of open-angle glaucoma. *Journal of Neural Transmission* , Vol. 109,pp. 1499-1504,ISSN 0300-9564.

Bleich, S; Roedl, J.; Von Ahsen, N.; Schlötzer-Scherardt, U.; Reulbach, U.; Beck, G., Kruse FE, Naumann, G.O.; Kornhuber, J. & Junemann, A.G. (2004). Elevated homocysteine levels in aqueous humor of patients with pseudoexfoliation glaucoma. *American Journal of Ophthalmology* , Vol. 138, pp. 162-164, ISSN 0002-9394.

Boveris, A.; Llesuy, S. & Fraga, C. (1985) Increased liver chemiluminescence in tumor-bearing mice. *Free Radical in Biology & Medicine*. Vol.1, pp.131-138, ISSN 0891-5849.

Brown, G. Reversible binding and inhibition of catalase by nitric oxide. (1995). *European Journal of Biochemistry*, Vol. 232, pp. 188-191, ISSN 0014-2956.

De la Paz, M. & Epstein, D. (1996). Effect of age on superoxide dismutase activity of human Trabecular Meshwork Invest. *Ophthalmology Vision Science*, Vol.6,No, 37,pp. 1849-1853, ISSN 0146-0404.

Enghild, J.; Thogersen, I.; Oury, T.; Valnickova, Z.; Hojrup, P. & Crapo J. (1999). The heparin binding domain of extracellular superoxide dismutase is proteolytically processed intracellulary during biosynthesis. *Journal of Biological Chemistry*, Vol 274,No 21, pp. 14818-14822, ISSN 0021-9258.

Evelson, P. & González Flecha B. (2000). Time course and quantitave analysis of the adaptive responses to 85% oxygen in the rat lung and heart. *Biochimica et Biophysica Acta.* Vol.1523, pp. 209-216, ISSN 0005-2736.

Evelson, P.; Travacio, M.; Repetto, M., Escobar, M.; Llesuy, S. & Lissi, E. (2001). Evaluation of total reactive antioxidant potential (TRAP) of tissue homogenates and their cytosols. *Archive of Biochemistry and Biophysisc*; Vol.388, pp. 261-266, ISSN 0003-9861.

Famulari,A.; Marschoff, E.; Llesuy, S.; Kohan, S.; Serra, J.; Dominguez, R.; Repetto, M.; Reides, C. & Lustig, E. (1996). The antioxidant enzymatic blood profile in Alzheimer´s and vascular diseases. Their association and a possible assay to differentiate demented subjects and controls. *Journal of Neurological Science.*, Vol 141, pp. 69-78. ISSN 0022-510X

Ferreira, S.; Lerner, F; Brunzini, R.; Evelson, P. & Llesuy, S. (2004). Oxidative stress markers in aqueous humor of glaucoma patients. *American Journal of Ophthalmology,* Vol.137,pp. 62-69, ISSN 0002-9394.

Ferreira, S.; Lerner, F.; Brunzini, R.; Evelson, P. & Llesuy, S. (2009). Antioxidant status in the aqueous humour of patients with glaucoma associated with exfoliation syndrome. *Eye*,Vol. 23, pp. 1691-1697, ISSN 0950-222X .

Ferreira, S.M.; Lerner, F.; Brunzini, R.; Reides, C.G.; Evelson, P.A. & Llesuy, S.F. (2010). Time course changes of oxidative stress markers in rat experimental glaucoma model. *Investigative Ophthalmology Visual Science,*Vol.51,pp. 4635- 4640, ISSN 0146-0404.

Foster, P.J.; Buhrmann, R.; Quigley, H.A. & Johnson, G.J. (2002). The definition and classification of glaucoma in prevalence surveys. *British Journal of Ophthalmology,* Vol.86,pp. 238-242, ISSN 0007-1161.

Garland, D.L. (1991). Ascorbic acid and the eye. *American Journal of Clinical Nutrition,* Vol 54,pp. 1193S-1202S, ISSN 1938-3207.

Gartaganis, S.P. ;Georgakopoulos, C.D.; Patsoukis, N.E.; Gotsis, S.; Gartaganis, V. & Georgiou C. (2005). Glutathione and lipid peroxide changes in pseudoexfoliation syndrome. *Current Eye Research* , Vol. 30,pp. 647-651, ISSN 0271-3683.

Giuseppe, L.; Squadrito, M., & Pryor, W. (1998). Oxidative chemistry of nitric oxide. The roles of superoxide peroxynitrite and carbon dioxide. *Free Radical Biology & Medicine*,Vol. 25, No 475,pp. 392-403, ISSN 0891-5849.

Halliwell, B. & Gutteridge J. (1989). *Free Radicals in biology and medicine* (3rd ed.), Oxford University Press Inc, Clarendon Press, ISBN 9780-19855, Oxford , England.

Heneka, M.T.; Loschmann, P.A.; Gleichmann, M.; Weller, M.; Schulz, J.B.; Wullner, U. & Klockgether, T. (1998) Induction of nitric oxide synthase and nitric oxide mediated apoptosis in neuronal PC12 cells after stimulation with tumor necrosis factor-alpha/lipopolysaccharide. *Journal of Neurochemistry*. Vol.71, pp.88-94, ISSN 1471-4159.

Hu, J, & Van Eldik, L.J. (1996). S100 beta induces apoptotic cell death in cultured astrocytes via nitric oxide-dependent pathway. *Biochimica et Biophysica Acta*. Vol. 1313, pp.239-245, ISSN 0005-2736.

Kasmala, L.T.; Ransom, N.L.; Conner, J.R. & Mc Kinno, S.J. (2004). Oral administration of SC-51, a nitric oxide synthase inhibitor, does not protect optic nerve axons in a hypertensive rat model of glaucoma. *Investigative Ophthalmology Visual Science*. Abstract 904. ISSN 0146-0404.

Koliakos, G.; Konstas, A.; Schlötzer-Scherardt, U.; Bufidis, N. & Ringvold, A. (2002). Ascorbic acid concentration is reduced in the aqueous humor of patients with exfoliation syndrome. *American Journal of Ophthalmology*,Vol. 134, pp. 879-883, ISSN 0002-9394.

Koliakos, G; Konstas, A.; Schlötzer-Schrehardt, U.; Hollo, G.; Katsimbris, I,; Georgiadis, N. & Ritch, R.(2003). 8-isoprostaglandin F2a and ascorbic acid concentration in the aqueous humor of patients with exfoliation syndrome. *British Journal of Ophthalmology*, Vol. 3,No. 87, pp. 353-356, ISSN 0007-1161.

Koliakos, G.; Konstas, A.; Triantos, A. & Ritch, R. (2000). Increased growth factor activity in the aqueous humor of patients with exfoliation syndrome. *Graefes Archive for Clinical and Experimental Ophthalmology*,Vol. 238, pp. 491-495, ISSN 0721-832X.

Koliakos, G.; Schöltzer-Schrehardt, U.; Konstas, A.G.; Bufidis, T.; Georgiadis, N. & Dimitriadou, A. (2001). Transforming and insulin-like growth factors in the aqueous humor of patients with exfoliation syndrome. *Graefes Archive for Clinical and Experimental Ophthalmology*,Vol. 239,pp. 482-487, ISSN 0721-832X.

Landers, M.B. (1982). *Glaucoma*. WB Saunders Co. Philadelphia, United States of America

Manning, P.; Cookson, M.R.; Mc Neil, C.; Figlewicz, D. & Shaw, P.J. (2001) Superoxide-induced nitric oxide release from cultured glial cells. *International Brain Research*. Vol.911,pp.203-210, ISSN 0306-4522.

Morrison, J.C.; Johnson, E.C.; Shepard, A.R.; Cepma, W.O. & Clark, A.F. (2003) Inducible nitric oxide synthase (iNOS) in a rat model of glaucoma with chronic elevated intraocular pressure resulting from aqueous humor outflow obstruction. *Investigative Ophthalmology Visual Science*. Vol.44, pp.2101-2007, ISSN 0146-0404.

Naumann, G.; Schlötzer-Schrehardt, U. & Küchle, M.(1998). Pseudoexfoliation Syndrome for the comprehensive ophthalmologist. Intraocular and systemic manifestations. *Ophthalmology* ,Vol. 105, pp. 951-968, ISSN 096-4488.

Neufeld, A.; Hernandez, M.R. & Gonzalez, M. (1997) Nitric oxide synthase in human glaucomatous optic nerve head. *Archives of Opthalmology*. Vol.115, pp. 497-503,ISSN: 1538-3601.

Neufeld, A.; Sawada, A. & Becker, B. (1999) Inhibition of nitric oxide synthase 2 by aminoguanidine provides neuroprotection of retinal ganglion cells in rat model of chronic glaucoma. *Proceedings of the National Academy of Sciences of the United States of America*. Vol.96, pp.9944-9948, ISSN 0027-8424.

Packer, J.E.; Slater, T.F. & Willson, R.L.(1997). Kinetic study of the reaction of vitamin C with vitamin E radicals (tocopheroxyls) in solutions. *Nature,* Vol. 278,pp. 737-738, ISSN 0028-0836.

Quigley, H.A.; West, S.K., Rodriguez, J.; Muñoz, .B; Klein, R. & Snyder, R. (2001). The prevalence of glaucoma in a population-based study of hispanic subjects. *Archive of Ophthalmology*, Vol. 119, pp. 1819-1826. ISSN 1538-3601.

Richer, S.P. & Rose, R,C. (1998). Water soluble antioxidants in mammalian aqueous humor. Interaction with UV and Hydrogen peroxide. *Vision Research.*, Vol. 38,No 19,pp. 2881-2888, ISSN 0042-9689.

Ritch, R. & Schlötzer-Schrehardt U. (2001). Exfoliation Syndrome. *Survey Ophthalmology,* Vol. 45,pp. 265-315, ISSN 0039-6257.

Ritch, R. (1994). Exfoliation syndrome: The most common identifiable cause of open-angle glaucoma. *Journal of Glaucoma,*Vol. 3, pp. 176-178, ISSN 1536-481X.

Schlötzer-Schrehardt, U. & Naumann, G. (2006). Ocular and systemic pseudoexfoliation syndrome. *American Journal of Ophthalmol*ogy, Vol. 141, pp. 921-937, ISSN 0002-9394.

Schöltzer-Schrehardt, U.; Lommatzsch, J.; Küchle, M.; Konstas, A. & Naumann G. (2003). Matrix metalloproteinases and their inhibitors in aqueous humor of patients with exfoliation syndrome glaucoma and primary open-angle glaucoma. *Investigation Ophthalmolology Vision &Science,* Vol. 44, pp. 1117-1125, ISSN 0146-0404.

Schlötzer-Schrehardt, U.; Koca, M.R. & Naumann, G. (1992). Pseudoexfoliation syndrome. Ocular manifestation of a systemic disorder?. *Archive of Ophthalmology* ,Vol. 110, pp. 1752-1756, ISSN 1538-3601.

Shareef, S.R.; Garcia-Valenzuela, E.; Salierno, A. ; Walsh, J. & Sharma, S.C. (1995) Chronic ocular hypertension following episcleral venous occlusion in rats. *Experimental Eye Research.* Vol.61, pp.379-382, ISSN 0014-4835.

Siu,A.W.; Leung, M.C.; To, C.H.; Siu, F.K.; Ji, J.Z. & So, K.F. (2002). Total retinal nitric oxide production is increased in intraocular pressure elevated rats. *Experimental Eye Research.* Vol.75, pp. 401-406, ISSN 0014-4835.

Tezel, G. (2006) Oxidative stress in glaucomatous neurodegeneration: Mechanisms and consequences). *Progress in Retin Eye Reesarch.*Vol.25, pp.490-513, ISSN 1350-9462.

Tezel, G. & Yang, X. (2004). Caspase - Inde pendent component of retinal ganglion cell death in vitro. *Investigative Ophthalmology Visual Science.*, 45, 4049. ISSN 0146-0404.

Varma, S.D. (1987) Ascorbic acid and the eye with special reference to the lens. Annals of the New York Academic of Sciences; 498: 280-306, ISSN 0077-8923.

Varma, S.D. (1991). Scientific basis for medical therapy of cataracts by antioxidants. *American Jounal of Clinical Nutrition* , Vol.53, pp. 335-345, ISSN 002-9165.

Vessani, R.; Ritch, R.; Liebmann, J. & Jofe, M. (2003). Plasma homocysteine is elevated in patients with exfoliation syndrome. *American Journal of Ophthalmology*, Vol 136,pp. 41-46, ISSN 0002-9394.

Vorwerk, C.K.; Hyman, B.T.; Miller, J.W.; Husain, D.; Zurakowiski, D.; Huang, P.l.; Fishman, M.C. & Dreyer, E.B.(1997). The role of neuronal and endothelial nitric oxide synthase in retinal excitotoxicity. *Investigative Ophthalmology Visual Science.* Vol. 38,pp2038-2044,ISSN 0146-0404.

Yimaz, A.; Adiguzel, U.; Tamer, L.; Yildirim, O.; Oz, O.; Vatansever, H; Ercan, B.; Degirmenci, U.S. & Atik, U. (2005). Serum oxidant/ antioxidant balance in exfoliation syndrome. *Clinical & Experimental Ophthalmology.* Vol.33, pp63-66, ISSN 1442-9071.

Zhou. L.; Higginbotham, E. & Yuc, B. (1998). Effects of ascorbic on levels of fibronectin, laminin and collagen type1 in bovine trabecular meshwork in organ culture. *Current Eye Research,*Vol 17, pp. 211-217, ISSN 1442-6404.

2

Differential Effects of Elevated Hydrostatic Pressure on Gene Expression and Protein Phosphorylation in Optic Nerve Head Astrocytes

Thomas J. Lukas, Pan Du, Haixi Miao and Simon Lin
Northwestern University, Feinberg School of Medicine, Chicago, IL
United States

1. Introduction

1.1 Primary Open Angle Glaucoma (POAG)

Elevated intraocular pressure (IOP) is the most important risk factor in POAG. Typically affecting older adults, in POAG the IOP exceeds the level that is tolerated by that individual's optic nerve head (ONH). However, many individuals with clinical ocular hypertension do not exhibit glaucomatous changes in the optic disk; whereas, some individuals will develop glaucomatous changes at clinically normal IOP levels. These clinical findings indicate that individual variability in susceptibility of the ONH to IOP is an important factor in glaucomatous optic neuropathy. However, the molecular and cellular factors that may underlie variability in susceptibility of the ONH to elevated IOP have not been elucidated.
The target of the mechanical stress generated by elevated IOP is the lamina cribrosa in the ONH (Bellezza et al., 2003). In the glaucomatous ONH, compression, stretching, and remodeling of the cribriform plates of the lamina cribrosa occur. In many POAG patients, these elevated IOP related changes result in remodeling of the extracellular matrix (ECM), altering the quantity and composition of several ECM macromolecules that significantly affect the biomechanical properties of the tissue supporting the nerve fibers (Hernandez, 2000; Bellezza et al., 2003). Alterations of ECM components of the ONH in glaucoma perhaps sets the stage for further optic nerve damage from IOP during the progression of the disease.

1.2 POAG in African Americans

Epidemiological and genetic studies indicate that ethnic/genetic background plays an important role in susceptibility to POAG. POAG is more prevalent in Black Americans of African ancestry (AA) than in White Americans of European ancestry (CA), with reported frequencies of 3-4% in the AA population over the age of 40 years, as compared with approximately 1% in CA populations (Friedman et al., 2004). The disease is particularly frequent in Afro-Caribbean populations, with prevalence of 7% in Barbados and 8.8% in St. Lucia (Nemesure et al., 2001). On average AAs have increased duration (Quigley and Vitale, 1997) and progression of disease (Broman et al., 2008) compared to other populations. A positive family history of POAG is a major risk factor for the disease in AA (Leske et al.,

2008). The Advanced Glaucoma Intervention Study (AGIS), which compared the glaucoma outcomes in AA and CA patients, concluded that after failure of medical therapy, surgical trabeculectomy delayed progression of glaucoma more effectively in CA than in AA patients (Beck, 2003; Ederer et al., 2004). AAs have significantly larger disc areas, larger cup areas, larger cup-to-disc ratios and smaller neural rim area-to-disc area ratios compared with CAs (Varma et al., 1994; Quigley et al., 1999). A morphometric study determined that AAs have a larger total area of the lamina cribrosa and a greater number of pores than CAs (Dandona et al., 1990). The cellular and molecular bases for these anatomic differences and disease prevalences have not been explored.

Our studies focus on how astrocytes in the lamina cribrosa of the human optic nerve head contribute to glaucomatous optic neuropathy that is associated with elevated IOP. There is mounting evidence that astrocytes are responsible for many of the pathological changes in the glaucomatous ONH and cells isolated from donors of different ethnic backgrounds vary in their gene expression (Miao et al., 2008; Hernandez et al., 2008). Cellular explanations for these population-related differences may be realized using primary ONH astrocytes as a source of differing cellular phenotypes and an *in vitro* system to simulate elevated IOP.

1.3 Astrocytes in the ONH

Astrocytes are the major glial cell type in the non-myelinated human ONH and provide cellular support functions to the axons while interfacing between connective tissue surfaces and surrounding blood vessels. In the normal ONH, astrocytes are quiescent, terminally differentiated cells. In the lamina cribrosa, quiescent astrocytes form lamellae oriented perpendicular to the axons surrounding a core of fibroelastic extracellular matrix (Hernandez, 2000). Astrocytes supply energy substrates to axons in the optic nerve and maintain extracellular pH and ion homeostasis in the periaxonal space (Fields and Stevens-Graham, 2002). ONH astrocytes express ECM proteins such as laminin, and proteoglycans, as well as bone morphogenetic proteins (Zode et al., 2007; Wordinger et al., 2002) neurotrophins and receptors (Lambert et al., 2004; Yang et al., 2007). Several of these may serve as neuroprotective factors for retinal ganglion cells (RGC). In addition to astrocytes, other cell types exist in the lamina cribrosa of humans and non human primates, including microglia, vascular endothelia and the lamina cribrosa cell. Lamina cribrosa cells can be distinguished from astrocytes because they do not express glial fibrillary acidic protein (GFAP) and they do not express vascular or microglial markers (Hernandez et al., 1988; Kirwan et al., 2005; Hernandez et al., 1989).

1.4 Reactive ONH astrocytes in glaucoma

Adult, quiescent astrocytes become "reactive" after injury or disease and participate in formation of a glial scar, which does not support axonal survival or growth (Sofroniew, 2005; McGraw et al., 2001; Hatten et al., 1991).The major hallmarks of a reactive astrocyte are an enlarged cell body and a thick network of processes with increased expression of GFAP and vimentin (Hatten et al., 1991). Similarly, reactive astrocytes in the glaucomatous ONH are large rounded cells with many thick processes and express increased amounts of GFAP, vimentin and HSP27 (Hernandez et al., 2008). The astrocytes are motile and migrate either to the edge of the laminar plates or to inside the nerve bundles (Hernandez et al., 2008). In glaucoma, reactive astrocytes exhibit putative neurodestructive and neuroprotective cellular cascades in the ONH (Hernandez and Pena, 1997). Previous studies demonstrated that the genomic responses of astrocytes in the glaucomatous ONH serve as the basis for these cascades (Hernandez et al., 2002). Damage to retinal ganglion cell axons and remodeling of the connective tissue plates in the lamina cribrosa appear to be mediated by astrocytes (Hernandez et al., 2008; Nickells, 2007). Reactive ONH astrocytes increase expression of various cell surface and extracellular matrix-related proteins such as laminin, tenascin C, and proteoglycans that play important roles in cell-cell recognition and in cell adhesion (Hernandez et al., 2002; Hernandez and Pena, 1997; Pena et al., 1999b). As might be expected there are also changes in signal transduction in reactive ONH astrocytes (Review (Hernandez et al., 2008)). For example, EGF receptors (Liu et al., 2006) and endothelin B receptors (Wang et al., 2006) are upregulated *in vitro and in vivo.* Finally differential gene expression analysis of human ONH astrocytes (Miao et al., 2008) (CA vs. AA) and astrocytes from AA compared to CA donors with glaucoma (Lukas et al., 2008) has revealed changes in multiple signaling systems that are also found in animal models of glaucoma (Johnson et al., 2007; Yang et al., 2007).

1.5 Susceptibility to glaucoma: Differential expression in the ONH astrocyte transcriptomes from glaucomatous AA and CA donors

Gene expression in primary cultures of ONH astrocytes obtained from age-matched normal and glaucomatous donors of CA and AA populations was done using Affymetrix GeneChip microarrays. Gene Ontology analysis and networks of interacting proteins were constructed using the BioGRID database (Stark et al., 2006). The differential gene expression data were distributed among three networks that include regulation of myosin, actin, and protein trafficking (Lukas et al., 2008). Remarkably, cultured glaucomatous astrocytes retain differential expression of genes that promote cell motility and migration, regulate cell adhesion, and are associated with structural tissue changes during neurodegeneration. Similar changes in gene expression were observed in glaucomatous optic nerve head tissues as assessed by immunohistochemistry (Lukas et al., 2008). Thus, the *in vitro* culture system "remembers" its origins from glaucomatous or control tissue. In these studies, the key differentially regulated genes included myosin light chain kinase (MYLK), TGFß receptor 2 (TGFBR2), Rho-family GTPase-2 (RAC2), and extracellular matrix protein, versican (VCAN). These differentially expressed components of integrated networks may reflect cellular and functional responses to chronic elevated IOP that are enhanced in the glaucomatous astrocytes from AA donors.

1.6 Model systems for glaucomatous astrocytes

One of the significant problems associated with work on glaucomatous astrocytes is that their availability is quite limited as the number of donors with glaucoma is much smaller than donors without eye disease. Therefore, we investigated methods to "transform" normal ONH astrocytes into a preglaucoma or glaucoma-like phenotype. In principle, mechanical stress applied to the cells by way of physical contact (as in the ONH) should mimic the *in vivo* phenotype. Such stress can be done using a mechanical device in which the cells are attached to a deformable surface. Trabecular meshwork (Liton et al., 2005), lamina cribrosa (Kirwan et al., 2004), and smooth muscle cells (Feng et al., 1999) have been studied in such systems to mimic forces of mechanical stretch. Some attempts have been made with astrocytes as well (Neary et al., 2003). However, high force stretch is more often associated with traumatic astrocyte injury (Ni et al., 1997) rather than the lower forces associated with increased IOP in glaucoma. Thus, our *in vitro* IOP model employs elevated hydrostatic pressure in an environmental chamber (Salvador-Silva et al., 2001) that compensates for gas composition and changes in media over time (Yang et al., 2004; Ricard et al., 2000). This model system has been used in a number of studies to study changes in bimolecular and cellular properties associated with this induced stress (Yang et al., 2004; Salvador-Silva et al., 2004; Salvador-Silva et al., 2001; Hernandez et al., 2000; Malone et al., 2007; Yang et al., 1993; Chen et al., 2009; Miao et al., 2010).

2. Results-gene expression studies in ONH astrocytes

2.1 Elevated hydrostatic pressure model system to simulate elevated IOP

We investigated the molecular bases of elevated hydrostatic pressure (HP) responses in primary cultures of ONH astrocytes derived from AA donors compared to CA donors. This model system simulates the mechanical stresses placed upon the optic nerve head by elevated IOP. Using high density microarrays we investigated global changes in gene expression in a cohort of three astrocyte cell lines from each group. We validated changes in expression induced by elevated HP in three to five additional AA and CA astrocyte lines using quantitative RT-PCR and/or Western Blotting. Using a global phosphoproteome approach, we also identified changes in protein phosphorylation associated with elevated HP. In both gene expression and proteome experiments, ONH astrocytes were subjected to elevated HP for periods of 3, 6, 24, and 48 hours. Control cells were cultured under ambient pressure (CP) for 6 or 48 hr. A custom made pressure chamber was used to subject cultured cells (6 well plates) to 60 mm (above atmospheric pressure) of HP for the desired periods of time. In order to compensate for potential changes in dissolved oxygen or pH, the gas mixture in the chamber was adjusted to 8% CO_2 and buffering capacity in the media increased (Yang et al., 2004). Under these conditions changes in dissolved oxygen and pH are negligible during the course of the experiment (Ricard et al., 2000). Messenger RNA and protein were extracted from the cells immediately after the experiment using standard published techniques (Lukas et al., 2008; Miao et al., 2010; Chen et al., 2009). Gene expression was measured using Illumina Human-6 beadchips following the manufacturer's protocols. These microarray chips have ~47,000 features representing ~31,000 human genes and expressed isoforms.

2.2 Microarray data analysis

To best utilize the unique features of Illumina BeadArray technology, we used the Bioconductor lumi package (Du et al., 2008; Lin et al., 2008; Du et al., 2007) to preprocess the raw data output by Illumina Beadstudio software. The data was preprocessed using variance stabilization transformation method (Lin et al., 2008) followed by quantile normalization. Probes with all samples "Absent" (lower or around background levels) were removed from further analysis to reduce false positives.

Two phases of analysis were done. First, to identify differentially expressed genes common to both the AA and CA groups, we applied routines implemented in limma package (Du et al., 2008) to fit linear models to the normalized expression values. The variance used in the t-score calculation was corrected by an empirical Bayesian method (Smyth, 2004) for better estimation with a small sample size. For each time point (3h, 6h, 24h and 48h), we compared all HP samples with the control samples, and defined the differentially expressed genes as fold-change higher than 1.3-fold ($p<0.01$). After this filtering we found 352 genes differentially expressed at least at one time point. In order to reduce variations across different clinical samples, we first normalized the pressure samples at each time point against the control sample from the same eye, then we standardized the normalized expression profile of each gene as one standard deviation and without centering (the fold-change direction is unchanged).

Hierarchical clustering was first applied to get an overview of the cluster distribution, and then we defined initial clusters with visually selected cutoff. Using these initial sets, we did K-Means clustering resulting in 4 clusters that include 67, 137, 56 and 93 genes, respectively. The average changes in expression for each cluster as a function of time of HP treatment are shown in Figure 1. The cluster profile is defined as the average of all gene time profiles in the cluster (solid lines in Figure 1). Clusters 1 and 4 exhibit a decreasing trend of expression, while clusters 2 and 3 have increased expression as a function of time of exposure to elevated HP. The profiles of clusters 3 and 4 exhibit a flattening at the 3 and 6 hr times followed by a continued increase or decrease at 24 and 48 hr. These data suggest that ONH astrocytes respond to elevated HP in a dynamic fashion that involves a fast (3-6 hr) and slower (or protracted) response that follows at 24-48 hr. These responses involve genes in different signaling pathways that define a transition to new cellular phenotypes. As we will demonstrate in subsequent sections, there is overlap between the pressure-induced phenotype and glaucomatous cellular profiles that have been described previously (Hernandez et al., 2002; Nickells, 2007). Similarly, we found that extended HP treatment of ONH astrocytes (72-120 hr) induces further changes in cellular phenotype with respect to the expression of genes that affect cell motility (Miao et al., 2010) and cell morphology (Yang et al., 1993).

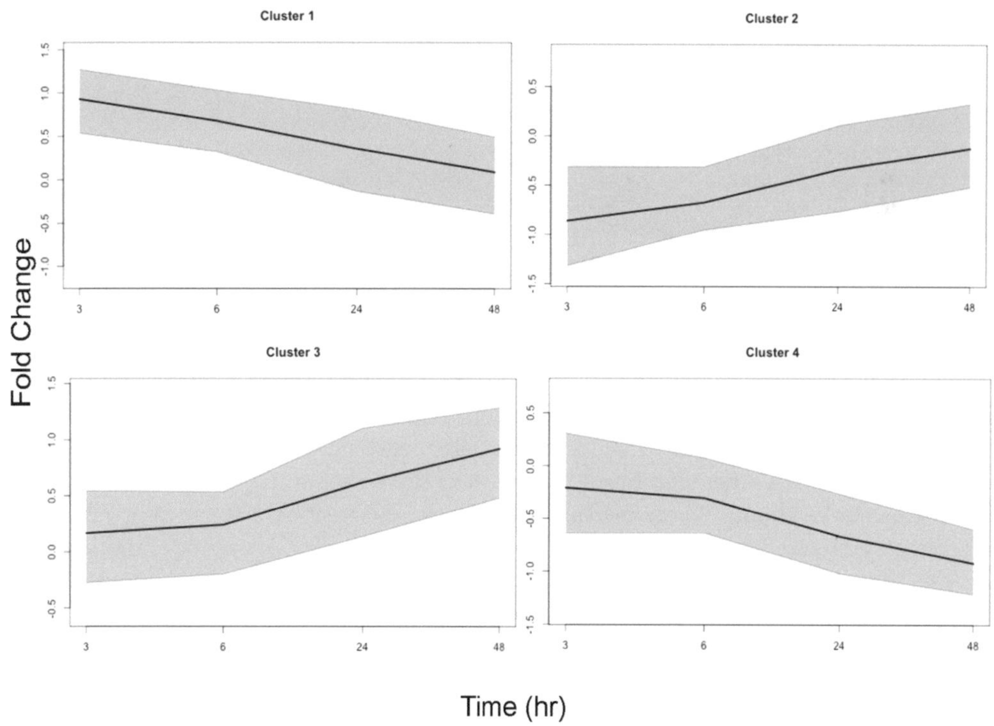

Fig. 1. **Time dependent expression of HP-induced gene clusters.** Solid lines are the fold-change (compared to cells at ambient pressure) average of all genes in the cluster while the gray areas indicate the 95% confidence interval of the averages.

2.3 HP-induced cellular processes in ONH astrocytes

For consistent comparison to the glaucomatous phenotype for ONH astrocytes (Nickells, 2007) we used the GeneGo suite to analyze the differential expression data for our elevated HP data. Using the gene clusters identified above, the genes were mapped onto existing canonical pathways that have been defined within GeneGo (Nikolsky et al., 2005). There are 650 such maps within the GeneGo library. The overrepresentation of genes within a pathway gives a p-value that estimates the significance of the mapped genes. The four top scoring maps for each cluster are summarized in Tables 1 and 2.

	Cluster 1			
	Map	Cell Process	p-value	Objects
1	Estradiol Metabolism		0.00007	3/19
2	Regulation of Triiodothryronine and thyroxine signaling	Transcription	0.0054	2/31
3	Ligand dependent transcription of retinoid target genes	Transcription	0.0047	2/32
4	Androgen receptor nuclear signaling	Transcription	0.0094	2/64
	Cluster 2			
1	Cell cycle-ESR1 regulation of G1/S transition	Response to hormone, extracellular stimulus	0.00001	6/32
2	BMP Signaling/ TGFβ inhibition	Cytokine mediated signaling	0.00033	3/33
3	Cell cycle regulation	Cell cycle	0.0063	3/29
4	Chemokines and cell adhesion	Cell Adhesion	0.0079	3/50

Table 1. **Pathway analysis for Gene Cluster s 1 and 2 ranked by p-value.** The number of objects refers to the enrichment of genes/total gene related objects in the map.

In the first two clusters, the activation of transcription and cytokine mediated signaling are among the most significant pathways. The transcriptional processes decline with increased time of HP suggesting that this is an early response that stabilizes to near control levels at 48 hr. As will be shown later this response also correlates with changes in protein phosphorylation. The other significant pathways in Clusters 1 and 2 are cytokine-related or other extracellular stimuli. These increase with time of HP treatment suggesting a transition to a phenotype associated with increased sensitivity to extracellular agents. In this regard, this cluster includes serotonin receptor 5B (Table 5), a receptor known to be upregulated by mechanical stress (Liang et al., 2006; Sanden et al., 2000).

Cluster 3 genes are found in pathways leading to cytoskeleton remodeling, transport, and other signaling processes. ONH astrocytes undergo changes in morphology after being subjected to elevated HP (Yang et al., 1993) and up-regulation of cytoskeletal signaling processes is consistent with these properties. Moreover, altered cytoskeletal , transport, and cell adhesion gene expression is also found in populations of glaucomatous astrocytes (Lukas et al., 2008).

	Map	Cell Process	p-value	Objects
	Cluster 3			
1	Cell contraction mediated by G-protein coupled receptors	Cytoskeleton	0.0019	3/15
2	Transport_RAB1A regulation pathway	ER-Golgi transport	0.0004	2/12
3	Cytoskeleton remodeling by Rho GTPases	Cytoskeleton	0.0053	4/23
4	Regulation of insulin pathway signaling	Receptor-mediated signaling	0.0050	2/42
	Cluster 4			
1	Transcription - Sin3 and NuRD in transcriptional regulation	Transcription	0.00059	3/38
3	G-protein receptor signaling via cyclic AMP pathways	Extracellular mediated signaling	0.0022	2/52
2	Regulation of lipid metabolism by transcription factor RXR via PPAR, RAR, and VDR pathways	Transcription	0.0075	2/30
4	Slit-Robo signaling in regulation of neuronal axon guidance	Development	0.0075	2/30

Table 2. **Pathway analysis of Cluster 3 and 4 ranked by p-value.** The number of objects refers to the enrichment of genes/total gene related objects in the map

Cluster 4 genes populate a distinct set of pathways in transcription, metabolism, and signal transduction. Inhibition of axonal guidance is altered under elevated HP due to secretion of Slit2/3 (Table 3) by astrocytes decreased with elevated HP over time. Further decreases in transcriptional pathways are evident in Cluster 4 with changes in the retinoid (RXR) based regulatory pathways. The latter involves changes in transcription through the post-translational modification of histones (Figure 2). Thus, besides the decrease in expression histones can undergo acetylation and methylation of lysine residues and phosphorylation of serine/threonine residues that alter chromatin structure and the transcription of specific DNA regions (Oki et al., 2007; Ito, 2007). As shown below we detected phosphorylation of lysine methyltransferase enzymes in ONH astrocytes at early time points of treatment with elevated HP. This is particularly interesting because there are few reports of epigenetic changes being induced by mechanical stress (Illi et al., 2005) and none by elevated HP. Thus, the transcriptome of ONH astrocytes may be undergoing reprogramming to accommodate this presence of this stress.

Other pathways represented in Cluster 4 genes that are altered by elevated HP include cyclic-AMP signaling. Our previous studies of short term elevated HP (30 min - 3 hr) treatment of ONH astrocytes revealed that cyclic-AMP signaling is differentially affected in astrocytes from African American donors (Chen et al., 2009). Upregulation of adenylate cyclases and parathyroid hormone-like hormone (PTHLH) that activates G-protein signaling to adenylate cyclases were detected (Chen et al., 2009). In the current work with longer term (24-48 hr) treatment both AA and CA astrocytes down regulate phosphodiesterases (PDE3A, PDE7B (Table 3.) which may result in higher levels of cyclic nucleotides and increased activity of transcription factors such as CREB that are activated by cyclic AMP-dependent phosphorylation (Johannessen et al., 2004; Delghandi et al., 2005).

Symbol	Description		HP3	HP6	HP24	HP48
		Cluster 1				
IL6	interleukin 6 (interferon, beta 2)		2.22	1.41	-1.15	-1.67
TAF5L	TAF5-like RNA polymerase II, p300/CBP-associated factor (PCAF)		1.59	1.24	1.44	1.38
PAG1	phosphoprotein associated with glycosphingolipid microdomains 1		1.44	1.11	-1.11	1.06
WNT5B	wingless-type MMTV integration site family, member 5B		1.38	1.26	1.22	1.08
ELF4	E74-like factor 4 (ets domain transcription factor)		1.37	1.15	1.10	-1.05
ITCH	itchy E3 ubiquitin protein ligase homolog		1.35	1.35	1.18	1.10
SULT1A3	sulfotransferase family, cytosolic, 1A 3		1.33	1.18	1.24	1.03
NCOR2	nuclear receptor corepressor 2		1.18	1.34	-1.02	1.02
		Cluster 2				
FOS	FBJ osteosarcoma viral oncogene homolog		-1.21	-1.74	-1.58	-1.44
MYC	v-myc myelocytomatosis viral oncogene homolog		-1.39	-1.37	-1.08	-1.03
SKP2	S-phase kinase-associated protein 2 (p45)		-1.30	-1.09	-1.00	1.03
CREB1	cAMP responsive element binding protein 1		-1.32	-1.42	-1.21	-1.16
OSMR	oncostatin M receptor		-1.16	-1.23	-1.53	-1.14
ITGA6	integrin, alpha 6		-1.39	-1.34	-1.76	-1.13
PITX1	paired-like homeodomain 1		-1.44	-1.25	-1.27	-1.37
BMP4	bone morphogenetic protein 4		-1.79	-1.35	1.04	1.06
SMAD5	SMAD family member 5		-1.34	-1.04	-1.00	-1.22
TGIF1	TGFB-induced factor homeobox 1		-1.10	-1.37	1.05	1.19
COL4A4	collagen, type IV, alpha 4		-1.56	-1.63	-1.32	-1.88
CFL2	cofilin 2		-1.12	-1.67	1.00	1.24
HTR2B	5-hydroxytryptamine receptor 2B		-1.61	-1.69	1.05	1.16
		Cluster 3				
MYL9	myosin, light chain 9, regulatory		1.05	1.04	1.11	1.42
PIK3IP1	phosphoinositide-3-kinase interacting protein 1		-1.04	1.22	1.04	1.39
IRS2	insulin receptor substrate 2		-1.04	-1.35	1.36	1.43
MYO1D	myosin ID		1.06	1.12	1.34	1.22
NAPA	N-ethylmaleimide-sensitive factor attachment protein, alpha		-1.02	-1.02	1.21	1.31
RUSC2	RUN and SH3 domain containing 2		1.17	1.03	1.39	1.23
RPS6KB2	ribosomal protein S6 kinase, 70kDa		1.10	1.17	1.15	1.39
PKN1	protein kinase N1		-1.28	-1.08	1.03	1.32
		Cluster 4				
PPARG	peroxisome proliferator-activated receptor gamma		-1.46	-1.28	-1.46	-1.28
PDE7B	phosphodiesterase 7B		-1.27	-1.20	-2.09	-2.06
HIST1H2BG	histone cluster 1, H2bg		-1.26	-1.19	-1.50	-1.31
THRA	thyroid hormone receptor, alpha		-1.24	-1.23	-1.30	-1.56
HIST1H2BD	histone cluster 1, H2bd		-1.23	-1.34	-1.63	-1.77
HIST1H4H	histone cluster 1, H4h		-1.18	-1.31	-1.38	-1.50

HIST1H4E	histone cluster 1, H4e	-1.16	-1.17	-1.33	-1.54
RARB	retinoic acid receptor, beta	-1.14	1.03	-1.39	-1.28
HIST2H4A	histone cluster 2, H4a	-1.11	-1.29	-1.45	-1.48
SLIT2	slit homolog 2 (Drosophila)	-1.08	-1.07	-1.22	-1.56
TGFBR2	transforming growth factor, beta receptor	-1.07	-1.08	-1.26	-1.37
HIST1H3D	histone cluster 1, H3d	-1.05	-1.25	-1.52	-1.49
HIST2H2AA3	histone cluster 2, H2aa3	1.04	-1.01	-1.31	-1.45
PDE3A	phosphodiesterase 3A, cGMP-inhibited	1.00	-1.62	-1.24	-1.54

Table 3. **Selected genes from clusters 1-4 that are found in relevant signaling pathway maps (Tables 1 and 2).** Fold change in expression (from controls) is indicated at each time point (HP3, HP6, HP24, HP48).

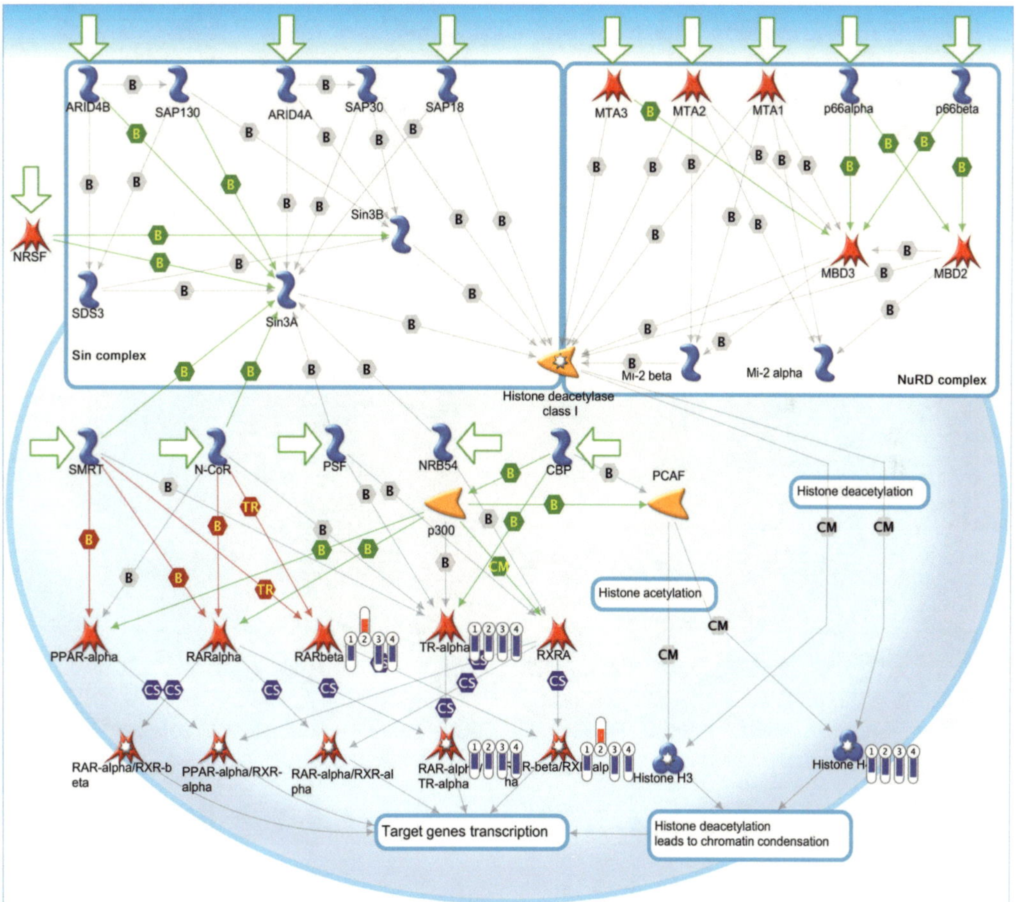

Fig. 2. Pathway map for differentially expressed transcription factors and histones in ONH astrocytes subjected to elevated HP. The genes with altered expression have a row of four "thermometers" adjacent to them that indicate the fold changes with time of exposure to elevated HP. (Blue thermometers are decreased fold-change, while red are increased fold-change.

2.4 Differential gene expression in ONH astrocytes from African American compared to Caucasian donors after treatment with elevated HP

Using the same gene selection and filtering criteria described above for the combined AA and CA data sets, we performed a cross comparison of gene expression at the same time points for genes differentially expressed by AA astrocytes. The 63 genes in Figure 3 were selected by satisfying these criteria: 1. a fold-change > 1.3, p-value < 0.01 of HP-AA vs. Ctrl at least at one time point, 2. a p-value < 0.01 of normalized HP-AA vs. normalized HP-CA at least at one time point (each time point was normalized against control).

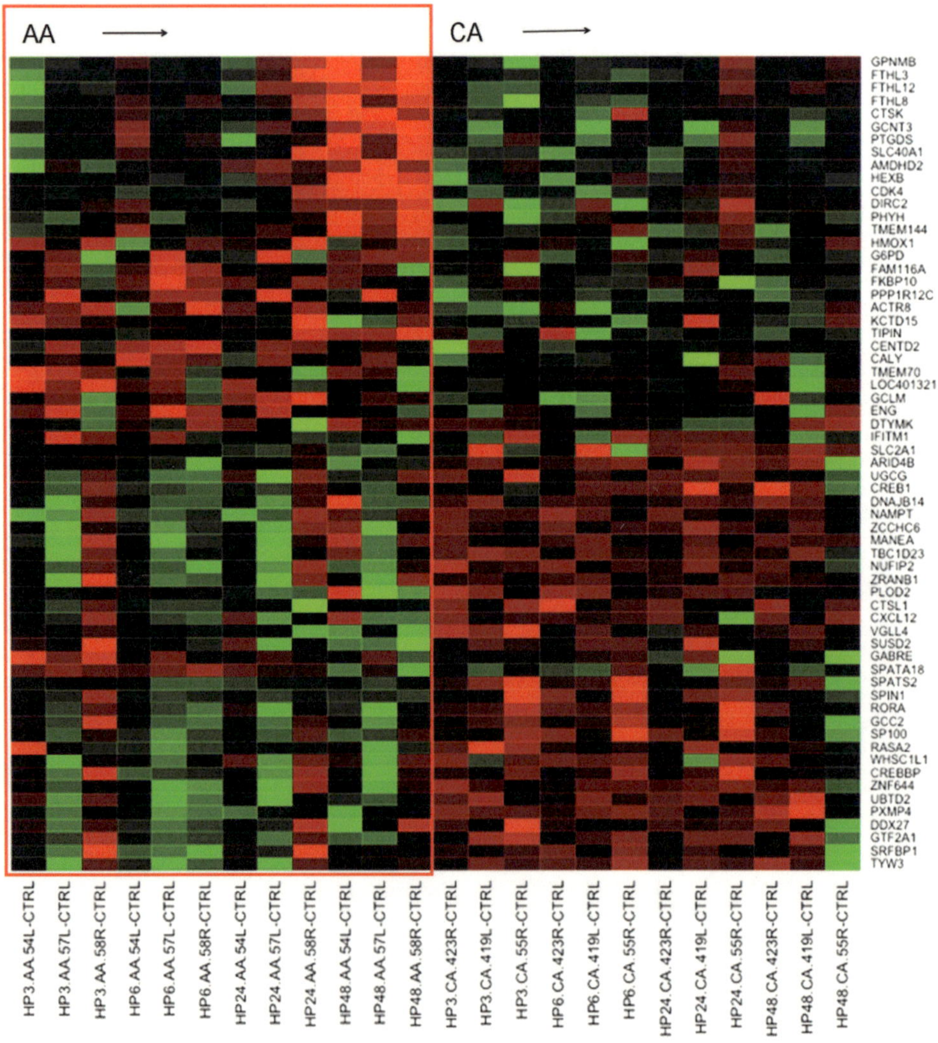

Fig. 3. **Heat map of gene expression within individual ONH cell lines as a function of time of elevated HP treatment.** The red, black and green colors represent higher than average, close to average and lower than average expression of the particular gene, respectively. The genes corresponding to each row of the heat map are on the right hand side of the picture.

To cluster the genes, we first standardized the normalized expression profile of each gene to one standard deviation and without centering (to keep the fold-change direction unchanged), then applied hierarchical cluster to get an overview of the cluster distribution. Based on the hierarchical clustering results, we defined initial clusters with visually selected cutoff value (5.5 for our case). Using these initial clusters, we did K-Means clustering. A total of 6 clusters were obtained. Two representative gene expression cluster patterns over the time course are shown in Figure 4. The early response genes (Figure 4A) increased significantly in AA (in red dotted line) after 3h exposure to HP compared to CA (black solid line). The late response genes (Figure 4B) increased significantly in AA (red dotted line) after 48h exposure to HP compared to CA (black solid line).

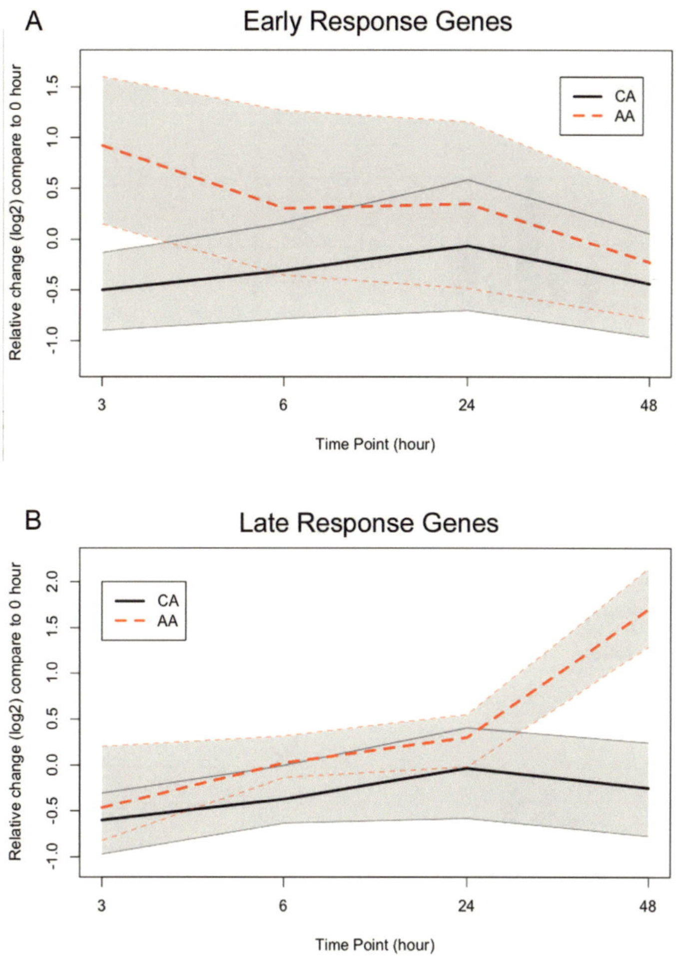

Fig. 4. **Altered gene expression in AA ONH astrocytes after elevated HP as a function of time**. A. Early response genes are those that differentially changed in AA compared to CA astrocytes after 3-6 hr of HP. B. Late response genes changed in AA or CA astrocytes at 24-48 hr of HP.

2.5 Validation of gene expression changes in ONH astrocytes subjected to elevated HP

Gene validation experiments were done primarily on the genes differentially expressed in the AA compared to CA ONH astrocytes as these were most likely to define some of the differences in sensitivity of AA cells to elevated HP. For validation, we tested GPNMB, CTSK, GCLM, HBEGF, and PLOD2. GPNMB is a late response gene. It has a requisite mutation (Anderson et al., 2008) in the hereditary glaucoma mouse model DBA-2J and is differentially expressed in ONH astrocytes in a primate ocular hypertension model (Kompass et al., 2008). Increased mRNA levels of GPNMB in AA correlate with the length of HP exposure (Figure 5A). Another late HP response gene is CTSK which is a lysosomal cysteine proteinase with strong degradative activity against the extracellular matrix and is suggested to play a role in tumor invasiveness. CTSK was significantly upregulated in AA

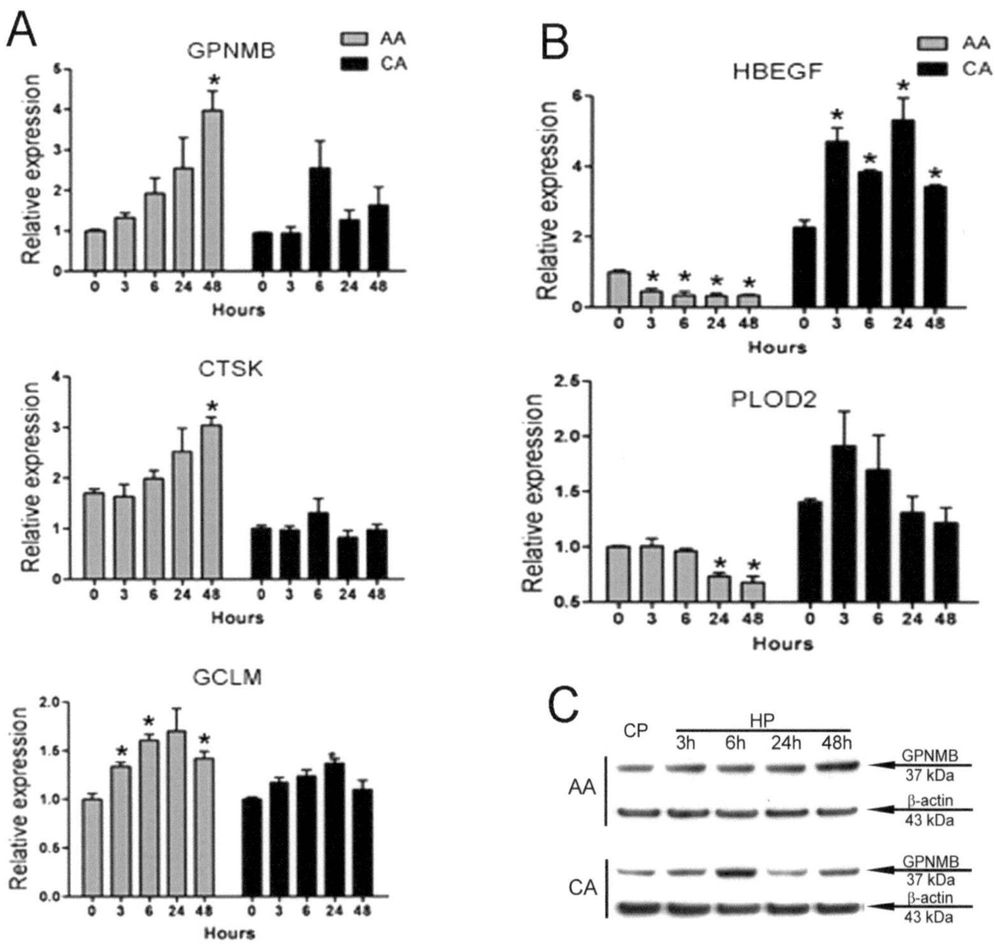

Fig. 5. **Validation experiments on selected genes from ONH astrocytes treated with elevated HP**. A. Quantitative real time PCR (qRT-PCR) of genes upregulated in AA astrocytes. B. qRT-PCR of Genes down regulated in ONH astrocytes. C. Western blot of GPNMB expression in ONH astrocytes.

astrocytes after 48 hr exposure to HP (Figure 5A). Two down regulated genes in the AA astrocytes compared to CA are HBEGF and PLOD2. In earlier work we found that HBEGF and PLOD2 were expressed significantly lower in native AA astrocytes compared to CA (Miao et al., 2008). When exposed to HP, HBEGF expression was further downregulated in AA, while upregulated in CA astrocytes (Figure 5B). PLOD2 encodes an enzyme which catalyzes the hydroxylation of lysyl residues in collagen-like peptides. It is important for the stability of intermolecular crosslinks in basement membranes. These data support our idea that the two populations of ONH astrocytes respond differently to elevated hydrostatic pressure with respect to changes in gene expression. Some responses may be due to intrinsically lower expression in the AA astrocyte population that is enhanced by elevated HP, while others appear to be specifically up-regulated in these cells.

2.6 Phosphoproteome profiling of ONH astrocytes subjected to elevated HP

Global phosphoproteome profiling was done using standard affinity-based methods to trap phosphopeptides coupled to high performance liquid chromatography-mass spectrometry (LC-MS) for detection and identification similar to our previous studies of changes in protein phosphorylation in the retina following optic nerve crush (Lukas et al., 2009). The strategy here was to determine whether changes in gene expression can be correlated with changes in protein phosphorylation in ONH astrocytes subjected to elevated HP. These studies were done on two pairs of ONH astrocytes- one pair from AA donors and the other

Time of HP (hr)	*GO category*	*p-value*	*#phosphoproteins*
0	Nuclear	0.0091	25
	Phosphorylation	0.029	6
	Cell Cycle	0.045	7
	Cytoskeleton	0.172	3
3	Nuclear	0.0025	25
	Phosphorylation	0.49	3
	Cell Cycle	0.04	5
	Cytoskeleton	0.02	8
6	Nuclear	0.0012	18
	Cell Cycle	0.04	5
	Cytoskeleton	0.02	6
	Phosphorylation	0.083	4
24	Nuclear	0.0013	19
	Cell cycle	0.004	7
	Cytoskeleton	0.029	6
	Phosphorylation	0.0085	6
48	Nuclear	0.231	12
	Cytoskeleton	0.003	8
	Cell cycle	0.47	2
	Phosphorylation	NS	0

Table 4. Gene Ontology categories enriched in phosphoproteins in AA and CA astrocytes at 0 (untreated), 3, 6, 24 and 48 hr of elevated HP treatment of ONH astrocytes.

from CA donors. As with the initial gene expression analysis, we combined all of the data at each time point to generate lists of the detected phosphoproteins. This was not a quantitative study, but rather a sampling of the phosphoproteome at each time point. This unbiased LC-MS method detects the most abundant phosphopeptides in the sample resulting in a limited survey of phosphoproteins. Phosphoproteome data were obtained at 3, 6, 12, and 24hr of elevated HP. These sets were individually submitted to Gene Ontology analysis using the GoMiner program (Zeeberg et al., 2003). During the time course of elevated HP, the number of detected nuclear and cell-cycle related phosphoproteins decreases and the cytoskeletal-associated phosphoproteins increase so as to make the differential enrichment significant (Table 4).

HP 3- 6hr	
Accession #	**Nuclear or Cell cycle Phosphoproteins**
IPI00448121	**CDC7 Cell division cycle 7-related protein kinase**
IPI00855998	**CENPF Centromere protein F**
IPI00103595	**CEP350 Centrosome-associated protein 350**
IPI00297851	**CHD1 chromodomain helicase DNA binding protein 1**
IPI00009724	**EFCAB6 EF-hand calcium-binding domain-containing protein 6**
IPI00015526	**EHMT1 Histone-lysine N-methyltransferase, H3 lysine-9 specific 5**
IPI00171903	**HNRPM Isoform 1 of Heterogeneous nuclear ribonucleoprotein M**
IPI00456887	**HNRPUL2 Heterogeneous nuclear ribonucleoprotein U-like protein 2**
IPI00299904	**MCM7 Isoform 1 of DNA replication licensing factor MCM7**
IPI00332499	**NASP nuclear autoantigenic sperm protein isoform 1**
IPI00470429	**PARK2 Isoform 5 of E3 ubiquitin-protein ligase parkin**
IPI00031627	**POLR2A DNA-directed RNA polymerase II subunit RPB1**
IPI00783392	**RB1CC1 RB1-inducible coiled-coil protein 1**
IPI00024710	**RGS10 Regulator of G-protein signaling 10**
IPI00004312	**STAT2 Signal transducer and activator of transcription 2**
IPI00044681	**UHRF2 Isoform 1 of E3 ubiquitin-protein ligase UHRF2**
IPI00783017	**ZEB2 Zinc finger E-box-binding homeobox 2**
IPI00003003	**ZNF385D Zinc finger protein 385D**
IPI00022177	**ZNF559 Zinc finger protein 559**
IPI00166972	**ZNF608 Isoform 1 of Zinc finger protein 608**
HP 24-48 hr	
IPI00747060	**ANKRD45 Isoform 1 of Ankyrin repeat domain-containing protein 45**
IPI00640320	**CDC25C Isoform 2 of M-phase inducer phosphatase 3**
IPI00009724	**EFCAB6 EF-hand calcium-binding domain-containing protein 6**
IPI00410079	**FAM82C Isoform 1 of Protein FAM82C**
IPI00171903	**HNRPM Isoform 1 of Heterogeneous nuclear ribonucleoprotein M**
IPI00307733	**SETD2 Isoform 1 of Histone-lysine N-methyltransferase SETD2**
IPI00025158	**STAG1 Cohesin subunit SA-1**
IPI00749005	**SYNE1 1011 kDa protein**
IPI00170921	**TIGD7 Isoform 1 of Tigger transposable element-derived protein 7**
IPI00217407	**UBR2 Isoform 4 of E3 ubiquitin-protein ligase UBR2**
IPI00796117	**ZMYND11 BS69 variant 1**
IPI00298731	**PPP1R10 Serine/threonine-protein phosphatase 1 regulatory subunit 10**

Table 5. Selected phosphoproteins found at early (3-6 hr) and late (24-48 hr) times of elevated HP in ONH astrocytes.

Summarized in Tables 5 and 6 are selected phosphoproteins identified in the early (3-6 hr) and late (24-48 hr) phases of elevated HP. Within the nuclear/cell cycle groups of phosphoproteins we find transcription factors, nuclear riboproteins, and ubiquitin ligases. Also notable are histone methyl transferase proteins that may be functioning to reprogram the ONH astrocyte gene expression in response to the stress induced by elevated HP. Phosphorylation of these proteins may function to activate epigenetic reprogramming of the ONH astrocyte in response to the stress induced by elevated HP.

HP 3-6 hr	Cytoskeletal Phosphoproteins
Accession#	**Name**
IPI00472779	**ANK3 Ankyrin-3**
IPI00011219	**ARHGAP24 Rho GTPase-activating protein 24**
IPI00008756	**DST Dystonin Isoform 1**
IPI00306929	**MYO18A Isoform 2 of Myosin-XVIIIa**
IPI00479962	**MYO5A Myosin-Va**
IPI00307155	**ROCK2 Rho-associated protein kinase 2**
IPI00289639	**VILL Isoform 1 of Villin-like protein**
HP 24-48 hr	
IPI00010448	**ARHGAP24 Rho GTPase-activating protein 24**
IPI00457243	**ARHGEF5 rho guanine nucleotide exchange factor 5**
IPI00792788	**DOCK5 Isoform 1 of Dedicator of cytokinesis protein 5**
IPI00216408	**DOCK9 Isoform 1 of Dedicator of cytokinesis protein 9**
IPI00642259	**DST Dystonin**
IPI00260090	**ELMO1/2 Engulfment and cell motility proteins**
IPI00452247	**KIF16B Isoform 2 of Kinesin-like motor protein C20orf23**
IPI00848334	**KIF2A Isoform 4 of Kinesin-like protein KIF2A**
IPI00306929	**MYO18A Isoform 2 of Myosin-XVIIIa**
IPI00479962	**MYO5A Myosin-Va**
IPI00303335	**NEB Nebulin**
IPI00071509	**PKP1 Isoform 2 of Plakophilin-1**

Table 6. Selected cytoskeletal phosphoproteins identified at early (3-6 hr) and late (24-48) times of elevated HP in ONH astrocytes.

Within the cytoskeletal group were several proteins associated with focal adhesions (Table 6). These include for example, DOCK5/9 and ELMO1/2. ELMO was detected at the 3hr HP time point and the detected phosphopeptide, RIAFDAESEPNNSSGpSMEKR, corresponds to residues 329-348 of ELMO1. ELMO1 interacts with DOCK-180 and other proteins in a large complex found at focal adhesions (Beausoleil et al., 2006). Specific antiphosphopeptide antibodies to ELMO1 were not available, but there are phosphorylation site antibodies to p130CAS, another known phosphoprotein in the DOCK protein complex (Menniti et al., 2006). p130CAS is known to become highly phosphorylated in response to mechanical stress (Sawada et al., 2006; Geiger, 2006). We found that p130CAS phosphorylation increases with HP, particularly at the 3 and 6 hr time points in AA astrocytes and at 24-48 hr in CA astrocytes (Figure 6). Thus, the AA astrocytes respond earlier to elevated HP than the CA astrocytes with respect to p130CAS phosphorylation. Phosphorylation of p130CAS and ELMO may modulate the dynamics of focal adhesions. To support this idea, we found that

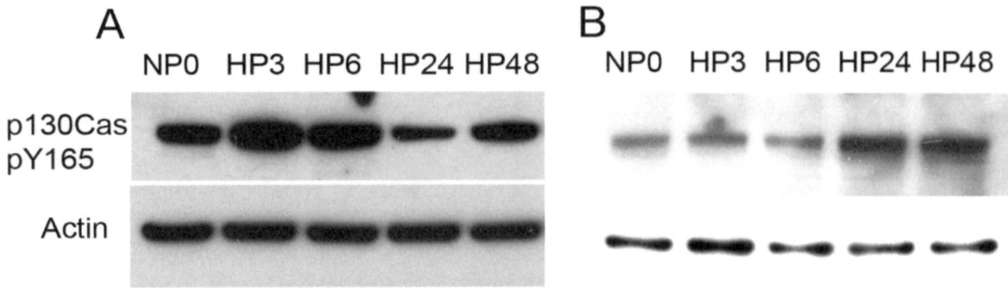

Fig. 6. **Phosphorylation of p130CAS in A. AA and B. CA astrocytes .** NP indicates cells at ambient pressure, while HP3-48 are cells exposed to elevated HP for those times. Antibodies specific for pY165 in p130CAS were used to probe Western Blots of cell extracts.

phosphorylation of focal adhesion kinase (FAK) was increased in CA astrocytes at 24-48 hr of elevated HP (Figure 7). Although FAK was phosphorylated in AA cells, its phosphorylation level was constant at each time point during elevated HP treatment (not shown).

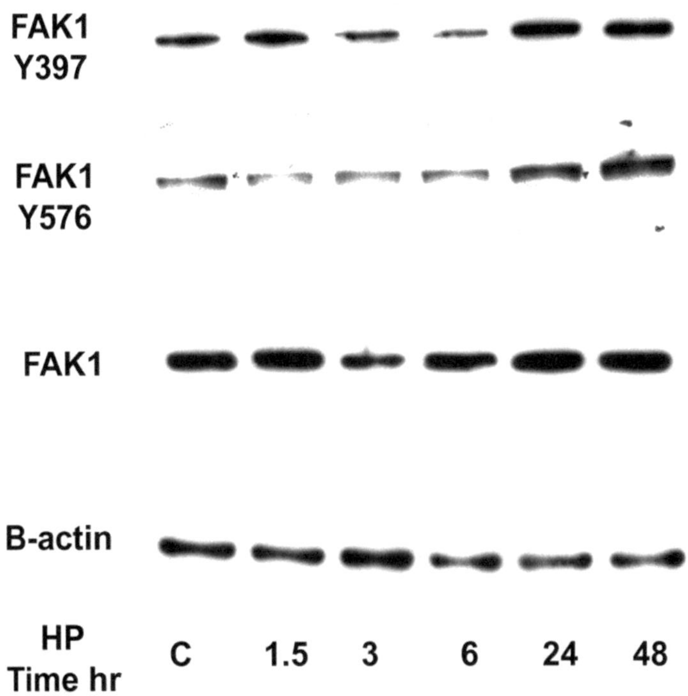

Fig. 7. **Phosphorylation of focal adhesion kinase (FAK) in CA ONH astrocytes exposed to elevated HP.** Antibodies specific to FAK phosphorylated at Y397 and Y576 were used to probe Western Blots of cell extracts.

2.7 Correlations of gene expression and protein phosphorylation in ONH astrocytes

The pattern of cytoskeletal protein phosphorylation is consistent with the differences in gene expression found in the late (24-48 hr) time of elevated HP treatment (Tables 1-3). Similarly, the pattern of protein phosphorylation at the early (3-6 hr) time of HP treatment is consistent with the transcriptional activity associated with this phase (Tables 1-3). Thus, the elevated HP system provides a potential "preglaucoma" state in ONH astrocytes because differential changes in expression of genes in the TGFβ pathways and cytoskeletal regulation are found in glaucomatous AA and CA astrocytes and in the glaucomatous ONH (Lukas et al., 2008). As shown earlier, elevated HP increases the expression of GPNMB protein in AA astrocytes compared to CA astrocytes (Figure 5C) consistent with the gene expression data. GPNMB is thought to function as a cell adhesion protein that connects the extracellular environment to downstream cellular signaling linked to gene transcription via TGFβ pathways that modulates the synthesis of extracellular matrix proteins in ONH astrocytes (Fuchshofer et al., 2005). Therefore, these pathways may be larger contributors to changes in cell adhesion in AA astrocytes compared to CA. On the other hand, the activation of focal adhesions complexes is linked to cytoskeletal remodeling and transcription through multiple pathways (Koyama et al., 2000). Thus, in signal transduction and gene expression, AA and CA astrocytes exhibit differential responses to elevated HP that can produce altered cell adhesion and morphology.

3. Conclusions

The types of experiments described in this report fall into the realm of systems biology. The guiding hypothesis is that subjecting a system such as cultured ONH astrocytes, to a stressor (elevated HP) will cause changes in gene expression and protein phosphorylation in a fashion that impacts multiple signaling networks and processes. We found that, indeed, elevated HP induces changes in gene expression patterns that are setting up new cellular phenotypes. Thus, the system is a model for what elevated IOP may induce in ONH astrocytes *in vivo*. However, the biological and mechanical properties of the lamina cribrosa are complex, defined by contributions from astrocytes, lamina cribrosa cells and blood vessels embedded in a three-dimensional extracellular matrix. Thus, astrocytes and lamina cribrosa cells respond not only to external stimuli such as IOP but to the stiffness of the matrix within which they reside (Bellezza et al., 2003). Therefore, a cultured cell system is not a perfect model. However, both *in vitro* and *in vivo* cells continuously sample their mechanical microenvironment by exerting internally generated tensile forces on the surrounding matrix and adjust their phenotype in a cell- and tissue-specific manner. These sorts of responses are clearly evident in the hydrostatic pressure model used herein. Moreover, the parallels between model and the glaucomatous optic nerve head are converging on the same cellular signaling systems and alterations in gene expression. However, additional validation studies that examine gene expression in the optic nerve head of control and glaucomatous tissues will be needed. These sorts of studies have already been done to validate selected unregulated genes such as the transcription factors Fos and Jun (Hashimoto et al., 2005), cell adhesion molecules (Kobayashi et al., 1997; Ricard et al., 1999), extracellular matrix (Pena et al., 1999b; Pena et al., 1998), TGFβ (Pena et al., 1999a) and TGFβ receptors (Lukas et al., 2008).

In the same realm, changes in protein phosphorylation may define dynamic cellular phenotypes which have characteristics of different cellular populations. The few differences we uncovered in protein phosphorylation of cytoskeletal proteins between CA and AA astrocytes after treatment with elevated IOP are likely just a small sampling of the entire signaling system. However, one of the exciting prospects revealed in this study is that elevated IOP might be inducing epigenetic changes in ONH astrocytes that are responsible, in part, for altering gene transcription programs. This opens up unexplored areas for future glaucoma research.

4. Acknowledgements

This work is dedicated to the memory of our colleague Dr. M. Rosario Hernandez. It was supported, in part, by a grant from the National Institutes of Health (EY06416) and unrestricted funds from Research to Prevent Blindness.

5. References

Anderson,M.G., Nair,K.S., Amonoo,L.A., Mehalow,A., Trantow,C.M., Masli,S., and John,S.W. (2008). GpnmbR150X allele must be present in bone marrow derived cells to mediate DBA/2J glaucoma. BMC Genet. *9*, 30.

Beausoleil,S.A., Villen,J., Gerber,S.A., Rush,J., and Gygi,S.P. (2006). A probability-based approach for high-throughput protein phosphorylation analysis and site localization. Nat. Biotechnol. *24*, 1285-1292.

Beck,A.D. (2003). Review of recent publications of the Advanced Glaucoma Intervention Study. Curr. Opin. Ophthalmol. *14*, 83-85.

Bellezza,A.J., Rintalan,C.J., Thompson,H.W., Downs,J.C., Hart,R.T., and Burgoyne,C.F. (2003). Deformation of the lamina cribrosa and anterior scleral canal wall in early experimental glaucoma. Invest Ophthalmol. Vis. Sci. *44*, 623-637.

Broman,A.T., Quigley,H.A., West,S.K., Katz,J., Munoz,B., Bandeen-Roche,K., Tielsch,J.M., Friedman,D.S., Crowston,J., Taylor,H.R., Varma,R., Leske,M.C., Bengtsson,B., Heijl,A., He,M., and Foster,P.J. (2008). Estimating the rate of progressive visual field damage in those with open-angle glaucoma, from cross-sectional data. Invest Ophthalmol. Vis. Sci. *49*, 66-76.

Chen,L., Lukas,T.J., and Hernandez,M.R. (2009). Hydrostatic pressure-dependent changes in cyclic AMP signaling in optic nerve head astrocytes from Caucasian and African American donors. Mol. Vis. *15*, 1664-1672.

Dandona,L., Quigley,H.A., Brown,A.E., and Enger,C. (1990). Quantitative regional structure of the normal human lamina cribrosa. A racial comparison. Arch. Ophthalmol. *108*, 393-398.

Delghandi,M.P., Johannessen,M., and Moens,U. (2005). The cAMP signalling pathway activates CREB through PKA, p38 and MSK1 in NIH 3T3 cells. Cell Signal. *17*, 1343-1351.

Du,P., Kibbe,W.A., and Lin,S.M. (2007). nuID: a universal naming scheme of oligonucleotides for illumina, affymetrix, and other microarrays. Biol. Direct. *2*, 16.

Du,P., Kibbe,W.A., and Lin,S.M. (2008). lumi: a pipeline for processing Illumina microarray. Bioinformatics. *24*, 1547-1548.

Ederer,F., Gaasterland,D.A., Dally,L.G., Kim,J., VanVeldhuisen,P.C., Blackwell,B., Prum,B., Shafranov,G., Allen,R.C., and Beck,A. (2004). The Advanced Glaucoma Intervention Study (AGIS): 13. Comparison of treatment outcomes within race: 10-year results. Ophthalmology *111*, 651-664.

Feng,Y., Yang,J.H., Huang,H., Kennedy,S.P., Turi,T.G., Thompson,J.F., Libby,P., and Lee,R.T. (1999). Transcriptional profile of mechanically induced genes in human vascular smooth muscle cells. Circ. Res. *85*, 1118-1123.

Fields,R.D. and Stevens-Graham,B. (2002). New insights into neuron-glia communication. Science *298*, 556-562.

Friedman,D.S., Wolfs,R.C., O'Colmain,B.J., Klein,B.E., Taylor,H.R., West,S., Leske,M.C., Mitchell,P., Congdon,N., and Kempen,J. (2004). Prevalence of open-angle glaucoma among adults in the United States. Arch. Ophthalmol. *122*, 532-538.

Fuchshofer,R., Birke,M., Welge-Lussen,U., Kook,D., and Lutjen-Drecoll,E. (2005). Transforming growth factor-beta 2 modulated extracellular matrix component expression in cultured human optic nerve head astrocytes. Invest Ophthalmol. Vis. Sci. *46*, 568-578.

Geiger,B. (2006). A role for p130Cas in mechanotransduction. Cell *127*, 879-881.

Hashimoto,K., Parker,A., Malone,P., Gabelt,B.T., Rasmussen,C., Kaufman,P.S., and Hernandez,M.R. (2005). Long-term activation of c-Fos and c-Jun in optic nerve head astrocytes in experimental ocular hypertension in monkeys and after exposure to elevated pressure in vitro. Brain Res. *1054*, 103-115.

Hatten,M.E., Liem,R.K., Shelanski,M.L., and Mason,C.A. (1991). Astroglia in CNS injury. Glia *4*, 233-243.

Hernandez,M.R. (2000). The optic nerve head in glaucoma: role of astrocytes in tissue remodeling. Prog. Retin. Eye Res. *19*, 297-321.

Hernandez,M.R., Agapova,O.A., Yang,P., Salvador-Silva,M., Ricard,C.S., and Aoi,S. (2002). Differential gene expression in astrocytes from human normal and glaucomatous optic nerve head analyzed by cDNA microarray. Glia *38*, 45-64.

Hernandez,M.R., Igoe,F., and Neufeld,A.H. (1988). Cell culture of the human lamina cribrosa. Invest Ophthalmol. Vis. Sci. *29*, 78-89.

Hernandez,M.R., Luo,X.X., Andrzejewska,W., and Neufeld,A.H. (1989). Age-related changes in the extracellular matrix of the human optic nerve head. Am. J. Ophthalmol. *107*, 476-484.

Hernandez,M.R., Miao,H., and Lukas,T. (2008). Astrocytes in glaucomatous optic neuropathy. Prog. Brain Res. *173*, 353-373.

Hernandez,M.R. and Pena,J.D. (1997). The optic nerve head in glaucomatous optic neuropathy. Arch. Ophthalmol. *115*, 389-395.

Hernandez,M.R., Pena,J.D., Selvidge,J.A., Salvador-Silva,M., and Yang,P. (2000). Hydrostatic pressure stimulates synthesis of elastin in cultured optic nerve head astrocytes. Glia *32*, 122-136.

Illi,B., Scopece,A., Nanni,S., Farsetti,A., Morgante,L., Biglioli,P., Capogrossi,M.C., and Gaetano,C. (2005). Epigenetic histone modification and cardiovascular lineage programming in mouse embryonic stem cells exposed to laminar shear stress. Circ. Res. *96*, 501-508.

Ito,T. (2007). Role of histone modification in chromatin dynamics. J. Biochem. (Tokyo) *141*, 609-614.

Johannessen,M., Delghandi,M.P., and Moens,U. (2004). What turns CREB on? Cell Signal. *16*, 1211-1227.

Johnson,E.C., Jia,L., Cepurna,W.O., Doser,T.A., and Morrison,J.C. (2007). Global changes in optic nerve head gene expression after exposure to elevated intraocular pressure in a rat glaucoma model. Invest Ophthalmol. Vis. Sci. *48*, 3161-3177.

Kirwan,R.P., Crean,J.K., Fenerty,C.H., Clark,A.F., and O'Brien,C.J. (2004). Effect of cyclical mechanical stretch and exogenous transforming growth factor-beta1 on matrix metalloproteinase-2 activity in lamina cribrosa cells from the human optic nerve head. J. Glaucoma. *13*, 327-334.

Kirwan,R.P., Leonard,M.O., Murphy,M., Clark,A.F., and O'Brien,C.J. (2005). Transforming growth factor-beta-regulated gene transcription and protein expression in human GFAP-negative lamina cribrosa cells. Glia *52*, 309-324.

Kobayashi,S., Vidal,I., Pena,J.D., and Hernandez,M.R. (1997). Expression of neural cell adhesion molecule (NCAM) characterizes a subpopulation of type 1 astrocytes in human optic nerve head. Glia *20*, 262-273.

Kompass,K.S., Agapova,O., Li,W., Kaufman,P.L., Rasmussen,C., and Hernandez,M.R. (2008). Bioinformatic and statistical analysis of the optic nerve head in a primate model of ocular hypertension. BMC Neuroscience in press.

Koyama,Y., Yoshioka,Y., Hashimoto,H., Matsuda,T., and Baba,A. (2000). Endothelins increase tyrosine phosphorylation of astrocytic focal adhesion kinase and paxillin accompanied by their association with cytoskeletal components. Neuroscience *101*, 219-227.

Lambert,W.S., Clark,A.F., and Wordinger,R.J. (2004). Effect of exogenous neurotrophins on Trk receptor phosphorylation, cell proliferation, and neurotrophin secretion by cells isolated from the human lamina cribrosa. Mol. Vis. *10*, 289-296.

Leske,M.C., Wu,S.Y., Hennis,A., Honkanen,R., and Nemesure,B. (2008). Risk Factors for Incident Open-angle Glaucoma The Barbados Eye Studies. Ophthalmology *115*, 85-93.

Liang,Y.J., Lai,L.P., Wang,B.W., Juang,S.J., Chang,C.M., Leu,J.G., and Shyu,K.G. (2006). Mechanical stress enhances serotonin 2B receptor modulating brain natriuretic peptide through nuclear factor-kappaB in cardiomyocytes. Cardiovasc. Res. *72*, 303-312.

Lin,S.M., Du,P., Huber,W., and Kibbe,W.A. (2008). Model-based variance-stabilizing transformation for Illumina microarray data. Nucleic Acids Res. *36*, e11.

Liton,P.B., Liu,X., Challa,P., Epstein,D.L., and Gonzalez,P. (2005). Induction of TGF-beta1 in the trabecular meshwork under cyclic mechanical stress. J. Cell Physiol *205*, 364-371.

Liu,B., Chen,H., Johns,T.G., and Neufeld,A.H. (2006). Epidermal growth factor receptor activation: an upstream signal for transition of quiescent astrocytes into reactive astrocytes after neural injury. J. Neurosci. *26*, 7532-7540.

Lukas,T.J., Miao,H., Chen,L., Riordan,S., Li,W., Crabb,A.M., Wise,A., Du,P., Lin,S.M., and Hernandez,M.R. (2008). Susceptibility to glaucoma: differential comparison of the astrocyte transcriptome from glaucomatous African American and Caucasian American donors. Genome Biol. *9*, R111.

Lukas,T.J., Wang,A.L., Yuan,M., and Neufeld,A.H. (2009). Early cellular signaling responses to axonal injury. Cell Commun. Signal. *7*, 5.

Malone,P., Miao,H., Parker,A., Juarez,S., and Hernandez,M.R. (2007). Pressure induces loss of gap junction communication and redistribution of connexin 43 in astrocytes. Glia *55*, 1085-1098.

McGraw,J., Hiebert,G.W., and Steeves,J.D. (2001). Modulating astrogliosis after neurotrauma. J. Neurosci. Res. *63*, 109-115.

Menniti,F.S., Faraci,W.S., and Schmidt,C.J. (2006). Phosphodiesterases in the CNS: targets for drug development. Nat. Rev. Drug Discov. *5*, 660-670.

Miao,H., Chen,L., Riordan,S.M., Li,W., Juarez,S., Crabb,A.M., Lukas,T.J., Du,P., Lin,S.M., Wise,A., Agapova,O.A., Yang,P., Gu,C.C., and Hernandez,M.R. (2008). Gene expression and functional studies of the optic nerve head astrocyte transcriptome from normal african americans and caucasian americans donors. PLoS. ONE. *3*, e2847.

Miao,H., Crabb,A.W., Hernandez,M.R., and Lukas,T.J. (2010). Modulation of factors affecting optic nerve head astrocyte migration. Invest Ophthalmol. Vis. Sci. *51*, 4096-4103.

Neary,J.T., Kang,Y., Willoughby,K.A., and Ellis,E.F. (2003). Activation of extracellular signal-regulated kinase by stretch-induced injury in astrocytes involves extracellular ATP and P2 purinergic receptors. J. Neurosci. *23*, 2348-2356.

Nemesure,B., He,Q., Mendell,N., Wu,S.Y., Hejtmancik,J.F., Hennis,A., and Leske,M.C. (2001). Inheritance of open-angle glaucoma in the Barbados family study. Am. J. Med. Genet. *103*, 36-43.

Ni,W., Rajkumar,K., Nagy,J.I., and Murphy,L.J. (1997). Impaired brain development and reduced astrocyte response to injury in transgenic mice expressing IGF binding protein-1. Brain Res. *769*, 97-107.

Nickells,R.W. (2007). From ocular hypertension to ganglion cell death: a theoretical sequence of events leading to glaucoma. Can. J. Ophthalmol. *42*, 278-287.

Nikolsky,Y., Ekins,S., Nikolskaya,T., and Bugrim,A. (2005). A novel method for generation of signature networks as biomarkers from complex high throughput data. Toxicol. Lett. *158*, 20-29.

Oki,M., Aihara,H., and Ito,T. (2007). Role of histone phosphorylation in chromatin dynamics and its implications in diseases. Subcell. Biochem. *41*, 319-336.

Pena,J.D., Netland,P.A., Vidal,I., Dorr,D.A., Rasky,A., and Hernandez,M.R. (1998). Elastosis of the lamina cribrosa in glaucomatous optic neuropathy. Exp. Eye Res. *67*, 517-524.

Pena,J.D., Taylor,A.W., Ricard,C.S., Vidal,I., and Hernandez,M.R. (1999a). Transforming growth factor beta isoforms in human optic nerve heads. Br. J. Ophthalmol. *83*, 209-218.

Pena,J.D., Varela,H.J., Ricard,C.S., and Hernandez,M.R. (1999b). Enhanced tenascin expression associated with reactive astrocytes in human optic nerve heads with primary open angle glaucoma. Exp. Eye Res. *68*, 29-40.

Quigley,H.A., Varma,R., Tielsch,J.M., Katz,J., Sommer,A., and Gilbert,D.L. (1999). The relationship between optic disc area and open-angle glaucoma: the Baltimore Eye Survey. J. Glaucoma. *8*, 347-352.

Quigley,H.A. and Vitale,S. (1997). Models of open-angle glaucoma prevalence and incidence in the United States. Invest Ophthalmol. Vis. Sci. *38*, 83-91.

Ricard,C.S., Kobayashi,S., Pena,J.D., Salvador-Silva,M., Agapova,O., and Hernandez,M.R. (2000). Selective expression of neural cell adhesion molecule (NCAM)-180 in optic nerve head astrocytes exposed to elevated hydrostatic pressure in vitro. Brain Res. Mol. Brain Res. *81*, 62-79.

Ricard,C.S., Pena,J.D., and Hernandez,M.R. (1999). Differential expression of neural cell adhesion molecule isoforms in normal and glaucomatous human optic nerve heads. Brain Res. Mol. Brain Res. *74*, 69-82.

Salvador-Silva,M., Aoi,S., Parker,A., Yang,P., Pecen,P., and Hernandez,M.R. (2004). Responses and signaling pathways in human optic nerve head astrocytes exposed to hydrostatic pressure in vitro. Glia *45*, 364-377.

Salvador-Silva,M., Ricard,C.S., Agapova,O.A., Yang,P., and Hernandez,M.R. (2001). Expression of small heat shock proteins and intermediate filaments in the human optic nerve head astrocytes exposed to elevated hydrostatic pressure in vitro. J. Neurosci. Res. *66*, 59-73.

Sanden,N., Thorlin,T., Blomstrand,F., Persson,P.A., and Hansson,E. (2000). 5-Hydroxytryptamine2B receptors stimulate Ca2+ increases in cultured astrocytes from three different brain regions. Neurochem. Int. *36*, 427-434.

Sawada,Y., Tamada,M., Dubin-Thaler,B.J., Cherniavskaya,O., Sakai,R., Tanaka,S., and Sheetz,M.P. (2006). Force sensing by mechanical extension of the Src family kinase substrate p130Cas. Cell *127*, 1015-1026.

Smyth,G.K. (2004). Linear models and empirical bayes methods for assessing differential expression in microarray experiments. Stat. Appl. Genet. Mol. Biol. *3*, Article3.

Sofroniew,M.V. (2005). Reactive astrocytes in neural repair and protection. Neuroscientist. *11*, 400-407.

Stark,C., Breitkreutz,B.J., Reguly,T., Boucher,L., Breitkreutz,A., and Tyers,M. (2006). BioGRID: a general repository for interaction datasets. Nucleic Acids Res. *34*, D535-D539.

Varma,R., Tielsch,J.M., Quigley,H.A., Hilton,S.C., Katz,J., Spaeth,G.L., and Sommer,A. (1994). Race-, age-, gender-, and refractive error-related differences in the normal optic disc. Arch. Ophthalmol. *112*, 1068-1076.

Wang,L., Fortune,B., Cull,G., Dong,J., and Cioffi,G.A. (2006). Endothelin B receptor in human glaucoma and experimentally induced optic nerve damage. Arch. Ophthalmol. *124*, 717-724.

Wordinger,R.J., Agarwal,R., Talati,M., Fuller,J., Lambert,W., and Clark,A.F. (2002). Expression of bone morphogenetic proteins (BMP), BMP receptors, and BMP associated proteins in human trabecular meshwork and optic nerve head cells and tissues. Mol. Vis. *8*, 241-250.

Yang,J.L., Neufeld,A.H., Zorn,M.B., and Hernandez,M.R. (1993). Collagen type I mRNA levels in cultured human lamina cribrosa cells: effects of elevated hydrostatic pressure. Exp. Eye Res. *56*, 567-574.

Yang,P., Agapova,O., Parker,A., Shannon,W., Pecen,P., Duncan,J., Salvador-Silva,M., and Hernandez,M.R. (2004). DNA microarray analysis of gene expression in human optic nerve head astrocytes in response to hydrostatic pressure. Physiol Genomics *17*, 157-169.

Yang,Z., Quigley,H.A., Pease,M.E., Yang,Y., Qian,J., Valenta,D., and Zack,D.J. (2007). Changes in gene expression in experimental glaucoma and optic nerve transection: the equilibrium between protective and detrimental mechanisms. Invest Ophthalmol. Vis. Sci. *48*, 5539-5548.

Zeeberg,B.R., Feng,W., Wang,G., Wang,M.D., Fojo,A.T., Sunshine,M., Narasimhan,S., Kane,D.W., Reinhold,W.C., Lababidi,S., Bussey,K.J., Riss,J., Barrett,J.C., and Weinstein,J.N. (2003). GoMiner: a resource for biological interpretation of genomic and proteomic data. Genome Biol. *4*, R28.

Zode,G.S., Clark,A.F., and Wordinger,R.J. (2007). Activation of the BMP canonical signaling pathway in human optic nerve head tissue and isolated optic nerve head astrocytes and lamina cribrosa cells. Invest Ophthalmol. Vis. Sci. *48*, 5058-5067.

3

Homocysteine in the Pathogenesis of Chronic Glaucoma

Mustafa R Kadhim[1] and Colin I Clement[2,3]
[1]*The Western Eye Hospital, London,*
[2]*Glaucoma Unit, Sydney Eye Hospital, Sydney,*
[3]*Central Clinical School, The University of Sydney, Sydney*
[1]*United Kingdom*
[2,3]*Australia*

1. Introduction

1.1 Metabolic pathway

Methionine is one of four amino acids that form succinyl CoA. This sulphur containing amino acid is the source of homocysteine (Hcy). It is converted to S-adenosylmethionine (SAM), the major methyl-group donor in one–carbon metabolism. The synthesis of SAM occurs when methionine condenses with adenosine triphosphate (ATP) by the hydrolysis of all three phosphate bonds. The methyl group attached to the tertiary group in SAM is activated and can be transferred to a variety of acceptor molecules, such as noradrenaline in the synthesis of adrenaline. The reaction product S-adenosylhomocysteine (SAH) is a simple thioether, analogous to methionine. The resulting loss of free energy accompanying the reaction makes the methyl transfer essentially irreversible. Next is the hydrolysis of SAH to Hcy and adenosine. Homocysteine has two fates. If there is a deficiency of methionine, Hcy may be re-methylated to methionine. If stores of methionine are adequate, Hcy may enter the trans-sulphuration pathway, where it is converted to cysteine. The re-synthesis of methionine occurs with the acceptance of a methyl group from N5-methyltetrahydrofolate (N5-methyl-THF) in a reaction that requires methyl-cobalamin, a coenzyme derived from cobalamin (vitamin B12). The methyl group is transferred from the B12 derivative to Hcy, and vitamin B12 is recharged from N5-methyl-THF. The synthesis of cysteine occurs when Hcy combines with serine, forming cystathionine, which is hydrolysed to α - ketobutyrate and cysteine. This sequence has the net effect of converting serine to cysteine and Hcy to α - ketobutyrate, which is oxidatively decarboxylated to form propionyl CoA. Because Hcy is synthesised from the essential amino acid methionine, cysteine is not an essential amino acid so long as methionine is available (Figure 1).

Under normal metabolic circumstances, there is a strict balance between Hcy formation and elimination. Usually about 50% of the Hcy formed is re-methylated to methionine. When protein or methionine intake is in excess, the trans-sulfuration pathway catabolises a larger proportion. If there is an increased formation of Hcy relative to its consumption, Hcy is excreted from the cells. This can be detected as an increased level of Hcy in plasma/serum or in the urine.

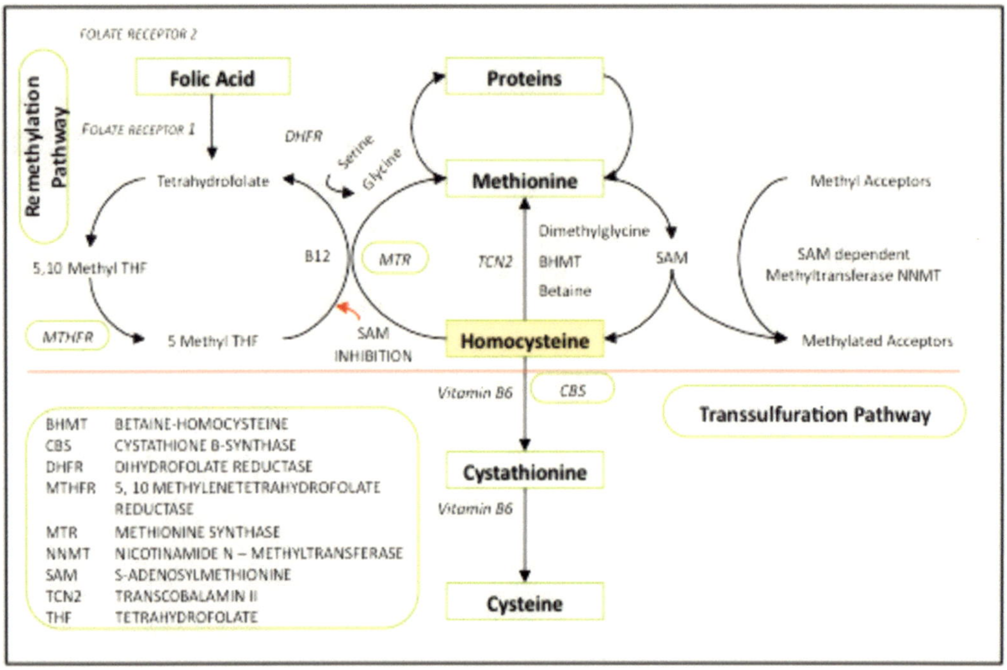

Fig. 1. Homocysteine Metabolism

1.2 Genetic influences

Homocysteine metabolism therefore has three key enzymes (Figure 1); methylenetetrahydrofolate reductase (MTHFR), cystathionine beta-synthase (CBS) and methionine synthesase (MTR).

The key enzyme in the remethylation pathway is MTHFR. Single nucleotide polymorphisms have been identified for this enzyme. The common C → T substitution at the 677 position results in decreased enzymatic function. This alanine to valine substitution, in heterozygotes, causes a 30% drop in function, and with homozygotes, a 60% reduction.[1] Deficiency of CBS deficiency likewise causes hyperhomocysteinaemia (HHcy), but the severity is less compared with vitamin B12 deficiency. This suggests the CBS enzyme is not as central to the total homocysteine (tHcy) level as the MTHFR enzyme.

The effect of the MTHFR genetic polymorphism has been scrutinized in a placebo controlled trial.[2] The TT homozygous group for the mutation had a 2.4 times greater reduction in tHcy compared to wild type after 1mg of folic acid was given daily for three months, owing to the elevated baseline tHcy of TT group compared to CC and CT subgroups. This means MTHFR TT groups can be targeted for therapy. However, a British study[3] of an older population described a regional difference in the tHcy even after adjustments for folate and vitamin B12 levels, smoking and the effect C677T polymorphism. This can only be explained by the effect of other unidentified genetic, systemic or environmental factors.

A secondary mutation of the MTHFR gene at position 1298 A→C also reduces function. Alone, this mutation confers no difference in the tHcy, but in combination with the 677 C→T mutation, unsurprisingly, there is an elevation in the tHcy and decreased folate levels.[4]

1.3 Systemic and environemental influences

The effect of systemic disease, medications and environmental exposures on Hcy has been described in detail.[5] A summary is provided in Table 1.

Reduced tHcy	*Moderate (15-30μmol/L)*	Intermediate *(30-100μmol/L)*	*Severe (>100μmol/L)*
Down syndrome	MTHFR C→T		
Pregnancy	homozygosity		
Folate excess	Male	Folate deficiency	Homocystinuria
B12 Excess	Post-menopausal		
B6 Excess	Smoking	Renal failure	Vitamin B12
Hyperthyroidism	Coffee		deficiency
Diabetes Mellitus	Alcohol		
Exercise	Diabetes Mellitus		

Table 1. Environmental and Systemic Influences on Homocysteine.

2. Homocysteine assays

Accurate measurement of Hcy requires a working knowledge of the plasma distribution. The vast majority is protein bound; the rest is free. This is further subdivided into Hcy-cysteine mixed disulphide, homocystine and Hcy. In combination they are tHcy.

Three types of assays have been used in Hcy-glaucoma studies: high performance liquid chromatography (HPLC), enzyme-linked immunoassays (EIA) and fluorescence polarization immunoassays (FPIA). The latter 2 give an estimation of the tHcy and are relatively easy to perform.[5] In contrast, HPLC is more difficult to run and may have a much lower through put, but has the advantage of a broader analytical range and lower cost per test. Results from all 3 are comparable although there can be significant differences between methods and even between laboratories using the same method.[6] Strategies to reduce the influence of inter-test variability should include running case and control assays simultaneously and using a single laboratory. Many Hcy-glaucoma studies have employed single laboratories but it is unclear whether testing was grouped or random. No method has demonstrated superiority over another.

3. Homocysteine and systemic disease

Injury to vascular endothelium, retinal ganglion cell apoptosis and extra-cellular matrix (ECM) remodelling of trabecular meshwork and/or lamina cribrosa may all contribute to optic nerve damage characteristic of glaucoma. All three events are linked with Hcy: the evidence is presented below.

3.1 Cardiovascular disease

In 1969, McCully[7] highlighted a potential link between Hcy and cardiovascular disease (CVD) by observing pathological changes to blood vessels in 2 children. In both cases, gross vascular damage to arteries (small, medium and large); focal narrowing due to intimal and medial fibrosis and focal proliferation of peri-vascular connective tissue in the small vessels was noted in the setting of raised Hcy and cystathione. Since then, further animal and human research has shown a link between tHcy elevation and bioavailablity of endothelium-derived nitric oxide.[8] Endothelium dependent vasodilation is significantly impaired in subjects with HHcy compared to controls.[9] The early pathogenesis of atherosclerosis is related to this impairment of vasodilation, and HHcy exacerbates this. Even in healthy adults, a methionine load that produces transiently raised tHcy levels, impairs flow mediated endothelium dependent vasodilation.[10]

In vitro, it has been demonstrated that HHcy may cause vessel dysfunction via induced endothelial apoptosis. Apoptotic cell death in the endothelium via the unfolded protein response [11] and the detachment-mediated process[12,13] are two possible mechanisms.

HHcy as a cardiovascular risk factor remains a contentious issue however. Observational studies have shown HHcy to be *associated* with an increased CVD risk,[14-17] though a causal role has been more difficult to confirm. A meta-analysis examining risk of ischaemic heart disease (IHD) and stroke found Hcy only a modest predictor in healthy populations.[18] With a 25% reduction in Hcy an 11% reduction in IHD and 19% reduction in stroke would occur if prospective data was used (the meta-analysis used retrospective data that may have suffered from reverse-causality) in the presence of adjustment for other known CVD risk and correction for regression dilution bias is performed.

Several randomized control trials (RCTs) on therapeutic reduction of Hcy in cardiovascular disease have been conducted; they typically use folate, vitamin B6 and B12 supplements as intervention. A meta-analysis of RCTs shows no significant difference between intervention and control groups.[19] Another large study[20] did not show a benefit in taking B group vitamins and folate verses placebo in those who has suffered a cerebrovascular event (ischaemic stroke, transient ischaemic attack or intracerebral haemorrhage). There was no reduction in the relative risk for non-fatal / fatal stroke, myocardial infarction or any other death from a vascular cause. The meta-analysis by Bazzano et al[21] similarly found all-cause mortality as well as CVD was not improved with folic acid supplementation amongst those with a prior history of vascular disease.

3.2 Homocysteine and apoptosis

As mentioned, evidence that Hcy induces vascular endothelial cell apoptosis exists.[11-13] Similar findings have been reported in neuronal tissue experiments as well. For example, Hcy stimulation of the N-methy-D-aspartate (NMDA) receptor of cerebellar granule cells has been shown to induce their death.[22] Importantly, this finding has been replicated for retinal ganglion cells (RGC). Moore et al[23] have shown intravitreal injection of homocysteine causes RGC apoptosis in vivo. Higher doses of homocysteine were associated with more widespread RGC apoptosis. In more recent work, Ganapathy et al[24] assessed mouse RGC cell culture response to Hcy exposure. They found marked RGC apoptosis in the presence of Hcy, a response that was significantly reduced by co-application of MK-801 (NMDA-receptor blocker). Homocysteine was also found to significantly increase intracellular calcium as well as reactive species superoxide, nitric oxide and peroxynitrite.

These studies in themselves do not constitute direct evidence that Hcy causes neuronal apoptosis. They do however suggest Hcy has the potential to do so through activation of NMDA-mediated intracellular pathways. Strategies that target Hcy and/or NMDA-receptors may potentially block this response and have therapeutic potential in glaucoma. Further work is need in this area.

3.2.1 Dementia and neurodegeneration

Given chronic glaucoma is characterised by progressive RGC apoptosis, it may be considered a form of neurodegeneration. Both chronic glaucoma and other neurodegenerative diseases, such as Alzheimer's disease (AD), similarly occur in predominantly elderly populations. A common aetiology is possible.

It is interesting to note the recent observation that Hcy is a biomarker for neurodegenerative disease and useful in identifying patients with B vitamin deficiency.[25] It has been shown that clinical symptoms of cognitive impairment and missing ankle tendon jerks are associated with patients with low vitamin B12 concentrations.[26]

A recent cohort study has demonstrated a correlation between polyneuropathy or dementia and increased tHcy in a geriatric population.[27] Similar findings were reported in an earlier study of neurodegenerative disorders, thus raising the possibility that Hcy has neurotoxic effects. These findings are consistent with laboratory data demonstrating neuronal apoptosis induced by Hcy as discussed above. However, given the apparent association between Hcy and CVD plus the role vascular disease plays in dementia and polyneuropathy,[28] it is difficult to know whether HHcy is causal or merely an association.

Evidence in support of a causal relationship between Hcy and neurodegeneration comes from a study examining central nervous system (CNS) atrophy with magnetic resonance imaging.[29] Patients aged over 70 years with mild cognitive impairment were randomised to receive either high-dose folic acid, vitamins B6 and B12 (n=85) or placebo (n=83) for 2 years. The mean rate of CNS atrophy per year was 0.76% [95% CI, 0.63–0.90] in the active treatment group and 1.08% [0.94–1.22] in the placebo group (P = 0.001). The treatment response was related to baseline Hcy levels: the rate of atrophy in participants with Hcy >13 µmol/L was 53% lower in the treatment group (P = 0.001). Whether the findings result from reduced Hcy, neuroprotective effects of folic acid, vitamin B6 and/or vitamin B12, improved CNS blood flow or some other mechanism is not clear. It does, however, raise the possibility that Hcy is involved in the neurodegenerative process.

3.2.2 Extracellular matrix remodelling

Extracellular matrix remodeling by Hcy is interesting because of implications for glaucoma pathogenesis. Effects on vascular tissues of the optic nerve head in addition to the trabecular meshwork or lamina cribrosa could result in glaucoma development or progression. There is no evidence to directly support this theory but findings in non-ocular tissue suggest a potential role. Human vascular smooth muscle cells from cardiomyopathic hearts demonstrate premature atherosclerosis when exposed to Hcy.[30] This is in association with significant up-regulation of collagen expression and α-actin. The response is potentially mediated through induced matrix metalloproteinase (MMP)-2, -4 and -9 activity as well as increased nitrotyrosine expression.[31-33]

4. Homocysteine and ocular vascular disease

Although the exact pathogenesis of glaucomatous optic neuropathy is unknown, impaired blood flow to the optic nerve head may play a role.[34,35]

Compromised optic nerve head perfusion may, in part, be due to the action of plasma Hcy. Raised tHcy causes overproduction of free radicals, intimal damage, matrix metalloproteinase up regulation and lysis of elastin or collagen in arterial media. [36,37] These effects are strongly linked with systemic vasculopathy including coronary artery disease,

aortic aneurysm, peripheral vascular disease and stroke. Similar events are likely to affect the microcirculation of the eye, including the optic nerve head.
Such associations have been described for a number of ocular vascular conditions. These are summarized below.

4.1 Retinal artery and vein occlusion

There have been numerous studies examining the association between raised plasma Hcy and retinal vascular occlusions. For instance, Moghimi et al[38] have demonstrated in an Iranian population, elevated plasma Hcy in retinal vein occlusion compared to control (14.76 vs 11.42 μmol/l). This is similarly the case in Indian,[39] North American,[40] Italian[41] and Chinese[42] studies. These findings are supported by data from the Blue Mountains Eye Study (Australia) demonstrating a significant correlation between vein occlusion and Hcy.[43]
Meta-analysis of Hcy in retinal vein occlusion has recently been performed.[44] In all, there were 1533 cases of retinal vein occlusion and 1708 controls where plasma Hcy was assessed. Individuals with vein occlusion had, on average, tHcy 2.8 μmol/L higher than the control group. It was concluded that evidence supports the role of Hcy in retinal vein occlusion but that publication bias and study heterogeneity were potential confounders. As for the cause for HHcy in these patients, the reason was not clear. The role of MTHFR mutation was examined but no correlation found. Environmental factors are likely to be important.
The literature on Hcy and retinal artery disease largely consists of small studies with fewer than 50 patients. One of the largest is a retrospective study of 105 patients with retinal artery occlusion.[45] This study found significant elevation of tHcy compared with the same number of controls. Mutation of MTHFR was also examined but no significant association could be found. Other notable studies[46,47] have reported similar findings and population based analysis from the Blue Mountains Eye Study also suggests HHcy and retinal artery emboli are weakly associated.[48] A small meta-analysis[49] suggests HHcy is more common in retinal artery occlusion but again no correlation with MTHFR mutation was found.

4.2 Choroidal neovascularization

Choroidal neovascularization (CNV), as seen in age-related macular degeneration (AMD), is a process of vascular proliferation beneath the retinal pigment epithelium and sub-retinal space. Risk factors are numerous and include cigarette smoking, lack of exercise, low fruit consumption, hypercholesterolaemia, increasing age and genetic susceptibility (eg: compliment factor H).[50,51]
A comprehensive epidemiological review shows links between CVD and AMD.[52] Analysis of data from the Framingham Eye Study and Beaver Dam Study, provides evidence that CVD and AMD share a similar risk profile (such as age, smoking, hypertension, hypercholesterolemia, post-menopausal estrogen use, diabetes, and dietary intake of fats, alcohol and antioxidants). In the same analysis, Hcy and vitamin B compounds were independent risk factors for both CVD and AMD.
Homocysteine as a risk factor for CNV development has been confirmed in a number of studies. Axer-Siegel et al[53] reported a significantly increased frequency of HHcy in patients with neovascular AMD (44.1%) compared to dry AMD (22.4%) and age-matched controls (21.4%). Several other groups have confirmed this finding.[54,55]

4.3 Diabetic retinopathy

The Wisconsin epidemiological study of diabetic retinopathy,[56] spanning from 1979 until 2007, looked at patients with type 1 diabetes mellitus. In the 1990-1992 prevalence data, Hcy was associated with increased odds of more severe diabetic retinopathy and presence of macular oedema. Many studies since have confirmed this association for type 2 diabetes mellitus as well.[57-59]

It is also true that severity of retinopathy correlates strongly with Hcy level, independent of glycaemic control.[60] Higher Hcy levels are observed in individuals with proliferative retinopathy compared to non-proliferative retinopathy, even though in both instances the levels are significantly elevated compared to control. This occurs despite similar baseline plasma glucose measurements and comparable frequencies of CVD (hypertension, ischaemic heart disease, cerebrovascular accident, thromboembolic event).

More recently, plasma and vitreous Hcy has been measured in patients with proliferative diabetic retinopathy.[61] Samples taken at the time of intra-ocular surgery showed mean elevation of both Hcy sample groups (plasma 16.04 ± 2.75 µmol/L; vitreous 3.64 ± 0.65 µmol/L) compared to non-diabetic controls. This both supports the outcomes of other studies on tHcy in diabetes and provides evidence of impaired blood-retina barrier in these patients. It is unclear what effect elevated vitreal Hcy has on disease progression.

There is conflicting evidence on the role of MTHFR mutation as a determinant of HHcy in diabetic retinopathy. A large study in Chinese patients[62] showed the MTHFR T allele was present in 49.09% of cases with diabetic retinopathy. This was significantly higher than in individuals with diabetes without retinopathy (33.16%) or no diabetes at all (31.58%). It has been suggested that homozygous mutation of MTHFR is associated with premature onset of diabetic retinopathy only in the presence of homozygous methionine synthase reductase mutation.[63] However, in a case series from Turkey,[64] no association between MTHFR C677T mutation and HHcy with retinopathy or neuropathy could be found. It is unclear whether such differences reflect ethnic variation, result from differences in study design or are influenced by other unidentified factors.

4.3.1 Non-Arteritic Ischaemic Optic Neuropathy (NAION)

In terms of pathophysiology, non-arteritic ischaemic optic neuropathy (NAION) and chronic glaucoma share a common mechanism. Both display deficiencies in optic nerve head perfusion although the mechanism is much less certain with chronic glaucoma. The event in NAION may represent a watershed infarct of retro-laminar optic nerve head tissue in individuals with compromised short posterior ciliary arteries and risk factors that include a crowded disc, poorly overlapping vascular fields, nocturnal hypotension and hypoxia.[65] Some risk factors are common to chronic glaucoma and typically ante cede both conditions by many years. However, whilst NAION is an acute condition, chronic glaucoma is not.

Given that impaired circulation is central to the development of NAION, it seems logical that HHcy might play a role. This has borne out in several studies examining associations between the two. Pianka et al[66] reported elevated levels in 45% of 40 NAION patients (mean age 66 years) but in only 9.8% of control subjects. Similar findings have been reported by Giambene et al[67] and Weger et al.[68]

However, some studies have questioned the association. Both Kawasaki et al[69] in a study of 17 patients and Biousse et al[70] in a study of 14 patients failed to find any significant association with Hcy. One might criticise these studies on the basis of small participant numbers but it is noteworthy that both patient cohorts were relatively young. This is interesting given plasma Hcy levels increase with age.[5] This raises the possibility that Hcy becomes increasingly important in NAION development with increasing age and again points to similarities with chronic glaucoma. Further research is required in this area.

4.4 Ocular Ischaemic Syndrome

Ocular ischemic syndrome (OIS) is the name given to the ocular symptoms and signs attributable to chronic, severe carotid artery obstruction, although chronic ophthalmic artery obstruction can cause a similar clinical picture. Atherosclerosis is the most common aetiology, but possible causes include Eisenmenger syndrome, giant cell arteritis, and other inflammatory conditions. Most patients are older than 55 years of age. Typically, a 90% or greater ipsilateral obstruction is necessary to cause the ocular ischemic syndrome. Both eyes are involved in about 20% of cases. Iris neovascularization is the most common anterior segment finding at diagnosis and typical fundus signs include retinal arteriole narrowing, retinal venous dilatation without tortuosity, midperipheral retinal haemorrhages and microaneurysms, and peripheral vascular closure.

Little information is available linking OIS with HHcy. A case described of bilateral OIS[71] without carotid artery stenosis and normal cardiovascular and biochemical markers had a markedly elevated tHcy of 20.8 μmol/l as the only abnormality. No larger studies have been published to confirm or deny this association.

5. Plasma homocysteine and chronic glaucoma

Chronic glaucoma may, in part, be the manifestation of abnormal optic nerve head perfusion. This is supported by evidence showing altered flow dynamics within the ophthalmic and retinal arteries of patients with glaucoma, an association between glaucoma and vascular disease, and acceleration of the glaucomatous process in the presence of nocturnal hypotension. Evidence also indicates glaucoma is a process of retinal ganglion cell apoptosis, which may in turn be related to or independent of optic nerve head perfusion.

Homocysteine potentially contributes to glaucoma pathogenesis via both mechanisms. Unsurprisingly, many studies have examined the role of Hcy in glaucoma over the past decade. However, there are inherent difficulties in comparing studies on tHcy. The work in relation to glaucoma is no exception. The main challenges relate to the way Hcy is measured, study design and differences in populations studied.

Despite the large number of Hcy-glaucoma studies, collectively they report on a relatively confined population. A significant number of studies have been in Turkish cohorts. German studies also contribute significantly to the overall number. The German studies are from the same group and presumably represent the same population.

There are also reports from Israel, Australia, USA, Italy and Pakistan. We have no results from populations in Asia, Africa or South America. Interestingly, there is also little data published from Scandinavia. Given the findings in pseudoexfoliation glaucoma (PXFG) and high prevalence of PXFG in this region, one would expect both interest and opportunity to conduct studies there. There has been a report on tHcy in pseudoexfoliation syndrome and PXFG combined from Finland;[72] we are not aware of any studies specifically reporting glaucoma.

The main determinants of mildly elevated plasma homocysteine remain poor diet, vegetarianism, low folate, low cobalamin, MTHFR mutation, renal impairment and medications[5]. Whilst the majority of Hcy-glaucoma studies control for the effects of medication and renal impairment, much less is known about the caloric intake of the study participants or folate/cobalamin status. Differences in diet are likely to be real but the impact is unknown in glaucoma research.

A few studies have reported folate and vitamin B status and point to significant differences between populations. Participants in an Italian study[73] were found to have high normal folate and mid normal vitamin B12 whereas 2 studies from Turkey have low normal vitamin B12 with normal[74] or depleted folate.[79] In at least 1 of these studies,[74] it is clear that some participants were vitamin B12 deficient as well. As the influence of folate and vitamin B12 on plasma homocysteine is non-linear,[5] these differences could amount to considerable variations in plasma homocysteine. For example, vitamin B12 in the mid normal range is associated with mean plasma homocysteine around 10 - 11 μmol/L compared to 14 μmol/L for vitamin B12 at the lower limit of normal.[5] Individuals that are vitamin B12 deficient can have plasma homocysteine near 20 μmol/L. Similarly, the difference in folate levels reported by Turgut[74] and Cumurcu[78] can amount to an almost doubling of plasma homocysteine.[5] Despite researchers best efforts, we are not comparing like with like.

Only a handful of the reports on Hcy and glaucoma are sufficiently powered to detect the outcome they describe. Sample size calculation, assuming the need to detect a 2 μmol/L difference, standard deviation of 3 μmol/L, a power of 90% and significance set at 0.05, requires a sample size of at least 48 cases per group. In studies where standard deviation exceeds 9 μmol/L (Table 2), 426 cases would be required to detect a significant difference. Clearly, these criteria have not been met in most studies.

Author	*Year*	*Design*	*Number*	*Location*	*Assay*	*Homocysteine (μmol/L)*	Elevated
Tranchina[73]	2011	Prospective	36	Italy	EIA	16.55 ± 7.23	Yes
Turgut[74]	2010	Prospective	34	Turkey	HPLC	15.46 ± 9.27	Yes
Clement[75]	2009	Prospective	48	Australia	FPIA	11.77 ± 4.18	Yes
Roedl[76]	2007	Prospective	30	Germany	HPLC	14.51 ± 4.43	Yes
Roedl[77]	2007	Prospective	70	Germany	HPLC	13.77 ± 4.13	Yes
Cumurcu[78]	2006	Prospective	24	Turkey	EIA	14.88 ± 3.26	Yes
Saricaoglu[79]	2006	Prospective	20	Turkey	EIA	18.50 ± 4.50	Yes
Turacli[80]	2005	Prospective	60	Turkey	FPIA	15.76 ± 5.55	No
Altinta[81]	2005	Prospective	22	Turkey	FPIA	14.96 ± 4.55	Yes
Bleich[82]	2004	Prospective	29	Germany	EIA	15.53 ± 7.76	Yes
Leibovitch[83]	2003	Prospective	30	*Israel*	HPLC	16.80 ± 3.20	Yes
Vessani[84]	2003	Prospective	50	*USA*	FPIA	10.1*	Yes
Bleich[85]	2002	Prospective	19	*Germany*	EIA	11.61± 3.74	Yes

* Standard Deviation not reported

Table 2. Homocysteine and Pseudoexfoliation Glaucoma (PXFG)

5.1 Pseudoexfoliation glaucoma

Pseudoexfoliation syndrome is a multi-system disorder of cellular metabolism resulting in random synthesis of extracellular fibrillar material. The main clinical manifestation is in the eye where fibrillar material can be seen on the lens capsule and pupil margin. Affected individuals have a weak lens capsule and zonules and have poor mydriasis. They are at

significant risk of developing raised IOP with associated glaucoma (PXFG) but glaucoma has also been reported despite apparently normal IOP.
PXFG shares many common associations with homocysteine. Cardioavascular disease [84], oxidative stress[87] increased prevalence with age and Alzheimer's disease [88,89] are common to both: a pathogenic link has been proposed.[90] This is supported by research showing exfoliation material contains laminin, elastin and fibrillin, components of extracellular matrix metabolism under the influence of homocysteine.
All studies looking at the association between PXFG and plasma homocysteine have demonstrated significant elevation with the exception of Turacli et al[80] (Table 2). This is the most consistent finding in homocysteine-glaucoma research and has occurred despite different assays and study populations across four continents. The control group in the Turacli et al study had the highest mean plasma homocysteine level (17.43 μmol/L; 67.6% with hyperhomocysteinaemia) of any study on glaucoma reported in the literature. Clearly this rate of hyperhomocysteinaemia in the general population is abnormal and makes detection of homocysteine elevation difficult in different cohorts.
The findings in PXFG are strongly suggestive that Hcy is a factor in its pathogenesis. Attention should shift now towards larger population-based studies and clinical trials to confirm this association and assess response to intervention (folate and vitamin B12). The prospect of an intervention that is taken orally, is cheap and with few side effects is an exciting prospect.

5.2 Primary open angle glaucoma

Studies are divided on the issue of plasma Hcy and POAG (Table 3). Equal numbers report a statistically significant correlation or no correlation at all. It is suggested that differences in Hcy assays, study design and populations sampled underlie these outcomes. The effect of assays can largely be discounted for 3 reasons: i) HPLC, EIA and FPIA are comparable tests,[5] ii) in each study POAG and control samples were analyzed using the same technique and laboratory, and iii) the findings for PXFG have been so consistent despite the use of different assays.

Author	*Year*	*Design*	*Number*	*Population*	*Assay*	*Homocysteine (μmol/L)*	*Elevated*
Tranchina[73]	2011	Prospective	40	Italy	EIA	13.91 ± 3.61	No
Turgut[74]	2010	Prospective	34	Turkey	HPLC	11.28 ± 4.80	No
Michael[90]	2009	Prospective	70	Pakistan	EIA	15.20 ± 1.28	Yes
Clement[75]	2009	Prospective	36	Australia	FPIA	11.21 ± 2.84	Yes
Roedl[91]	2008	Prospective	36	Germany	HPLC	13.43 ± 3.53	Yes
Roedl[92]	2007	Prospective	39	Germany	HPLC	13.93 ± 4.59	Yes
Cumurcu[78]	2006	Prospective	25	Turkey	EIA	9.22 ± 3.70	No
Altinta[81]	2005	Prospective	19	Turkey	FPIA	11.91 ± 4.38	No
Wang[93]	2004	Retrospective	55	USA	HPLC	14.90 ± 6.45	No
Bleich[85]	2002	Prospective	18	Germany	EIA	12.52 ± 3.62	Yes

Table 3. Homocysteine and Primary Open Angle Glaucoma (POAG)

It is however, quite reasonable to suggest study design and population sampled are significant factors. Given the sample size calculations already mentioned, it seems hardly surprising some studies have had a negative outcome. In this respect, it is interesting to note that 3 of 5 studies reporting no significant association actually demonstrated small[78] or considerable[74,81] differences in plasma homocysteine between POAG and control. This is confounded by large variance in the population (as shown by standard deviation) and high mean plasma homocysteine in controls.

5.3 Normal tension glaucoma

Non-IOP dependent factors are of particular interest in normal tension glaucoma (NTG). Work has focused on optic nerve head perfusion and its influences including atherosclerotic disease, systemic hypertension, use of anti-hypertensive agents and vasospastic disorders (eg: migraine, Raynaud's phenomenon). Similarly, retinal ganglion cell apoptosis might play a role. Homocysteine has the potential to contribute to NTG pathogenesis via both pathways: as a mediator of vascular injury leading to impaired optic nerve head perfusion and as an excitatory amino acid triggering RGC apoptosis.[23,24]

Five studies have reported on plasma homocysteine in NTG (Table 4). With the exception of Clement et al,[75] none have found a statistically significant association. However, closer examination of these data is needed. Both Turgut et al[74] and Cumurcu et al[78] reported increased plasma homocysteine in NTG though it did not reach statistical significance. Levels in NTG were 29.8% and 23.7% higher than control compared to 19.6% as reported by Clement et al. Again, sample size plays a role here. Both studies are significantly underpowered to detect a difference given the high standard deviation reported.

It may be the case that homocysteine is not associated with NTG. However, based on the scope and quality of research currently available, no conclusions can be made yet. Further work is needed to clarify this issue.

Author	*Year*	*Design*	*Number*	*Population*	*Assay*	*Homocysteine (μmol/L)*	*Elevated*
Rossler[94]	2010	Prospective	42	Germany	FPIA	10.95 ± 2.65	No
Turgut[74]	2010	Prospective	48	Turkey	HPLC	11.27 ± 4.91	No
Clement[75]	2009	Prospective	34	Australia	FPIA	11.74 ± 3.79	Yes
Cumurcu[78]	2006	Prospective	19	Turkey	EIA	10.39 ± 3.89	No
Vessani[84]	2003	Prospective	25	*USA*	FPIA	9.1*	No

* Standard Deviation not reported

Table 4. Homocysteine and Normal Tension Glaucoma (NTG)

5.4 Primary angle closure glaucoma

The proposed mechanism by which raised homocysteine contributes to primary angle closure glaucoma (PACG) differs significantly from PXFG, POAG and NTG. Much less emphasis has been placed on the role of homocysteine in ocular circulation, RGC apoptosis and trabecular meshwork remodelling. Instead, the effect on extracellular matrix remodelling of other anterior segment structures has been promoted.[90] This is on the basis that patients with PACG have reduced MMP-2 and MMP-9 expression in Tenon's capsule and Hcy has demonstrable effects on MMP expression.

The only study reporting plasma Hcy in PACG (Table 5) showed significant elevation compared with POAG and control.[90] The same report demonstrated increased frequency of

C677T and A1298C MTHFR polymorphisms. However, closer analysis shows MTHFR mutations are frequent in 1 ethnic group (Punjabi) but not the other (Pathan). Unfortunately, Hcy levels within each ethnic group are not stated. A difference between the two would suggest i) Hhcy is not associated with PACG but may occur in parallel in some populations due to certain factors (eg: MTHFR polymorphisms) ii) the anterior segment remodelling theory is unlikely. In the absence of such data we can only speculate. We await other studies with interest.

Author	*Year*	*Design*	*Number*	*Population*	*Assay*	*Homocysteine (µmol/L)*	*Elevated*
Michael[90]	2009	Prospective	48	Pakistan	EIA	20.8 ± 4.8	Yes

Table 5. Homocysteine and Primary Angle Closure Glaucoma (PACG)

6. MTHFR mutation and chronic glaucoma

MTHFR mutation is of interest given its role as the major genetic determinant of raised plasma Hcy. Increased mutation rates could help explain the finding of raised plasma Hcy in some glaucoma patients. Studies have reported on the frequency of MTHFR C677T mutation, and to a lesser extent A1298C, in different types of glaucoma (Table 6).

Author	*Year*	*Glaucoma*	Increased Frequency
Clement[75]	2009	PXFG	No
Fan[95]	2008	PXFG	No
Fingert[96]	2006	PXFG	No
Mossbock[97]	2006	PXFG	No
Fan[98]	2010	POAG	No
Michael[90]	2009	POAG	No
Clement[75]	2009	POAG	No
Michael[99]	2008	POAG	No
Zetterberg[100]	2007	POAG	No
Mabuchi[101]	2006	POAG	No
Fingert[96]	2006	POAG	No
Mossbock[97]	2006	POAG	No
Junemann[102]	2005	POAG	Yes
Bleich[85]	2002	POAG	Yes
Clement[75]	2009	NTG	No
Woo[103]	2009	NTG	Yes
Mabuchi[101]	2006	NTG	No
Michael[90]	2009	PACG	Yes
Michael[99]	2008	PACG	Yes

Table 6. MTHFR Mutation and Chronic Glaucoma

Although, there is a large body of evidence supporting a role for Hcy in the pathogenesis of PXFG, there are few studies on MTHFR mutation in this condition. Despite this, the findings have been universal: MTHFR mutation is not a risk factor for PXFG. Raised plasma Hcy is due to other factors in these patients.

Most MTHFR mutation research in glaucoma has been on POAG. Despite the inconsistent findings regarding Hcy, studies generally agree MTHFR mutation does not occur at an increased rate in POAG. Two studies[85,102] have reported MTHFR C677T mutation is a risk factor for POAG. Both are from the same research group. It is unclear whether this data is from the same cohort of patients.

Fewer studies have examined MTHFR mutation in NTG. For this reason, it is hard to make a sensible conclusion. At this stage, it seems MTHFR is not likely to be a risk factor for NTG but further research is needed.

Two reports on PACG suggest an association. In both studies[90,99] from the same group, the association was seen in only one ethnic subgroup (Pakistani Punjabi). The significance of this is uncertain without corroborating evidence from other groups examining different populations.

7. Conclusion

There is now a substantial body of literature on Hcy and glaucoma. Although there is general agreement that Hcy is raised in patients with PXFG, the findings have been less consistent for other types of chronic glaucoma. The reason for this is not entirely clear but may, in part, relate to study design and population differences.

The findings in PXFG, and to a lesser extent with other chronic glaucoma, suggest therapeutic intervention might be an option in these patients. Plasma Hcy may be lowered by supplemental folate and vitamin B12: both are readily available, cheap and have few side effects. Benefit is likely to be derived from positive effects on vascular health, in particular optic nerve head perfusion. Reduced RGC apoptosis is another potential outcome. No studies have yet examined the effect of taking these supplements on glaucoma progression.

With respect to treating raised Hcy in glaucoma, there are two areas of concern. First, the level of Hcy required to start treatment is ill defined. Although raised compared to control, most research quotes mean Hcy levels within the normal reference range. For example, our study[75] found HHcy (female > 12 μmol/L; male > 14 μmol/L) in 27.6%, 30.6% and 29.4% of patients with PXFG, POAG and NTG respectively. This means two-thirds of patients return what is considered a normal Hcy reading. What do we do here? Options include treating only those with raised Hcy by laboratory definition, reducing the threshold for treatment or treating everyone irrespective of Hcy level. Clinical trials measuring glaucoma progression following folate and vitamin B12 supplementation relative to Hcy level will help define this better.

Secondly, and more worrying, is the observation in the cardiovascular literature that interventions that reduce Hcy have little benefit.[19] This is despite the consistent observation that raised Hcy is a risk factor for CVD. This points to a similar outcome in glaucoma research. However, glaucoma pathogenesis is multi-factorial and optic nerve head perfusion is only part of the story. Homocysteine, and strategies to lower it, can potentially have direct actions on the optic nerve (ie: apoptosis of RGCs) and structures that support it (ie: ECM remodeling). We have been encouraged by the outcomes in AD research[29] showing benefit from supplemental folate and vitamin B12 intake.

8. Acknowledgment

The authors wish to thank Mr Haider Twaij for assistance with Figure 1.

9. References

[1] Miyaki K. Genetic polymorphisms in homocysteine metabolism and response to folate intake: A comprehensive strategy to elucidate useful genetic information. *J Epidemiol.* 2010; 20: 266-70.

[2] Miyaki K, Murata M, Kikuchi H et al. Assessment of tailor-made prevention of atherosclerosis with folic acid supplementation: Randomized, double-blind, placebo-controlled trials in each MTHFR C677T genotype. *J Hum Genet* 2005; 50: 241-8.

[3] Dekou V, Whincup P, Papacosta O et al. The effect of the C677T and A1298C polymorphisms in the methylenetetrahydrofolate reductase gene on homocysteine levels in elderly men and women from the british regional heart study. *Atherosclerosis.* 2001; 154: 659-66.

[4] Van Der Put NMJ, Gabreëls F, Stevens EMB et al. A second common mutation in the methylenetetrahydrofolate reductase gene: An additional risk factor for neural-tube defects? *Am J Hum Genet.* 1998; 62:1044-51.

[5] Refsum H, Smith AD, Ueland PM et al. c *Clin Chem* 2004 50: 3-32.

[6] Pfeiffer CM, Huff DL, Smith SJ et al. Gunter Comparison of Plasma Total Homocysteine Measurements in 14 Laboratories: An International Study *Clin Chem* 1999; 45: 1261-8

[7] McCully KS. Vascular pathology of homocysteinemia: Implications for the pathogenesis of arteriosclerosis. *Am J Pathol.* 1969; 56: 111-28

[8] Zhang X, Li H, Jin H et al. Effects of homocysteine on endothelial nitric oxide production. *Am J Physiol - Renal Physiol.* 2000; 279: F671-8

[9] Tawakol A, Omland T, Gerhard M et al. Hyperhomocysteinemia is associated with impaired endothelium- dependent vasodilation in humans. *Circulation.* 1997; 95:1119-21

[10] Bellamy MF, McDowell IFW, Ramsey MW et al. Hyperhomocysteinemia after an oral methionine load acutely impairs endothelial function in healthy adults. *Circulation.* 1998; 98:1848-52

[11] Austin RC, Lentz SR, Werstuck GH. Role of hyperhomocysteinemia in endothelial dysfunction and atherothrombotic disease. *Cell Death Differ.* 2004; 11: S56-64

[12] Di Simone N, Maggiano N, Caliandro D et al. Homocysteine induces trophoblast cell death with apoptotic features. *Biol. Reprod.* 2003; 69: 1129–34

[13] Hultberg B, Andersson A, Isaksson A. Metabolism of homocysteine, its relation to the other cellular thiols and its mechanism of cell damage in a cell culture line (human histiocytic cell line U-937). *Biochem. Biophys. Acta* 1995; 1269: 6–12

[14] Faeh D, Chiolero A, Paccaud F. Homocysteine as a risk factor for cardiovascular disease: Should we (still) worry about it? *Swiss Medical Weekly.* 2006; 136: 745-56

[15] Ueland PM, Refsum H, Beresford SA et al. The controversy over homocysteine and cardiovascular risk. *Am J Clin Nutr.* 2000; 72: 324–32

[16] Kaplan ED. Association between homocysteine levels and risk of vascular events. *Drugs Today.* 2003; 39: 175–92

[17] Cacciapuoti F. Hyper-homocysteinemia: a novel risk factor or a powerful marker for cardiovascular diseases? Pathogenetic and therapeutical uncertainties. *J Thromb Thrombolysis*. 2011 Jan 14. [Epub ahead of print]

[18] Clarke R, Collins R, Lewington S et al. Homocysteine and risk of ischemic heart disease and stroke: A meta-analysis. JAMA. 2002; 288: 2015-22

[19] Mei W, Rong Y, Jinming L et al. Effect of homocysteine interventions on the risk of cardiocerebrovascular events: A meta-analysis of randomised controlled trials. *Int J Clin Pract*. 2010; 64: 208-15

[20] Graeme J. B vitamins in patients with recent transient ischaemic attack or stroke in the VITAmins TO prevent stroke (VITATOPS) trial: A randomised, double-blind, parallel, placebo-controlled trial. *Lancet Neurol*. 2010; 9: 855-65

[21] Bazzano LA, Reynolds K, Holder KN et al. Effect of folic acid supplementation on risk of cardiovascular diseases: A meta-analysis of randomized controlled trials. *JAMA*. 2006; 296: 2720-6

[22] Kim W, Pae Y. Involvement of N-methyl-D-aspartate receptor and free radical in homocysteine-mediated toxicity on rat cerebellar granule cells in culture. *Neurosci Lett*. 1996; 216: 117-20.

[23] Moore P, El-sherbeny A, Roon P, Schoenlein PV, Ganapathy V, Smith SB. Apoptotic cell death in the mouse retinal ganglion cell layer is induced in vivo by the excitatory amino acid homocysteine. *Exp Eye Res*. 2001; 73: 45-57.

[24] Ganapathy PS, White RE, Ha Y, Bozard BR, McNeil PL, Caldwell RW, Kumar S, Black SM, Smith SB. The Role of N-Methyl-D-Aspartate Receptor Activation in Homocysteine-Induced Death of Retinal Ganglion Cells. *IOVS* 2011 Mar 24. [Epub ahead of print].

[25] Herrmann W, Obeid R. Homocysteine: A biomarker in neurodegenerative diseases. *Clin Chem Lab Med*. 2011; 49: 435-41

[26] Hin H, Clarke R, Sherliker P et al. Clinical relevance of low serum vitamin B12 concentrations in older people: The banbury B12 study. *Age Ageing*. 2006; 35: 416-22

[27] Kim J, Park MH, Kim E et al. Plasma homocysteine is associated with the risk of mild cognitive impairment in an elderly korean population. *J Nutr*. 2007; 137: 2093-7

[28] Leblhuber F, Schroecksnadel K, Beran-Praher M et al Polyneuropathy and dementia in old age: Common inflammatory and vascular parameters. *J Neural Transm*. 2011 [Epub ahead of print].

[29] Smith AD, Smith SM, de Jager CA et al. Homocysteine-lowering by b vitamins slows the rate of accelerated brain atrophy in mild cognitive impairment: A randomized controlled trial. *PLoS ONE*. 2010; 5:1-10

[30] Tyagi SC. Homocysteine redox receptor and regulation of extracellular matrix components in vascular cells. *Am J Physiol - Cell Physiol*. 1998; 274: C396-405.

[31] Bescond A, Augier T, Chareyre C et al. Influence of homocysteine on matrix metalooproteinase-2: activation and activity. *Biochem Biophys Res Commun* 1999: 263; 205-16

[32] Sood HS, Cox MJ, Tyagi SC. Generation of Nitrotyrosine Precedes Activation of Metalloproteinase in Myocardium of Hyperhomocysteinemic Rats. *Antiox Redox Signal.* 2002: 4; 799-804

[33] Moshal KS, Sen U, Tyagi N et al. Regulation of homocysteine-induced MMP-9 by ERK1/2 pathway *Am J Physiol Cell Physiol,* 2006: 290; C883-C891

[34] Flammer J, Orgul S, Costa VP et al. The impact of ocular blood flow in glaucoma. *Prog Retin Eye Res* 2002: 21:359-93

[35] Hayreh SS: Blood flow in the optic nerve head and factors that may influence it. *Prog Retin Eye Res* 2001: 20:595-624

[36] Finkelstein JD: The metabolism of homocysteine: pathways and regulation. *Eur J Pediatr* 1998: 157; 40-44

[37] Brunelli T, Prisco D, Fedi S et al. High prevelance of mild hyperhomocysteinemia in patients with abdominal aortic aneurysm. *J Vasc Surg* 2000: 32; 531-536

[38] Moghimi S, Najmi Z, Faghihi H et al. Hyperhomocysteinemia and central retinal vein occlusion in Iranian population. *Int Ophthalmol.* 2008; 28; 23-8

[39] Narayanasamy A, Subramaniam B, Karunakaran C et al. Hyperhomocysteinemia and low methionine stress are risk factors for central retinal venous occlusion in an Indian population. *IOVS* 2007: 48; 1441-6

[40] Glueck CJ, Ping W, Hutchins R et al. Ocular vascular thrombotic events: central retinal vein and central retinal artery occlusions. *Clin Appl Thromb Hemost.* 2008: 14; 286-94

[41] Ferrazzi P, Di Micco P, Quaglia I et al. Homocysteine, MTHFR C677T gene polymorphism, folic acid and vitamin B 12 in patients with retinal vein occlusion. *Thromb J.* 2005: 7; 3-13

[42] Gao W, Wang YS, Zhang P et al. Hyperhomocysteinemia and low plasma folate as risk factors for central retinal vein occlusion: a case-control study in a Chinese population. *Graefes Arch Clin Exp Ophthalmol.* 2006: 244; 1246-9

[43] Chua B, Kifley A, Wong TY et al. Homocysteine and retinal vein occlusion: a population-based study. *Am J Ophthalmol.* 2005: 139; 181-2

[44] McGimpsey SJ, Woodside JV, Cardwell C et al. Homocysteine, methylenetetrahydrofolate reductase C677T polymorphism, and risk of retinal vein occlusion: a meta-analysis. *Ophthalmology.* 2009: 116; 1778-87

[45] Weger M, Stanger O, Deutschmann H, Leitner FJ, Renner W, Schmut O, Semmelrock J, Haas A. The role of hyperhomocysteinemia and methylenetetrahydrofolate reductase (MTHFR) C677T mutation in patients with retinal artery occlusion. *Am J Ophthalmol.* 2002: 134; 57-61

[46] Marcucci R, Sodi A, Giambene B et al. Cardiovascular and thrombophilic risk factors in patients with retinal artery occlusion. *Blood Coagul Fibrinolysis.* 2007: 18; 321-6

[47] Martin SC, Rauz S, Marr JE et al. Plasma total homocysteine and retinal vascular disease. *Eye* 2000: 14; 590-3

[48] Chua B, Kifley A, Wong TY et al. Homocysteine and retinal emboli: the Blue Mountains Eye Study. *Am J Ophthalmol.* 2006; 142: 322-4

[49] Cahill MT, Stinnett SS, Fekrat S. Meta-analysis of plasma homocysteine, serum folate, serum vitamin B(12), and thermolabile MTHFR genotype as risk factors for retinal vascular occlusive disease. *Am J Ophthalmol.* 2003: 136; 1136-50

[50] Williams PT. Prospective study of incident age-related macular degeneration in relation to vigorous physical activity during a 7-year follow-up. *IOVS*. 2009: 50; 101-6.
[51] Magnusson KP, Duan S, Sigurdsson H et al. CFH Y402H confers similar risk of soft drusen and both forms of advanced AMD. *PLoS Med.* 2006: 3; e5.
[52] Snow KK, Seddon JM. Age-related macular degeneration and cardiovascular disease share common antecedents? *Ophthalmic Epidemiol.* 1999: 6; 125-43.
[53] Axer-Siegel R, Bourla D, Ehrlich R et al. Association of neovascular age-related macular degeneration and hyperhomocysteinemia. *Am J Ophthalmol.* 2004: 137; 84-9.
[54] Javadzadeh A, Ghorbanihaghjo A, Bahreini E. Plasma oxidized LDL and thiol-containing molecules in patients with exudative age-related macular degeneration. *Molecular Vis.* 2010; 16: 2578-84
[55] Coral K, Raman R, Rathi S et al. Plasma homocysteine and total thiol content in patients with exudative age-related macular degeneration. *Eye.* 2006; 20: 203-7
[56] Klein BEK, Knudtson MD, Tsai MY et al. The relation of markers of inflammation and endothelial dysfunction to the prevalence and progression of diabetic retinopathy: Wisconsin epidemiologic study of diabetic retinopathy. *Arch Ophthalmol.* 2009; 127: 1175-82
[57] Hoogeveen EK, Kostense PJ, Eysink PE et al. Hyperhomocysteinemia is associated with the presence of retinopathy in type 2 diabetes mellitus: the Hoorn study. *Arch Intern Med.* 2000 23; 160: 2984-90
[58] Brazionis L, Rowley K Sr, Itsiopoulos C et al. Homocysteine and diabetic retinopathy. *Diabetes Care.* 2008; 31: 50-6.
[59] Aydin E, Demir HD, Ozyurt H et al. Association of plasma homocysteine and macular edema in type 2 diabetes mellitus. *Eur J Ophthalmol.* 2008; 18: 226-32
[60] Goldstein M, Leibovitch I, Yeffimov I et al. Hyperhomocysteinemia in patients with diabetes mellitus with and without diabetic retinopathy. *Eye* 2004; 18: 460-5
[61] Aydemir O, Türkçüoğlu P, Güler M et al. Plasma and vitreous homocysteine concentrations in patients with proliferative diabetic retinopathy. *Retina.* 2008; 28: 741-3
[62] Sun J, Xu Y, Zhu Y et al. The relationship between MTHFR gene polymorphisms, plasma homocysteine levels and diabetic retinopathy in type 2 diabetes mellitus. *Chin Med J.* 2003; 116: 145-7
[63] Wiltshire EJ, Mohsin F, Chan A. Methylenetetrahydrofolate reductase and methionine synthase reductase gene polymorphisms and protection from microvascular complications in adolescents with type 1 diabetes. *Pediatr Diabetes.* 2008; 9: 348-53
[64] Ukinc K, Ersoz HO, Karahan C, et al. Methyltetrahydrofolate reductase C677T gene mutation and hyperhomocysteinemia as a novel risk factor for diabetic nephropathy. *Endocrine.* 2009; 36: 255-61.
[65] Hayreh SS. Acute ischemic disorders of the optic nerve: pathogenesis, clinical manifestations and management. *Ophthal Clin North Am* 1996; 9: 407–42
[66] Pianka P, Almog Y, Man O, et al. Hyperhomocysteinemia in patients with non-arteritic anterior ischaemic neuropathy, central retinal artery occlusion and central retinal vein occlusion. *Ophthalmology* 2000; 107: 1588–92

[67] Giambene B, Sodi A, Sofi F et al. Evaluation of traditional and emerging cardiovascular risk factors in patients with non-arteritic anterior ischemic optic neuropathy: A case-control study. *Graefe Arch Clin Exp Ophthal.* 2009; 247: 693-7

[68] Weger M, Stanger O, Deutschmann H, et al. Hyperhomocysteinaemia, but not MTHFR C677T mutation, as a risk factor for nonarteritic ischemic optic neuropathy. *Br J Ophthalmol* 2001; 85: 803–6

[69] Kawasaki A, Purvin VA, Burgett RA. Hyperhomocysteinaemia in young patients with non-arteritic anterior ischaemic optic neuropathy. *Br J Ophthalmol* 1999; 83: 1287–90

[70] Biousse V, Kerrison JB, Newman NJ. Is non-arteritic anterior ischaemic optic neuropathy related to homocysteine? *Br J Ophthalmol* 2000; 84: 555

[71] Imrie FR, Hammer HM, Jay JL. Bilateral ocular ischaemic syndrome in association with hyperhomocysteinaemia. *Eye.* 2002; 16: 497-500.

[72] Puustjärvi T, Blomster H, Kontkanen M et al. Plasma and aqueous humour levels of homocysteine in exfoliation syndrome. *Graefes Arch Clin Exp Ophthalmol.* 2004; 242: 749-54.

[73] Tranchina L, Centofanti M, Oddone F et al. Levels of plasma homocysteine in pseudoexfoliation glaucoma. *Graefes Arch Clin Exp Ophthalmol* 2011 249; 443-448

[74] Turgut B, Kaya M, Arslan S et al. Levels of circulating homocysteine, vitamin B6, vitamin B12, and folate in different types of open-angle glaucoma *Clin Interventions Aging* 2010:5 133–9

[75] Clement CI, Goldberg I, Healey P *et al* Plasma Homocysteine, MTHFR Gene Mutation, and Open-angle Glaucoma *J Glaucoma* 2009: 18; 73-8

[76] Roedl JB, Bleich S, Reulbach U et al. Homocysteine in tear fluid of patients with pseudoexfoliation glaucoma. *J Glaucoma.* 2007; 16: 234-9

[77] Roedl JB, Bleich S, Reulbach U et al. Vitamin deficiency and hyperhomocysteinemia in pseudoexfoliation glaucoma. *J Neural Transm.* 2007; 114: 571-5

[78] Cumurcu T, Sahin S, Aydin E. Serum homocysteine, vitamin B12 and folic acid levels in different types of glaucoma. *BMC Ophthalmol.* 2006; 6: 6.

[79] Saricaoglu MS, Karakurt A, Sengun A et al. Plasma homocysteine levels and vitamin B status in patients with Pseudoexfoliation syndrome. *Saudi Med J.* 2006; 27: 833-7.

[80] Turaci ME, Tekeli O, O¨zdemir F, et al. Methylenetetrahydrofolate reductase 677 C-T and homocysteine levels in Turkish patients with pseudoexfoliation. *Clin Exp Ophthalmol.* 2005; 33: 505–8.

[81] Altinta O, Maral H, Yüksel N et al. Homocysteine and nitric oxide levels in plasma of patients with pseudoexfoliation syndrome, pseudoexfoliation glaucoma, and primary open-angle glaucoma. *Graefes Arch Clin Exp Ophthalmol.* 2005; 243: 677-83

[82] Bleich S, Roedl J, Von Ahsen N, et al. Elevated homocysteine in aqueous humor of patients with pseudoexfoliation glaucoma. *Am J Ophthalmol.* 2004; 138: 162–4

[83] Leibovitch I, Kurtz S, Shemesh G et al. Hyperhomocystinemia in Pseudoexfoliation Glaucoma *J Glaucoma* 12: 36–9

[84] Vessani RM, Ritch R, Liebmann JM, et al. Plasma homocysteine is elevated in patients with exfoliation syndrome. *Am J Ophthalmol.* 2003; 136: 41–6

[85] Bleich S, Jünemann A, von Ahsen N et al. Homocysteine and risk of open-angle glaucoma. *J Neural Transm.* 2002; 109:1499-504

[86] Mitchell P, Wang JJ, Smith W. Association of pseudoexfoliation syndrome with increased vascular risk. *Am J Ophthalmol* 1997; 124: 685–687
[87] Koliakos GG, Konstas AG, Schlötzer-Schrehardt U et al. Endothelin-1 concentration is increased in aqueous humour of patients with exfoliation syndrome. *Br J Ophthalmol* 2004: 88; 523-7
[88] Linner E, Popovic V, Gottfries CG et al The exfoliation syndrome in cognitive impairment of cerebrovascular or Alzheimer's type. *Acta Ophthalmolo Scand* 2001: 79; 283 - 5
[89] Leblhuber F, Walli J, Artner-Dworzak E et al Hyperhomocysteinemia in dementia. *J Neural Transm* 2000: 107 1469 - 74
[90] Micheal S, Qamar R, Akhtar F et al. MTHFR gene C677T and A1298C polymorphisms and homocysteine levels in primary open angle and primary closed angle glaucoma. *Mol Vis.* 2009;15: 2268-78.
[91] Roedl JB, Bleich S, Schlötzer-Schrehardt U et al. Increased homocysteine levels in tear fluid of patients with primary open-angle glaucoma. *Ophthalmic Res.* 2008; 40: 249-56
[92] Roedl JB, Bleich S, Reulbach U et al. Homocysteine levels in aqueous humor and plasma of patients with primary open-angle glaucoma. *J Neural Transm.* 2007; 114: 445-50
[93] Wang G, Medeiros FA, Barshop BA et al. Total plasma homocysteine and primary open-angle glaucoma. *Am J Ophthalmol.* 2004; 137: 401-6
[94] Rössler CW, Baleanu D, Reulbach U et al. Plasma homocysteine levels in patients with normal tension glaucoma. *J Glaucoma.* 2010; 19: 576-80
[95] Fan BJ, Liu K, Wang DY et al. Association of polymorphisms of tumor necrosis factor and tumor protein p53 with primary open-angle glaucoma. *IOVS* 2010; 51: 4110-6
[96] Fingert JH, Kwon YH, Moore PA et al. The C677T variant in the methylenetetrahydrofolate reductase gene is not associated with disease in cohorts of pseudoexfoliation glaucoma and primary open-angle glaucoma patients from Iowa. *Ophthalmic Genet.* 2006; 27: 39-41
[97] Mossbock G, Weger M, Faschinger C et al. Methylenetetrahydrofolatereductase (MTHFR) 677C>T polymorphism and open angle glaucoma. *Mol Vis.* 2006 17; 12: 356-9
[98] Fan BJ, Chen T, Grosskreutz C et al. Lack of association of polymorphisms in homocysteine metabolism genes with pseudoexfoliation syndrome and glaucoma. *Mol Vis.* 2008; 14: 2484-91
[99] Michael S, Qamar R, Akhtar F et al. C677T polymorphism in the methylenetetrahydrofolate reductase gene is associated with primary closed angle glaucoma. *Mol Vis.* 2008; 14: 661-5
[100] Zetterberg M, Tasa G, Palmér MS et al. Methylenetetrahydrofolate reductase genetic polymorphisms in patients with primary open-angle glaucoma. *Ophthalmic Genet.* 2007; 28: 47-50
[101] Mabuchi F, Tang S, Kashiwagi K et al. Methylenetetrahydrofolate reductase gene polymorphisms c.677C/T and c.1298A/C are not associated with open angle glaucoma. *Mol Vis.* 2006; 12: 735-9

[102] Jünemann AG, von Ahsen N, Reulbach U et al. C677T variant in the methylentetrahydrofolate reductase gene is a genetic risk factor for primary open-angle glaucoma. *Am J Ophthalmol.* 2005; 139: 721-3
[103] Woo SJ, Kim JY, Kim DM et al. Investigation of the association between 677C>T and 1298A>C 5,10-methylenetetra- hydrofolate reductase gene polymorphisms and normal-tension glaucoma. *Eye.* 2009; 23: 17-24

4

Expression of Metabolic Coupling and Adhesion Proteins in the Porcine Optic-Nerve Head: Relevance to a Flow Model of Glaucoma

Francisco-Javier Carreras[1], David Porcel[2], Francisco Rodriguez-Hurtado[3], Antonio Zarzuelo[4], Ignacio Carreras[1] and Milagros Galisteo[4]
[1]Department of Surgery (Ophthalmology), Faculty of Medicine, University of Granada
[2]Center of Scientific Instrumentation, University of Granada,
[3]Division of Ophthalmology, Licinio de la Fuente University Hospital, Granada,
[4]Department of Pharmacology, Faculty of Pharmacy, University of Granada,
Spain

1. Introduction

Astrocytes perform several well-established homeostatic functions in the maintenance of a nervous system that is viable for neurons. These functions include: the provision of metabolic support for neurons; maintenance of the blood-brain barrier (BBB); absorption of K+ and neurotransmitters from extracellular spaces; and participation in the processes of synaptogenesis and angiogenesis (Wanga & Bordey, 2008)

Astrocytic processes send out projections towards blood vessels that terminate in prolongations called endfeet. These express on the membrane a specific form of glucose transporter, GLUT1 (Morgello et al., 1995; Yu & Ding, 1998). Astrocytes take glucose from blood and transfer it to neurons, but it is also now known that an O_2 limitation is not a requirement for the formation of l-lactate in the cell metabolism. It is becoming increasingly clear that neurons utilize different substrates (glucose, glycogen, and lactate) to support their metabolism (Brown et al., 2004; Brooks, 2009), although this process may depend on the surrounding conditions. Lactate is an important intermediary in aerobic glucose metabolism, and a mediator of the redox state in intracellular and extracellular compartments (Brown et al., 2004). Specifically, l-lactate and molecular transporters (monocarboxylate translocator isoforms or MCT) play an important role in the metabolism of mitochondria (Pasarella et al. 2008). It has been proposed that l-lactate is the main product of glycolysis in the brain, regardless of the presence of oxygen (Brooks, 2002; Schurr, 2006)).

It has been shown that all isoenzymes of LDH, LDH1-LDH5 are present in varying proportions in synaptic terminals and cultured neurons and astrocytes taken from the brain. In rats, there is a selective enrichment of LDH1 in synaptosomes and LDH5 in astrocytes, although there is no exclusive localization of isoenzymes. The production of lactate by astrocytes and its subsequent use by nerve endings for energy production and neurotransmitter synthesis has been suggested (O'Brien et al., 2007).

A model known as the astrocyte-neuron lactate shuttle hypothesis (Pellerin & Magistretti, 1994) proposes that glucose taken up by astrocytic GLUT1 is partly processed oxidatively (via the tricarboxylic acid cycle pathway), partly converted to lactate, and then carried to extracellular spaces via monocarboxylate transporters (MCT1). Once in an extracellular space, l-lactate is then transported into neurons via MCT2 and converted to pyruvate (which can be used in the tricarboxylic acid cycle (Pellerini et al., 2007a)). The production and release of lactate by Müller cells in the retina has been found to fuel the mitochondrial oxidative metabolism and glutamate resynthesis in photoreceptors. Lactate has been found to be a better substrate than glucose for the oxidative metabolism *in vitro* for the Müller cell-photoreceptor complex (Poitry-Yamate et al., 1995). Recent *in vivo* studies in humans suggest that lactate may be preferred to glucose as fuel for neuronal metabolism (Brooks, 2009; Smith et al., 2003). Alternative approaches for improving energy metabolism in neurons based on astrocyte-neuron interactions, such as enhancing lactate uptake in neurons, or confronting challenges to these vias, may constitute the basis for new therapeutic strategies for neuroprotection (Smith et al.,2003).

Except for vessels and microglia, the anterior surface of the optic nerve head is formed by only one type of astrocyte with slight though significant differences that depend on the zone of settlement in relation to axons. The main difference between two subgroups of stellate astrocytes that form the anterior part of the optic nerve head may be their relative commitment either to envelope axons or merely to become part of the contingent surrounding vessels where axons are absent. Membrane adhesion is a critical feature of the astrocyte-astrocyte and axon-astrocyte relationship. Membrane-adhesion molecules are key to the axon-astrocyte proximity that enable metabolic enzymes and transport molecules to function in the nutrition chain of the neuron. N-cadherin has been described as a major linking protein for the two subgroups of stellate astrocytes in the prelaminar tissue of the optic nerve during development (Redies & Takeichi, 1993). N-cadherin participates both in complex and in simple attachments between membranes in the adult optic nerve head (Carreras et al., 2009, 2010a).

In the study of the pathology of the circulation of aqueous humor, clinically manifested in distinct types of glaucoma, considerable emphasis has been placed on changes in intraocular pressure. As a consequence of less outflow ease through conventional pathways, a redirection of flow towards alternative pathways reportedly occurs. The resulting pharmacological possibilities have been exploited by a group of drugs that reduce intraocular pressure by increasing uveoscleral outflow(Alma & Nilsson, 2009). However, deviation of flow towards the posterior pole has not been thoroughly investigated. Recently, a pathogenic role for a postulated greater outflow through the optic nerve head has been proposed, and N-cadherin has been suggested as a possible target for ionic stress in the optic nerve head (Carreras et al., 2009). In support of this, permeability of the optic-nerve head to tracers has also been recently corroborated (Carreras et al., 2010b).

Neurons have different types of self-destruct programs that are spatially compartmentalized, and one of these programs is located in the axon. Compartmentalized autonomous axonal self-destruction has been proposed as an optic-nerve occurrence in glaucoma (Whitmore et al., 2005). Local noxae constricted to the prelaminar tissue would suffice to interrupt the continuity of axons. Here we explore possible mechanisms through which a reduced extracellular concentration of calcium in the prelaminar tissue caused by the occasional (pathological) flow of aqueous humor through the optic nerve head could interfere with axon metabolism. The maintenance of narrow spaces between the membranes of the astrocytes and axons is essential for the interchange of metabolic fuel mediated by transport molecules. Research on the kinetics of lactate uptake in the brain (Aubert et al., 2005) has shown that this transport depends on the lactate concentration itself in the extracellular space.

We reasoned that the reinforced presence of N-cadherin may be linked to the presence of the monocarboxylic acid transport chain in the same area. If so, in areas where axons are not present, such as the perivascular region, which is composed only of astrocytes, we would expect to find no evidence of a monocarboxylic acid transport chain, and the concentration of N-cadherin would also be lower. If evidence for the lactate-transport chain in the axonal region of the prelaminar optic nerve head is concurrent with the presence of increased amounts of N-cadherin, compared to that of the perivascular areas, this could reinforce the suggestion that the deviation of bulk aqueous flow through the optic nerve could be harmful. The aqueous humor, low in calcium, would interfere with cell-cell adhesion and the transmembrane metabolic shuttle.

In this paper, we study the presence of enzymes involved in the lactate shuttle in the optic nerve head, seeking to colocalize the main molecule responsible for the maintenance of tight extracellular spaces. The study focuses on N-cadherin distribution in the prelaminar optic nerve head tissue, with the aim of colocalizing the MCT1 and MCT2 transport molecules, as well as LDH 1 and LDH 5, the main enzymes responsible for lactate metabolism in astrocytes and neurons. MCT1 and MCT2 are transmembrane proteins expressed in small amounts on the cell surface. Compared to prevalent proteins in axons and astrocytes as neurofilament and glial fibrillary acidic protein fluorescence of MCTs is expected to be very reduced, and prior identification by Western blot is helpful. Once its presence is determined in the tissue, histological localization with immunofluorescence allows comparisons of the tissue distribution of both N-cadherin and MCTs.

We found MCT1 and 2 in astrocytes and neurons, but membrane localization with TEM immunolabeling, although suggestive, by itself is not informative of the precise distribution of the two isoforms among the two cellular types, astrocytes, and neurons. Organotypic culture of the excised prelaminar region of the optic-nerve head can be useful in ascertaining the distribution of MCTs: first, the survival of astrocytes in organotypic culture is established; simultaneously the timing of axonal destruction is monitored; and, finally, MCTs are quantitatively determined by Western blot in control tissue and after axon disintegration. Comparisons of the amount of MCTs both in the presence an absence of axons elucidates the distribution of those transport molecules between the astrocytes and neurons (axons).

2. Methods

2.1 Animals

For this study, a total of 83 eyes from six-month-old domestic pig were collected at an abattoir soon after the animals were killed. The time between the death of the animals and processing of the tissue averaged less than 3 h. Eyes for the morphological study were processed in the first hour after death. The procedures followed in this research adhered to the tenets of the Helsinki Declaration.

Five eyes were used to determine the presence of MCT1 and MCT2 in normal tissue by Western blot.

Fresh eyes were dissected with blades and scissors. The optic nerve was prepared for transmission electron microscopy (TEM) and confocal laser scanning microscopy (CLSM). Immunostaining was performed for CLSM and TEM. For TEM, 8 eyes were prepared: 4 for immunogold staining, and another 4 for conventional TEM. Five eyes were used for CLSM. Thirty-six eyes were used for the organotypic culture of the prelaminar optic nerve head and processed for morphological assessment by immunolabeling and CLSM.

Finally, 28 pig eyes were used for the organotypic culture of the prelaminar optic nerve head and processed for Western blot of MCT 1, MCT 2 and a control protein (β-actin). Additionally, 4 eyes from 4 normal Wistar rats (from a different experiment), were used as positive controls for the detection of MCT1 and MCT in the optic disc in order to test the efficacy of the antibodies. Results were positive (not shown).

2.2 Antibodies and staining reagents

The following specific primary antibodies were used: anti-neurofilament, anti- GFAP (Glial Fibrillary Acidic Protein), anti-N-cadherin, anti-LDH5, anti-LDH1, anti-MCT1, and anti-MCT2. Secondary antibodies were labeled with fluorescent dyes (FITC or Texas red) for CLSM, or with colloidal gold for TEM. Secondary antibody for Western blot was labeled with horseradish peroxidase and revealed with luminol as substrate (ECL Western Blotting Substrate kit from abcam lab). Information on the antibodies used is presented in Table 1. Several assays were performed until operative working solutions were obtained. The most used dilutions are listed in table 1. Nuclear counterstaining for CLSM was performed with mounting media using DAPI (Vectashield, Vector Laboratories, CA, USA).

2.3 Confocal laser scanning microscopy (CLSM)

General procedure: The tissues were immunostained by fixing in glyoxal (Shandon Lipshaw, Pittsburgh, PA, USA) and then processed for paraffin embedding. Sections 5 μm thick were cut and mounted on polylysine-coated plates. Serial sections were washed in PBS after deparaffinization with xylene and graded alcohol. The sections were incubated in pre-diluted block serum for 1 h, and then incubated with the primary antibody diluted overnight in PBS containing 1.5% blocking serum, at4ºC. Control sections that did not receive the primary antibody were maintained with block serum. Primary antibodies were monoclonal antibodies against neurofilament, N-cadherin, LDH5, LDH1, MCT1, and MCT2. The secondary antibody was chosen as shown in Table 1, and incubation was performed for 1 h at room temperature. After being mounted with Vectashield, the sections were observed and photographed using a Leica SP5 confocal laser microscope.

2.4 Statistical analysis of immunofluorescent density

The first step was to study the distribution of the axons in the prelaminar optic nerve head with anti-neurofilament. Ten sections from 5 eyes (from different animals) were then incubated with anti-N-cadherin antibody as detailed above. The secondary antibody was marked with FITC. Two additional sections received only the secondary antibody and were used as controls. The sections were examined and photographed in such a way that at least one major vessel was present in each photograph. Low magnification (200 x) was used to include the vessel and the fiber layer in the same picture. Digital images were collected by adjusting the sensitivity of the photomultiplier according to the fluorescent intensity of the negative control section incubated with the secondary antibody, but not with the primary antibody. Once established, the same parameters were used to explore the sections incubated with the primary and secondary antibodies. Selection of the areas was based on the morphology of the tissue and the distribution of the DAPI-stained nuclei . Using the results of the anti-neurofilament labeling as reference, we distinguished areas with axons and astrocytes (axonal areas) as well as areas with only astrocytes (perivascular). Fluorescent intensity was measured in three or (mainly) four locations in each region of each picture (depending on the area available).

Antibody	Laboratory	Species	Label	Final dilution	Proven reactivity
Anti-GFAP	Abcam	Mouse IgG	Alexa Fluor 594	Prediluted	human, rat, pig
Anti-GFAP	eBioscience	Mouse IgG	Alexa Fluor 488	2.5 μg/ml	chicken, monkey, rabbit, human, mouse, rat, pig
Anti-N Cadherin Secondary antib.	Sigma-Aldrich Sigma-Aldrich	Mouse IgG Goat anti-mouse	 FITC	1/100 1/200	chicken, monkey, rabbit, human, mouse, rat
Anti-Neurofilament Secondary antib.	Sigma-Aldrich Sigma-Aldrich	Mouse IgG Goat anti-mouse	FITC	1/50 1/100	wide range
Anti-Neurofilament	Santa Cruz Tech	Goat anti-human		1/50	human, mouse, rat
Secondary antib.	Santa Cruz Tech	Mouse-antigoat		1/100	
Anti-LDH 1 Secondary antib.	Sigma-Aldrich Sigma-Aldrich Abcam	Mouse IgG Anti-mouse IgG Anti-mouse IgG	FITC Texas Red	1/100 1/200 1/500	human
Anti-LDH 5 Secondary antib.	Abcam Abcam	Sheep IgG Rabbit anti-sheep	Texas Red	1/100 1/500	
Anti-MCT 1 Secondary antib.	Santa Cruz Tech Santa Cruz Tech Sigma-Aldrich	Goat IgG Donkey anti-goat Rabbit anti-goat	FITC Gold	1/100 1/100 1/75	mouse, rat, cow, human
Anti-MCT 2 Secondary a.	Santa Cruz Tech Santa Cruz Tech Santa Cruz Tech	Rabbit IgG Goat anti-rabbit Goat anti-rabbit	Texas Red Gold 10 nm	1/100 1/100 1/75	mouse, rat

Table 1. List of antibodies for Immunostaining

Image Pro Plus 6.3 (Media Cybernetics, MD, USA) was used to analyze the photographs. The "line profile" command was used to plot the intensity values of a single circular line within the image (along a single line of pixels). It is important to note that the line profile measures pixel values as they appear in the bitmapped image. After selecting only the green channel, the program plots only the values for FITC fluorescence. Because part of the spectrum of DAPI can overlap the green channel, care was taken to avoid placing the line (circumference) on top of the blue-stained nuclei. Pooled data from each area in each section was recorded as ± SE, and statistical differences were assessed using the Student's t-test.

2.5 Transmission electron microscopy

The prelaminar region of the optic nerve head and the adjacent retina were sectioned with a Parker blade and deposited in fixative. For a simple TEM, 2% glutaraldehyde and 2% formaldehyde in a PBS buffer were used as a fixative. After fixation, the specimens were rinsed several times with a buffer solution followed by post-fixation with 1% osmium tetroxide for 1 h. After rinsing again with PBS buffer for 15 min, the tissue specimens were dehydrated with a series of graded ethyl alcohols ranging from 70% to 100%. The blocks were embedded in epoxy resin. The resin blocks were initially thick-sectioned at 1-2 microns with glass knives, using an Ultramicrotome Leica Ultracut S, and stained with Toluidine blue. These sections were used as a reference to trim blocks for thin sectioning. The appropriate blocks were then thin sectioned with a diamond knife at 70-90 nm, and the sections were placed on nickel mesh grids. After drying on filter paper, the sections were stained with uranyl acetate and lead citrate for contrast. After drying, the grids were then viewed and photographed using a Zeiss EM 10C electronic microscope.

For immune procedures, tissue was fixed with 2% paraformaldehyde and 0.2% glutaraldehyde in PBS. For better preservation of antigenicity, no osmium tetroxide was used. London White embedding resin was used. The grids were incubated with the secondary antibody as a control, but they were not incubated with the primary antibody. The grids were incubated in block serum for 10 min. The sections were then incubated overnight with the primary antibody (anti-MCT1 and anti-MCT 2; see Table 1). The same primary monoclonals were used for TEM and confocal laser microscopy. The washed grids were then incubated with the secondary antibody labeled with nanogold 10 nm. After drying on filter paper, the sections were stained with uranyl acetate for contrast. No lead citrate was used so as to avoid masking the gold marker.

2.6 Organotypic culture of prelaminar optic-nerve explants

Explants of the dissected prelaminar region of the optic nerve head of recently enucleated pig eyes were cultured *in vitro* following the method described by Stoppini et al. (1991) as adapted by Carrasco et al. (2010).

Briefly, optic discs were dissected with a surgical blade in a sterile environment and placed in a Petri dish containing the same culture medium as detailed below. Explants were subsequently placed on 30-mm Millicell CM culture plate inserts (Millipore, Billerica, MA, USA; pore size 0.4 µm) in 6-well plates containing 1 ml/well culture medium and incubated *in vitro* for different time periods (see below) at 37°C in a humidified atmosphere with 5% CO2. The face of the explant in contact with the membrane was not controlled. The medium was replaced after 24 or 48 h, coinciding with the harvesting of the samples. The culture medium was composed of 50% basal medium with Earle's salts (BME), 25% Hank's balanced salt

solution, 10% horse serum (HS), 1 mM L-glutamine, 10 IU-µg/ml penicillin-streptomycin (all purchased from Invitrogen, Paisley, United Kingdom), and 5 mg/ml glucose (BME+25%HS). A total of 64 eyes were used in this phase of the study. Optic-nerve explants were incubated in groups of variable number of samples.
For morphological studies of viability of axons and astrocytes a total of 36 eyes were studied, including 6 control eyes (0 days of culture). Initially, explants were retired daily for the first 4 days an then every 2 days up to day 12. After experience concerning the rate of desintegration of the axons in the culture was gained, we cultured 6 explants for 24 h and then prepared for histological study. Samples were fixed in Glyoxal for 24 and then either immersed in 30% glucose and included in OCT and frozen. Another similar culture was alternatively processed for paraffin embedding. In both cases, sections of the embedded tissue were labeled with fluorescent antibodies against Neurofilament or GFAP and observed in the CLSM. Counterstaining was consistently DAPI, as stated above.

Antibody	Laboratory	Species	Label	Final dilution	Proven reactivity
Anti-MCT 1	Abcam	mouse		1/400	mouse, rat, cow, human
Anti-MCT 2	Abcam	mouse		1/400	mouse, rat, cow, human
Secondary antib.	Sigma	goat	HRP	1/1000	

Table 2. List of antibodies for Western blot.

2.7 Western-blot analysis for MCT1 and MCT2 expression in prelaminar optic nerve

For protein immunoblot determination, an initial Western-blot analysis was performed in 5 fresh samples to determine the presence or absence of MCT1 and MCT2 in the prelaminar optic nerve of the pig.
To determine the distribution of MCT isoforms, we processed an additional group of 28 eyes, including 6 controls (not cultured) and 22 cultured eyes. Samples were harvested at days 1 (24 h), 2, and 5 . From prior immunolabeling histological results, we knew that axons disintegrated after one day of culture. A quantitative comparison between cultured and control samples was calculated to determine the proportional distribution of MCT1 and MCT2 between axons and neurons. Western-blot analysis was performed in control tissue from untreated normal pigs. The analysis was repeated after organotypic culture of the prelaminar optic nerve for a number of days (1, 2 and 5) until the disintegration of the axons was tested with immunolabeling of neurofilament, as discussed above.
Samples of the prelaminar region of the optic nerve head, control or cultured, were homogenized in buffer (20 mmol/L Tris-HCl, 5mmol/L EDTA, pH 7.5, 10mmol/L sodium pyrophosphate, 100 mmol/L sodium fluoride, 1% (v/v) Igepal, 2 mmol/L sodium orthovanadate, 1 mmol/L phenylmethylsulfonyl fluoride, 10 µg/ml aprotinin and 10 µg/ml leupeptin). Homogenates were centrifuged at 14,000 rpm for 10 min at 4°C. Protein concentrations in homogenates were measured by the bicinchoninic acid protein assay. Thirty µg of protein of each sample were subjected to 10% SDS-PAGE and electrophoretically transferred to nitrocellulose membranes overnight. The membranes were blocked with 5% non-fat dry milk in TBST for 2 h at room temperature and subsequently

blotted with the appropriate antibodies in 5% non-fat dry milk-TBST. The antibodies anti-MCT1, and anti-MCT2, were purchased from Abcam (Cambridge, UK) and were used at manufacturer-recommended dilutions (1/400). Incubations with primary antibodies were performed overnight at4ºC. Following incubation, membranes were washed 3 times with TBST for 10 min each, before incubation for 2 h at room temperature with secondary peroxidase conjugated anti-mouse antibody, in the case of MCT1 (Santa Cruz Biotechnology, Santa Cruz, CA, USA), or anti-rabbit antibody, in the case of MCT2 (Santa Cruz Biotechnology, Santa Cruz, CA, USA) diluted at 1:2000 in 5% non-fat dry milk-TBST. Membranes were then washed 5 times with TBST for 10 min each, and the bound antibodies were visualized by an ECL system. Films were scanned and densitometric analysis was performed on the scanned images using Scion Image-Release Beta 4.02 software (*http://www.scioncorp.com*). Antibodies used are summarized in table 2.

Aquantitative comparison between cultured an control sample was calculated in the following manner: relative values were expressed as means, indicating the values from densitometric analysis normalized to Ponceau red staining, relative to control measurements, which were assigned a value of 100.

3. Results

3.1 Protein immunoblot of complete tissue

The Western-blot results from normal fresh tissue for MCt1 and MCT2 rendered specific positive results for both molecules. A stained band in the region below the mark of 50 KDa indicated the presence of types 1 and 2 of the monocarboxylate transporter (Fig. 1).

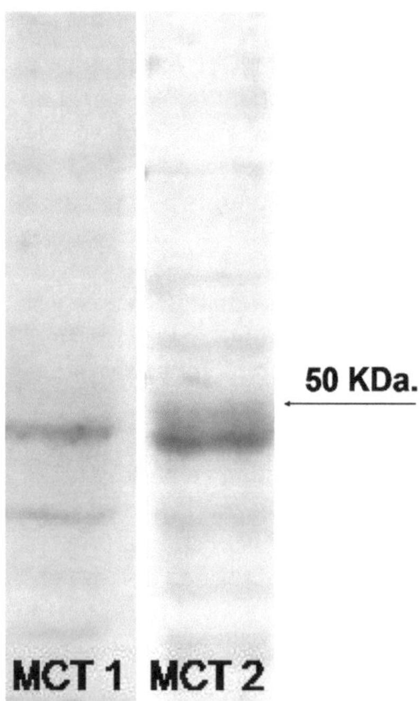

Fig. 1. Western blot detection of MCT-1 and MCT2 in the bands well under 50 k Daltons from fresh tissue samples of the prelaminar region of the porcine optic-nerve head.

3.2 Normal histology

Qualitative assessment. Fluorescence intensity was scored on a **qualitative** scale: - negative; +/- borderline; + weakly positive; + + positive; +++ strongly positive.

3.2.1 Immunolabeling of the neurofilament and GFAP

Qualitative assessment of neurofilament staining was strongly positive. Immunolabeling for the neurofilament clearly separated areas with and without axons in the optic nerve head sections (Figure 2a). Apart from the vessel walls, perivascular tissue was formed almost exclusively of astrocytes and no axons were present. The perivascular tissue was composed of Elschnig's astrocytes, which also formed the superficial Elschnig's "membrane" and the astrocytes of the meniscus of Kuhnt in the center of the optic disc. Figure 2a shows the course of axons in the optic nerve head and the nuclei of the astrocytes. Some of the astrocytes tended to gather in columns on each side of the axon bundles. Another group of astrocytes was situated around the main vessels. No immunofluorescence was found in the spaces near the vessels. Two arrangements of astrocytes - from the standpoint of their relationship to axons - could be distinguished using neurofilament immunofluorescence: perivascular astrocytes and axon-related astrocytes.

Qualitative assessment of GFAP staining was strongly positive (Figure 2b). Of particular interest in our work was the determination of whether the segment of the fiber bundles piercing the *lamina cribrosa* was still the domain of axon-wrapping astrocytes, because the most intense staining of MCT molecules was rendered in this area. Our results show that astrocytes, and consequently not oligodendrocytes, were present in the tunnels of the *lamina cribrosa* (Fig 2b, long arrow).

3.2.2 TEM of zonulae adherens

A conventional TEM of the prelaminar tissue of the optic nerve head shows important structural differences in the perivascular and axonal layers. Perivascular astrocytes, unrelated to axons, formed a mesh of astrocytic projections, with ample extracellular spaces (Figure 3). Periaxonal astrocytes sent out projections that tightly wrapped around nerve fibers, leaving barely discernible extracellular spaces (Figure 4). Figures of zonulae adherens were found among the astrocytic projections in both areas, but not in the same numbers. The vast majority of the membrane contacts among projections in the perivascular area were simple membrane apposition (Figure 3b). Union complexes of the zonula adherens type were structured unions with extracellular and intracellular elements that produced a characteristic five-layered image in TEM. Zonulae adherens were occasionally found among perivascular astrocytes (Figure 3c), but were more numerous among periaxonal astrocytes where cellular contact was close. Zonulae adherens were seen to predominate near the axons joining thin astrocytic processes in several layers around the neural fibers (Figures 4b and c).

3.2.3 Immunolabeling of N-cadherin

Qualitative assessment of N-cadherin staining was strongly positive. Since the main extracellular component of zonula adherens is N-cadherin, the immunolabeling of N-cadherin is a suitable method for studying the distribution of zonulae adherens at the CLSM level. After the immunostaining of sections of the optic nerve head, N-cadherin staining was positive in areas of the prelaminar region, but intense fluorescence occurred in the

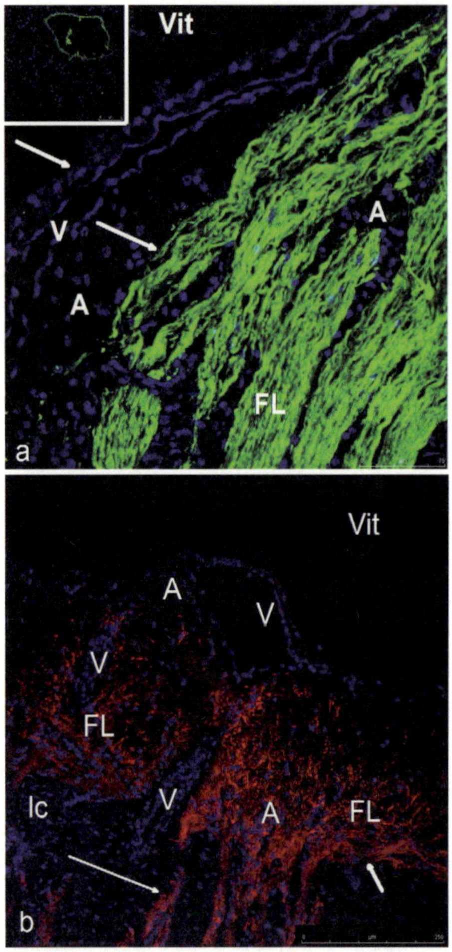

Fig. 2. a) Confocal laser scanning micrograph of a section of the anterior part of the optic nerve head in contact with the vitreous body stained with fluorescent antibodies directed against an anti-neurofilament antibody. The result is a clear indication of the flow of axons in the optic nerve head. Axons are shown to form clearly delimited bundles interspersed with columnar astrocytes. The astrocytes are only detected above by the blue counterstaining of their nuclei (DAPI). A vessel is present in the upper third if the micrograph shows that no green dye is present, thereby indicating the absence of axons in this area. Astrocytic nuclei are numerous in the proximity of the vessel. These are the astrocytes described by Elschnig as responsible for the formation of the incomplete inner limiting membrane of the optic nerve. White arrows indicate the limits between the vitreous surface and the fiber layer. b) Confocal laser scanning micrograph of a section optic nerve head, including the lamina cribrosa, stained with fluorescent antibodies directed against an anti-GFAP antibody. Astrocytes strongly express GFAP. The short arrow points to the upper limit of the sclera where the horizontal portion of the fiber layer lies. The long arrows point towards the bundles piercing the holes of the lamina where intense GFAP staining shows that the axons at the lamina are still wrapped by astrocytes instead of oligodendrites. (**Vit**: Vitreous body; **V**: Vessel; **A**: Astrocytes; **FL**: Fiber layer).

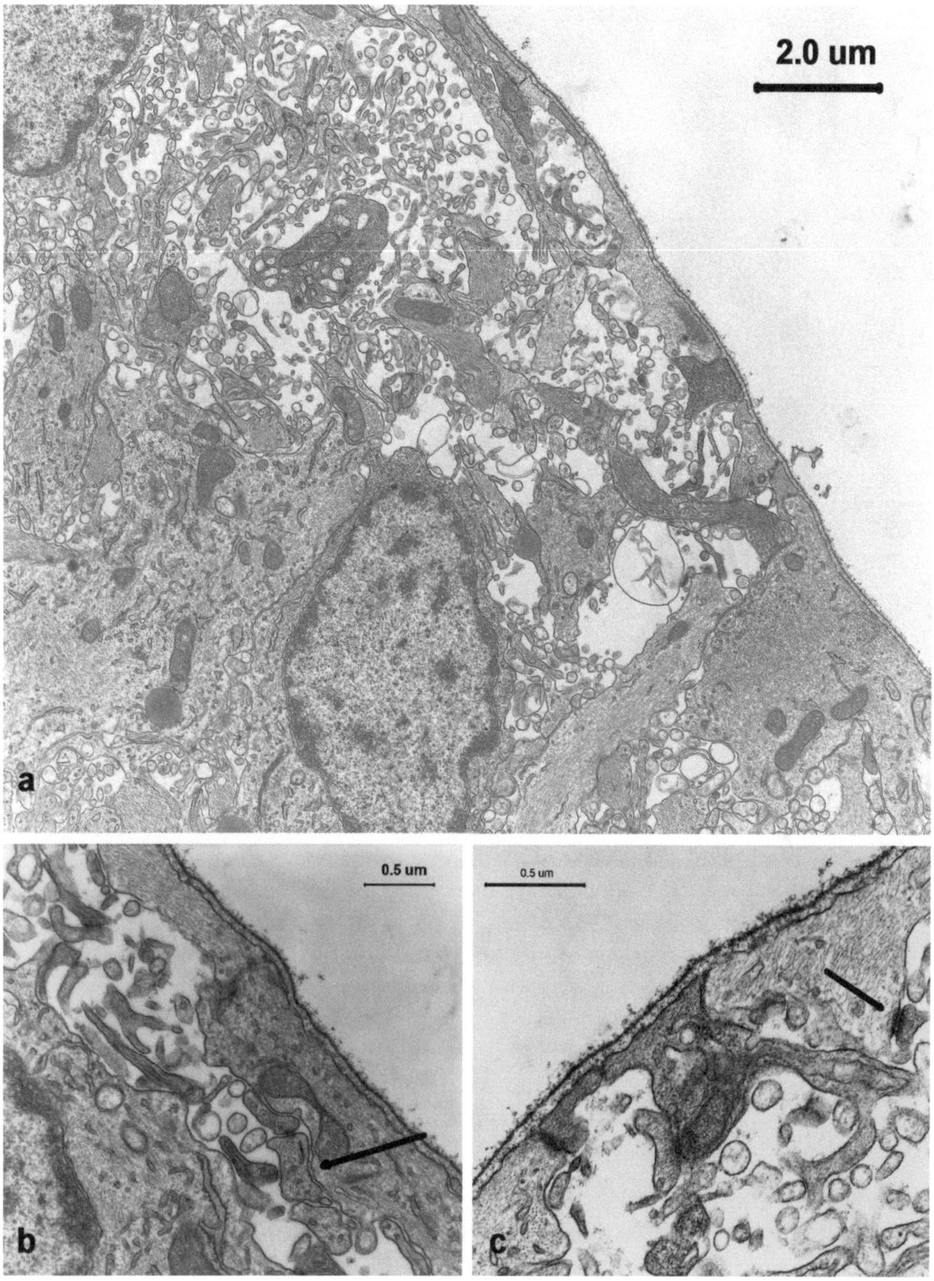

Fig. 3. TEM micrograph of Elschnig's perivascular astrocytes . a) Astrocytes forming the vitreous interface. Ample extracellular spaces are present among the astrocytic prolongations; and it is from these spaces that free-floating lesser projections arise. No axons are present in the area near the vessel wall. b) A close view of the membrane-to-membrane contact. The most common form of attachment between membranes is simple membrane apposition (arrow). c) This micrograph shows that structured forms of attachment, such as zonulae adherens, are occasionally found in this area (arrow). (**Vit**: Vitreous body; **A**: Astrocytes).

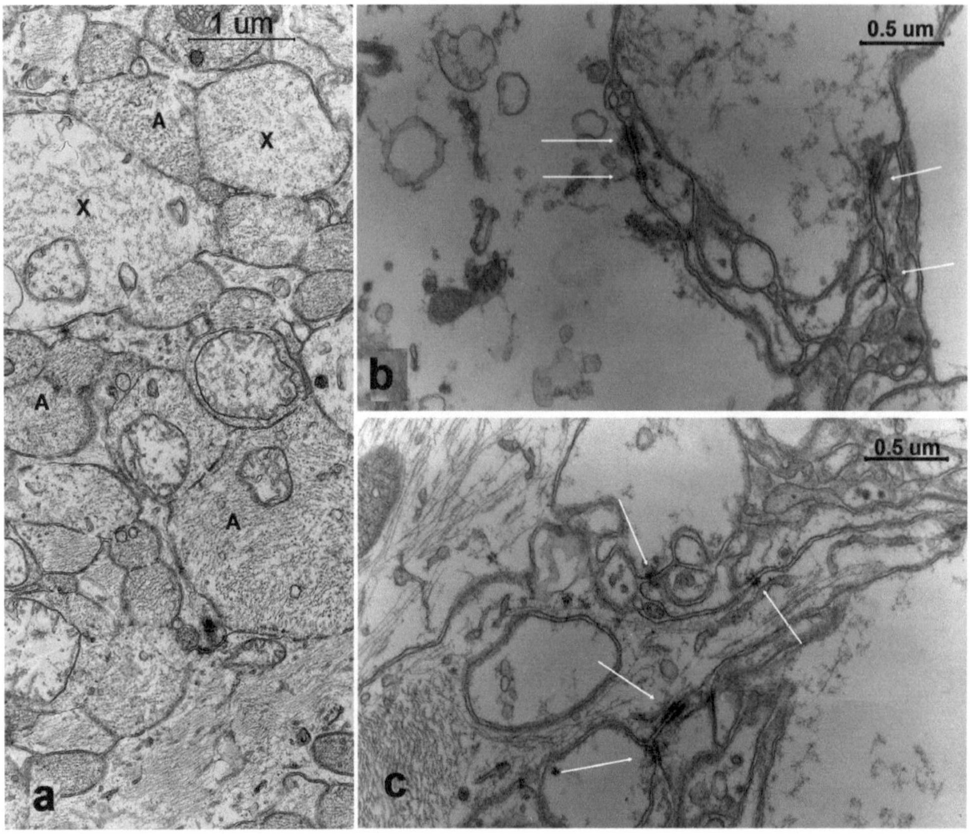

Fig. 4. TEM micrograph of the periaxonal astrocytes in the nerve-fiber layer. a) A general view of the axon-astrocyte relationship. All the spaces unoccupied by axons (X) are filled with thin astrocytic processes (A). Extracellular spaces are slit-like and scarce. b) and c) A close-up view of the membrane-to-membrane contact between axons and astrocytes. Astrocytic prolongations form multi-layered structures surrounding axons. Zonulae adherens are frequently found. (Compare with Figure 2, in which only isolated and scarce figures of zonulae adherens are found.) Figures of zonulae adherens are grouped together, and the thin-layered astrocytic prolongations are tightly wrapped around axons (arrows). These details should be taken into account when interpreting the non-contrasted immunogold micrographs shown in Figures 9 and 10.

nerve-fiber layer. The distribution of N-cadherin suggests a moderate presence of zonulae adherens among perivascular astrocytes (Elschnig's cover and Kuhnt's meniscus), pointing to an increased concentration in the ganglion cell-fiber columns (Figure 5). These results concur with previous findings with TEM.

Due to the uncertainties inherent in TEM immunolabeling, a quantitative approach using this technique is fraught with difficulties. However, quantitative immunofluorescence has been greatly facilitated by the development of image-analysis software. Accordingly, a quantitative approach to the relative concentration of N-cadherin labeling was used as a method to discern the relative concentration of zonulae adherens among astrocytes in the perivascular area and those in the fiber layer.

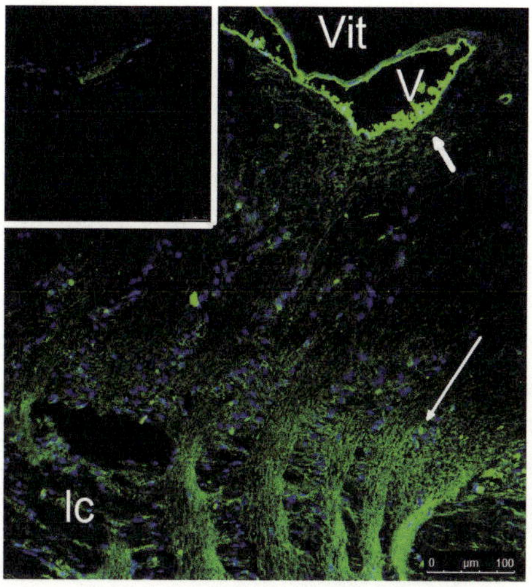

Fig. 5. CLSM of distribution of N-cadherin in the prelaminar region. N-cadherin is present in Elschnig's perivascular astrocytes (short arrows) and in periaxonal astrocytes (long arrows). Background noise has been eliminated. Magnification is shown in the figure. (**V**: vessel; **ca**: columnar astrocytes; **lc**: lamina cribrosa; and **sc**: sclera).

3.2.4 Statistical comparison of the intensity of N-cadherin immunofluorescence between perivascular astrocytes and axon-wrapping astrocytes

A statistical analysis examined data on fluorescent intensity along lines drawn in the two areas under comparison: namely, the perivascular area and the nerve-fiber layer. Figure 6 shows an example of the preparations used in the statistical analysis. The squares show the areas where the labeling intensity was measured. Figure 6a shows the intensity profiles for the selected lines of two identical squares, at a random location situated in each of the anatomically defined areas under comparison, and shown in Figure 6b. This figure is a sample photograph of one of the sections which was immunolabeled for N-cadherin.
Circular lines instead of straight lines were used for statistical calculations (this is a constraint of the software). Circular lines of the same length and traced with the "line profile" command in the software package were randomly placed in both regions and the average intensities compared. The results of the statistical labeling analysis are shown in Table 3. Statistical analysis of the measurements of fluorescent intensity along the lines

Parameter:	PERIVASCULAR	FIBER LAYER
Mean:	31.047	66.246
N. of points:	39	39
Std deviation:	11.168	33.527
Std error:	1.788	5.369
Minimum:	17.117	27.251
Maximum:	60.181	156.69
Median:	26.656	63.456
Lower 95% CI:	27.425	55.373
Upper 95% CI:	34.668	77.118

Table 3. Data summary from the comparison in N-Cadherin content between perivascular and periaxonal astrocytes.

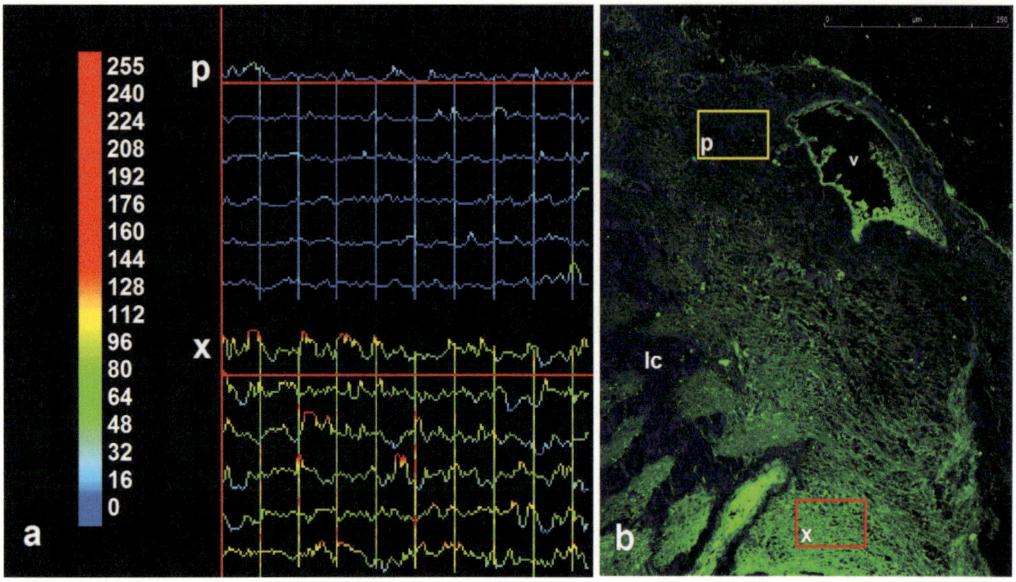

Fig. 6. a) False color scale and curves from data measured in b. Data taken from six lines in squares p and x is printed graphically as a curve where the color hue indicates the pixel intensity according to the conventional scale that is depicted on the far left. b) CLSM photograph of immunofluorescence staining against N-cadherin in the optic-nerve head. At the top, the image shows one of the central vessels (v) surrounded by Elschnig's astrocytes; and, on the left, part of the lamina cribrosa sclerae (lc). The squares show two typical locations where fluorescent intensity is measured along six lines. The square marked p is located in the perivascular region where Elschnig's astrocytes are found. The square marked x is located in the area of axon bundles. The measurements on the squares are represented graphically in a). (Vit: Vitreous body; V: Vessel; A: Astrocytes; FL: Fiber layer; lc: lamina cribrosa).

drawn in the perivascular area and fiber layer showed that the N-cadherin concentration was greater in the fiber area (Figure 7). The two-tailed p-value was < 0.0001 (considered extremely significant).

In summary, the axon-laden region of the prelaminar tissue was rich in N-cadherin compared to the perivascular region. This confirms the impression conveyed by the TEM micrographs, which show more numerous figures of zonulae adherens among the astrocytic projections surrounding axon fibers.

3.2.5 The presence of four molecules related to the lactate shuttle in the prelaminar region of the optic nerve head

Qualitative assessment of LDH 1 staining was positive. The presence of the molecule was best denoted in the fiber layer, indicating its presence in the astrocyte-axon couple. Figure 8a shows a case of LDH 1 and the corresponding negative control.

Qualitative assessment of LDH 5 staining was positive. Fluorescence is detected in the astrocyte-axon in the region of the tightly packed axon bundles. Figure 8b shows a case of LDH 1 and the corresponding negative control.

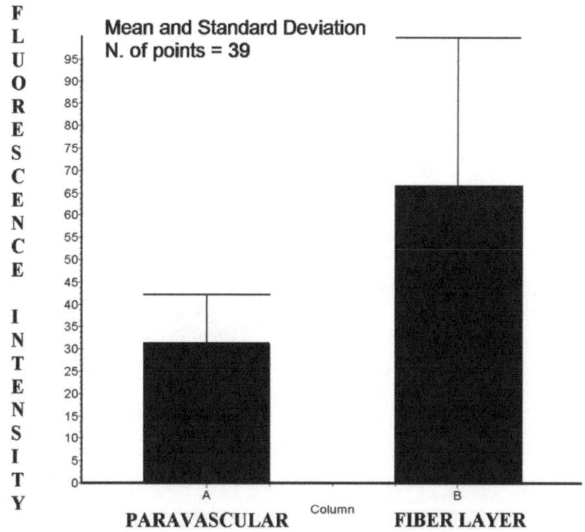

Fig. 7. Comparison of the fluorescent intensity of anti-N-cadherin antibodies in the perivascular area and in the nerve-fiber layer: the bars represent the mean of the fluorescence intensity in each area. The standard deviation is also included. The y-axis depicts the intensity scale in arbitrary units.

CLSM immunofluorescent labeling of MCT 1 was weakly positive in the astrocyte-axon of the prelaminar tissue. This presence of this molecule was best denoted in the fiber layer, while in other areas it was barely detectable (Figure 8c). The same labeling of MCT 2 was also weakly positive in the prelaminar tissue and its presence was clearest in the fiber layer, indicating its presence in the axon-astrocyte couple (Figure 8d). Due to the weak fluorescence of MCTs, we used the optic nerve from Wistar rats as a positive control and confirmed the correct labeling of the targets while excluding species disparity in the specificity of the primary antibodies (not shown).

3.2.6 TEM immunogold of MCT1 and MCT2

After the detection of MCT1 and 2 under light microscopy, it was necessary to localize the molecules in the plasma membranes to confirm their metabolic role in the lactate shuttle between astrocytes and neurons. Both molecules were localized mainly in the plasma membranes in both cell types. MCT1 was also localized in the inner mitochondrial membrane (not shown). TEM immunogold labeling of MCT1 showed the distribution of MCT1 molecules in the astrocyte membrane near the axon membrane (Figures 9a, b, c). TEM immunogold labeling of MCT2 revealed the distribution of MCT2 molecules in the axon membrane near the astrocyte membrane, as well as in the astrocyte membranes surrounding the axons (Figures 10a and b). Immunogold was also present in the numerous thin astrocytic projections that filled extra-axonal spaces and which were not in contact with the axon membrane. This occurred with both MCT1 and MCT2 (Figures 9c and 10b).

In summary, the enzyme isoforms, LHD 1 and LDH 5 were detected in the prelaminar tissue, and the staining was more intense in areas where axons joined to pierce the lamina cribrosa sclerae. Both of the monocarboxylate transporters studied here (MCT1 and 2) were located in the plasma membrane of the astrocyte-axon couple. Together, these four molecules formed part of a chain in the metabolic link between astrocytes and neurons.

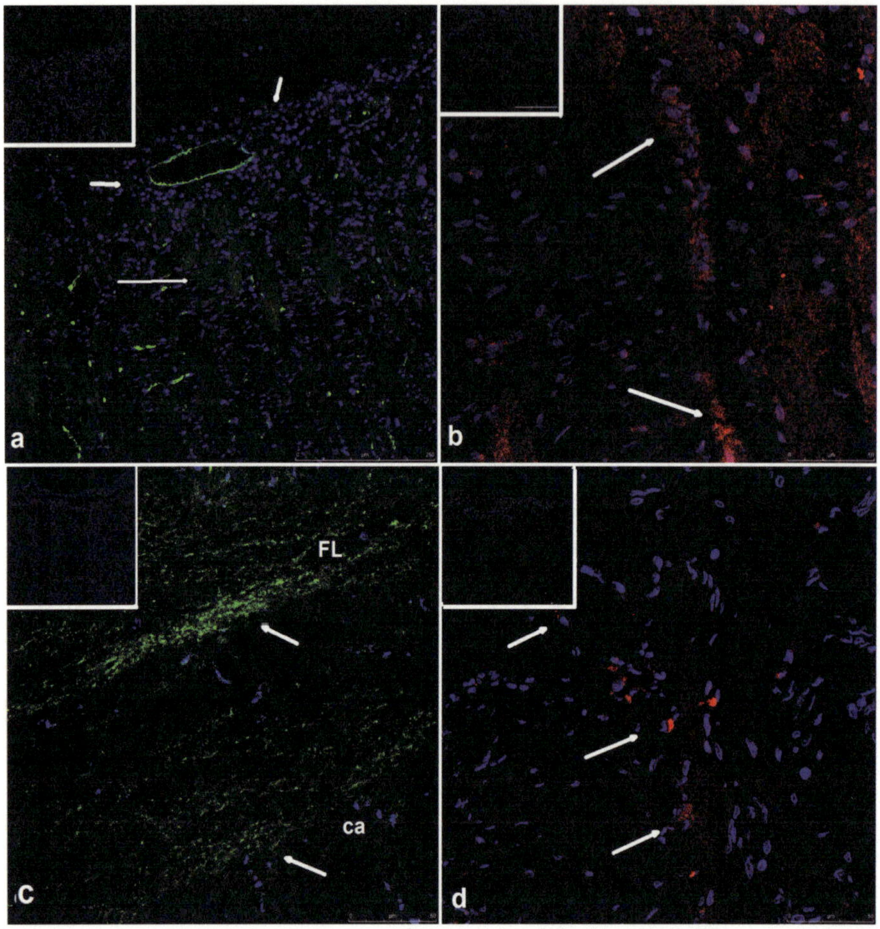

Fig. 8. a) CLSM micrograph of the optic-nerve-head-labeling LDH1 with fluorescein (green color, FITC). Immunostaining is positive in the nerve-fiber layer (long arrow) and less intense in the perivascular astrocytes (short arrows). (Insert) Negative control of LDH1 antibody. Secondary fluorescent anti-FC fraction antibody is used without previous incubation with the primary antibody. Both images have been taken with the same parameters of laser intensity and aperture. b) CLSM micrograph of the optic-nerve-head-labeling LDH 5 (red color, TR). Labeling is intense in the fiber bundles near and inside the cribrosa lamina (arrows). (Insert) Negative control of LDH5 antibody. (**Vit**: Vitreous body; **V**: Vessel; **ca**: Columnar astrocytes; **lc**: Lamina cribrosa). c) CLSM micrograph of the optic-nerve-head-labeling MCT1 with fluorescein (green color, FITC). Green immunostaining is positive in the astrocytes-axon couple (arrowed) and located in the nerve-fiber layer. (Insert) Negative control of MCT1 antibody. Secondary fluorescent anti-FC fraction antibody is used without previous incubation with primary antibody. Both images were taken with the same laser intensity and aperture to the change in magnification. d) CLSM micrograph of the optic-nerve-head-labeling MCT 2 (red color, TR). Red immunostaining positive in the astrocytes-axon couple. Staining was more detectable at the level of the lamina cribrosa. Insert: Negative control of MCT 2 antibody. (**FL**: Fiber layer; **ca**: Columnar astrocytes; **lc**: Lamina cribrosa).

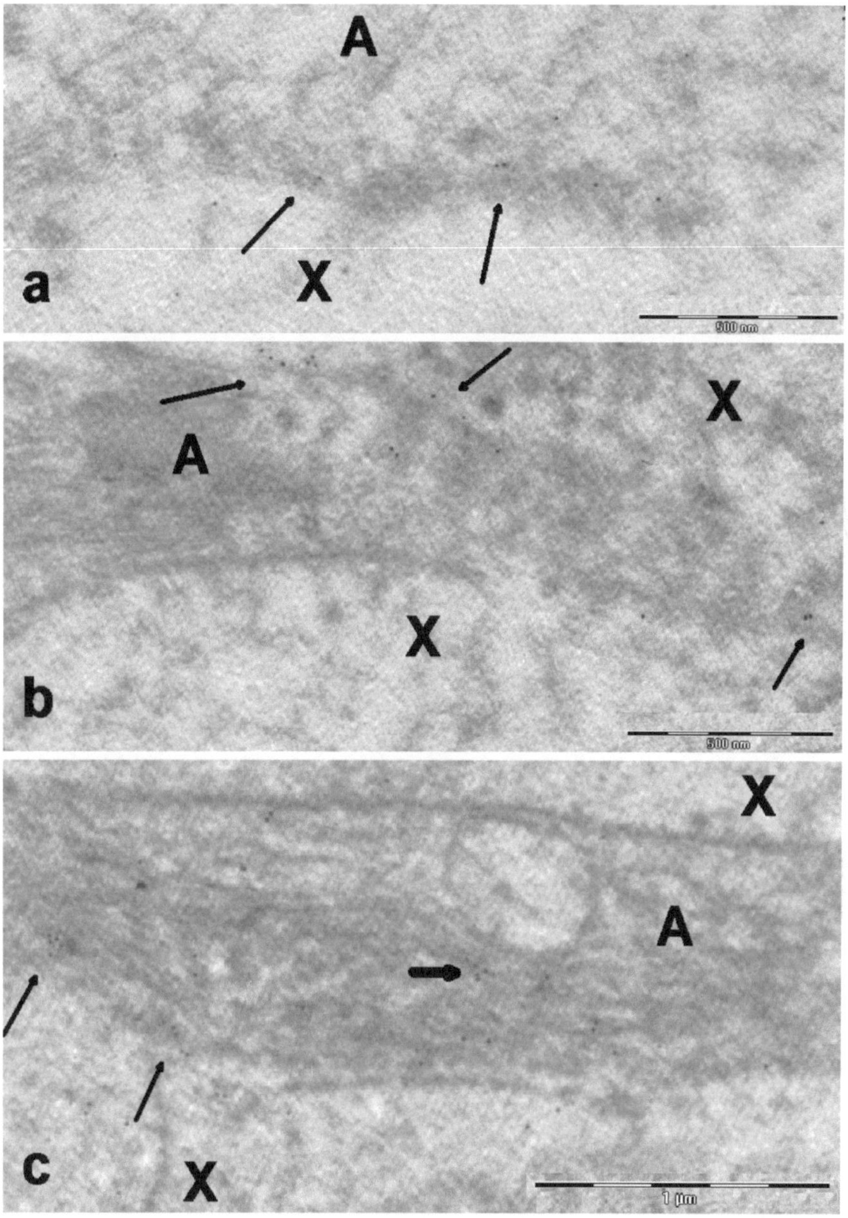

Fig. 9. TEM micrograph of the fiber layer of the optic-nerve head immunolabeled with anti-MCT1 antibody and immunogold. Membranes are not easily seen with this technique, as electron-dense contrast is avoided so that the gold micelles are not masked. **a**, **b**, and **c** are different samples in which specific markings of MCT1 are deduced from the delineation of the membranes by the marker (long arrows). The short arrow points to the multi-layered projections as seen in Figure 4b and c. X indicates axon; and A indicates astrocyte. A distinction between astrocytic projections and axons is established by the shape and presence of intermediate filaments. Ultra-thin sections, as well as osmium tetroxide-free and uranyl acetate, counterstain without lead citrate. Magnification is shown in the figure.

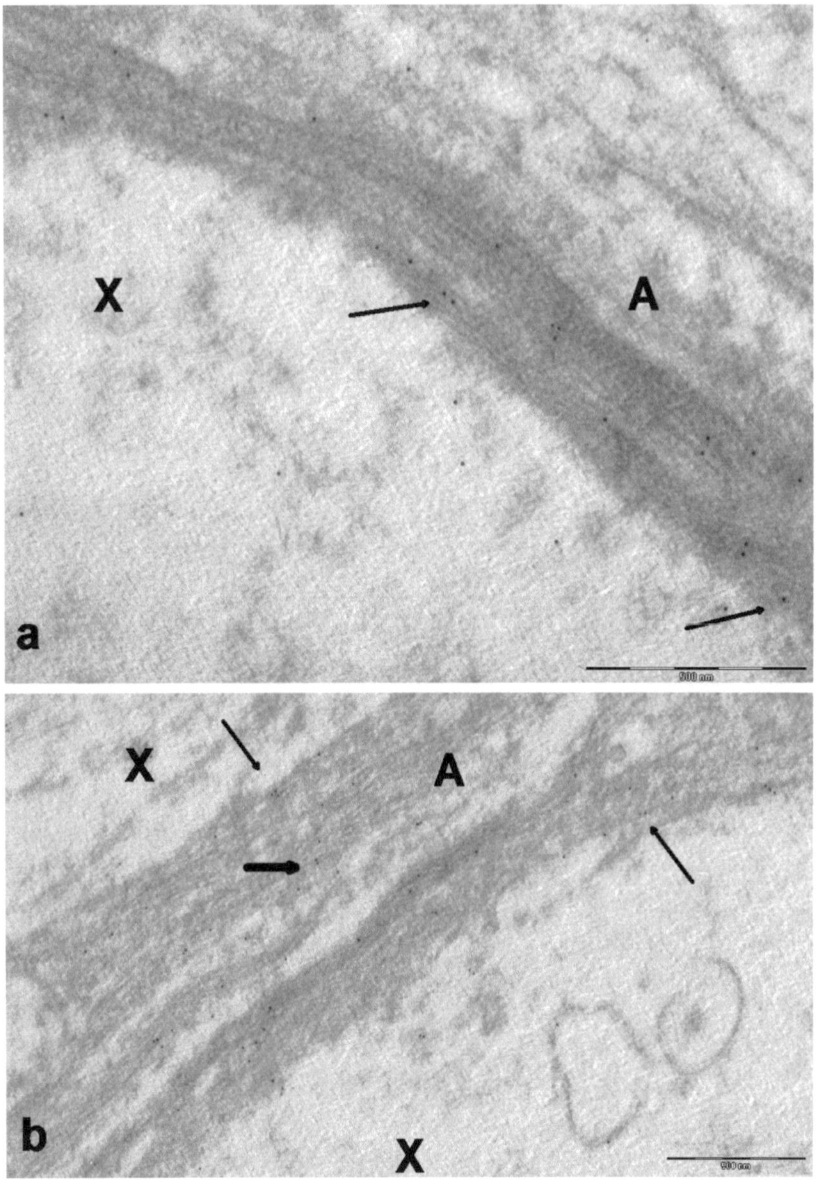

Fig. 10. TEM micrograph of the fiber layer of the optic-nerve head immunolabeled with anti-MCT2 antibody and immunogold. As in Figure 10, membranes are not easily seen in these sections because they have been processed without electron-dense contrast (so as not to mask the gold micelles). **a** and **b** are different samples in which specific markings of MCT2 are deduced by the delineation of the membranes by the marker (long arrows) in the astrocytic membrane. The short arrow points to the presence of MCT2 in the membrane of multi-layered projections that fill extra-axonal spaces. This suggests lactate re-uptake on the part of the astrocytes, the **X** axon, and the A astrocyte. Ultra-thin sections, as well as osmium tetroxide-free and uranyl acetate, counterstain without lead citrate. Magnification is shown in the figure.

3.3 Organotypic culture

3.3.1 Morphology

We cultured samples of the prelaminar optic nerve up to 12 days. The samples were studied and labeled for neurofilament and GFAP daily for the first 6 days of culture and twice daily afterwards.

The persistence of healthy astrocytes in organotypic culture of the prelaminar optic nerve is illustrated in Figure 11 a to c. Even on day 12 of the culture, astrocytes were found with regular features of nuclei and GFAP labeling (Fig 11 c). The mass reduction of the culture tissue detected over the culture process indicates that astrocytes are also regularly lost, as confirmed by the presence of pycnotic nuclei in some portions of the sections (Figure 11e

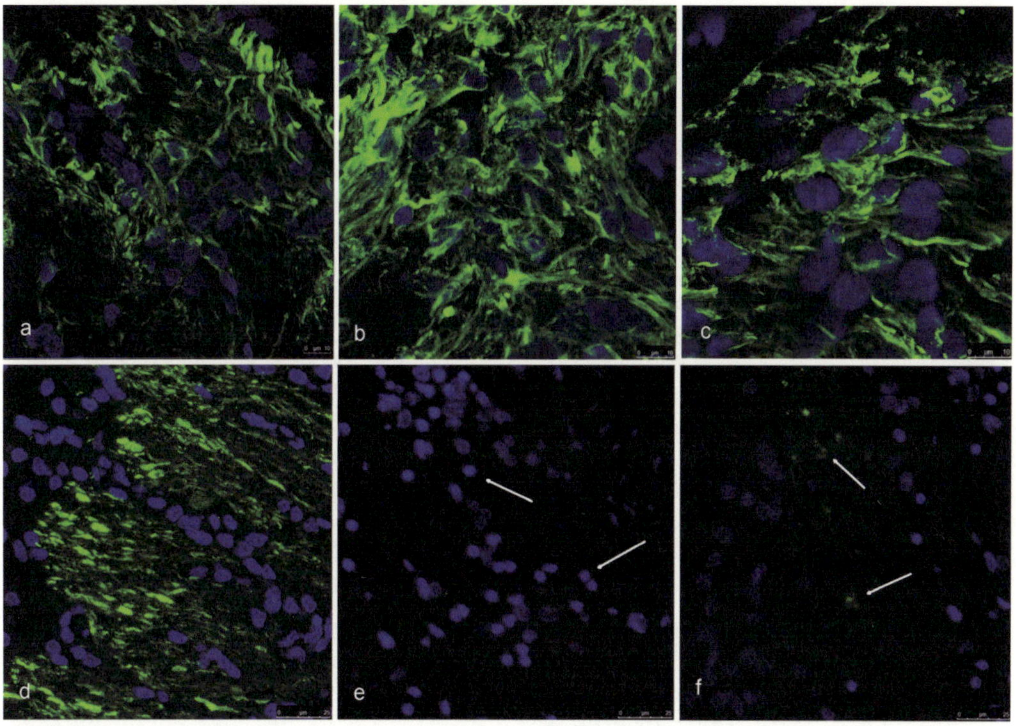

Fig. 11. CLSM micrographs of immunolabeled tissue. Upper row shows the fate of astrocytes in culture by the morphology of GFAP filaments and nuclear staining with DAPI. The lower row shows the fate of axons after one day of culture by the labeling of neurofilament. Nuclear staining with DAPI. a) GFAP Control, in cultured tissue. b) GFAP after 4 days of culture. Normal appearance of nuclei and GFAP filaments. c) GFAP after 12 days of culture. Normal aspect of remaining nuclei. GFAP is still abundant in the cytoplasm with signs of clumping is some areas. d) CLSM micrography Control preparation of prelaminar optic-nerve head in a non-cultured sample. Immunolabeling with anti-neurofilament. Secondary antibody labeled with FITC. Paraffin embedding. d) Same immunolabeling in a prelaminar optic disc cultured for 24 h. Axons have completely disintegrated as shown by the absence of staining in the major part of the sample. f) Same preparation. Only traces of neurofilament are visible in some regions (arrows). Figures b and c show some nuclei are undergoing pycnosis (arrow head). Magnification shown in the figures.

and f) and aggregated GAFP in the cytoplasm of cells with pycnotic (not shown) or normal-appearing nuclei (Fig 11 c).
Neurofilament staining in cultured and control tissues showed that neurofilament was practically absent from the samples after one day culture onwards (Figure 11 d to e).

3.3.2 Protein immunoblotting

Western-blot analysis of MCT1 and MCT 2 after 1, 2, and 5 days of culture, when axons had already disintegrated allowed a quantitative comparison between cultured and control samples of both MCT1 and MCT2. An instance of the bands obtained are represented in figure 12. Astrocytes express 42±6% of the total amount of MCT1. Astrocytes express 57±17% of the total amount of MCT2. See Figure 12 for a sample of the Western blot's bands for MCT1 and MCT 2 along with thePonceau' protein staining.
Although the standard deviation is not small in the case of MCT2 (17%), due to intrinsic limitations in the methodology of western blot we cannot deduce those results exactly show the real expresion of MCT in axons and astrocytes in the normal tissue. Then we will discuss those results assigning to astrocytes around 40% of the total MCT1 and to axons the remaining 60%. In like manner, we can round up MCT2 content attributing to astrocytes 60% of the total and to axons the remaining 40% (Table 4).

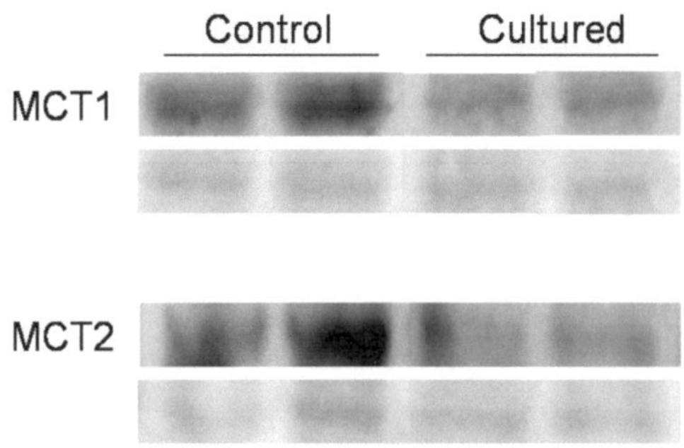

Fig. 12. Samples from Western blot analysis of cultured vs. uncultured prelaminar optic nerve of MCT1 and MCT2. Upper row shows immunolabeling and lower row shows protein staining with the Ponceau method to show the amount of protein content in the sample. Both figures show a reduction of the molecule in cultured tissue after axon removal. Both MCT1 and MCT2 are consequently expressed in axons and astrocytes alike. For quantitative results, see text.

	ASTROCYTE	AXON
MCT1 (percentage)	40%	60%
MCT2 (percentage)	60%	40%

Table 4. Distribution of MCT1 and MCT2 between astrocytes and axons after comparing fresh to cultured prelaminar optic nerve tissue (figures rounded up).

4. Discussion

We determined the presence of monocarboxylate transporters MCT1 and MCT2 in the prelaminar optic nerve head by Western blot, indicative of the activity of the lactate shuttle in the area. Then, as the fluorescence and ultrastructural observation of the prelaminar optic nerve suggested that zonulae adherens and its main constituent, N-cadherin, were more prevalent in the bundles of nerve fibers and columnar astrocytes than in the perivascular astrocytes, we performed a statistical study of the distribution of N-cadherin in images of CLSM with fluorescent immunolabeling. This study showed N-cadherin to concentrate in the axon-astrocyte bundles. With the idea that adhesion structures such as zonulae adherens would contribute to the feasibility of the transport of lactate across the astrocyte-axons boundary, we colocalized in this area MCT isoforms 1 and 2 as well as LDH isoenzymes 1 and 5. Finally, culturing the prelaminar optic nerve for 1 to 5 days, we separated the population of astrocytes of the optic nerve head from the sectioned axons that disintegrated in the culture. Western-blot analysis of cultured vs. control prelaminar tissue rendered the proportion of MCT isoforms present in each cellular type, astrocytes and neurons (axons). Both MCT1 and MCT2 were present in astrocytes as well as the axons but in different proportions.

4.1 Western-blot bands

Information regarding the localization of the bands of porcine MCTs is somewhat conflicting. Welter and Claus (2008) point to the band of 41 kDa for MCT1 of porcine origin, while Santa Cruz Biotechnology situates MCT1 of human origin between 43 and 50 Kda, and Abcam Laboratories around 52 Kda. For MCT2 of human origin, Santa Cruz biotechnologies predicts a band in the 43 KDa mark, and Abcam in the band of 52 KDa. Our bands coincide with the data of Santa Cruz Technologies. The resulting bands were neatly marked, indicating a specific detection (Figures 1 and 12)

4.2 Morphology

The tissue structure of the fiber layers of the prelaminar optic nerve head is intricate. Numerous thin astrocytic projections intermingle with axons and other astrocyte projections, forming a mesh that defies the resolution power of fluorescent confocal laser microscopy. In this particular region, it is not possible to identify the type of cell in paraffin sections, even with the help of double-labeling. Target molecules are normally colocalized using an ancillary antibody directed against a molecule that helps identify the type of cell involved. A second problem arises when this technique is attempted in paraffin sections of our area of interest when the molecule to detect is present in small amounts in the tissue: if an intracellular target such as GFAP is used for astrocytes, or neurofilament for axons, the staining is so intense that it masks the weak fluorescence of the primary target molecule. As a result, instead of singling out individual cells with co-labeling, we considered the astrocyte-neuron couple as a functional unit from the standpoint of the lactate shuttle. For our purposes, it is sufficient to detect whether the molecules are present or absent in particular areas of the optic nerve head.

Accordingly, here we present our results with the single-staining technique. Our method was to use the control section without a primary antibody, to set the acquisition parameters of the microscope so that there was no background and the image was completely dark. Any fluorescence found when exploring the specimen with primary and secondary antibodies was considered positive if the anatomical distribution of the labeling was specific. The background was eliminated because the parameters were identical to control. This method enabled a qualitative evaluation of the results. The results were classified as negative or positive (weak, moderate or intense). We interpreted weak positives to mean that the molecules being detecting were present in the tissue in very small amounts. We are dealing, in part, with transporting molecules floating in the cell membrane in very tiny amounts, surrounded by many different molecules sharing the membrane. Consequently, the resulting fluorescence were small.

Our results can be briefly described as showing that zonulae adherens in pig eyes are more abundant at sites having both the presence of astrocytes and axons than at astrocyte-only sites (perivascular astrocytes of Elschnig and Kuhnt). The areas of astrocyte-axon contact gave more intense results than did the perivascular areas when evidence of enzymes related to the lactate shunt was searched for. All four proteins —LDH 1, LDH 5, MCT 2, and MCT 1— were detected in the areas where astrocytes and neural fibers were densely packed, as occurs in the fiber layer of the optic nerve head near the lamina cribrosa. As shown in the TEM micrographs, astrocytic projections were firmly maintained in place around axons by closely situated zonulae adherens. This arrangement suggests that axon-wrapping astrocytic prolongations may play a role in facilitating the lactate shuttle, for which a narrow and stable (in relation to space) extracellular gap is a precondition. Disruption of this equilibrium may have pathological consequences. As suggested above, a misdirection of the aqueous humor outflow that subsequently interferes with N-cadherin attachments may alter the relationship between the lactate shuttle and the narrow intercellular spaces (Carreras et al., 2009).

Optic-nerve-head astrocytes are believed to be controllers of the development of the retinal vasculature in mammals. Around birth, astrocytes in the optic-nerve head spread across the inner surface of the retina (Watanabe, 1998) and act as a template for the developing retinal vasculature. This retinal development (Fruttiger, 2002) is controlled by a hierarchy of interactions among retinal neurons, astrocytes, and blood vessels. Retinal neurons stimulate a proliferation of astrocytes which in turn stimulate blood-vessel growth, and the developing vessels then provide feedback signals that trigger astrocyte differentiation, and vessel growth is stopped (West et al., 2005). The astrocytes in the center of the disc and accompanying the main central trunks (known as the meniscus of Kuhnt and Elschnig's astrocytes) surround the central branches and form the incomplete inner limiting membrane (ILM). These astrocytes can be considered as a functional unit. Axon-wrapping astrocytes form another functional group, providing support for the neurons.

In the TEM micrographs, we found that the figures for zonula seemed to be more numerous among those astrocyte projections that tightly surround axons in the fiber layers of the optic nerve head. To test this hypothesis, we performed many immunolabeling sections using eyes from different pigs and comparing the immunolabeling intensity among perivascular astrocytes with axon-related astrocytes. The possibility that the difference between the groups was due to sampling has a probability of less than one in 10,000 ($p < 0.0001$). Our results show that N-cadherin, and consequently zonulae adherens, were more numerous in the proximity of the axons. This may indicate the importance of membrane contact and narrow extracellular spaces in the axon-astrocyte relationship.

4.3 Lactate shuttle enzymes

The results of this study demonstrate that the isozymes LDH1 and LDH5 were present in the astrocyte-axon of the prelaminar tissue of the optic nerve head. From what is known about the kinetics of LDH, these results are compatible with the concept of the participation of such a group of isozymes in lactate production in astrocytes and energy metabolism in axons.

The interconversion of lactate and pyruvate is catalyzed by the enzyme lactate dehydrogenase. The LDH-5 subunit (muscle type) tends to favor the formation of lactate from pyruvate. The LDH-I subunit (heart type) preferentially leads toward the production of pyruvate. Isozymes of LDH, LDH1, and LDH5 are easy to separate antigenically because LDH1 is formed by four H subunits and LDH5 by four M subunits. All isoenzymes are present in different proportions in all the processes, but the differences may be sufficient to be brought about by immunostaining. It has been found (using immunohistochemistry techniques on the occipital cortex of rats) that neurons contain mainly the LDH1 subunit, while astrocytes contain both isozymes. These observations support the notion of a regulated lactate flux between astrocytes and neurons (Bittar et al, 1996).

The concept of the cell-cell lactate shuttle implies that the production and exchange of lactate is a major means of providing energy to the cell. A related notion, the intracellular lactate shuttle, states that the mitochondria are sites of lactate oxidation by lactate dehydrogenase (LDH) (Passarella et al., 2008). Examples of cell-cell shuttles include lactate exchanges between astrocytes and neurons. Lactate exchange between production sites and removal is facilitated by monocarboxylate transport proteins, of which there are several isoforms. The presence of cell-cell and intracellular lactate shuttles shows that glycolytic and oxidative pathways are linked processes, in which lactate is the product of one pathway and the substrate for the other pathway (Brooks, 2009).

4.4 Organotypic culture and MCT distribution

Early destruction of axons in tissue culture of the prelaminar optic nerve is consequence of the sectioning of axons at the level of the peripapillary neuroretinal rim and at the level of the lamina cribrosa. In less than 24 h the remains of the axons were merely testimonial. Astrocytes may persist with normally distributed GFAP even after 12 days of culture, but nuclear pycnosis and GFAP clumping, probably a sign of blebbing, was present in the cultured tissue in variable amounts from day 1 with the method followed here. Because of the preservation of a large enough proportion of the astrocytes, a comparison of the relative amount of MCTs of a cultured prelaminar tissue relative to non-cultured fresh tissue is a means of ascertaining the distribution of the two molecular types between the two cell types involved, astrocytes and neurons. After one day of culture, one population of astrocytes was well preserved, while axon membranes were completely absent. Only scant remains of neurofilaments dispersed in some regions of the sample ensured that one-day-old cultures were adequate to quantify the expression of MCTs in the membrane of astrocytes (Figure 11).

Fourteen MCT isoforms and their specific tissue distribution have previously been identified in mammals. Four of these isoforms, MCT1-4, have also been shown experimentally to act as transmembrane transporters of lactate, pyruvate, and ketone bodies (Halestrap & Meredith, 2004). Distribution of MCT variants among cell types is not even. Broer et al. (1997) showed that cultures of astroglial cells contained mRNA encoding MCT1, but little mRNA encoding MCT2. Hanu et al. (2000) reported that neonate rat astrocytes in primary culture express significant levels of both MCT1 and MCT2, and confirmed previous results indicating that the expression of the two transporters is restricted to specific populations of astrocytes in the mature brain. The same cell may contain MCT1 and MCT2, as occurs with Müller cells. Gerhart et al. (1999), working on rat retinas, found that MCT-1 was expressed by the apical processes of the retinal pigment epithelium as well as in endothelial cells, Müller-cell microvilli and in inner rod segments. MCT-2 was found to be expressed by Müller's cells and by glial cell processes surrounding retinal microvessels.

Debernardi et al. (2003) reported that in mouse-brain cortical-cell cultures that astrocytes strongly expressed MCT1 but had very little if any MCT2, at both the mRNA and the protein levels. By contrast, neurons had high amounts of MCT2 and low to moderate levels of MCT1. Thus, studies of cells *in vitro* and *in vivo* have yielded somewhat different results and, on the other hand, astrocytes and neurons can express different isomorphs of MCT in specific areas of the CNS. Consequently, each region of the CNS demands its specific study of the distribution of MCT. That distribution would speak of the role of both the neuron and the astrocyte in the regulation of lactate (and other monocarboxylates) in the intercellular cleft. The extracellular lactate pool is increased by MCT 1 release and decreased by MCT2 intake, as the extracellular lactate concentration has been found to be approx. 1 mM in both rats and humans (Abi-Saab et al., 2002; Pellerin, 2005b).

Western-blot analysis of MCT1 and MCT 2 after 1, 2, and 5 days of culture, when axons had already disintegrated showed that both MCT1 and MCT2 were still present in the tissue. It indicated that MCT1 and MCT2 were present in the membrane of the astrocytes. Both MCT isoforms were present in equivalent proportions in astrocytes and axons alike. As indicated in Table 4, a 40-60% for MCT1 and a 60-40% for MCT2 are present in astrocytes and axons respectively.

In our results, astrocytes anchored MCT1 and MCT2 in their plasma membrane, and accordingly had the ability to move lactate into the extracellular spaces and also the resources to re-uptake it. Astrocytes were thus able to control the extracellular concentration of lactate near the axon. This is corroborated in Figures 9 and 10, in which the membranes of the axon and the astrocytic prolongations in direct contact with the axons are labeled in gold. Discrepancies between the strong presence of MCT2 in optic-nerve astrocytes and not in cortical astrocytes, as reported by Debernardi (2003), may be partially related to the coupling of synaptic activity to glucose utilization in the astrocyte. This role is marked by the presence of receptors for a variety of neurotransmitters in the astrocytic processes near synapses that can influence the intake of glucose by the vascular feet of the astrocytes (Pellerin, 2005b). In the white matter, as in the prelaminar optic nerve, where synapses are absent, the regulatory ability to control the pool of monocarboxylates in the intercellular cleft appears to be permanently shared by both sides, astrocytes and neurons (axons).

Whether it is the astrocyte or the neuron that is responsible for maintaining a stable lactate pool can be deduced from the presence the two transporter molecules in the membrane of each cell type . Our results indicate that, in the optic nerve head astrocytes, neurons express similar amounts of MCT1 and MCT2 in their membranes. Although it could seem improbable that the neuron returns the lactate that it uses as fuel back to the intercellular cleft under normal conditions, the possibility of this return exists, and a reverse neuron-to-astrocyte lactate shuttle has recently been proposed (Mangia et al., 2009). It bears mentioning here that, in addition to lactic acid transport, MCTs also mediate the transport of many other metabolically important monocarboxylates such as pyruvate, the branched-chain oxo acids derived from leucine, valine, and isoleucine as well as the ketone bodies (acetoacetate, hydroxybutyrate and acetate (Halestrap & Meredith, 2004)). Having the ability to expel unwanted metabolites via MCT1 is a plausible role for this molecule in the axonal membrane.

The fact that MCT 1 is present in the astrocyte and MCT2 appears in the axon membrane agrees with the results of Pellerin et al. (2005a) and other authors on cortical neurons (see Pellerin 2005b and 2007b for a review). However, the abundance (up to 60%) of MCT2 in astrocytes and MCT1 in neurons may be a feature of the optic nerve and perhaps white matter. It has been shown that, in the gray matter, levels of expression of MCT2 in the membrane can change in response to variable situations in order to adjust for energy requirements (Pellerin et al., 2007a). Metabolic requirements of cortical-cell activity are presumably more complex that mere axonal conduction, and the expression of similar amounts of MCT isoforms in the membranes of both astrocytes and neurons can be a regular feature, but this point needs to be assessed. In the optic nerve, Tekkok et al. (2005) corroborated previous works by their group that L-lactate is released from astrocytes and taken up by axons in an experimental setting with mice. In addition, immunocytochemical staining localized MCT2 predominantly in axons, and MCT1 predominantly in astrocytes. The limitations of immunolabeling alone, and even supplemented with TEM, discussed previously in this paper, prompted us to complement the morphological approach with tissue culture. Our results, although slightly divergent, do not contradict previous results but show that MCT2 is also present in astrocytes and MCT1 also present in neurons in considerable proportion. Previously, MCT2 had been localized on glial foot processes surrounding retinal vessels (Gerhart et al., 1999).

The conclusion that there is a coincidental distribution of metabolic coupling molecules and N-cadherin suggests a close relationship between the functions of both sets of molecules intervening in the metabolism of lactate. The presence of four essential components of the l-lactate metabolic chain suggests that the survival of the axon depends on the close membrane contact brought about by N-cadherin-mediated zonulae adherens. Closely apposed membranes are an important requisite for the transfer of lactate from astrocytes to neurons, and on this feature depends partially the concentration of lactate in intercellular spaces. These features are represented on the left side of Figure 13.

4.5 N-cadherin and apoptosis

Astrocytes support neurons by means of the uptake and release of neurotrophic factors and cytokines, such as NGF, TNFa, and bFGF, which are fundamental for the viability of neurons. In addition, astrocytes prevent neurotoxic levels of neuron-released glutamate and K^+ from accumulating in extracellular spaces (Tsacopoulos & Magistretti, 1996). Cell-adhesion complexes act as sensors and at the same time contribute to the adhesive process and to the transmission of signals that result in a variety of cellular responses. Indeed, adhesion receptors can modulate or activate intracellular signal-transduction pathways in several ways, such as by interacting with proteins that link adhesive structures to cellular cytoskeletal networks, or by directly activating enzymes on the inner surface of the plasma membrane (Brunton & McPherson, 2004).

N-cadherin is a calcium-dependent molecule because calcium ions occupy positions in the extracellular domain of the molecule that enable the homo-engagement of similar molecules in the opposite membrane. Attachment does not take place when there are low levels of calcium in extracellular spaces. The separation of zonulae adherens may have two important consequences: 1) The separation of the membranes may negatively affect the transport of lactate (and other molecules) that are fundamental for the neuronal metabolism.

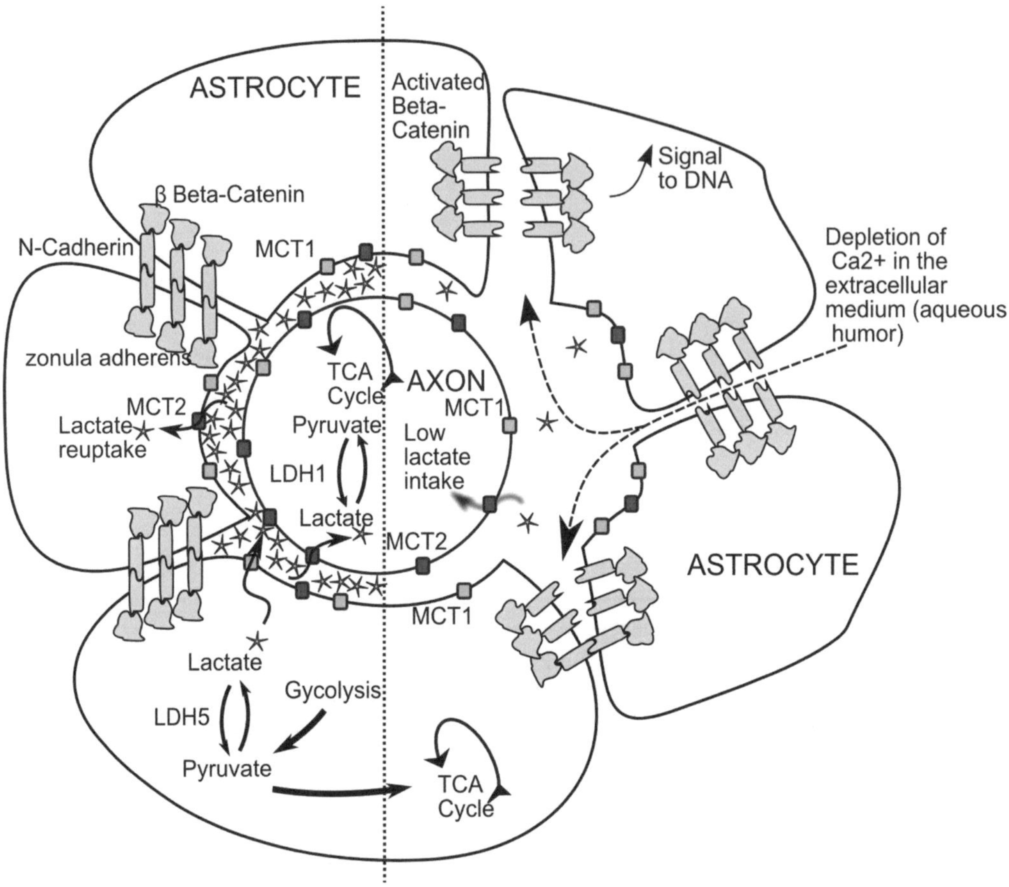

Fig. 13. Diagram of the relationships between the lactate shuttle and the membrane position through zonulae adherens in the axon and astrocytic projections. The left side shows physiological relationships: membranes are closely apposed by zonulae adherens. The main attachment complex is formed by N-cadherin, which is responsible for homotypic adhesion between the external surfaces of facing membranes. Beta catenin is known to be present on the inner side of the membrane. Catenins link the adherens junctions with the actin cytoskeleton. However, the catenins also transfer signals into and out of the cells, thereby mediating a variety of cell behavior such as proliferation, migration, differentiation, and death. Both carboxylate transporters MCT1 and MCT2 are present in axons and astrocytes. The right half of the diagram represents the hypothetical effects of aqueous humor flowing through the fiber layer of the optic nerve. The low calcium content of aqueous humor (roughly half the plasma concentration) could hypothetically wash away the calcium from sites in the N-cadherin molecule and lead to a separation of the zonulae adherens. Here the icon of beta catenin rotates to represent the activation of the signaling activity after the detachment of N-cadherin. Beta catenin signaling may trigger molecular cascades conducive to cell migration and/or apoptosis of the astrocyte. Increased extracellular spaces interfere with the dynamics of the lactate shuttle. Low lactate intake and the absence of astrocytes eventually determine the fate of the axon. This mechanism may play a role in the pathogeny of glaucomas, but a confirmation that the concentration of calcium ion in the aqueous is low enough to cause astrocytic detachment and/or apoptosis needs to be experimentally tested.

Extracellular spaces must have a critical volume for the adequate exchange of lactate. Abnormally increased extracellular spaces may interfere with the correct concentration of lactate and other molecules that must be incorporated into the cell (neuron) at a sustained rate, the dynamic of which is concentration dependent. The interruption of this chain may trigger axonal compartmentalized self-destruction (Whitmore, 2005). 2) Loosening the intermembrane attachment might compromise the information capabilities of this type of junction (Gumbiner, 1996). It has been shown that the blocking of N-cadherin-mediated intercellular interaction increases the number of cells undergoing apoptosis (Li et al., 2001). Messages are carried to the nucleus of the astrocyte and these may precipitate the mechanisms of cell migration (Nakagawa & Takeichi, 1998) and/or apoptosis (Makrigiannakis et al. 2000; Peluso et al., 1996). This doubly harmful effect could explain the disappearance of axons as well as astrocytes by two separate mechanisms related to the depletion of calcium ions. These features are represented on the right side of Figure 13.

5. Conclusion. Optic nerve architecture and glaucoma

Unlike epithelial-type cells, mesenchymal cells, of which astrocytes are an example, do not form impermeable barriers. Cell unions are invariably lax and therefore fluid can circulate between them (Adams & Nelson, 1998). Astrocytes and axons of the retinal ganglion cells are the main components of the optic nerve head. The structure of the anterior interface of the optic nerve has recently been revised. Simple membrane apposition is the main cell-attachment mechanism in the vitreous interface, and zonulae adherens is the only attachment junction among astrocytes (Carreras et al., 2009). The cell architecture enables the unimpeded passage of fluids from the vitreous cavity because of the complete absence of tight junctions (Carreras et al., 2010a 2010b).

The surface of the optic nerve in contact with the vitreous is uneven with respect to the penetration of fluids. As mentioned above, no sealed membrane exists and the entire surface is permeable. However, the presence of preferential flow routes in the perivascular region suggests that small quantities of fluid follow the perivascular route. (Carreras et al., 2010a). If the flow of fluid supersedes the ability of the preferential (or lymphatic-like) routes to evacuate, then aqueous humor from the anterior segment would reach the axon layers and interfere with the intermembrane contacts and its signaling activities. The pattern of visual field defects in glaucoma has been reproduced in a computer model that simulates progressive damage affecting the optic-nerve head from the vitreous (anteroposteriorly), as would be caused by the diverted flow of aqueous humor (Carreras et al., 2011).

In summary, the aqueous flow through the prelaminar tissue may interfere with the astrocyte-axon relationship in more than one way. An increase in the intermembrane gap and a simple washout of the extracellular lactate would directly interfere with the kinetics of monocarboxylate uptake. Low calcium-ion concentration, a hallmark of aqueous composition, may interfere with the cadherin attachments and increase separation. Moreover, messenger activity by zonulae adherens may trigger signals conducive to apoptosis. This mechanism may play a role in the pathogeny of glaucomas, but a confirmation that the concentration of calcium ion in the aqueous is low enough to cause astrocytic detachment and/or apoptosis needs to be experimentally tested.

6. Acknowledgments

Authors wish to thank Carmen Ruiz and Juan de Dios Bueno for their technical assistance.

7. References

Abi-Saab WM, Maggs DG & Jones T. Striking differences in glucose and lactate levels between brain extracellular fluid and plasma in conscious human subjects: effects of hyperglycemia and hypoglycemia. Journal of Cerebral Blood Flow & Metabolism. 2002; 22: 271–279.

Adams CL & Nelson WJ. Cytomechanics of cadherin-mediated cell-cell adhesion. Current Opinion in Cell Biology. 1998; 10:572-7.

Alma A & Nilsson SFE. Uveoscleral outflow - A review. Experimental Eye Research. 2009; 88:760-768

Aubert A, Costalat R, Magistretti PJ & Pellerin L. Brain lactate kinetics: Modeling evidence for neuronal lactate uptake upon activation. PNAS. 2005; 102:16448–16453

Bittar PG, Charnay Y, Pellegrin L, Bouras C & Magistretti PJ. Selective distribution of lactate dehydrogenase isoenzymes in neurons in astrocytes of human brain. . Journal of Cerebral Blood Flow & Metabolism. 1996; 16:1079-1089

Broer S, Rohman B, Pellegri G, Pellerin L, Martin JL, Verleysdonk S, Hamprecht B, & Magistretti PJ. Comparison of lactate transport in astroglial cells and monocarboxylate transporter 1 (MCT1) expressing Xenopus laevis oocytes. The Journal of Biological Chemistry 272: 30096–30102, 1997.

Brooks GA. Lactate shuttles in nature. Biochemical Society Transactions. 2002; 30:258–264.

Brooks GA. Cell–cell and intracellular lactate shuttles. The Journal of Physiology. 2009; 587: 5591–5600.

Brown AM, Tekkök S B & Ransom BR. Energy transfer from astrocytes to axons: the role of CNS glycogen. Neurochemistry International. 2004; 45:529-536.

Brunton VG, MacPherson IRJ & Frame MC. Cell adhesion receptors, tyrosine kinases and actin modulators: a complex three-way circuitry. Biochimica et Biophysica Acta. 2004; 1692: 121-144

Carrasco MC, Navascués J, Cuadros MA, Calvente R, Martín-Oliva D, Santos AM, Sierra A, Ferrer-Martín RM & Marín-Teva JL. Migration and ramification of microglia in quail embryo retina organotypic cultures. Developmental Neurobiology. 2010 OI:10.1002/dneu.20860

Carreras FJ, Porcel D, Alaminos M & Garzon I. Cell-cell adhesion in the prelaminar region of the optic nerve head: a possible target for ionic stress. Ophthalmic Research 2009; 42:106-111.

Carreras FJ, Porcel D & Muñoz-Avila JI. Mapping the Surface Astrocytes of the Optic Disc: A Fluid-conducting Role of the Astrocytic Covering of the Central Vessels. Clinical & Experimental Ophthalmology. 2010; 38:300-308.

Carreras FJ, Porcel D, Guerra- Tschuschke I & Carreras I. Fenestrations and preferential flow routes in the prelaminar optic nerve through wet-SEM and perfusion of tracers. Clinical & Experimental Ophthalmology. 2010 ; 38:705-717.

Carreras FJ, Rica R, Delgado A. Modeling the patterns of visual field loss in glaucoma. Optometry and Vision Science. 2011; 88:63-79.

Fruttiger M. Development of the mouse retinal vasculature: angiogenesis versus vasculogenesis. Invest Ophthalmol Vis Sci. 2002; 43:522-527.

Debernardi R, Pierre K, Lengacher S, Magistretti PJ, Pellerin L. Cell-specific expression pattern of monocarboxylate transporters in astrocytes and neurons observed in different mouse brain cortical cell cultures. J Neurosci Res 200; 373:141–155

Gerhart DZ, Leino RL, Drewes LR. Distribution of monocarboxylate transporters MCT1 and MCT2 in rat retina. Neuroscience. 1999; 92:367-375.

Gumbiner BM. Cell adhesion: the molecular basis of tissue architecture and morphogenesis. Cell. 1996; 84:345-57.

Halestrap, A. P.; Meredith, D. The SLC16 gene family —from monocarboxylate transporters (MCTs) to aromatic amino acid transporters and beyond. Pflugers Arch. 2004, 447, 619–628.

Halestrap AP, Meredith D. The SLC16 gene family-from monocarboxylate transporters (MCTs) to aromatic amino acid transporters and beyond. Pflugers Arch. 2004; 447:619-628.

Hanu R, McKenna M, O'Neill A, Resneck WG, Bloch RJ. Monocarboxylic acid transporters, MCT1 and MCT2, in cortical astrocytes in vitro and in vivo. Am J Physiol Cell Physiol May 2000; 278:C921-C930

Li G, Satyamoorthy K, Herlyn M. N-Cadherin-mediated Intercellular Interactions Promote Survival and Migration of Melanoma Cells. Cancer Res. 2001; 61:3819-3825Morgello S, Uson RR, Schwartz EJ, Haber RS. The human blood-brain barrier glucose transporter (GLUT1) is a glucose transporter of gray matter astrocytes. Glia. 1995; 14: 3–54.

Makrigiannakis A, Coukis G, Blaschuk O, Coutifaris C: Follicular atresia and luteolysis. Evidence for a role for N-Cadherin. Ann NY Acad Sci. 2000; 900: 46-55.

Mangia S, Simpson IA, Vannucci SJ, Carruthers A. The in vivo neuron-to-astrocyte lactate shuttle in human brain: evidence from modeling of measured lactate levels during visual stimulation. J Neurochem. 2009; 109 Suppl 1:55-62.

Nakagawa S, Takeichi M. Neural crest emigration from the neural tube depends on regulated cadherin expression. Development. 1998; 125:2963-71.

O'Brien J, Kla KM , Hopkins IB, Malecki EA, McKenna MC. Kinetic Parameters and Lactate Dehydrogenase Isozyme Activities Support Possible Lactate Utilization by Neurons. Neurochem Res. 2007; 32:597-607

Passarella S, Bari L de, Valenti D, Pizzuto R, Paventi G, Atlante A. Mitochondria and L-lactate metabolism. FEBS Letters. 2008; 582:3569-3576

Pellerin L, Magistretti PJ.Glutamate uptake into astrocytes stimulates aerobic glycolysis: a mechanism coupling neuronal activity to glucose utilization. Proc Natl Acad Sci USA.1994; 91:10625–10629.

Pellerin L, Begersen L, Halestrap AP, Pierre K. Cellular and subcellular distribution of monocarboxylate transporters in cultured brain cells and in the adult brain. J. Neurosci. Res,2005a;. 79: 55–64.

Pellerin L. How astrocytes feed hungry neurons. Molecular Neurobiology2005b; 32: 59–72.

Pellerin L, Bouzier-Sore AK, Aubert A, et al. Activity-dependent regulation of energy metabolism by astrocytes: an update. Glia. 2007a; 55:251–1262.

Pellerin L, Bouzier-Sore AK, Aubert A, Serres S, Merle M, Costalat R and Magistretti PJ. Activity-dependent regulation of energy metabolism by astrocytes: an update. Glia 2007b; 55:1251-1262.

Peluso JJ, Pappalardo A and Trolice MP. N-cadherin-mediated cell contact inhibits granulosa cell apoptosis in a progesterone-independent manner. Endocrinology. 1996; 137:1196-1203.

Poitry-Yamate CL , Poitry S. Tsacopoulos M. Lactate Released by Miiller Glial Cells Is Metabolized by Photoreceptors from Mammalian Retina. J Neurosci. 1995; 15:5179-5191.

Redies C, Takeichi1 M. N- and R-cadherin expression in the optic nerve of the chicken embryo. Glia. 1993; 8: 161–171.

Schurr A. Lactate: the ultimate cerebral oxidative energy substrate? J Cereb Blood Flow Metab. 2006; 26:142–152.

Smith D, Pernet A, Hallett WA, Bingham E, Marsden PK, Amiel SA. Lactate: a preferred fuel for human brain metabolism in vivo. J Cerb Blood Flow Metab. 2003; 23:658-64.

Stoppini, L., Buchs, P. A., Muller, D., "A simple method for organotypic cultures of nervous tissue" J Neurosci Meth. 1991; 37:173–82.

Tekkok SB, Brown AM, Westenbroek R, Pellerin L, Ransom BR (Sep 2005) Transfer of glycogen-derived lactate from astrocytes to axons via specific monocarboxylate transporters supports mouse optic nerve activity., Journal of Neuroscience Research, 81 (5), 644-52.

Tsacopoulos M and Magistretti PJ. Metabolic coupling between glia and neurons. J. Neurosci. 1996; 16:877-885

Wanga DD, Bordey A. The astrocyte odyssey. Progress in Neurobiology. 2008; 86:342–367.

Watanabe T, Raff MC. Retinal astrocytes are immigrants from the optic nerve. Nature. 1988; 332:834-837.

Welter H, Claus R. Expression of the monocarboxylate transporter 1 (MCT1) in cells of the porcine intestine. Cell Biol Internat. 2008; 32:638-645.

Whitmore AV, Libby RT, John SWM. Glaucoma: Thinking in new ways--a rôle for autonomous axonal self-destruction and other compartmentalised processes? Prog Ret Eye Res. 2005; 24:639-662.

West H, Richardson WD, Fruttiger M. Stabilization of the retinal vascular network by reciprocal feedback between blood vessels and astrocytes. Development 2005; 132:1855-1862.

Yu S, Ding WG,. The 45 kDa form of glucose transporter 1 (GLUT1) is localized in oligodendrocyte and astrocyte but not in microglia in the rat brain. Brain Res. 1998; 797:65–72.

5

Anatomical and Molecular Responses Triggered in the Retina by Axonal Injury

Marta Agudo-Barriuso[1], Francisco M. Nadal-Nicolás[1,2], Guillermo Parrilla-Reverter[1,2], María Paz Villegas-Pérez[2] and Manuel Vidal-Sanz[2]
[1]*Unidad de Investigación. Hospital General Universitario Virgen de la Arrixaca, Fundación para la Formación e Investigación Sanitarias de la Región de Murcia,*
[2]*Departamento de Oftalmología. Facultad de Medicina, Universidad de Murcia, Spain*

1. Introduction

After receiving their visual input from photoreceptors via the intermediate neurons (bipolar, horizontal and amacrine cells), retinal ganglion cells (RGCs) relay this intraretinally pre-processed visual information to the centres in the brain for further processing. Thus, RGCs are the only projecting neurons in the retina, and their axons form the optic nerve. These central nerve axons originate at the RGC bodies located in the neural retina, travel along the nerve fibre layer converging to the optic disk and finally exit the eye through the optic nerve head (ONH).

Glaucomatous optic neuropathy is a complex, multifactorial and heterogeneous human chronic neurodegenerative disease that characteristically affects the RGC population and their axons. It is a slowly progressive form of optic nerve damage and blindness that begins with loss of peripheral vision and is followed by gradual narrowing of the remaining central vision.

Glaucoma currently affects over 70 million people (Quigley, 1996). Second only to cataract is the leading cause of irreparable blindness. This disease affects all age groups, but is more frequent in the elderly (Quigley & Vitale, 1997). Glaucoma is broadly classified into three main groups, i) primary open glaucoma (POAG); ii) primary acute closed angle glaucoma; and iii) primary congenital glaucoma. Among these, the most frequent is POAG (Shields et al., 1996). In this type of glaucoma the main risk factors are age and an elevated intraocular pressure (IOP). In most cases, lowering the IOP has a beneficial effect on RGC survival. However, some individuals with low or even normal IOP develop this disease with associated RGC loss, yet others with high IOP do not develop glaucoma or lose these neurons. Because of this, it has been proposed that there are genetic variants in humans that affect the relative susceptibility or resilience of RGCs to the same insult. This hypothesis is based on recent works showing that RGCs from different mice strains have an intrinsically different resistance to optic nerve injury. Li et al (2007) analyzed the survival of RGCs in 15 mice strains after optic nerve crush, and found that RGCs from the DAB/2J strain were the most resistant, while the ones from BALB/cByJ were the most susceptible. Interestingly, this

rank of relative vulnerability to optic nerve crush does not translate to other lesions or regions of the CNS, which means that the genetic background has a complex effect on the resistance to injury of specific neurons from specific areas. In addition to this putative implication of the different human genotypes on developing glaucoma, there are 25 loci that have been found linked to POAG. However, only 3 genes are known to cause glaucoma if mutated (*Myocilin, WDR36* and *Optineurin*), though at least 30 more genes have been reported to be associated with this neuropathy (for reviews see Ray & Mookherjee, 2009; Fuse, 2010). This is further complicated by the fact that environmental factors and systemic disorders play a role in glaucoma, making it a multifactorial disease. Because, to date, there is not a cure for this neurodegenerative disease many efforts are being devoted to understand its molecular, cellular and etiological causes.
Two of the more popular hypotheses to explain the initial glaucomatous damage to the ONH are the mechanical and the vascular theory of glaucoma. The mechanical theory states that the raised IOP obstructs RGC axons, thus causing their degeneration and death. With respect to the vascular theory, there is evidence of vascular dysregulation in some forms of glaucoma (Flammer & Mozaffarieh, 2007) that may endanger ONH blood flow. Thus, this might induce an ischemia-reperfusion nerve injury. Additionally, the role of glial cells at the ONH has received increasing attention (Ramirez et al., 2010; Nguyen et al., 2011).

2. Animal models of glaucoma

The high incidence of glaucoma, and the lack of non-invasive approaches to study in humans the subjacent neuronal responses, make necessary the use of animal models to understand the pathogenesis of this neuropathy (for a more detailed account of these models see Morrison et al., 2010).

2.1 Spontaneous, transgenic or deficient mice

Some mice strains have spontaneously developed mutations that produce a chronic elevation of the IOP, and result in a phenotype similar to chronic age-related glaucoma. The best studied is the DAB/2J inbred line (John et al., 1997, 1998). This strain is homozygous for two mutations related to melanosomes accumulation. Thus, it has been suggested that the initial pathology of the anterior chamber is due to an abnormal iris pigmentation and melanosome structure (John, 1998) though it is not the only cause as there is also an immune component involved (Chang et al., 1999). These mice start to exhibit increased IOP by 8-13 months old. The course of the disease, however, varies on individual colonies and environmental factors.
Mice can be genetically manipulated, and so transgenic mice have been generated targeting proteins implicated in the aqueous outflow or those for which human mutations related to glaucoma have been described. Examples of such transgenic mice are the ones with the targeted mutation in the $\alpha 1$ subunit of collagen type 1 (Aihara et al., 2003) or the ones expressing the Tyr437His mutation in myocilin (Zhou et al., 2008), associated with human patients developing early onset glaucoma (Alward et al., 1998). Recently, it has been reported that mice deficient of Vav 2 and/or Vav 3 proteins (guanine nucleotides exchange factors for Rho guanosine triphosphatases) show early onset of iridocorneal angle changes and elevated intraocular pressure (Fujikawa et al., 2010). Interestingly, *VAV2* and *VAV3* genes seem to be candidates for associated genes in Japanese open-angle glaucoma patients.

2.2 Induced

The majority of the induced animal models of glaucoma are based on experimental elevation the IOP. Most of these models are carried out in rats and in mice. There are some advantages of these experimental models over the spontaneous models. First, the onset of the elevated IOP is predictable, making possible to determine the temporal course of the degenerative events in retina and optic nerve. Second, unilateral IOP elevation leaves the fellow eye as internal control, hence accounting for inter-individual variability. Third, IOP increase occurs soon after the treatment, and thus it is not necessary to wait long periods for the animal to develop the symptoms. However, these models have in common a high variability, in terms of the IOP reached and the damage induced.

The goal of any experimental procedure to elevate the IOP is to inhibit aqueous humour outflow without interfering with the eye's ability to produce this humour. There are four main approaches, scarring the anterior angle chamber by hypertonic saline injection (rats, Johnson et al., 1996; Morrison et al., 1997; mice, Kipfer-Kauer et al., 2010) laser photocoagulation (rats and mice, Salinas-Navarro et al., 2009a, 2010, Cuenca et al., 2010), venous cautery (Shareef et al., 1995) and injection of microbeads in the anterior chamber (mice, Cone et al., 2010; Chen et al., 2011; rats and mice, Sappington et al., 2010).

Laser photocoagulation, a method first described in monkeys (Gaasterland & Kupfer, 1974) and later in rats (Ueda et al., 1998), is based on the photocoagulation of the trabecular mesh alone or in combination with episcleral veins and/or perilimbar vessels (WoldeMussie et al., 2001; Levkovitch-Verbin et al., 2007; Salinas-Navarro et al., 2009a, 2010, Cuenca et al., 2010). The IOP increase occurs because the drainage of the aqueous humour is obstructed by the closure of the intratrabecular spaces and of the majority of drainage channels. In this model, RGC loss occurs mainly in pie-shaped sectors located in the dorsal retina, with their apex pointing to the optic nerve disk. It has been described that there is first an impairment of the anterograde active axonal transport, followed by a retrograde degeneration of RGCs (Salinas-Navarro et al., 2009a, 2010).

3. Intraorbital optic nerve crush (IONC)

Another good approach is to study separately the RGC response to axotomy. Intraorbital optic nerve crush (IONC) is based on crushing the entire retinofugal pathway at the exit of the eye. This model specifically injures all the RGC axons, avoiding any ischemic insult. Thus, as a model to study the underlying causes of RGC death by axonal injury, IONC is clean and predictable.

Traumatic axonal injury to the optic nerve, either by complete transection or crush, is a well established model (Bray et al., 1987) that can be evaluated morphologically (Nadal-Nicolas et al., 2009; Parrilla-Reverter et al., 2009a, 2009b), molecularly (Agudo et al., 2008, 2009) and functionally, and has been thoroughly analyzed by our group, both in rats and mice (Alarcon-Martinez et al., 2009, 2010). These lesions induce a quick and massive death of RGCs (Peinado-Ramon et al., 1996; Chidlow et al., 2005; Sobrado-Calvo et al., 2007; Agudo et al., 2008, 2009; Galindo-Romero et al., 2011; Sanchez-Migallon et al., 2011). After IONC, the whole RGC population is injured and degenerates within a short period of time. In addition, as long as the lesion is inflicted at the same distance from the optic disk (Villegas-Perez et al., 1993), there is a small variability among different animals.

IONC has several advantages: i) the insult affects the whole RGC population. This is important because the population of RGCs only represents approximately 1% of the retinal cells, thus, there is a dilution effect that may hinder the study of protein or transcript regulation in the affected RGCs. This dilution effect is higher if only part of the RGC population is affected by the lesion, as it happens in the increased IOP models (Guo et al., 2010); ii) the temporal course of RGC degeneration is well established; iii) there is a body of reports in which the molecular correlates associated to this injury have been studied (Agudo et al., 2008, 2009). Importantly, this lesion mimics the crush-like injury observed in the optic nerve after IOP increase (Salinas-Navarro et al., 2009a, 2010) but leaves aside the possible ischemic insult, thus easing the understanding of the obtained data.

3.1 Early signs of retinal ganglion cell degeneration

Degeneration of CNS axons after a traumatic insult was first described by Ramón y Cajal (Ramón y Cajal 1914) and his co-workers (Tello 1907; Leoz y Arcuate 1914). They observed many degenerative changes such as axons that broke up rapidly and axons ending in club-like shapes known as terminal swellings, ganglioform swellings or cytoid bodies. Later, in 1967, Reimer and Wolter (Reimer & Wolter, 1967) after analyzing the retinas of 3 patients with ocular or systemic diseases and the cordotomized spinal cord of a fourth patient, concluded that these degenerative events were the common reaction of CNS axons to damage. These authors stained the axons with the silver-carbonate or silver nitrate methods. Nowadays axons are identified by immunodetecting proteins specifically expressed by them. Furthermore, because specific proteins (or their isoforms) are expressed in specific neuronal compartments, it is possible to study them separately. Neurofilaments (NF) are the main cytoskeletal proteins in mature axons. They are assembled from three subunits, high (H), medium (M) or low (L). NF suffer post-translational modifications wherein the most relevant is phosphorylation. Phosphorylation of NF, particularly of NFH (pNFH) is considered to decrease their transport rate (for review see Perrot et al., 2008). Thus, highly phosphorylated isoforms of pNFH are found in the mature axons while dephosphorylated isoforms are expressed in the soma and dendrites (Perrot et al., 2008). Degenerating neurons insulted by either disease or trauma show an altered organisation and/or metabolism of pNFH that is associated with several human neurodegenerative diseases or experimental paradigms (for review see Al Chalabi & Miller, 2003). The levels of NF transcripts decrease after different retinal injuries, such as ischemia, excitotoxicity or optic nerve injury (McKerracher et al., 1990a, 1990b; Chidlow et al., 2005b; Agudo et al., 2008). This regulation correlates, after optic nerve transection, with an impairment of the axonal transport if the RGCs are committed to death, but not if RGCs are allowed to regenerate along peripheral nerve grafts (McKerracher et al., 1990a, 1990b; Vidal-Sanz et al., 1991, 2000). In healthy retinas pNFH expression is circumscribed to the mature portion of the intrarretinal axons, i.e. in the central-medial retina, while in the periphery few, thin pNFH positive axons ($pNFH^+$) are observed. In fact, quantitative analyses show that $pNFH^+$ axons occupy 61%, 14% and 0.37% of the central, medial and peripheral retinal surface, respectively (Parrilla-Reverter et al., 2009a). In addition, few or none RGC somas express this isoform. After optic nerve injury this pattern changes dramatically (Drager & Olsen, 1981; Vidal-Sanz et al., 1987; Villegas-Perez et al., 1988, Parrilla-Reverter et al., 2009). Three days after IONC the expression pattern of pNFH resembles that of a control retina when analyzed at low magnification. However, at high magnification two aberrant patterns emerge. Firstly, pNFH signal in the medial and peripheral retina increases significantly, occupying 24% and 9% of the middle and peripheral retinal surface, respectively. Secondly, some RGCs somas, preferentially in these retinal areas, become pNFH positive ($pNFH^+$RGCs) (Figure 1A). With time, these abnormalities progress further (Figure 1B-D). The distribution of pNFH⁺RGCs widens, their number increases, peaking at 14 dpl, and the intensity of their staining augments. pNFH⁺RGCs appear first in the medial and peripheral retina, then they spread centripetally throughout the whole retinal surface. In general, pNFH⁺somas are weakly stained (Figure 1A arrow), but from day 14 onwards strongly stained ones appear, mainly in the temporal retina (Figures 1B-C arrows).

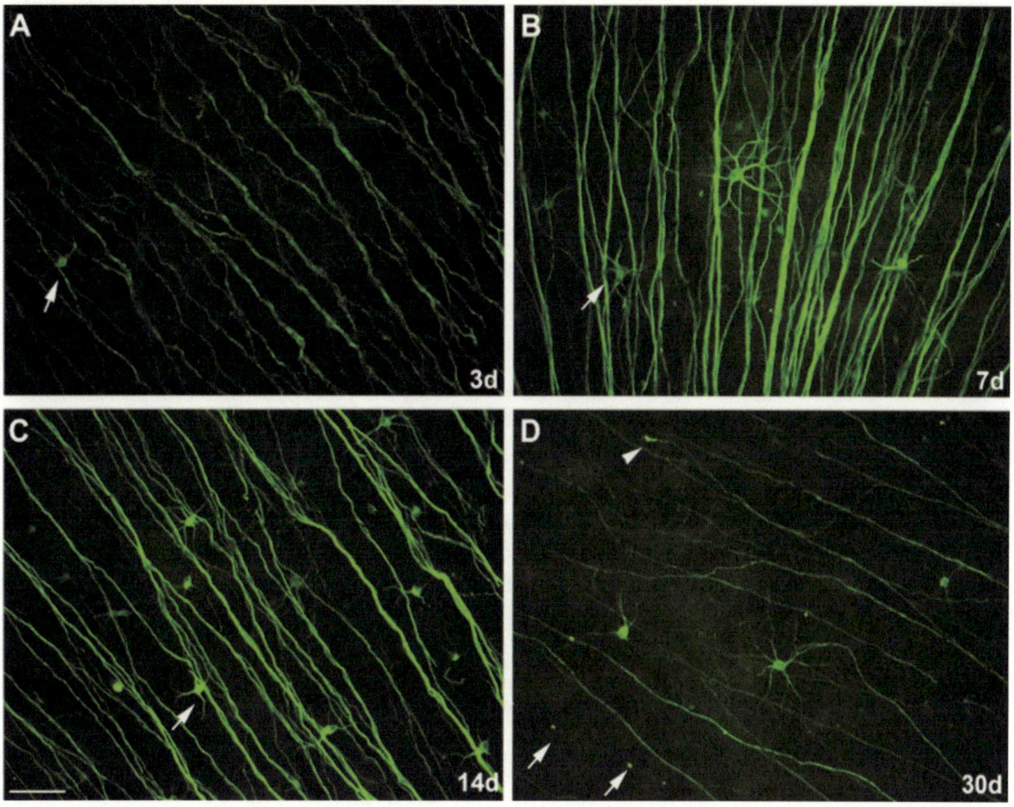

Fig. 1. Aberrant expression of pNFH after IONC. Microphotographs acquired from the retinal periphery of IONC-injured retinas at increasing days post-lesion (dpl). A: As soon as 3 dpl pNFH signal is observed in the retinal periphery and in some RGCs' bodies that have become pNFH positive (arrow). This abnormal expression progresses (B, C), and at 7 and 14dpl there are more pNFH⁺RGCs somas with variable signal intensity (weak as arrow in A, medium as arrow in B, or strong as arrow in C). D. 30 dpl the general intensity of pNFH signal has decreased, there are fewer axons but still scattered pNFH⁺somas are observed. In addition, club-like degenerating axonal tips (arrow-head) and axons with rosary-like pNFH accumulations are observed (arrows). Bar: 100μm.

With respect to the axonal expression of pNFH, in the medial and peripheral retina is maintained above the control levels at least till 30dpl. In the central retina, where the RGC axonal bundles converge to exit the eye, pNFH expression decreases gradually. At late times post-lesion axonal degenerative events similar to those described by Ramón y Cajal are observed, such as rosary-like intra-axonal accumulations and club-like axonal ends (Figure 1D, arrows and arrowhead).

The aberrant expression of pNFH in the ganglion cell layer is common to other insults that affect the RGC either primarily, like optic nerve transection or IOP increase (Salinas-Navarro et al., 2009a, 2010; Parrilla-Reverter et al., 2009a; Nguyen et al., 2011), or secondarily, like phototoxicity (Villegas-Pérez et al., 1996, 1998; Marco-Gomariz et al., 2006; Garcia-Ayuso et al., 2010). It is worth noting than even though all these insults cause the same aberrant patterns, their quantity and time course differs. For example after intraorbital nerve transection there are fewer pNFH$^+$somas but in turn, early after the injury, there are more axons showing rosary-like accumulations of pNFH. These differences allow the correlation of different retinal diseases with a crush or transection-like temporal course of degeneration. In relation to this, our group has shown that after increasing the IOP in mice and rats, the RGCs located in the sectors of RGC loss express pNFH in their soma in a pattern closer to that observed after optic nerve crush than after optic nerve transection (Salinas-Navarro et al., 2009a; 2010). In conclusion, the pathological expression of pNFH is an early event that marks RGC degeneration and it is observed as early as 3 days following the insult.

3.2 Retinal ganglion cell loss after IONC

3.2.1 RGC identification and quantification

RGCs share their location in the ganglion cell layer with the equally numerous population of displaced amacrine cells (Drager & Olsen, 1981). In order to study the RGC population is then, necessary to distinguish them from the amacrine neurons. There are several techniques that specifically label RGCs. These are based either on tracing them from their projection areas, which in rodents are mainly the superior colliculi (SCi) (Linden & Perry, 1983; Thanos et al., 1987) or by detecting proteins or transcripts specifically expressed by these neurons (Barnstable & Drager, 1984; Chidlow et al., 2005). Retrograde tracing is based on applying onto the retinorecipient areas in the brain a fluorescent tracer, among which fluorogold is the most utilized. This tracer is taken up by the RGC terminals and transported actively through their axons till their somas in the retina (Figure 2A). In mice or rats, fluorogold applied onto the SCi detects 97.5% or 98.4% of the total RGC population, respectively (Salinas-Navarro et al., 2009b, 2009c).

Few proteins are known to be specifically expressed by RGCs, among them are γ-synuclein, Bex1/2, Thy1, NeuN or Brn3a (Barnstable & Drager, 1984; Quina et al., 2005; Bernstein et al., 2006; Soto et al., 2008; Buckingham et al., 2008; Nadal-Nicolas et al., 2009). Detection of γ-synuclein mRNA (Soto et al., 2008; Nguyen et al., 2011) has been used to investigate the fate of mice RGCs after ocular hypertension. Immunodetection of the transcription factor Brn3b has been used to estimate RGCs in a mice model of ocular hypertension (Fu & Sretavan, 2010). Detection of another member of this family of transcriptions factors, Brn3a, is a reliable method to identify the whole population of rats and mice RGCs in control retinas, after insults such as optic nerve axotomy, ocular hypertension or photoreceptor degeneration (Nadal-Nicolas et al., 2009; Salinas-Navarro et al., 2009a, 2010; Garcia-Ayuso et al., 2010; Galindo-Romero et al., 2011) and importantly, to test the efficacy of neuroprotective therapies (Sanchez-Migallon et al., 2011).

Quantification of RGCs can be done by sampling and manual counting, or by automated routines. Automated quantification is an objective routine that allows counting the whole population of a given cell (Soto et al., 2008; Nadal-Nicolas et al., 2009; Salinas-Navarro et al., 2009b, 2009c; Ortin-Martinez et al., 2010) while avoiding the tiresome and time consuming

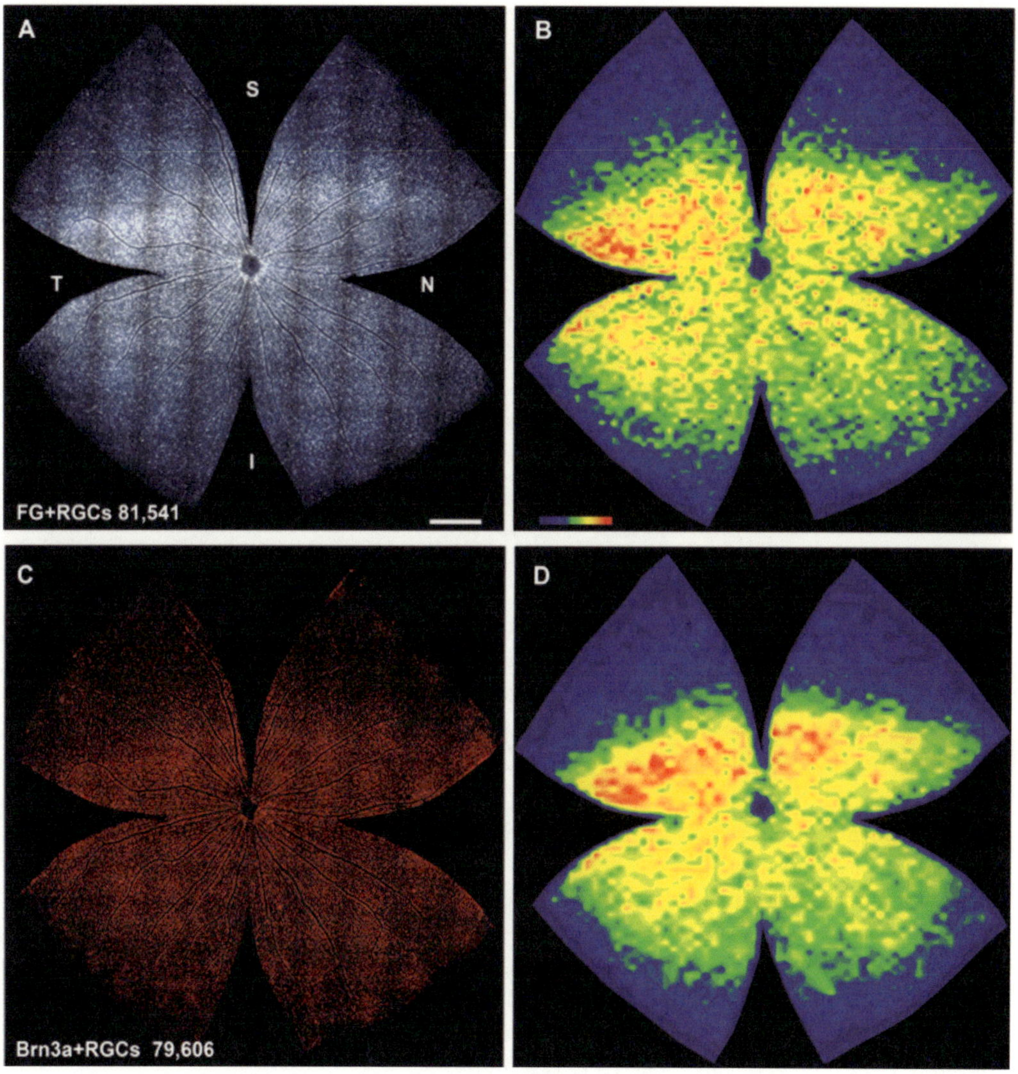

Fig. 2. Retinal ganglion cell distribution in the adult rat. In A and C is shown the same whole-mounted control rat retina where RGCs have been identified by retrograde tracing with fluorogold (A) or immunodetection of Brn3a (C). In this retina, the number of FG or Brn3a positive RGCs has been automatically quantified (A and C bottom left). In B and D are shown the isodensity maps generated from these quantitative data showing the spatial distribution of $FG^{+}RGCs$ (B) and of $Brn3a^{+}RGCs$ (D). The density colour-scale goes from 0 (purple) to 3,500 or higher (red) RGCs/mm^2 (B, bottom left). S: superior I: inferior, N: nasal, T: temporal. Scale bar: 1mm.

effort of sampling and manual-counting. These routines have been shown to be successful to quantify RGCs identified by their Brn3a (Figure 2C) or γ-synuclein expression and can be applied to control or injured retinas (Soto et al., 2008; Nadal-Nicolas et al., 2009; Nguyen et al., 2011). In addition, automated routines allow the generation of detailed isodensity maps (Figure 2 B,D). These maps are useful to assess the distribution and densities of the studied cells in control retinas as well as to understand their topographical loss after an insult (Nadal-Nicolas et al., 2009; Salinas-Navarro et al., 2009a, 2009b, 2009c, 2010 Garcia-Ayuso et al., 2010; Ortin-Martinez et al., 2010; Galindo-Romero et al., 2011; Sanchez-Migallon et al., 2011).

By using this approach our group has reported that RGCs are not homogenously distributed in the retina (Figure 2 B,D). In fact, their lower densities are located in the periphery (blue colours) while their higher ones are found in the superior retina (red-oranges), along the nasotemporal axis, wherein the highest densities are located in the superotemporal quadrant. Furthermore, because in this retinal area L-cones reach their maximum densities, paralleling the RGC distribution, and the S cones reach their lowest, this area of high RGC density has been proposed to be the visual streak of rats (Nadal-Nicolas et al., 2009; Salinas-Navarro et al., 2009b, 2009c; Ortin-Martinez et al., 2010).

Both, tracing and immunodetection of RGCs have advantages and disadvantages. For instance, by retrograde tracing is possible to assess the number of RGCs that maintain a functional retrograde axonal transport. However, if the lesion impairs the axonal flow only the RGCs that have a competent axonal transport will be detected and the alive but impaired ones will be missed. On the other hand, while Brn3a or γ-synuclein detect those RGCs that are still alive independently of their axonal transport state, they are not useful to identify transport failures. Combination of tracing and Brn3a immunodetection has served to demonstrate that after IOP increase there is first a loss of the retrograde active transport that is followed by the death of the affected RGCs (Salinas-Navarro et al., 2009a, 2010).

3.2.2 Temporal course of RGC loss after IONC.

RGC loss after axonal injury depends on two main factors. The type of lesion, crush or transection and the distance from the eye where the lesion is inflicted (Villegas-Perez et al., 1993). In albino Sprague Dawley rats, when the optic nerve is completely crushed 3mm away from the eye, the loss of Brn3a$^+$RGCs is first significant 5 days later (Nadal-Nicolas et al., 2009). At this time point the percentage of surviving RGCs is a 48% of the original population. This loss progresses quickly, decreasing to 28 and 14% of the original population at 9 and 14 days, respectively (Figure 3).

If the population of RGCs is identified by tracing, the loss of RGCs is significant later, at 7 dpl, and by day 14pl the percentage of survival is 29% (Nadal-Nicolas et al., 2009; Parrilla-Reverter et al., 2009b). This discrepancy is explained by the different nature of each marker. While Brn3a is an endogenous protein that is expressed as long as the RGC is alive (Sanchez-Migallon et al., 2011), fluorogold is an exogenous molecule that persists in the retina for at least 3-4 weeks after application (Selles-Navarro et al., 1996; Gomez-Ramirez et al., 1999). This means that fluorogold positive but already dead RGCs will be detected and will only disappear from the retina when the phagocytic microglia clears them.

Comparing these results with the time course of RGC loss in our model of IOP increase by laser photocoagulation (LP), it is observed that there is a massive death of these neurons

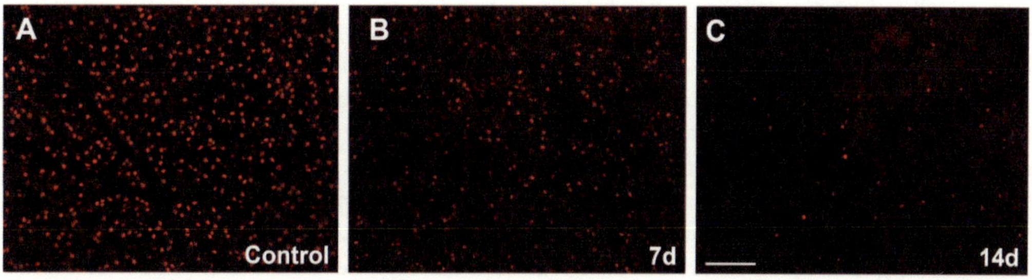

Fig. 3. Temporal loss of Brn3a⁺RGCs after optic nerve crush. Microphotographs from flat mounted retinas in which RGCs have been detected by their expression of Brn3a. A: control; B: 7 days after IONC, C: 14 days after IONC. Bar: 200 μm.

within the first 2 weeks post-LP, which accounts for 53% and 81% of the RGC population at 8 and 14 days post-LP, respectively (Nadal-Nicolas et al., 2009; Parrilla-Reverter et al., 2009b; Salinas-Navarro et al., 2010). Thus, the mean number and course of RGC loss in both models are similar. However there are two important differences. First, in terms of the damage caused IONC induces a consistent injury, while LP insult is highly variable among animals and so, in some retinas the RGC loss accounts for almost 80% of the RGCs, whilst in others only 40% of the original RGC population is affected. Second, after IONC, RGC death is diffuse and affects the whole retina (Figure 4) whereas after LP, RGC death occurs mainly in the dorsal retina in pie-like sectors which are devoid of RGCs, though it has been also observed a diffuse RGC loss in the rest of the retina.

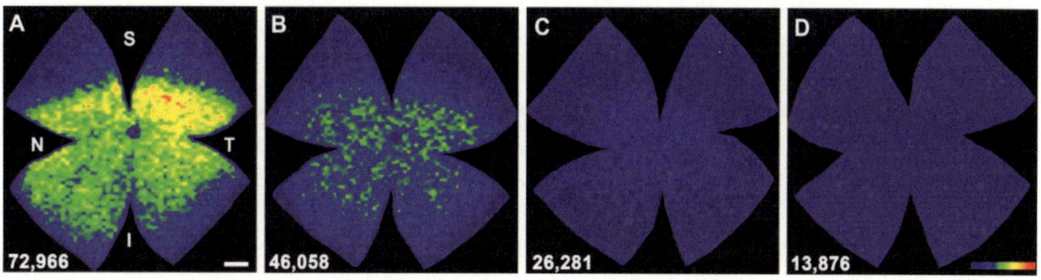

Fig. 4. Temporal loss of RGCs after intraorbital nerve crush. Isodensity maps from IONC-injured retinas analyzed at 2 (A), 5 (B), 9 (C) and 14 (D) days post-lesion. This injury induces a quick and diffuse loss of RGCs that affects the whole retina. At the bottom of each map is shown the number of Brn3a⁺RGCs quantified in the retina wherefrom the map has been generated. Colour-scale goes from 0 (purple) to 3,500 or higher (red) RGCs/mm^2 (D, bottom right). S: superior I: inferior, N: nasal, T: temporal. Scale bar: 1mm.

3.3 Molecular causes underlying RGC loss after IONC

Why do RGC degenerate upon axonal injury? The main theory is that there is a withdrawal of trophic factors from the retinorecipient areas in the brain once the retina is deafferented. That is the reason why many neuroprotective therapies have been based on trophic factors delivery (see below). However, these therapies are only successful to a point, since the best protection only lasts up to 9 days post-lesion wherefrom the RGCs decay quickly.

This prompted us to do an extensive array analysis comparing the transcriptome regulation in naive retinas with retinas extracted at different times post-IONC (12h, 24h, 48h, 3d and 7d) (Agudo et al., 2008). This analysis rendered plenty of data, in fact over a thousand of genes along time showed an altered regulation compared to control retinas. Clustering of the regulated sequences revealed that they were related to several biological processes. Among them, the most significant were: cytoskeleton and associated processes (pEASE: 8,20E-13), primary metabolism (pEASE: 7,80E-14), protein metabolism (pEASE: 1,8E-29), immune response and inflammation (pEASE: 4,80E-11), RNA metabolism (processing and translation pEASE: 3,90E-25), cell cycle (pEASE: 1,20E-05), extracellular matrix remodelling (pEASE: 4,10E-07) and sensory perception of light (pEASE: 1,40E-09). Cell death, as expected, was highly regulated (97 genes, pEASE 2,20E-7). It was surprising to observe a transient down-regulation of genes related to phototransduction such as opsins, rhodopsins and phosducin, since IONC only affects RGCs. The down-regulation of photorreceptor genes may be a reflection of the arrest in transcription observed in the retina soon after injury (Lindqvist et al., 2002; Casson et al., 2004). Thus, while IONC specifically injures RGCs, also induces a retinal response that, even though is not lethal for other retinal neurons, has an effect on them.

Because the more dramatic effect of IONC is the RGC death, we focused our array analyses on the 97 death-related regulated genes. These were further clustered, and the most relevant sub-clusters were inflammation and death receptors, both implicated in triggering the extrinsic pathway of apoptosis and DNA damage, caspases, cell cycle deregulation and stress response, all of which are linked to the induction of the intrinsic pathway of apoptosis (Figure 5). There was a seventh group of death-related genes clustered under lysosomal cell death. A current body of evidence points to a role of lysosomes, and more specifically of cathepsins, in apoptosis. In fact, the "lysosomal pathway of apoptosis" is a phenomenon widely recognized (reviewed in Guicciardi et al., 2004) which would act through caspase activation, and hence activating the intrinsic pathway of apoptosis. However, it has been reported the role of autophagy in RGC death triggered by axotomy (Koch et al., 2010).

Autophagy is a highly regulated pathway that involves the degradation of cytoplasmic organelles or cytosolic components by the lysosomes, thus it is possible that the activation of the lysosomal cell death observed in our arrays analysis is in fact playing a part in autophagy and apoptosis (Figure 5). This is based on the fact that there is a crosstalk between both processes (Zhou et al., 2011) which is complex, and sometimes opposing. Indeed, autophagy can be a cell survival pathway to suppress apoptosis (Yang et al., 2010) or can lead to cell death, either in collaboration with apoptosis or as an alternative mechanism when apoptosis is defective. This crosstalk is mediated, in part, by calpains, which are activated in axotomized RGCs (Paquet-Durand et al., 2007; Agudo et al., 2008, 2009). Calpains cleave and activate Atg5, which is one of the autophagy effectors (Zhou et al., 2011).

Several of these death-effectors have been shown to be expressed by the primarily injured neurons, the RGCs (Cheung et al., 2004; Agudo et al., 2009). Among them, Tnfr1, Caspases 3 and 11, Calpain 1 and Cathepsins B and C are of special interest because each is linked to a different pathway that ends in cell death. The majority of these proteins showed an up-regulation as soon as 12h post-IONC, peaking at 48h, well before the time point when the anatomical RGC loss is first significant (5 days, see above). Thus, these data indicate that axotomized RGCs enter the path to death quickly after the injury, and even though pro-survival or protective mechanisms are concomitantly activated (Schwartz 2004; Levkovitch-Verbin et al., 2007) they are not enough to overcome the death signals. It is worth highlighting that Tnfr1 is up-regulated in our IONC model and in glaucomatous retinas from human patients (Tezel et al., 2001).

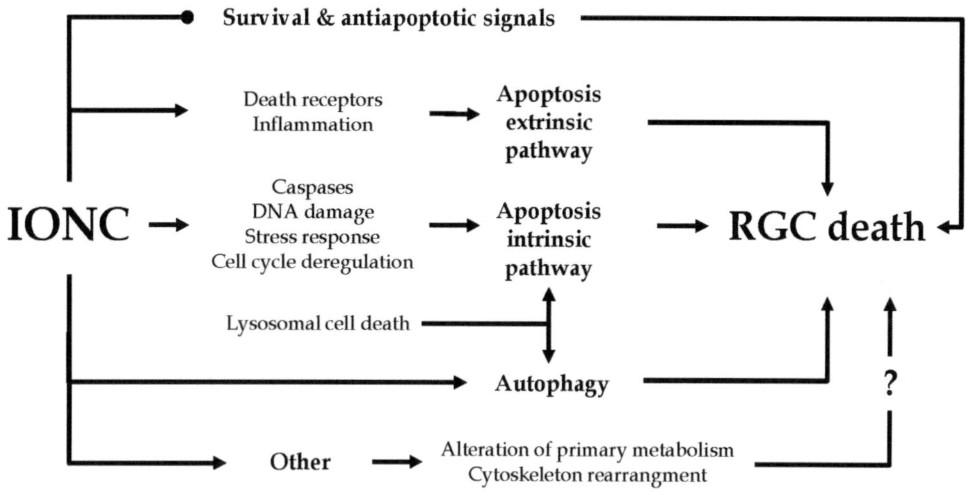

Fig. 5. Scheme summarizing the retinal response to IONC leading to death. After IONC, several pathways ending in cell death are up-regulated. This is accompanied by a down-regulation of survival signals, which, in turn may end in cell death. In addition, there are changes that affect the maintenance of basic cellular functions, such as the cytoskeleton or primary metabolism (catabolism, transcription, biosynthesis), that may tip the scale against survival.

Finally, we have compared our array results with the array analyses of Guo et al, 2010 (Table 1). These data show that there is a common response to both types of injuries. In fact all the altered genes follow the same trend (up or down-regulation). These genes are mainly related to inflammation, apoptosis, cytoskeleton and extracellular matrix remodeling. Guo et al, (2010) analyzed the gene expression patterns occurring in the retina in response to elevated IOP induced by hypertonic saline injection. Their big contribution has been that the analysis was performed in extracts from whole retinas and in extracts from cells isolated from the ganglion cell layer. They observed that several genes were regulated in the whole retina and in the isolated cells (both, in the table) while others where only detected in the whole-retinal extracts (retina, in the table) and *vice versa.* The latter will be genes regulated only in the RGC layer, whose regulation might be lost in a whole-retinal extract due to the dilution effect. The main differences found among both sets of experiments were that in the isolated cells there was not regulation of inflammation, which was the leading process observed in whole retinal extracts. In turn, protein biosynthesis and metabolism were the most regulated categories in the isolated cells. This does not mean that inflammation does not take part on RGC death, but rather that cell isolation helps the determination of RGC specific mechanisms.

In conclusion, even though IONC only mimics part of the pathogenesis of glaucoma only by compiling data from different models will be possible to understand the retinal response to injury. Given the complexity of these molecular events, the development of neuroprotective therapies must, probably, be combinatory. This panorama might be further complicated because basic cellular functions, such as primary metabolism and cytoskeleton maintenance are highly altered after IONC and IOP increase, opening up the possibility that the failure to preserve the cellular homeostasis might be the actual trigger of this complex regulation.

Gene name	Gene Symbol	Gene Ontology	IOP increase	IONC
Growth arrest and DNA-damage-inducible 45 gamma	Gadd45g	Activation p38/JNK pathway	↑ (both)	↑
Clusterin	Clu	Apoptosis and cell survival	↑ (retina)	↑
Suppressor of cytokine signaling 3	Socs3	Apoptosis and cell survival	↑ (both)	↑
Tumor necrosis factor receptor superfamily, member 12a	Tnfrsf12a	Apoptosis and cell survival	↑ (both)	↑
Lysozyme	Lyz	Cell wall catabolism, cytolysis	↑ (both)	↑
Ceruloplasmin	Cp	CNS iron homeostasis and neuroprotection	↑ (retina)	↑
Neurofilament, light polypeptide	Nfl	Cytoskeleton	↓ (both)	↓
Transgelin 2	Tagln2	Development	↑ (retina)	↑
Olfactomedin 1	Olfm1	Development	↓ (both)	↓
Secreted acidic cysteine rich glycoprotein	Sparc	Extracellular matrix	↑ (both)	↑
Alpha-2-macroglobulin	A2m	Immune response and inflammation	↑ (retina)	↑
Beta-2 microglobulin	B2m	Immune response and inflammation	↑ (retina)	↑
Interferon-inducible protein variant 10	Ifitm3	Immune response and inflammation	↑ (retina)	↑
Signal transducer and activator of transcription 3	Stat3	JAK/STAT cascade	↑ (both)	↑
Signal transducer and activator of transcription 1	Stat1	JAK/STAT cascade	↑ (retina)	↑
Cd63 antigen	Cd63	Lysosomal protein	↑ (both)	↑

Gene name	Gene Symbol	Gene Ontology	IOP increase	IONC
Synuclein, gamma	Sncg	Nervous system development	↓ (retina)	↓
Carbonic anhydrase 14	Car14	Primary metabolism	↓ (retina)	↓
Carnitine o-octanoyltransferase	Crot	Primary metabolism	↑ (retina)	↑
Udp glycosyltransferase 1 family, polypeptide a1	Ugt1a	Primary metabolism	↑ (both)	↑
Lipocalin 2	Lcn2	Protection of MMP-9, iron transport	↑ (both)	↑
Arginyl aminopeptidase	Rnpep	Proteolysis	↑ (both)	↑
Corneal wound healing related protein	Mak10	Response to injury	↑ (retina)	↑
Hnrnp-associated with lethal yellow	Raly	RNA metabolism	↓ (retina)	↓
Tax1 binding protein 3	Tax1bp3	Signalling	↑ (both)	↑
Potassium voltage gated channel, member 2	Kcnd2	Synapsis	↓ (both)	↓
Solute carrier family 6, member 6	Slc6a6	Transport	↓ (retina)	↓
ATPAse, NA+/K+ transporting, beta 1 polypetide	Atp1b1	Transport	↓ (both)	↓

Table 1. Genes commonly regulated in glaucoma and after IONC.
↑ gene upregulation, ↓ gene downregulation. See text for further explanations.

4. RGC neuroprotection

Neuroprotection refers to therapies aimed to prevent, stop or at least delay the degeneration that follows CNS trauma. For a neuroprotective agent to be successful it must be directed to a target in the retina, it must be applied before the death of the neurons, it should be safe and it should work on animal models. Once fulfilled these criteria, the next steps are to design the pharmaceutical forms to deliver the compound to the human retina at the appropriate concentrations and to conduct the clinical trials.

After the injury, which cells are the candidates for neuroprotection? Obviously, not the neurons already dead, thus, it is important to know the temporal course of RGC degeneration to narrow the temporal window to intervene. Those cells in the process of degeneration are candidates if their somas are still healthy. In this case, function will only be restored if protection of the cell bodies is followed by regeneration and reconnection. Having this in mind, neuroprotection can be attained by preventing the degeneration of the healthy fibres, or by delaying it in the cell bodies of the damaged fibres.

Neuroprotection can be divided into two main groups: therapies that target specific genes or proteins related to cell death or therapies that increase the resistance of the injured neurons to the trauma. The former approach, though more specific, is very difficult for several reasons: i) it would be necessary to identify all the implicated signals; ii) some of these signals are pleiotropic, playing roles in survival or death depending on the delicate balance of other proteins; iii) some proteins while pathological if over-expressed, are essential for survival; thus, blocking their expression might be deleterious for the neurons that are not yet compromised; iv) signalling pathways are interconnected. Consequently, to tailor an effective therapy all this must be taken into account, and probably should imply the manipulation of several proteins. This requires careful analyses of the pathways and their interactions. Furthermore, the targeted proteins/genes should be head of pathways, provided that the downstream signals do not bifurcate into survival or death. Alternative targets could be the effectors, either proteins (i.e. caspases) or metabolites (i.e. ceramide).

4.1 Targeting specific signals

One way of targeting specific pathways is the use of inhibitors. Rho Kinase (ROCK) is a serine-threonine kinase that regulates the organization of the actin cytoskeleton (Mueller et al., 2005). Its activation is linked to the morphological changes observed during the execution phase of apoptosis (Coleman & Olson, 2002). Tura et al, (2009) showed that after IONC, the intravitreal administration of the ROCK inhibitor H-1152P produced two effects: a significant reduction of apoptosis in the ganglion cell layer and a reduction of the reactive gliosis.

Among the best characterized pro-death proteins is BAX. This protein associates with the permeability transition pore of the mitochondrial inner membrane opening it and thus inducing a series of events such as a disruption of the electrochemical membrane gradient, a disruption in ATP production and release of cytochrome C (Marzo et al., 1998). The released cytochrome C in turn, activates the caspase cascade. Li et al. (2000) demonstrated that in Bax deficient mice 2 weeks after optic nerve crush, there was less than a 10% of cell loss in the ganglion cell layer, which was significantly lower than the 41.3% observed in wild type mice. This survival was not due to a slower death-rate in the Bax-/- mice, since 4 weeks after the lesion there was not further cell loss. However, the lack of BAX did not prevent the ganglion cells to undergo early changes in response to optic nerve crush, such as a decrease in the average size of their nuclei. It is worth noting, that the deficiency in this gene protected cells in the ganglion layer after optic nerve crush but not after experimentally induced excitotoxicity. This means that in response to different insults, ganglion cells activate different pathways of cell death.

The discovery of RNA interference (RNAi) has opened new avenues to investigate in neuroscience. RNAi is an endogenous mechanism that silences gene expression after translation. Silencing is highly sequence-specific and ends with the targeted mRNA cleaved into smaller fragments which results in the inhibition of protein synthesis (for review see Sontheimer, 2005). RNAi is mediated by small interference RNA (siRNA). The use of RNAi to knock-down specific pro-death proteins in axotomized RGCs has been only used after complete transection of the optic nerve (Lingor et al., 2005). Lingor et al. showed that in retinas treated with siRNAs against Apaf-1 (component of the apoptosome) or c-Jun (immediate response gene) there was a significant RGC survival compared to control ones.

However, anti-Bax siRNAs did not increase RGC survival; this does not correlate with the experiments carried out on Bax-deficient mice. This discrepancy might be due to the different species (rats *vs* mouse) used and on the lesion, because even though crush and transection are both axonal traumas and there are many commonly regulated genes (Agudo et al., 2008, 2009) there are differences in the temporal course and amount of these regulations.

In glaucoma, RNAi has been directed mainly to lower the IOP (for review see Mediero et al., 2009) rather than to induce a direct RGC survival. Targeting adrenergic receptors, acetylcholinesterase and ATPases, decreases the IOP. This approach has minimal side effects and the reduction of IOP lasts almost 5 days. This is important at the clinical level because the regime is simpler than pharmacological treatments, particularly eye drops that may require several administrations at day. In addition to lower the IOP, RNAi is been tested in vitro to knock-down the gain of function of mutated genes associated to glaucoma, such as myocilin (Li et al., 2009).

4.2 Therapies to increase the resistance of the injured neurons

Administration of neurotrophins to the injured retina is one of the most successful therapies. Our group has shown that a single intravitreal injection of neurotrophin 4 (NT-4), ciliary neurotrophic factor (CNTF), or brain derived neurotrophic factor (BDNF) at the moment of the injury delays IONC-induced RGC death (Parrilla-Reverter et al., 2009b). At 7dpl all of them prevent almost completely the loss of RGCs. However, while at 12 dpl NT-4 and BDNF still protect, CNTF does not. Nevertheless, none of these factors were able to rescue the injured RGCs permanently. It is possible that a single injection is not sufficient. To solve this there are strategies to achieve a sustained expression of neurotrophins: transfection by viral vectors, cell based delivery approaches or microspheres loaded with the neurotrophin of choice (reviewed in Dahlmann-Noor et al., 2010). Another approach consists on the selective stimulation of trophic factor receptors using specific agonists. Thus, it has been shown that a selective agonist of TrkB (BDNF receptor) causes a long term TrKB activation and significantly delays RGC degeneration after IOP increase and after optic nerve transection (Bai et al., 2010).

Brimonidine, an α-2 adrenergic agonist, has been shown to neuroprotect RGCs after retinal ischemia (Lafuente et al., 2001,2002; Lafuente Lopez-Herrera et al., 2002; Vidal-Sanz et al., 2001a,b, 2007; Aviles-Trigueros et al., 2003; Mayor-Torroglosa et al., 2005; Lonngren et al., 2006), after optic nerve crush (Wheeler et al., 1999) and after laser-induced ocular hypertension (Wheeler & WoldeMussie, 2001; Lambert et al., 2011). A randomized trial comparing brimonidine and timolol (β-adrenergic antagonist) in low tension glaucomatous patients, has shown that the loss of visual field is statistically lower in brimonidine treated-patients than in those treated with timolol, thus documenting, for the first time, its neuroprotective effect in human diseases (Krupin et al., 2011).

5. Conclusions

Optic nerve injury induced either by IOP increase or by direct trauma, causes profound structural, functional and molecular alterations in the primarily injured neurons, the RGCs, as well as in the rest of the retina. The consequences of these alterations are permanent as the CNS neurons die upon injury and the surviving ones fail to spontaneously regenerate their axons till their targets (Aguayo et al., 1987). Research is being focused in understanding the network of changes occurring in the traumatized retina and, more importantly, the effect of one upon another. To date, it is clear that numerous mechanisms are involved; some of them are common to different insults while others are injury-specific, some of them depend on inherited tracts, others implicate the glial and immune response and many reflect the commitment to death of the injured neurons. Only by gathering and unifying all these data we will be able to understand the common responses of the CNS to injury and to decipher the specific ones. With this knowledge it will be possible to design broad-spectrum and tailored therapies to successfully rescue the wounded system.

6. Acknowledgments

This work was supported by research grants from Fundación Séneca 04446/GERM/07; Spanish Ministry of Education and Science SAF-22010-10385; Spanish Ministry of Science and Innovation and ISCIII-FEDER: PI10/00187, PI006/0780 and Red Temática de Investigación Cooperativa en Oftalmología RD07/0062/0001.

7. References

Aguayo AJ, Vidal-Sanz M, Villegas-Perez MP, Bray GM. 1987. Growth and connectivity of axotomized retinal neurons in adult rats with optic nerves substituted by PNS grafts linking the eye and the midbrain. Ann N Y Acad Sci 495:1-9.

Agudo M, Perez-Marin MC, Lonngren U, Sobrado P, Conesa A, Canovas I, Salinas-Navarro M, Miralles-Imperial J, Hallbook F, Vidal-Sanz M. 2008. Time course profiling of the retinal transcriptome after optic nerve transection and optic nerve crush. Mol Vis 14: 1050-63.

Agudo M, Perez-Marin MC, Sobrado-Calvo P, Lonngren U, Salinas-Navarro M, Canovas I, Nadal-Nicolas FM, Miralles-Imperial J, Hallbook F, Vidal-Sanz M. 2009. Immediate upregulation of proteins belonging to different branches of the apoptotic cascade in the retina after optic nerve transection and optic nerve crush. Invest Ophthalmol Vis Sci 50 (1): 424-31.

Aihara M, Lindsey JD, Weinreb RN. 2003. Ocular hypertension in mice with a targeted type I collagen mutation. Invest Ophthalmol Vis Sci 44 (4): 1581-5.

Al Chalabi A, Miller CC. 2003. Neurofilaments and neurological disease. Bioessays 25 (4): 346-55.

Alarcon-Martinez L, Aviles-Trigueros M, Galindo-Romero C, Valiente-Soriano J, Agudo-Barriuso M, de la Villa P, Villegas-Perez MP, Vidal-Sanz M. 2010. ERG changes in albino and pigmented mice after optic nerve transection. Vision Res 50 (21): 2176-87.

Alarcon-Martinez L, de la Villa P, Aviles-Trigueros M, Blanco R, Villegas-Perez MP, Vidal-Sanz M. 2009. Short and long term axotomy-induced ERG changes in albino and pigmented rats. Mol Vis 15: 2373-83.

Alward WL, Fingert JH, Coote MA, Johnson AT, Lerner SF, Junqua D, Durcan FJ, McCartney PJ, Mackey DA, Sheffield VC, Stone EM. 1998. Clinical features associated with mutations in the chromosome 1 open-angle glaucoma gene (GLC1A). N Engl J Med 338 (15): 1022-7.

Aviles-Trigueros M, Mayor-Torroglosa S, Garcia-Aviles A, Lafuente MP, Rodriguez ME, Miralles d, I, Villegas-Perez MP, Vidal-Sanz M. 2003. Transient ischemia of the retina results in massive degeneration of the retinotectal projection: long-term neuroprotection with brimonidine. Exp Neurol 184 (2): 767-77.

Bai Y, Xu J, Brahimi F, Zhuo Y, Sarunic MV, Saragovi HU. 2010. An agonistic TrkB mAb causes sustained TrkB activation, delays RGC death, and protects the retinal structure in optic nerve axotomy and in glaucoma. Invest Ophthalmol Vis Sci 51 (9): 4722-31.

Barnstable CJ, Drager UC. 1984. Thy-1 antigen: a ganglion cell specific marker in rodent retina. Neuroscience 11 (4): 847-55.

Bernstein SL, Koo JH, Slater BJ, Guo Y, Margolis FL. 2006. Analysis of optic nerve stroke by retinal Bex expression. Mol Vis 12: 147-55.

Bray GM, Villegas-Perez MP, Vidal-Sanz M, Carter DA, Aguayo AJ. 1991. Neuronal and nonneuronal influences on retinal ganglion cell survival, axonal regrowth, and connectivity after axotomy. Ann N Y Acad Sci 633:214-28.

Buckingham BP, Inman DM, Lambert W, Oglesby E, Calkins DJ, Steele MR, Vetter ML, Marsh-Armstrong N, Horner PJ. 2008. Progressive ganglion cell degeneration precedes neuronal loss in a mouse model of glaucoma. J Neurosci 28 (11): 2735-44.

Casson RJ, Chidlow G, Wood JP, Vidal-Sanz M, Osborne NN. 2004. The effect of retinal ganglion cell injury on light-induced photoreceptor degeneration. Invest Ophthalmol Vis Sci 45(2):685-93.

Chang B, Smith RS, Hawes NL, Anderson MG, Zabaleta A, Savinova O, Roderick TH, Heckenlively JR, Davisson MT, John SW. 1999. Interacting loci cause severe iris atrophy and glaucoma in DBA/2J mice. Nat Genet 21 (4): 405-9.

Chen H, Wei X, Cho KS, Chen G, Sappington R, Calkins DJ, Chen DF. 2011. Optic neuropathy due to microbead-induced elevated intraocular pressure in the mouse. Invest Ophthalmol Vis Sci 52 (1): 36-44.

Cheung ZH, Chan YM, Siu FK, Yip HK, Wu W, Leung MC, So KF. 2004. Regulation of caspase activation in axotomized retinal ganglion cells. Mol Cell Neurosci 25 (3): 383-93.

Chidlow G, Casson R, Sobrado-Calvo P, Vidal-Sanz M, Osborne NN. 2005a. Measurement of retinal injury in the rat after optic nerve transection: an RT-PCR study. Mol Vis 11: 387-96.

Coleman ML, Olson MF. 2002. Rho GTPase signalling pathways in the morphological changes associated with apoptosis. Cell Death Differ 9 (5): 493-504.

Cone FE, Gelman SE, Son JL, Pease ME, Quigley HA. 2010. Differential susceptibility to experimental glaucoma among 3 mouse strains using bead and viscoelastic injection. Exp Eye Res 91 (3): 415-24.

Cuenca N, Pinilla I, Fernandez-Sanchez L, Salinas-Navarro M, Alarcon-Martinez L, Aviles-Trigueros M, de l, V, Miralles d, I, Villegas-Perez MP, Vidal-Sanz M. 2010. Changes in the inner and outer retinal layers after acute increase of the intraocular pressure in adult albino Swiss mice. Exp Eye Res 91 (2): 273-85.

Dahlmann-Noor A, Vijay S, Jayaram H, Limb A, Khaw PT. 2010. Current approaches and future prospects for stem cell rescue and regeneration of the retina and optic nerve. Can J Ophthalmol 45 (4): 333-41.

Drager UC, Olsen JF. 1981. Ganglion cell distribution in the retina of the mouse. Invest Ophthalmol Vis Sci 20 (3): 285-93.

Flammer J, Mozaffarieh M. 2007. What is the present pathogenetic concept of glaucomatous optic neuropathy? Surv Ophthalmol 52 Suppl 2: S162-S173.

Fu CT, Sretavan D. 2010. Laser-induced ocular hypertension in albino CD-1 mice. Invest Ophthalmol Vis Sci 51 (2): 980-90.

Fujikawa K, Iwata T, Inoue K, Akahori M, Kadotani H, Fukaya M, Watanabe M, Chang Q, Barnett EM, Swat W. 2010. VAV2 and VAV3 as candidate disease genes for spontaneous glaucoma in mice and humans. PLoS One 5 (2): e9050.

Fuse N. 2010. Genetic bases for glaucoma. Tohoku J Exp Med 221 (1): 1-10.

Gaasterland D, Kupfer C. 1974. Experimental glaucoma in the rhesus monkey. Invest Ophthalmol 13 (6): 455-7.

Galindo-Romero C, Aviles-Trigueros M, Jimenez-Lopez M, Valiente-Soriano FJ, Salinas-Navarro M, Nadal-Nicolas F, Villegas-Perez MP, Vidal-Sanz M, Agudo-Barriuso M. 2011. Axotomy-induced retinal ganglion cell death in adult mice: Quantitative and topographic time course analyses. Exp Eye Res. 92(5):377-87

Garcia-Ayuso D, Salinas-Navarro M, Agudo M, Cuenca N, Pinilla I, Vidal-Sanz M, Villegas-Perez MP. 2010. Retinal ganglion cell numbers and delayed retinal ganglion cell death in the P23H rat retina. Exp Eye Res 91 (6): 800-10.

Gomez-Ramirez AM, Villegas-Perez MP, Miralles d, I, Salvador-Silva M, Vidal-Sanz M. 1999. Effects of intramuscular injection of botulinum toxin and doxorubicin on the survival of abducens motoneurons. Invest Ophthalmol Vis Sci 40 (2): 414-24.

Guicciardi ME, Leist M, Gores GJ. 2004. Lysosomes in cell death. Oncogene 23 (16): 2881-90.

Guo Y, Cepurna WO, Dyck JA, Doser TA, Johnson EC, Morrison JC. 2010. Retinal cell responses to elevated intraocular pressure: a gene array comparison between the whole retina and retinal ganglion cell layer. Invest Ophthalmol Vis Sci 51 (6): 3003-18.

John SW, Hagaman JR, MacTaggart TE, Peng L, Smithes O. 1997. Intraocular pressure in inbred mouse strains. Invest Ophthalmol Vis Sci 38 (1): 249-53.

Johnson EC, Morrison JC, Farrell S, Deppmeier L, Moore CG, McGinty MR. 1996. The effect of chronically elevated intraocular pressure on the rat optic nerve head extracellular matrix. Exp Eye Res 62 (6): 663-74.

Kipfer-Kauer A, McKinnon SJ, Frueh BE, Goldblum D. 2010. Distribution of amyloid precursor protein and amyloid-beta in ocular hypertensive C57BL/6 mouse eyes. Curr Eye Res 35 (9): 828-34.

Koch JC, Knoferle J, Tonges L, Ostendorf T, Bahr M, Lingor P. 2010. Acute axonal degeneration in vivo is attenuated by inhibition of autophagy in a calcium-dependent manner. Autophagy 6 (5).

Krupin T, Liebmann JM, Greenfield DS, Ritch R, Gardiner S. 2011. A Randomized Trial of Brimonidine Versus Timolol in Preserving Visual Function: Results From the Low-pressure Glaucoma Treatment Study. Am J Ophthalmol 151 (4): 671-81.

Lafuente Lopez-Herrera MP, Mayor-Torroglosa S, Miralles d, I, Villegas-Perez MP, Vidal-Sanz M. 2002. Transient ischemia of the retina results in altered retrograde axoplasmic transport: neuroprotection with brimonidine. Exp Neurol 178(2):243-58.

Lafuente MP, Villegas-Perez MP, Mayor S, Aguilera ME, Miralles d, I, Vidal-Sanz M. 2002. Neuroprotective effects of brimonidine against transient ischemia-induced retinal ganglion cell death: a dose response in vivo study. Exp Eye Res 74 (2): 181-9.

Lafuente MP, Villegas-Perez MP, Sobrado-Calvo P, Garcia-Aviles A, Miralles d, I, Vidal-Sanz M. 2001. Neuroprotective effects of alpha (2) -selective adrenergic agonists against ischemia-induced retinal ganglion cell death. Invest Ophthalmol Vis Sci 42 (9): 2074-84.

Lambert WS, Ruiz L, Crish SD, Wheeler LA, Calkins DJ. 2011. Brimonidine prevents axonal and somatic degeneration of retinal ganglion cell neurons. Mol Neurodegener 6 (1): 4.

Leoz O and Arcuate LR. 1914. Procesos regenerativos del nervio óptico y retina, con ocasión de injertos nerviosos. Trab Lab Invest Biol 11: 239-54.

Levkovitch-Verbin H, Harizman N, Dardik R, Nisgav Y, Vander S, Melamed S. 2007. Regulation of cell death and survival pathways in experimental glaucoma. Exp Eye Res 85 (2): 250-8.

Li M, Xu J, Chen X, Sun X. 2009. RNA interference as a gene silencing therapy for mutant MYOC protein in primary open angle glaucoma. Diagn Pathol 4: 46.

Li Y, Schlamp CL, Poulsen KP, Nickells RW. 2000. Bax-dependent and independent pathways of retinal ganglion cell death induced by different damaging stimuli. Exp Eye Res 71 (2): 209-13.

Li Y, Semaan SJ, Schlamp CL, Nickells RW. 2007. Dominant inheritance of retinal ganglion cell resistance to optic nerve crush in mice. BMC Neurosci 8: 19.

Linden R, Perry VH. 1983. Massive retinotectal projection in rats. Brain Res 272 (1): 145-9.

Lindqvist N, Vidal-Sanz M, Hallbook F. 2002. Single cell RT-PCR analysis of tyrosine kinase receptor expression in adult rat retinal ganglion cells isolated by retinal sandwiching. Brain Res Brain Res Protoc 10 (2): 75-83.

Lingor P, Koeberle P, Kugler S, Bahr M. 2005. Down-regulation of apoptosis mediators by RNAi inhibits axotomy-induced retinal ganglion cell death in vivo. Brain 128 (Pt 3): 550-8.

Lonngren U, Napankangas U, Lafuente M, Mayor S, Lindqvist N, Vidal-Sanz M, Hallbook F. 2006. The growth factor response in ischemic rat retina and superior colliculus after brimonidine pre-treatment. Brain Res Bull 71 (1-3): 208-18.

Marco-Gomariz MA, Hurtado-Montalban N, Vidal-Sanz M, Lund RD, Villegas-Perez MP. 2006. Phototoxic-induced photoreceptor degeneration causes retinal ganglion cell degeneration in pigmented rats. J Comp Neurol 498 (2): 163-79.

Marzo I, Brenner C, Zamzami N, Jurgensmeier JM, Susin SA, Vieira HL, Prevost MC, Xie Z, Matsuyama S, Reed JC, Kroemer G. 1998. Bax and adenine nucleotide translocator cooperate in the mitochondrial control of apoptosis. Science 281 (5385): 2027-31.

Mayor-Torroglosa S, de la Villa P, Rodriguez ME, Lopez-Herrera MP, Aviles-Trigueros M, Garcia-Aviles A, de Imperial JM, Villegas-Perez MP, Vidal-Sanz M. 2005. Ischemia results 3 months later in altered ERG, degeneration of inner layers, and deafferented tectum: neuroprotection with brimonidine. Invest Ophthalmol Vis Sci 46 (10): 3825-35.

McKerracher L, Vidal-Sanz M, Aguayo AJ. 1990a. Slow transport rates of cytoskeletal proteins change during regeneration of axotomized retinal neurons in adult rats. J Neurosci 10 (2): 641-8.

McKerracher L, Vidal-Sanz M, Essagian C, Aguayo AJ. 1990b. Selective impairment of slow axonal transport after optic nerve injury in adult rats. J Neurosci 10 (8): 2834-41.

Mediero A, Alarma-Estrany P, Pintor J. 2009. New treatments for ocular hypertension. Auton Neurosci 147 (1-2): 14-9.

Morrison JC, Cepurna W, Guo Y, Johnson EC. 2010. Pathophysiology of human glaucomatous optic nerve damage: Insights from rodent models of glaucoma. Exp Eye Res. E-pub ahead of print doi:10.1016/j.exer.2010.08.005.

Morrison JC, Moore CG, Deppmeier LM, Gold BG, Meshul CK, Johnson EC. 1997. A rat model of chronic pressure-induced optic nerve damage. Exp Eye Res 64 (1): 85-96.

Mueller BK, Mack H, Teusch N. 2005. Rho kinase, a promising drug target for neurological disorders. Nat Rev Drug Discov 4 (5): 387-98.

Nadal-Nicolas FM, Jimenez-Lopez M, Sobrado-Calvo P, Nieto-Lopez L, Canovas-Martinez I, Salinas-Navarro M, Vidal-Sanz M, Agudo M. 2009. Brn3a as a marker of retinal ganglion cells: qualitative and quantitative time course studies in naive and optic nerve-injured retinas. Invest Ophthalmol Vis Sci 50 (8): 3860-8.

Nguyen JV, Soto I, Kim KY, Bushong EA, Oglesby E, Valiente-Soriano FJ, Yang Z, Davis CH, Bedont JL, Son JL, Wei JO, Buchman VL, Zack DJ, Vidal-Sanz M, Ellisman MH, Marsh-Armstrong N. 2011. Myelination transition zone astrocytes are constitutively phagocytic and have synuclein dependent reactivity in glaucoma. Proc Natl Acad Sci USA 108 (3): 1176-81.

Ortin-Martinez A, Jimenez-Lopez M, Nadal-Nicolas FM, Salinas-Navarro M, Alarcon-Martinez L, Sauve Y, Villegas-Perez MP, Vidal-Sanz M, Agudo-Barriuso M. 2010. Automated quantification and topographical distribution of the whole population of S- and L-cones in adult albino and pigmented rats. Invest Ophthalmol Vis Sci 51 (6): 3171-83.

Paquet-Durand F, Johnson L, Ekstrom P. 2007. Calpain activity in retinal degeneration. J Neurosci Res 85 (4): 693-702.

Parrilla-Reverter G, Agudo M, Nadal-Nicolas F, Alarcon-Martinez L, Jimenez-Lopez M, Salinas-Navarro M, Sobrado-Calvo P, Bernal-Garro JM, Villegas-Perez MP, Vidal-Sanz M. 2009a. Time-course of the retinal nerve fibre layer degeneration after complete intra-orbital optic nerve transection or crush: a comparative study. Vision Res 49 (23): 2808-25.

Parrilla-Reverter G, Agudo M, Sobrado-Calvo P, Salinas-Navarro M, Villegas-Perez MP, Vidal-Sanz M. 2009b. Effects of different neurotrophic factors on the survival of retinal ganglion cells after a complete intraorbital nerve crush injury: a quantitative in vivo study. Exp Eye Res 89 (1): 32-41.

Peinado-Ramon P, Salvador M, Villegas-Perez MP, Vidal-Sanz M. 1996. Effects of axotomy and intraocular administration of NT-4, NT-3, and brain-derived neurotrophic factor on the survival of adult rat retinal ganglion cells. A quantitative in vivo study. Invest Ophthalmol Vis Sci 37 (4): 489-500.

Perrot R, Berges R, Bocquet A, Eyer J. 2008. Review of the multiple aspects of neurofilament functions, and their possible contribution to neurodegeneration. Mol Neurobiol 38 (1): 27-65.

Quigley HA. 1996. Number of people with glaucoma worldwide. Br J Ophthalmol 80 (5): 389-93.

Quigley HA, Vitale S. 1997. Models of open-angle glaucoma prevalence and incidence in the United States. Invest Ophthalmol Vis Sci 38 (1): 83-91.

Quina LA, Pak W, Lanier J, Banwait P, Gratwick K, Liu Y, Velasquez T, O'Leary DD, Goulding M, Turner EE. 2005. Brn3a-expressing retinal ganglion cells project specifically to thalamocortical and collicular visual pathways. J Neurosci 25 (50): 11595-604.

Ramirez AI, Salazar JJ, de Hoz R, Rojas B, Gallego BI, Salinas-Navarro M, Alarcon-Martinez L, Ortin-Martinez A, Aviles-Trigueros M, Vidal-Sanz M, Trivino A, Ramirez JM. 2010. Quantification of the effect of different levels of IOP in the astroglia of the rat retina ipsilateral and contralateral to experimental glaucoma. Invest Ophthalmol Vis Sci 51 (11): 5690-6.

Ramón y Cajal S. 1914. Estudios sobre la degeneración y regeneración del sistema nervioso. In: Hijos de Nicolás Moyá M, editor. p 203-17.

Ray K, Mookherjee S. 2009. Molecular complexity of primary open angle glaucoma: current concepts. J Genet 88 (4): 451-67.

Reimer J, Wolter MD. 1967. Axonal enlargments in the nerve-fiber layer of the human retina. American Journal of Ophthalmology 65 (1): 12.

Salinas-Navarro M, Alarcon-Martinez L, Valiente-Soriano FJ, Jimenez-Lopez M, Mayor-Torroglosa S, Aviles-Trigueros M, Villegas-Perez MP, Vidal-Sanz M. 2010. Ocular hypertension impairs optic nerve axonal transport leading to progressive retinal ganglion cell degeneration. Exp Eye Res 90 (1): 168-83.

Salinas-Navarro M, Alarcon-Martinez L, Valiente-Soriano FJ, Ortin-Martinez A, Jimenez-Lopez M, Aviles-Trigueros M, Villegas-Perez MP, de l, V, Vidal-Sanz M. 2009a. Functional and morphological effects of laser-induced ocular hypertension in retinas of adult albino Swiss mice. Mol Vis 15: 2578-98.

Salinas-Navarro M, Jimenez-Lopez M, Valiente-Soriano FJ, Alarcon-Martinez L, Aviles-Trigueros M, Mayor S, Holmes T, Lund RD, Villegas-Perez MP, Vidal-Sanz M. 2009b. Retinal ganglion cell population in adult albino and pigmented mice: a computerized analysis of the entire population and its spatial distribution. Vision Res 49 (6): 637-47.

Salinas-Navarro M, Mayor-Torroglosa S, Jimenez-Lopez M, Aviles-Trigueros M, Holmes TM, Lund RD, Villegas-Perez MP, Vidal-Sanz M. 2009c. A computerized analysis of the entire retinal ganglion cell population and its spatial distribution in adult rats. Vision Res 49 (1): 115-26.

Samsel PA, Kisiswa L, Erichsen JT, Cross SD, Morgan JE. 2010. A novel method for the induction of experimental glaucoma using magnetic microspheres. Invest Ophthalmol Vis Sci.

Sanchez-Migallon MC, Nadal-Nicolas FM, Jimenez-Lopez M, Sobrado-Calvo P, Vidal-Sanz M, Agudo-Barriuso M. 2011. Brain derived neurotrophic factor maintains Brn3a expression in axotomized rat retinal ganglion cells. Exp Eye Res 92 (4): 260-7.

Sappington RM, Carlson BJ, Crish SD, Calkins DJ. 2010. The microbead occlusion model: a paradigm for induced ocular hypertension in rats and mice. Invest Ophthalmol Vis Sci 51 (1): 207-16.

Schwartz M. 2004. Optic nerve crush: protection and regeneration. Brain Res Bull 62 (6): 467-71.

Selles-Navarro I, Villegas-Perez MP, Salvador-Silva M, Ruiz-Gomez JM, Vidal-Sanz M. 1996. Retinal ganglion cell death after different transient periods of pressure-induced ischemia and survival intervals. A quantitative in vivo study. Invest Ophthalmol Vis Sci 37 (10): 2002-14.

Shareef SR, Garcia-Valenzuela E, Salierno A, Walsh J, Sharma SC. 1995. Chronic ocular hypertension following episcleral venous occlusion in rats. Exp Eye Res 61 (3): 379-82.

Shields M, Ritch R, Krupin T. 1996. Classfication of the glaucomas. Mosby, St Louis, USA.

Sobrado-Calvo P, Vidal-Sanz M, Villegas-Perez MP. 2007. Rat retinal microglial cells under normal conditions, after optic nerve section, and after optic nerve section and intravitreal injection of trophic factors or macrophage inhibitory factor. J Comp Neurol 501 (6): 866-78.

Sontheimer EJ. 2005. Assembly and function of RNA silencing complexes. Nat Rev Mol Cell Biol 6 (2): 127-38.

Soto I, Oglesby E, Buckingham BP, Son JL, Roberson ED, Steele MR, Inman DM, Vetter ML, Horner PJ, Marsh-Armstrong N. 2008. Retinal ganglion cells downregulate gene expression and lose their axons within the optic nerve head in a mouse glaucoma model. J Neurosci 28 (2): 548-61.

Tello F. 1907. La régeneration dans les voies optiques. Trabajos de Laboratorio en Investigación Biológica: 237-48.

Tezel G, Li LY, Patil RV, Wax MB. 2001. TNF-alpha and TNF-alpha receptor-1 in the retina of normal and glaucomatous eyes. Invest Ophthalmol Vis Sci 42 (8): 1787-94.

Thanos S, Vidal-Sanz M, Aguayo AJ. 1987. The use of rhodamine-B-isothiocyanate (RITC) as an anterograde and retrograde tracer in the adult rat visual system. Brain Res 406 (1-2): 317-21.

Tura A, Schuettauf F, Monnier PP, Bartz-Schmidt KU, Henke-Fahle S. 2009. Efficacy of Rho-kinase inhibition in promoting cell survival and reducing reactive gliosis in the rodent retina. Invest Ophthalmol Vis Sci 50 (1): 452-61.

Ueda J, Sawaguchi S, Hanyu T, Yaoeda K, Fukuchi T, Abe H, Ozawa H. 1998. Experimental glaucoma model in the rat induced by laser trabecular photocoagulation after an intracameral injection of India ink. Jpn J Ophthalmol 42 (5): 337-44.

Urcola JH, Hernandez M, Vecino E. 2006. Three experimental glaucoma models in rats: comparison of the effects of intraocular pressure elevation on retinal ganglion cell size and death. Exp Eye Res 83 (2): 429-37.

Vidal-Sanz M, Aviles-Trigueros M, Whiteley SJ, Sauve Y, Lund RD. 2002. Reinnervation of the pretectum in adult rats by regenerated retinal ganglion cell axons: anatomical and functional studies. Prog Brain Res 137: 443-52.

Vidal-Sanz M, Bray GM, Villegas-Perez MP, Thanos S, Aguayo AJ. 1987. Axonal regeneration and synapse formation in the superior colliculus by retinal ganglion cells in the adult rat. J Neurosci 7 (9): 2894-909.

Vidal-Sanz M, de la Villa P, Aviles-Trigueros M, Mayor-Torroglosa S, Alarcon-Martinez L, Villegas-Perez MP. 2007. Neuroprotection of retinal ganglion cell function and their central nervous system targets. Eye 21:S42-S45.

Vidal-Sanz M, Lafuente MP, Mayor S, de Imperial JM, Villegas-Perez MP. 2001a. Retinal ganglion cell death induced by retinal ischemia. neuroprotective effects of two alpha-2 agonists. Surv Ophthalmol 45 Suppl 3: S261-S267.

Vidal-Sanz M, Lafuente MP, Mayor-Torroglosa S, Aguilera ME, Miralles d, I, Villegas-Perez MP. 2001b. Brimonidine's neuroprotective effects against transient ischaemia-induced retinal ganglion cell death. Eur J Ophthalmol 11 Suppl 2: S36-S40.

Vidal-Sanz M, Villegas-Perez MP, Carter DA, Julien JP, Peterson A, Aguayo AJ. 1991. Expression of Human Neurofilament-light Transgene in Mouse Neurons Transplanted into the Brain of Adult Rats. Eur J Neurosci 3 (8): 758-63.

Villegas-Perez MP, Lawrence JM, Vidal-Sanz M, Lavail MM, Lund RD. 1998. Ganglion cell loss in RCS rat retina: a result of compression of axons by contracting intraretinal vessels linked to the pigment epithelium. J Comp Neurol 392 (1): 58-77.

Villegas-Perez MP, Vidal-Sanz M, Bray GM, Aguayo AJ. 1988. Influences of peripheral nerve grafts on the survival and regrowth of axotomized retinal ganglion cells in adult rats. J Neurosci 8 (1): 265-80.

Villegas-Perez MP, Vidal-Sanz M, Rasminsky M, Bray GM, Aguayo AJ. 1993. Rapid and protracted phases of retinal ganglion cell loss follow axotomy in the optic nerve of adult rats. J Neurobiol 24 (1): 23-36.

Villegas-Perez MP, Vidal-Sanz M, Lund RD. 1996. Mechanism of retinal ganglion cell loss in inherited retinal dystrophy. Neuroreport 7(12):1995-9.

Wheeler LA, Lai R, WoldeMussie E. 1999. From the lab to the clinic: activation of an alpha-2 agonist pathway is neuroprotective in models of retinal and optic nerve injury. Eur J Ophthalmol 9 Suppl 1: S17-S21.

Wheeler LA, WoldeMussie E. 2001. Alpha-2 adrenergic receptor agonists are neuroprotective in experimental models of glaucoma. Eur J Ophthalmol 11 Suppl 2: S30-S35.

WoldeMussie E, Ruiz G, Wijono M, Wheeler LA. 2001 Neuroprotection of retinal ganglion cells by brimonidine in rats with laser-induced chronic ocular hypertension. Invest Ophthalmol Vis Sci. 2001 Nov;42(12):2849-55.

Yang Y, Xing D, Zhou F, Chen Q. 2010. Mitochondrial autophagy protects against heat shock-induced apoptosis through reducing cytosolic cytochrome c release and downstream caspase-3 activation. Biochem Biophys Res Commun 395 (2): 190-5.

Zhou F, Yang Y, Xing D. 2011. Bcl-2 and Bcl-xL play important roles in the crosstalk between autophagy and apoptosis. FEBS J 278 (3): 403-13.

Zhou Y, Grinchuk O, Tomarev SI. 2008. Transgenic mice expressing the Tyr437His mutant of human myocilin protein develop glaucoma. Invest Ophthalmol Vis Sci 49 (5): 1932-9.

6

Neuroprotective Agents in Glaucoma

Eleni Bagli and George Kitsos
Department of Ophthalmology, Medical School, University of Ioannina
Greece

1. Introduction

1.1 Glaucoma as a neurodegenerative disorder

Glaucoma is a multifactorial disease in which multiple genetic, systemic and environmental factors interact to precipitate the disease. Increased intraocular pressure (IOP) is believed to be one of the major factors responsible for glaucomatous cell death. (Guo et al., 2005). The axons of the optic nerve make a twisting exit through the fenestrated collageneous barrier (the lamina cribrosa) before entering the brain. It has been proposed that increased IOP causes mechanical stress to the lamina cribrosa, which in turn exerts pressure on the axons that pass through it. This pressure may block the passage of essential material through the axons; which would lead to a slow degeneration of the axons of the retinal ganglion cells (RGCs) (Howell et al., 2007). With increased IOP, gradual withdrawal of trophic factor from RGCs has been observed in a mouse model. Also apoptosis was observed to be a significantly delayed in RGCs in such conditions (Johnson et al., 2000). It was therefore proposed that with increased IOP and mechanical stress on the lamina cribrosa, axons of RGCs are lost much earlier than the cell body of the RGCs. Thus RGCs become ineffective in their visual function much earlier than actual phenotypic changes are observed in the retina/optic disc, as they are incapable of sending visual signals to the visual center of the brain (Whitmore et al., 2005).

The primary goal of glaucoma treatment is to preserve vision. Elevated IOP as an important risk factor for glaucoma has continued to be a clinical focus for several reasons, including limited knowledge of the factors causing optic nerve damage, ease of measurement, the number of available IOP-reducing therapies, and the relationship of elevated IOP to disease progression. However, the relationship between IOP reduction and glaucoma damage is less clear, and such ambiguities suggest that factors other than IOP may be responsible for some of the long-term damage from glaucoma. Ocular blood flow in various tissues (e.g. retina, iris, optic nerve and choroid) was found to be reduced in glaucoma patients (Flammer et al., 2002). The blood flow reduction was more pronounced in Normal Tension Glaucoma (NTG) patients (Mozaffarieh et al., 2008). Interestingly, reduction of blood flow was also observed in the nail-bed capillaries of fingers in glaucoma patients; suggesting that global vascular dysregulation is involved in Primary Open Angle Glaucoma (POAG) especially in NTG cases.

Glaucoma is therefore no longer diagnosed by elevated IOP levels, and is now recognized as a neuropathy defined by characteristic optic disc and visual field change (Walland et al., 2006). IOP level is no longer relied on as a diagnostic criterion because 20% to 30% of glaucoma patients have IOP in the normal range (typically 10-21 mm Hg) (Sommer et al., 1991). Furthermore, there is annual progression even in patients treated with IOP-lowering medical, laser, or surgical therapy. The Early Manifest Glaucoma Trial (Heijl et al., 2002; Leske et al., 2003) found that although the mean IOP during follow-up was significantly associated with the risk of progression, this risk was highly variable, and several other baseline factors were significant independent predictors whose combined effect might be as important as IOP. These additional independent predictors included presence of bilateral disease, worse mean deviation, degree of baseline exfoliation, age older than 68 years, presence of frequent disc hemorrhages, and duration between follow-up visits. The Ocular Hypertension Treatment Study found a relationship between IOP reduction and glaucoma incidence (Kass et al., 2002); however, progression was not confirmed in 85% of cases. (Greenfield & Bagga, 2005). The Collaborative Normal- Tension Glaucoma Study (1998a, 1998b) found that visual field progression could occur in both treated and untreated NTG patients, and no analyses of studies detected a relationship between a changes in the IOP and visual field progression. This clinical evidence of continued disease progression despite IOP management has provided the basis for proposed alternative risk factors and treatment approaches that could modify the clinical course of glaucoma.

Recent observations suggest that, in addition to RGCs, glaucoma patients have neurodegenerative lesions deep in the brain, supporting the hypothesis that it is a neurodegenerative disorder. In fact there are certain similarities between common neurodegenerative disorders and glaucoma (Ray & Mookherjee, 2009) which include:

- Loss of specific neuronal population. A common feature shared by neurodegenerative disorders is the loss of specific groups of neurons. For example, loss of cortical and hippocampal neurons in Alzheimer disease can be correlated with the loss of memory and cognitive function. After exiting from the eye, the axons of RGCs cross each other at the optic chiasm and terminate at the lateral geniculate nucleus (LGN). The LGN of each hemisphere represents the contrallateral half of the visual field. Definite degenerative changes were observed in the optic tracts of the brains of glaucomatous patients and in the LGN. Also axonal loss was found in the intracranial optic tract and progressive degeneration in the visual cortex was observed along with the degeneration of RGCs (Gupta et al., 2006). Using Conventional MRI and magnetisation transfer imaging of the brain and optic pathway we also reached the same conclusion in our previous study (Kitsos et al., 2009). Thus, as in other neurodegenerative disorders a loss of specific groups of neurons involved in vision was observed in the glaucoma patients (Gupta et al., 2006, 2009; Yucel et al., 2001).
- Trans-synaptic spreading of neurodegeneration from RGC to cells deep in the brain. In neurodegenerative disorders, the disease spreads from sick neuron to healthy neurons through synaptic connections along functional and anatomical neural pathways, a process called *trans*-synaptic degeneration. Such degeneration is well known in Alzheimer disease and has also been found in human and experimental glaucoma cases (Gupta & Yucel, 2001). Studies have shown that RGCs damage in glaucoma is not confined to the primary insulted neurons, but that secondary injury follows which affects neighboring neurons as well. It is therefore believed that in glaucoma, treatment modalities that directly target both primary and secondary degeneration of the RGCs are required.
- Deposition of protein aggregates in glaucomatous RGCs as observed in other neurodegenerative disorders like Alzheimer's disease, Parkinson disease etc. Like other neurodegenerative disorders, deposition of unfolded or misfolded protein aggregates has been found in RGCs of glaucoma patients and there are indications that β-amyloid

is involved in glaucoma pathogenesis (Gupta et al., 2008; Wang et al., 2008). Abnormal Tau protein, AT8 which is a hallmark of many neurodegenerative disorders has also been reported in glaucomatous RGCs (Gupta et al., 2008).

- Drugs administered in neurodegenerative disorders, treat glaucoma. Neuroprotective agents approved for the treatment of neurodegenerative diseases such as Alzheimer disease (Reisberg et al., 2003), are being assessed for the treatment of glaucoma to maximize recovery of injured RGCs and minimize secondary insults (Ettaiche et al., 1999).

1.2 The rationale of neuroprotection in Glaucoma

Neuroprotection refers to the use of any therapeutic modality that prevents, retards, or reverses neuronal cell death resulting from primary neuronal lesions. While neuroprotection refers to any therapy that prevents the death of existing RGCs after injury, neuroregeneration refers to any strategy that stimulates regrowth of an injured RGC axon. The idea of neuroprotection as a treatment strategy for glaucoma was borrowed from the neurological field, where the limitation of neuronal injury and protection from secondary insults spares neurons and improves clinical outcomes. This strategy has, however, not been successful in acute clinical neuronal injury, particularly with stroke. Nevertheless, for chronic neurodegenerative conditions, the strategy has made some small but important breakthroughs. Neuroprotection is similar to other cytoprotective therapies (eg, cardioprotection) in which the loss of the cell is targeted, not the disease process by which the loss occurs. For example, in cardioprotection, the cardiomyocyte itself is treated rather than the atheromatous plaque within a coronary artery that leads to myocardial infarction. Analogously, in glaucoma, an optic nerve disease, the RGC is treated rather than elevated IOP or other etiologies that indirectly cause the death of the RGC. Although IOP lowering and other such therapies can be considered indirectly neuroprotective, by strict definition and by comparison with other cytoprotective therapies, a neuroprotective therapy is directed at the neuron itself.

Glaucoma as all optic nerve diseases has an irreversible effect on vision because it causes death of RGCs and loss of their axons. As with all other neurons, once death of the RGC occurs, it is irreversible because mammalian neurons do not ordinarily replace themselves. Although the possibility of non–IOP-lowering therapy for glaucoma it was first recognized in 1972 (Becker et al., 1972) with the use of diphenylhydantoin for treatment of visual field loss in POAG, only recently have significant advances in the understanding of the mechanisms for death of retinal neurons occurred.

2. Potential neuroprotective strategies and agents in glaucoma

Several mechanisms, which are believed to initiate the apoptotic cascade in glaucoma and therefore are potential targets for neuroprotection include excitotoxicity, mitochondrial dysfunction, protein misfolding, oxidative stress, inflammation and neurotrophin deprivation (Baltmr et al., 2010). Therapeutic strategies targeting the mechanisms of cell damage listed above or the apoptotic cascade itself are reviewed.

2.1 Excitotoxicity

Most neurons (and also glia) contain high concentrations of glutamate (~10 mm) (Lipton & Rosenberg, 1994) after sequestration inside synaptic vesicles, glutamate is released for very brief periods of time (milliseconds) to communicate with other neurons via synaptic endings. Once it is released in the pre-synaptic terminals it binds to a variety of receptor linked channels in the post-synaptic membrane, resulting in the influx of Ca2+ and the initiation of the action potential (Pin & Duvoisin, 1995). Glutamate is a major excitatory neurotransmitter in the central nervous system, including the retina (Thoreson & Witkovsky, 1999).

However, because glutamate is so powerful, its presence in excessive amounts or for excessive periods of time can literally excite cells to death. This phenomenon named glutamate receptor-mediated excitotoxicity has been associated with various diseases of the brain including Alzheimer's disease. Several studies have confirmed the neurotoxic effect of glutamate in the retina, while others have suggested glutamate-mediated RGC injury and death in glaucoma (Guo et al., 2006; Salt & Cordeiro, 2006). Increased buildup of glutamate was observed at the posterior aspect of the glaucomatous eye in monkeys with elevated IOP and in human glaucoma patients (Dreyer et al., 1996). Glutamate released from the apoptotic cell can trigger necrotic death of surrounding cells that have been spared from the original insult, initiating a cascade of autodestruction, further cellular injury and death (Casson, 2006; Cheung et al., 2008).

Once released from the pre-synaptic membrane, glutamate binds to specific postsynaptic receptors. There are three classes of glutamate-gated ion (or ionotropic) channels, known as (α-amino-3-hydroxy-5-methyl-4-isoxazolepropionic acid AMPA), kainate, and N-methyl-D-aspartate (NMDA) receptors. Among these, the ion channels coupled to classical NMDA receptors are generally the most permeable to Ca2+. Conventional NMDA receptors consist of two subunits (NR1 and NR2A-D), and more rarely NR3A or B subunits. There are binding sites for glutamate, the endogenous agonist, and glycine, which is required as a co-agonist for receptor activation (Johnson & Ascher, 1987). The receptor is probably composed of a tetramer of these subunits. The subunit composition determines the pharmacology and other parameters of the receptor-ion channel complex. Alternative splicing of some subunits, such as NR1, further contributes to the pharmacological properties of the receptor. Furthermore, the subunits are differentially expressed both regionally in the brain and temporally during development. Thus, developing antagonists selective for a particular subunit could be crucial in clinical practice.

Prolonged activation of glutamate receptors by increased levels of glutamate leads to high Ca++ level in the cytosol and thus facilitates the opening of mitochondrial permeability transition pore complex (PTPC) (Crompton et al., 1999). Opening of the PTPC will lead to apoptotic cell death (Kroemer et al., 2007). Increased activity of the enzyme nitric oxide synthase (NOS) is also associated with excitotoxic cell death. The neuronal isoform of the enzyme is physically tethered to the NMDA receptor and activated by Ca2+ influx receptor-associated ion channel, leading to increased nitric acid (NO) production. Increased levels of NO and the formation of toxic peroxynitrite (ONOO−) have been detected in animal models of stroke and neurodegenerative diseases (Lipton et al., 1993). Importantly, elevations in extracellular glutamate are not necessary to invoke an excitotoxic mechanism. Excitotoxicity can come into play even with normal levels of glutamate, if NMDA receptor activity is increased, e.g., when neurons are injured and thus become depolarized (more positively charged); this condition relieves the normal blocking of the ion channel by Mg2+ and thus abnormally increases NMDA receptor activity (Zeevalk & Nicklas, 1992).

The role of energy expense in excitoxicity has gained a lot of attention. With the disruption of energy metabolism during acute and chronic neurodegenerative disorders, glutamate is not cleared properly and may even be inappropriately released. Elevated levels of glutamate subsequently results in increased concentrations of cytosolic Ca2+ and inorganic phosphate as well as decreased cellular ATP. (Crompton, 1999). This cellular state results in cell death; however, it has been observed that cells can remain viable in the presence of elevated Ca2+, provided that ATP levels remain relatively unchanged (Broderick & Somlyo, 1987). Furthermore, extended elevation of cytosolic Ca2+ concentrations in the absence of exogenous adenine nucleotides can result in opening of the mitochondrial permeability pore (Crompton, 1999). Action potentials, consisting predominantly of the transport of Na+ by Na K ATPases, have been shown to consume approximately 50% of the total cellular energy used in the rabbit retina (Ames et al., 1992). As a result, energy compromised neurons cannot maintain ionic homeostasis and become depolarized.

Modulation of the NMDA receptor has been constituted a major area of research in glaucoma neuroprotection (Dong et al., 2008; Guo et al., 2006). In vivo and in vitro studies have suggested that blocking both the NMDA and the non-NMDA receptors simultaneously offers optimal protection against ischemic neurodegeneration (Mosinger et al., 1991). However, to be clinically acceptable, an anti-excitotoxic therapy must block excessive activation of the NMDA receptor while leaving normal function relatively intact to avoid side effects. Drugs that simply compete with glutamate or glycine at the agonist binding sites block normal function and therefore do not meet this requirement, and have thus failed in clinical trials to date because of side effects (drowsiness, hallucinations and even coma) (Lipton, 1993; Palmer, 2001).

MK801, is a non-competitive antagonist of the NMDA receptor and has demonstrated neuroprotective potential in the CNS for many years. MK-801 has also been found to protect RGCs both in vitro and in vivo in hypertensive rat models (Guo et al., 2006). Unfortunately, MK801 is not used clinically because of its neurotoxic effect, which are believed to be due to high affinity to the NMDA receptors and its long dwell time in the channel (Lipton, 1993).

Memantine also known as 1-amino-3,5-dimethyl-adamantane, is a moderate affinity, uncompetitive NMDA receptor antagonist. It is an 'open channel blocker', which means it can only bind within the NMDA ion channel if glutamate has previously bound to its receptor and induced the channel to open. Hence, when extracellular glutamate levels are elevated excessively, as is thought to occur in glaucoma, memantine becomes effective by having access to a site within the open NMDA (Osborne, 2009). Preliminary research into memantine as a neuroprotective agent in glaucoma demonstrated a reduction in NMDA-induced neuronal death in vitro and a protection of RGCs in several animal models of glaucoma (Lagreze et al., 1998) , potentially via reduced cytochrome c release in the glaucomatous mouse retina (Ju et al., 2009). It appears that the compound enters the channel preferentially when it is (pathologically) activated for long periods of time, i.e., under conditions of excessive glutamate exposure (Chen & Lipton, 1997). Treatment with memantine also resulted in a reduction in the shrinkage of neurons within the contra-lateral LGB relay (layers 1, 4, and 6), a major target for RGCs (Yucel et al., 2006). So memantine had favorable activity in the channel to provide neuroprotection, while displaying minimal adverse effects, when administrated to patients (Lipton, 1993). Memantine is Food and Drug Administration (FDA) approved for treating moderate to severe Alzheimer's disease (Reisberg et al., 2003) and is the only neuroprotective agent that has completed phase III clinical trial in patients with OAG. The trial showed that memantine was ineffective by the primary end point, with the variable mechanisms of retinal ganglion apoptosis being offered as an explanation (Osborne, 2008), although inadequate study design and inappropriate end point could be additional reasons for this result.

Bis(7)-tacrine a noncompetitive NMDA receptors antagonist had beneficial effect on glutamate-induced rat RGCs damage in vitro and in vivo (Fang et al., 2010)
Topiramate, a drug used clinically as an anti-epileptic was also shown to be protective against excitotoxic and ischemic retinal-neuron damage in vitro and in vivo (Yoneda et al., 2003).
Riluzole (2-amino-6-trifluoromethoxy benzothiazole) is a neuroprotective drug, which has been shown to block glutamatergic neurotransmission in the central nervous system (Martin et al., 1993), probably as a consequence of its action on ion channels. Riluzole could also prevent or decrease pressure-induced apoptosis and enhance ERG wave recovery in a pressure-induced ischemia animal model, highlighting the benefits of targeting multiple receptors in excitotoxic cell death (Ettaiche et al., 1999).
Galantamine, a small molecule acetylcholinesterase (AChE), which is used for the symptomatic treatment of Alzheimer's disease, protected RGCs in a rat glaucoma model. The neuroprotective effect of galantamine was superior to that conferred by memantine and occurred by activation of types M1 and M4 muscarinic acetylcholine receptors (Almasieh et al., 2010).

2.2 Mitochondrial dysfunction

Neurons, because of their high energy requirement, are heavily dependent on mitochondria for survival. Mitochondria not only constitute an energy-generating system, but are also critically involved in calcium signaling and apoptosis. Any malfunction of the mitochondrial electron transport chain results in an excessive generation of free radicals. When this overwhelms the intrinsic antioxidant capacity, amplified generation of free radicals results in the state of oxidative stress, which is evident in glaucomatous tissues. Mitochondria are morphologically dynamic organelles exhibiting a precise balance of ongoing fission and fusion during development and aging, which can be modified by disease (Santel & Frank, 2008). Mitochondrial fission is characterized by the conversion of tubular fused mitochondria into isolated small organelles, translocation of dynamin-related protein 1, and reduction of cellular ATP (Santel & Frank, 2008).
IOP elevation in vivo has been linked to mitochondrial damage in the optic nerve head by the promotion of mitochondrial fission, cristae depletion, and alterations in the expression and distribution of optic atrophy type 1 in DBA/2J mice (Ju et al., 2008). Intra-mitochondrial accumulation of Ca2+, decrease in mitochondrial membrane potential and increase in membrane permeability have been implicated as a causative factor for RGCs apoptosis in glaucoma (Tatton et al., 2001; Tezel & Yang, 2004). Moreover, glaucoma-related stimuli such as hypoxia, TNF-a and oxidative stress can trigger the mitochondrial-mediated RGC death pathway.
Several compounds, have been proposed to enhance the available energy within the cell and prevent mitochondrial depolarization.
Nicotinamide is a non-toxic precursor of NADH, which is a substrate for complex I in the electron transport chain, a free radical scavenger and an inhibitor of poly-ADP-ribose polymerase (PARP). Dietary supplementation of nicotinamide in conjunction with creatine supplementation was shown to decrease the lesion volume induced by intracerebral injections of NMDA. PARP is a nuclear enzyme that is activated by breaks in the DNA chain and aids in minor DNA repair. The presence of excessive DNA damage initiates a PARP-mediated apoptotic response. The action of PARP results in the depletion of NAD and ATP, and ultimately cell death (Pieper et al., 1999). PARP inhibition, by 3-aminobenzamide, has

been shown to reduce neuronal damage in a high-pressure retinal ischaemia model. Of particular interest with regard to glaucoma, nicotinamide has recently been shown to attenuate ischaemic and phototoxic injuries to RGCs (Ji et al., 2008). It is important now to ascertain whether nicotinamide is equally beneficial in chronic models of RGC injury.

CoQ10, also known as Ubiquinone, plays an indispensable role in energy metabolism and offers the greatest potential as a neuroprotectant. It serves as a co-factor within the respiratory chain, carrying electrons and facilitating ATP production. It has been found to be highly effective as a neuroprotectant in animal models of neurodegenerative diseases such as Parkinson's disease (Beal, 2003). Its neuroprotective effect, demonstrated on RGCs both in vivo and in vitro, is believed to be multifactorial (Nakajima et al., 2008;,) exerted not only through mediation of electron transport from complex I and II to complex III within the electron transport chain but also through its antioxidant properties, regulation of gene expression, and inhibition of PTP (Cheung et al., 2008).

There is increasing evidence in a variety of models that creatine may provide neuroprotection through metabolic energy buffering (Beal, 2003). Creatine is a guanidine compound that is found in meat and is also endogenously produced. Neuronal tissue has a very high ATP requirement for the generation of action potentials through the axonal ATP-dependent Na+/K+ ion transport system as stated previously. In order to replenish ATP levels, the phosphoryl-group from phosphocreatine is donated to ADP via the action of mitochondrial and cytosolic creatine kinase to produce ATP and creatine (Wallimann & Hemmer, 1994). There are two main isoforms of creatine kinase: cytosolic creatine kinase that balances energy distribution in the cytosol, and mitochondrial creatine kinase (Mi-Ck) that buffers energy between the mitochondria and the cytosol. (Brdiczka & Wallimann, 1994) There are several possible explanations for the neuroprotective qualities of creatine. First, creatine supplementation, which results in increased levels of phosphocreatine, may cause greater energy buffering during cell repair processes that occur during injury. Second, creatine may reduce cerebral ischemia infarct volume by improving cerebral blood flow (Prass et al., 2007). Third, the administration of creatine could result in a decreased release of glutamate. This may be achieved either through increased glutamate uptake into synaptic vesicles, which is an energy-dependent process, (Xu et al., 1996) or by an increased conversion of glutamate to glutamine (Bender et al., 2005). Finally, creatine supplementation may inhibit the opening of the PTP through the action of Mi-Ck (Beal, 2003; Kroemer et al., 2007). Creatine supplementation has provided significant neuroprotection against in vivo models of traumatic brain injury (Scheff and Dhillon, 2004), cerebral ischaemia (Lensman et al., 2006), Huntington's and Parkinson's disease. Concerning the neuroprotective effects of creatine against retinal/optic nerve neurodegenerative disorders, intravitreal injection of creatine partially rescues RGCs from NMDA-induced excitotoxcity (Schober et al., 2008).

2.3 Protein misfolding treatments

Amyloid deposits, consisting of aggregates of Ab, are a characteristic feature of several neurodegenerative diseases such as Alzheimer's, Parkinson's disease and mild cognitive impairment. They have also been recently implicated in the pathogenesis of retinal damage (Shimazawa et al., 2008), age-related macular degeneration (AMD) (Johnson et al., 2002) and glaucoma (Gupta et al., 2008; Wang et al., 2008; Guo et al., 2007).

Drugs designated to target b-Amyloid (Ab) include b-secretase inhibitors (BSI) such as N-benzyloxycarbonyl-Val-Leu-leucinal (Z-VLL-CHO) which has been found to reduce RGC apoptosis in vitro and in vivo, as well as Congo red and Anti-Ab antibodies (Guo et al., 2007

). Triple therapy, targeting different stages of the Ab pathway using BSI, Anti-Ab antibodies and Congo red, showed a superior neuroprotective effect on RGC apoptosis in a rat ocular hypertension model compared to mono-therapy (Guo et al., 2007).

Also of interest with regards to protein misfolding are Heat shock proteins (HSPs), a group of specialized molecular chaperones which are upregulated in stressful conditions and mediate various physiological functions inside cells such as restoration of normal structural integrity (Soti et al., 2005). Several families of HSP have been implicated in neurodegenerative diseases, and glaucomatous RGC apoptosis (Guo et al., 2007) , with increased levels of circulating autoantibodies to alpha-crystallins and HSP27 (Tezel et al., 1998), and increased immunostaining of HSP-60, HSP-27 in RGCs and the retinal blood vessels in glaucoma patients (Tezel et al., 2000). Considerable evidence also supports the involvement of HSPs, including HSP27, in intrinsic protection mechanisms of retinal cells in glaucoma. HSP27 is upregulated in experimental models of glaucoma, as well as in human glaucoma and the phosphorylation state of HSP27 is a critical determinant of its ability to act in a protective capacity as detected in glial cells. However, the exact biological mechanism is still unclear. HSP72 is an anti-apoptotic chaperone protein that may interfere with multiple stages of the apoptotic pathway. (Mosser et al., 2000). The preinduction of HSP72 in RGCs enhances the survival of RGCs under hypoxic, excitotoxic, and glaucomatous stress (Park et al., 2001). Systemic administration of Geranylgeranylacetone, an agent that has been used clinically for the treatment of gastric ulcers and gastritis, in the rat glaucoma model has been shown to increase the expression of HSP-72 with a marked reduction in RGC loss (Ishii et al., 2003).

2.4 Oxidative stress

Oxidative stress is a pathological condition in which the rate of reactive oxygen species (ROS) production exceeds the body's antioxidative capacity. Any malfunction of the mitochondrial electron transport chain results in an excessive generation of free radicals. When this overwhelms the intrinsic antioxidant capacity, amplified generation of free radicals results in the state of oxidative stress, which is evident in glaucomatous tissues.

Ischemia, potentially caused by vascular dysregulation and reperfusion injury to cells are critical inducers of oxidative stress (Flammer et al., 1999), leading to further ROS generation with ATP depletion and mitochondrial failure, triggering the caspase-dependent and caspase-independent mitochondrial cell death pathways. The increased levels of ROS enhance lipid peroxidation, protein peroxidation and single strand breaks in nucleic acids (Finkel & Holbrook, 2000). It has been proposed that after an initial insult to RGC axons at the optic nerve head, besides neurotrophin insufficiency, increased superoxide generation may also signal apoptosis of the RGC soma. Evidently, there is an increase in mitochondrial superoxide production within RGCs after axonal injury that is further amplified by oxidative stress (Nguyen et al., 2003). It is also evident that a shift to a reduced intracellular redox state induced by the use of sulfhydryl-reducing agents markedly prolongs RGC survival in in vitro and in vivo models of axonal injury (Swanson et al., 2005). RGC mitochondria regulate superoxide production differently from other neuronal cells, most likely as a result of differential expression and function of the mitochondrial electron transport chain components.

There is an increasing body of clinical as well as experimental evidence that oxidative stress contributes to the pathology of glaucoma (Izzotti et al., 2006; Tezel, 2006). Increased levels of free radicals have been measured in the retina and optic nerve head of animals with experimental glaucoma. Free radical scavengers have been shown to protect against RGC death in various models of injury, while clinically glaucoma patients have been shown to have reduced antioxidant defenses (Izzotti et al., 2006). ROS have also been found to induce Muller cell activation and dysfunction, generating further oxidative material (Neufeld & Liu, 2003;). Furthermore, many retinal proteins exhibit oxidative modifications in experimental glaucoma, which may lead to important structural and functional alterations (Tezel et al., 2005).

Melatonin, a potent naturally occurring antioxidant with free radical scavenging activity, displays a critical role in aqueous humour circulation and demonstrated a neuroprotective effect on RGCs in vivo (Siu et al., 2004; Tang et al., 2006) via multiple mechanisms.

Derived from leaves of the G. biloba tree, Ginkgo biloba extract (GBE) has been used in traditional Chinese medicine for thousands of years, and has been one of the most prescribed drugs in Europe (Mahadevan & Park, 2008). It has been effectively used to treat diseases such as peripheral vascular disease (Mahadevan & Park, 2008), Alzheimer's disease (Yancheva et al., 2009), AMD (Rhone & Basu, 2008) and low-tension glaucoma (Quaranta et al., 2003). Ginkgo biloba extract (EGb761) contains two major compounds: 24% flavones glycoside and 6% terpenoids. The exact mechanism of the neuroprotective effect of EGb 761 is still unknown. However EGb 761 was found to be an excellent antioxidant, effectively inhibiting chemically induced apoptosis (Thiagarajan et al., 2002), as well as possessing both anti-inflammatory and antiplatlet activating factor activities. EGb 761 also enhances the cerebral blood flow and increases the ocular blood flow velocity (Chung et al., 1999). In a model of chronic glaucoma, GBE was shown to be neuroprotective for the pre-treatment and early post-treatment phases of glaucoma (Hirooka et al., 2004) and the few studies that have evaluated whether GBE may improve visual function, have produced promising results (Quaranta et al., 2003; Cheung et al., 2002). However, a National Health Interview study showed that there was no significant association between glaucoma patients and Gingko biloba use (Khoury et al., 2009).

2.5 Anti-inflammatory and immunological strategies

Growing evidence in clinical and experimental studies over the past decade strongly suggests the involvement of the immune system in glaucoma. Serum and tissue findings, including chronic activation of resident immunoregulatory glial cells, altered T-cell repertoires, increased autoantibody production, retinal immunoglobulin deposition, and complement activation, support the hypothesis that both innate and adaptive immune activity accompany glaucomatous neurodegeneration (Tezel & Wax, 2007).

Regarding T-cell cytotoxicity to RGCs, there is in vitro evidence that activated T cells may be directly cytotoxic to RGCs and induce RGC apoptosis mainly through death receptor-mediated signaling. Recent in vivo studies also support the feasibility of eliciting a T-cell-mediated experimental autoimmune model of glaucomatous neurodegeneration. In rats immunized with HSPs, RGCs progressively die, exhibiting a pattern with similarities to human glaucoma, including topographic specificity of cell loss. (Wax et al., 2008)

It is evident that the glial activation response in glaucomatous eyes involves activation of glial immunoregulatory functions and antigen-presenting ability. The expression of MHC class II molecules on glial cells, required for antigen presentation to T cells, is upregulated in glaucomatous eyes. Not only microglial cells, but also astrocytes exhibit HLA-DR immunolabeling in the glaucomatous human retina and optic nerve head (Tezel et al., 2003; Yang et al., 2001). Up-regulation of MHC class II molecules on rat glial cells and stimulation

of T cell activation in cultured retinal and optic nerve tissue have been demonstrated (Tezel et al., 2007). Glial MHC class II molecules are also upregulated in experimental animal models of glaucoma which may have neurosupportive and neurodestructive consequences.
Increased expression of HSPs28 and ROS-dependent controlling pathways seem to be critical for the initiation of an activated immune response (Tezel et al., 2007, 2005). In addition to T-cell–mediated injury, autoantibody-mediated retinal damage has been associated with the pathogenesis of retinal diseases (Khan et al., 2006) .Increased serum autoantibodies to various retina and optic nerve proteins have also been identified in patients with glaucoma over the past decade (Grus et al., 2008; Tezel & Wax, 2007) and retinal immunoglobulin deposition was seen in glaucomatous human donor eyes.There is evidence supporting the hypothesis that exogenously applied antibodies, including HSP antibodies, which exhibit increased serum titers in many patients with glaucoma, can be internalized by retinal neurons. At concentrations similar to those found in the patient serum, these antibodies can facilitate neuronal apoptosis (Tezel and Wax, 2000b) . However, despite many immunologic associations, there is presently no direct evidence to confirm that neurodegenerative injury in glaucoma occurs as the direct result of aberrant cellular or humoral immunity.
Growing evidence implicates the involvement of the complement cascade in the neurodegenerative injury in glaucoma. Recent histopathologic studies of human tissues as well as in vivo studies using animal models have demonstrated that various complement components are synthesized during glaucomatous neurodegeneration (Stasi et al., 2006; Kuehn et al., 2006). In addition, terminal complement complex has been shown to be formed in the retina in both human and rat glaucoma (Kuehn et al., 2006).
Ongoing studies are testing an increasing number of innovative immunomodulatory strategies as a promising alternative to classic immunosuppressive treatments (Smith & Rosenbaum, 2000). One of the most efficient and specific ways to treat organ-specific autoimmune diseases has been based on systemic administration of native autoantigen or its altered peptide variants. Such strategies have been considered to be an important therapeutic option for the treatment of autoimmune diseases, because they selectively aim to deplete disease-inducing T cells in blood circulation or to trap these cells in peripheral lymphoid organs, thereby preventing them from invading the target organ. Antigen-based immunomodulatory treatments aiming to elicit immunogenic tolerance to tissue-specific antigens may also induce regulatory T cells. It has also been suggested that the loss of immunity to certain self-antigens or its insufficiency in the presence of increased levels of risk factors play an important role in neurodegenerative processes. For that reason, it has been proposed that vaccination could be a means of inducing the immune system to help eliminate many adverse factors associated with glaucomatous neurodegeneration and perhaps also supporting cell renewal and repair. Such a vaccine is thought to induce a beneficial immune response that recruits immune effector cells to counteract or neutralize some destructive factors, thereby preventing disease progression, although not its onset. Augmentation of immune system by passive transfer of T cells directed against myelin basic proteins or active immunization with the myelin-derived peptide reduces RGC loss after optic nerve injury (Schwartz, 2001).
Minocycline, a neuroprotective tetracycline derivative that suppresses chronic neuroinflammation and microglial activation, was shown to protects RGCs after optic nerve transection and in optic neuritis models (Maier et al., 2007). Furthermore, long-term and systemic treatment of DBA/2J mice with minocycline, commencing before clinical evidence

of glaucoma, suppressed retinal microglial activation and improved ganglion cell integrity (Bosco et al., 2008).

Copolymer-1 (Cop-1), also known as glatiramer acetate is a promising drug. It has been approved by the FDA to treat the Multiple sclerosis (MS). Cop-1 is a low affinity synthetic non-encephalitogenic analogue to myelin basic protein, triggering a neuroprotective autoimmune response, by binding to MHC proteins and cross reacting with various T cell and CNS myelin. Cop-1 displayed neuroprotective activity on RGCs in vivo in the rat model of optic nerve crush (Kipnis et al., 2000), in animal models of high IOP (Bakalash et al., 2003) and against glutamate-induced excitotoxicity (Schori et al., 2001). The neuroprotective effect in the rat model of glaucoma is believed to be mediated by increasing the number of T-Lymphocytes.

T-cell/glia/macrophage interactions should be well-controlled and synchronized and precise control mechanisms of the immune activity should be identified, so that these strategies will be clinical successful. For example, Monocyte chemoattractant protein-1 (MCP-1)/CCL2 (chemokine involved in the activation and recruitment of monocytic cells) was able to protect RGCs in experimental glaucoma. However, the appropriate dose of the drug was crucial for the neuroprotective effect (Chiu et al., 2010).

Targeting specific immunomediators involved in immunogenic injury constitutes another strategy for immunomodulation. It has been proposed that pro-inflammatory cytokines like TNF-α, which is produced in the brain and in the eye by microglial cells, play an important role in glaucomatous neurodegeneration (Tezel et al., 2001). Increased expression of TNF-α and its receptor were observed in the optic nerve heads of glaucoma patients. TNF-α, a potent proinflammatory cytokine, induces the production of NO which can be cytotoxic to the RGC (Tezel & Wax, 2000a). TNF-α activities are mediated via interaction with two distinct receptors, the death domain-containing TNF-receptor 1 (TNF-R1) which mediate the majority of TNF-α biological activity, and the non-death domain-containing TNF-receptor 2 (TNF-R2). The release of TNF-α and its subsequent binding to TNR-R1, triggers a caspase-dependant and a caspase-independent component of mitochondrial death-promoting pathways (Tezel et al., 2004). TNFR1 was shown to be involved in the neurodegenerative process of glaucoma (Tezel et al., 2001), neuronal cell loss and retinal ischemia, whereas TNF-R2 showed neuroprotective activity, reducing retinal ischemia (Fontaine et al., 2002).

Anti-inflammatory drugs, which target the TNF-α signaling pathway and display neuroprotective activity, have become an area of increasingly active investigation. Blocking TNF-α with anti-TNF-α neutralizing antibody or deleting the genes encoding TNF-α or its receptor prevented the effects of ocular hypertension in a mouse model (Nakazawa et al., 2006a). Opioid-receptor activation using morphine could reduce retinal ischemic/reperfusion-injury in vivo via suppression of TNF-α production (Husain et al., 2011). Finally, an antioxidant enzyme, peroxiredoxin 6 has shown to reduce TNF-α-induced and glutamate-induced RGC death in a rat model by reducing levels of reactive oxygen species, NF-kB activation and intracellular calcium influx (Tulsawani et al., 2010).

2.6 Neurotrophin deprivation

Neurotrophic factors, small molecular weight peptides, which are widely expressed in RGCs, have an indispensable role in growth, differentiation and survival. They include: nerve growth factor (NGF), brain-derived neurotrophic factor (BDNF), Neurotrophins 3, 4 and 5 (NT3, NT4 and NT5), which exert their effects through tropomyosin related kinases (Trk). Several research studies demonstrated that the flow of neurotrophic factors from the superior colliculus in the CNS to the RGCs is markedly reduced in the animal model of glaucoma, where both retrograde and anti-retrograde axonal transport are compromised (Hayreh et al., 1979; Rudzinski et al., 2004). This leads to a reduction in neuronal trophic support, which in turn compromises neuronal survival and triggers apoptosis, as seen in RGCs following transection of the optic nerve (Berkelaar et al., 1994).

There is substantial evidence that exogenous neurotrophic factors have a powerful survival effect on injured RGCs. Several groups have investigated the effect of intraocular injection of BDNF in models of RGC death. Intraocular delivery of BDNF protein (Ko et al., 2001) or gene transfer using adeno-associated virus (AAV) (Martin et al., 2003) led to RGC neuroprotection in experimental glaucoma induced by chronic intraocular pressure elevation. However, the effect of exogenous BDNF is temporary: it delays, but does not prevent, the onset of RGC death. (Di Polo et al., 1998; Mansour-Robaey et al., 1994). Administration of BDNF by repeated intravitreal injections or osmotic minipumps failed to extend the time-course of RGC neuroprotection (Mansour-Robaey et al., 1994). Delivery of BDNF by adenovirus-infected Muller cells provided a sustained source of NT, but led to only transient rescue of RGCs (Di Polo et al., 1998) which could be explained by the fact that TrkB mRNA and protein levels are markedly down-regulated in experimental glaucoma. These results suggest that reduced TrkB expression in injured RGCs contributes to their desensitization to exogenous, and possibly endogenous, BDNF. Based on this, a neuroprotective strategy was developed involving up-regulation of endogenous TrkB in RGCs by AAV-mediated gene transfer (Cheng et al., 2002). This study demonstrated a marked increase in the duration and level of BDNF-induced neuroprotection of axotomized RGCs upon up-regulation of TrkB. Specifically, TrkB gene transfer into RGCs, combined with exogenous BDNF administration, increased survival by 76% at 2 weeks after axotomy, a time frame in which 90% of these neurons are lost without treatment. This strategy substantially extended RGC survival compared with the shorter effect of BDNF protein alone (Di Polo et al., 1998; Mansour-Robaey et al., 1994). Recently, it has also been shown that the co-injection of an antagonist to leucine-rich repeat protein, LINGO-1, a known negative regulator of neuronal survival, with BDNF had a greater neuroprotective effect on RGCs than with BDNF alone (Fu et al., 2008a). Agonistic TrkB mAb causing sustained TrkB activation also delayed RGC death, and protected the retinal structure in optic nerve axotomy and in glaucoma animal models (Bai et al., 2010).

In addition to BDNF, other neurotrophic factors have shown efficacy in models of RGC injury. For example, exogenous ciliary neurotrophic factor (CNTF) protein enhanced RGC survival during elevated intraocular pressure (Ji et al., 2004). Intraocular injection of glial cell line-derived neurotrophic factor (GDNF) or neurturin was neuroprotective for axotomized RGCs, albeit with less efficacy than BDNF (Koeberle & Ball, 2002; Yan et al., 1999). Combined treatment of BDNF and GDNF resulted in increased RGC survival compared to independent administration of each neurotrophic factor (Koeberle & Ball, 2002; Yan et al., 1999). Interestingly, adenovirus-mediated CNTF gene transfer was reported to increase retinal CNTF and CNTF receptor levels, which correlated with increased survival of axotomized RGCs (van Adel et al., 2005). A novel approach to deliver CNTF in vivo involves the use of encapsulated cell intraocular implants. Cells transfected with the human CNTF gene are sequestered within capsules that can then be surgically implanted into the vitreous chamber of the eye. A semipermeable membrane in the implant allows CNTF to diffuse out and nutrients to diffuse in, while preventing immune cells from destroying CNTF-producing cells. A phase I safety clinical trial of this technology in patients with retinal degeneration was recently completed without apparent ocular or systemic complications (Sieving et al., 2006). Thus, the use of encapsulated cell implants is a novel approach for retinal delivery of neurotrophic factors that may have future applications for glaucomatous and other optic neuropathies as well as other retinal diseases. Similarly, GDNF gene transfer using adenovirus or electroporation conferred protection of RGCs after optic nerve transection. (Ishikawa et al., 2005; Straten et al., 2002). More recently, intraocular injection of slow-release poly(DL-lactide-co-glycolide) microspheres containing GDNF was shown to promote RGC survival in an animal model of inherited glaucoma. (Ward et al., 2007).

Finally in a recent study it was shown that administration of eyedrops containing NGF was able to prevent RGC loss in an animal glaucoma model and furthermore to improve visual function in patients with advanced glaucoma. Although only three patients were included, the results are promising (Lambiase et al., 2009).

2.7 Apoptosis cascade

The structure and function of mitochondria are critical determinants of neuronal health, whereas mitochondrial dysfunction leads to RGC death through caspase-dependent and caspase-independent pathways, initiated by the loss of mitochondrial membrane potential, release of cell death mediators, and oxidative stress.

Mitochondria-related neuroprotective strategies were focused on the control of mitochondrial function by targeting the Bcl2 family. A caveat in the therapeutic targeting of mitochondria-mediated events is the reversal of the early steps of the cell death cascade. Most importantly, once the mitochondrial lipid bilayer is compromised after the mitochondrial translocation of Bax, cell death is inevitable, because already triggered events, the disruption of oxidative phosphorylation, loss in ATP production, increased generation of ROS, and release of cytochrome c constitute the crucial step that represents the point of no return for apoptotic cell death.

A promising agent for glaucoma therapy is BIRC-4, also known as XIAP (IAP: inhibitor of apoptosis protein). Intravitreal injection of adeno-associated viral vector using chicken-b-actin (AAV-CBA) coding for human BIRC4 in the rat model of chronic glaucoma resulted in marked reduction in RGC apoptosis that was sustained for 12 weeks. This neuroprotective effect is believed to be mediated either via direct inhibition of caspase-3 and caspase-8, indirectly by maintaining the neurotrophin production from Muller cells and influencing aqueous humour circulation or a combination of both (McKinnon et al., 2002).

Synthetic IQACRG peptide was delivered in vivo in order to work as an enzymatically inactive caspase mimetic which binds to caspase substrates as a pseudoenzyme and protects them from proteolysis by caspases. IQACRG significantly reduced NMDA-induced RGC death in culture and in vivo by inhibiting NMDA-triggered MMP-9 activity and preventing cleavage of MEF2C protein that would otherwise have been engendered by caspase activation preceding RGC death. (Seki et al., 2010)

2.8 Compounds with multiple/novel mechanisms of action

Brimonidine tartrate, is a third generation α2 adrenergic agonist with weak α1 activity. Animal studies demonstrated the presence of α2 receptors in the retina or optic nerve head, laying the foundation for the potential neuroprotective role of brimonidine (Wheeler et al., 2001). Experimental models suggest that brimonidine confers neuroprotection in several types of ocular injury, including ischemia-induced injury, (Aktas et al., 2007; Danylkova et al., 2007) optic nerve compression or optic nerve crush injury (Levkovitch-Verbin et al.,

2000),. photoreceptor degeneration, (Wen et al., 1996) and ocular hypertension and glaucoma (Hernandez et al., 2008; Wheeler et al., 2001). The mode of action of Brimonidine however remains unclear with various proposed mechanisms. The positive effect of Brimonidine on RGC survival, that includes a reduction in their soma size in a rat model of ocular hypertension, is believed to be mediated through the attenuation of glutamate toxicity by inhibition of NMDA receptor function (Dong et al., 2008) and/or the upregulation of brain-derived neurotrophic factors (Hernandez et al., 2008). However, in a rat model of pressure- induced retinal ischemia, it was suggested that Brimonidine's neuroprotective effect is mediated via the inhibition of the apoptotic cascade, possibly through the induction of anti-apoptotic genes such as bcl-2 and bcl-x, as well as extracellular-signal regulated kinases (ERKs) and phosphatidylinositol-30 kinase/ protein kinase Akt pathways (Lai et al., 2002).While Brimonidine's effect on RGCs in isolated rat retinas, as well as in vivo in rat and rabbit glaucoma models was also shown to be mediated through the reduction of a2-adrenoceptor mediated reduction of intracellular cAMP (Dong et al., 2008). A clinical trial assessing the non-IOP-related effects of Brimonidine, demonstrated reduced visual field deterioration in comparison to 360° laser trabeculoplasty (Gandolfi et al., 2003) . The results of Brimonidine treatment in Low-Pressure Glaucoma Treatment Study are pending (Krupin et al., 2005).

Estrogens, cholesterol derived steroid hormones, maintain the normal function of various organs, with estrogen receptors ERa and ERb widely expressed in human and animal retinal tissues (Kobayashi et al., 1998). Estrogen has demonstrated neuroprotective effects in animal models of Alzheimer's and other neurological diseases (Hoffman et al., 2006). The neuroprotective effect of estrogen is believed to be mediated mainly via estrogen receptors ERa (Dubal et al., 2001;) and icludes multiple mechanisms of action. 17b-estradiol treatment of rat cortical neurons exposed to glutamate demonstrated increased neuronal integrity and function, mediated possibly by a reduction in the levels of caspase-3 and calpain (Sribnick et al., 2004). An estradiol analogue also demonstrated protective on the RGCs in vitro and in vivo (Nakazawa et al., 2006b;.)

Endogenous erythropoietin/erythropoietin receptor (EPO/EPOR) system was shown to participate in intrinsic recovery mechanisms after retina injury. ERO, in addition to being a hematopoietic cytokine, demonstrated neuroprotective effect in various models of neurodegeneration. Furthermore, exogenous erythropoietin could rescue RGCs in an experimental ocular hypertension model (Fu et al., 2008b).

Candesartan an angiotensin II type 1 receptor (AT1-R) blocker showed significant neuroprotection against RGC loss in a rat chronic glaucoma model. (Yang et al., 2009) According to the same study, upregulation of AT1-R was associated with chronic elevated IOP . Consistent with that, the long-term use of angiotensin-converting enzyme (ACE) inhibitors, which are widely used as antihypertensive drugs, are believed to have a favorable effect on the visual fields in patients with normal-tension glaucoma (Hirooka et al., 2006) and angiotensin II receptor gene polymorphisms have been found in humans, and may be associated with the risk for glaucoma (Hashizume et al., 2005).

3. Challenges, limitations, clinical perscpectives of neuroprotection

The treatment of glaucoma is no longer restricted to managing vision loss related to elevated IOP. The focus has shifted to reducing disease progression and loss of visual function that result from neurodegeneration. Alternative strategies that include neuroprotectants may be useful in preventing optic nerve damage, thereby improving the structural, functional, and other patient-reported outcomes.

There is however substantial evidence that the results of preclinical neuroprotection studies fail to correlate with their clinical counterparts. Although numerous neuroprotective agents have been shown to limit neuronal damage in animal models of disease these encouraging preclinical results almost invariably fail to translate into clinical success. This lack of correlation between preclinical and clinical results could be due to various reasons (Danesh-Meyer & Levin, 2009).

A. Issues concerning the preclinical studies

- Lack of perfect animal model of glaucoma. Although animal models are useful tools for elucidating pathogenic mechanisms and testing the neuroprotective ability of new treatments, it is very likely that the initiating insults and pathogenic pathways vary between different experimental models and even more compared to humans. Because of this, animal models may not mirror human disease accurately since they often lack the heterogeneity inherent in human pathologic conditions. When an animal model for glaucoma is first designed, the goal is to produce a homogeneous reproducible optic nerve injury meaning loss of RGCs. However, the ideal model should produce focal injury to RGC axons at the optic nerve head, death of groups of RGCs in sectors in the retina with no loss of other retinal neurons. In clinical trials there is considerable heterogeneity, compounded by comorbidities, risk factors, polypharmacy, and minimal if any control over physiologic parameters. These variables may influence the efficacy of the potentially neuroprotective agent under investigation. These limitations are further exemplified by the contrast between the slow and multifactorial progressive onset of glaucoma in humans and its rapid or subacute induction in young healthy laboratory animals by pharmacologic agents or one particular intervention (for example obliteration of episcleral vessels). Furthermore, factors associated with glaucoma in humans, such as chronicity of injurious conditions and age-dependent dysregulation of tissue response mechanisms, may play a role in the cumulative deterioration of the homeostatic balance, thereby promoting the spread of neuronal damage, rather than favoring retained cell survival. As new biological pathways participating in glaucoma damage are discovered (for example activation of the glia), a critical question that arises, is which experimental model(s) accurately mimic various conditions in human glaucoma and are therefore useful for testing neuroprotective treatments, and for generating sufficient and compelling preclinical evidence in order to justify testing new agents in well-designed clinical trials.
- Dose. The appropriate dose of a potential neuroprotective drug for use in human subjects is difficult to extrapolate from animal studies due to differences in CNS microcirculation and structure, receptor and postreceptor signaling. The presence of the blood barrier in the nervous system makes bioavailability prediction more difficult. Furthermore, many neuroprotective drugs exhibit U-shaped curves in which concentrations higher or lower than optimum are toxic or ineffective. Lack of a complete dose-response curve, insufficient data on CNS penetration, inadequate assessment of therapeutic index, or a combination of these in preclinical studies could be responsible for clinical studies failure.
- Timing. Differences between preclinical and neuroprotection clinical trials relate also to the timing of the intervention. In animal models, the neuroprotective agent is

introduced relatively soon after induction of the disease, when neuroprotection may have its greatest effects, in contrast to human clinical trials, in which the patient is enrolled after glaucoma is well established and irreversible RGC loss is manifested by visual field defects. It is suggested that a window of time exists between the initial phases of injury and the final phases of cell death and only during this time frame, treatment with a neuroprotective agent could rescue injured neurons. Hence, the treatment drug may reach the neural tissue only after death of the neurons is already inevitable and because of this may be ineffective.

- Study Design. The methodology of preclinical study design and the statistical analysis of the results also differ significantly from clinical studies. For example, although randomization and masking are standard practices in phase III clinical trials, these techniques are not always applied to animal experimentation. When such methods are incorporated into animal studies, a treatment effect is less likely to be reported. Also, if a drug is administered in error or at the wrong dose, or if injury seems inadequate, animals typically are dropped from the study and replaced. Finally, a minority of neuroprotective agents have been evaluated by more than one research group using consistent methodologies. For these reasons, basic research on neuroprotective agents should adopt more rigorous methods, analogous to those in clinical trials, such as randomization, masking, prespecified analysis plans, and replication of findings and reproducibility of results in more than one laboratory.
- Premature Initiation Of Clinical Trials. It seems that clinical trials frequently are initiated with insufficient preclinical data. For example, preclinical studies rarely demonstrate long-lasting neuroprotective effects. Studies that evaluate only one time point (which may be a relatively short interval after the injury) may actually represent a delay, but not an arrest, of cell death. Assessments at later time points are necessary to prove sustained neuroprotection (Fisher M et al.,1999).

B. Issues concerning clinical trials

- Problems In The Execution Of Neuroprotection Clinical Trials. Clinical trials have inherent limitations. To encourage enrollment, inclusion criteria may result in discrepancies between the patient's injury and that studied in the animal model. Heterogeneous levels of injury may preclude identifying a benefit for more strictly defined and homogenous subgroup of patients. More carefully selected subgroups may be more likely to identify a benefit, but have the disadvantage of requiring a longer study time in order to recruit adequate numbers.
- Choice Of Clinical Endpoints. The decision of primary endpoints is critical to demonstrating that a therapeutic intervention is efficacious (Fisher et al., 2001). A major difference between animal and clinical studies is choice of outcome measures. Most animal studies use pathologic endpoints such as number of preserved retinal ganglion cell bodies or axons to classify successful treatment responses. Clinical trials of glaucoma, however, judge efficacy by using imaging or functional outcomes (visual field-VF testing), or both, most often months after the initial insult. However, VF testing is limited by the variability in results, and usually multiple tests are used to reduce the variability and increase specificity. Structural biomarkers in optic nerve and retinal disease include new technologies such as optical coherence tomography which could quantitatively evaluate RGC layers, nerve fiber layer and focal thickness, size of the neuroretinal rim, and number of RGCs or axons. Such tools may provide an endpoint

that potentially can be used in both preclinical and clinical studies. However, significant research needs to be carried out to determine how changes in these parameters correlate with visual function and whether they can be used as a surrogate for visual outcome.

4. Conclusion

Glaucoma is a multifactorial disease in which multiple factors interact to precipitate the disease. Various genes and pathways are involved in glaucoma pathophysiology. Incidentally, a recent report has identified a potential regulatory network operating in astrocyte-mediated neurotoxicity in cases of glaucomatous neurodegeneration (Nikolskaya et al., 2009). Their data on genetics, gene expression and proteomics provide a more detail network of genes involved in glaucomatous neurodegeneration and have led to the identification of some key network hubs involved in astrocytes-mediated neurotoxicity in glaucoma. Their analyses have also indicated the involvement of the immune system, oxidative stress, alteration of the extracellular matrix structure and glutamate excitotoxicity in glaucomatous neurodegeneration. Moreover, it was found that over two thirds of the genes linked to glaucoma by genetic analysis can be functionally interconnected into one epistatic network via experimentally-validated interactions. It is more obvious now that it is very hard to inhibit glaucomatous damage by inhibiting one particular pathophysiologic mechanism. It is becoming clear that novel neuroprotectants should be characterized by multiple modes of actions targeting key biological network modules. Along these lines, combinations of medications with different mechanisms of action are more likely to produce better results with fewer adverse effects. Thus, a multidrug approach may be useful, which includes agents targeted toward lowering IOP as well as an agent directed at preserving and protecting the optic nerve from different mechanisms of glaucomatous damage (targeting both cellular energy metabolism and excitoxicity).

Tools such as new imaging technologies have been developed and may be incorporated into studies providing endpoints that potentially can be used in both preclinical and clinical studies. In this way premature initiation of clinical trials could be avoided. Furthermore, development of minimally invasive (subconjunctival injection, eyedrops) biotechnical or prolonged methods of drug delivery might increase the efficiency and safety of neuroprotectants. In addition, intense research in gene therapy has made it an emerging therapeutic possibility in glaucoma management. Intraocular transfer of genes expressing neurotrophic factors or their receptors and antiapoptotic proteins has demonstrated neuroprotective capacity in vivo.

Despite the challenging history of neuroprotectants in various disease states, there is a convincing rationale for the use of neuroprotection as a therapy for glaucoma. Clearly, the concept of neuroprotective agents playing a major role in glaucoma management continues to be an exciting area of research within the glaucoma field. However, a better understanding of the pathophysiological mechanisms involved in glaucoma and better designed randomized clinical trials will undoubtedly lead us to new, safe and effective neuroprotective therapy.

5. References

Aktas, Z., Gurelik, G., Akyurek, N., Onol, M., & Hasanreisoglu, B. (2007). Neuroprotective effect of topically applied brimonidine tartrate 0.2% in endothelin-1-induced optic nerve ischaemia model. *Clinical and Experimental Ophthalmology* Vol.35, No6, pp.527-534, ISSN 1442-6404

Almasieh, M., Zhou, Y., Kelly, M.E., Casanova, C., & Di Polo, A. (2010). Structural and functional neuroprotection in glaucoma: role of galantamine-mediated activation of muscarinic acetylcholine receptors. *Cell Death and Disease* Vol.1, No.2, pp.e27, ISSN 2041-4889

Ames, A., 3rd, Li, Y.Y., Heher, E.C., & Kimble, C.R. (1992). Energy metabolism of rabbit retina as related to function: high cost of Na+ transport. *Journal of Neuroscience* Vol.12, No.3, pp.840-853, ISSN 0270-6474

Bai, Y., Xu, J., Brahimi, F., Zhuo, Y., Sarunic, M.V., & Saragovi, H.U. (2010). An agonistic TrkB mAb causes sustained TrkB activation, delays RGC death, and protects the retinal structure in optic nerve axotomy and in glaucoma. *Investigative Ophthalmology & Visual Science* Vol.51, No.9, pp.4722-4731, ISSN 0146-0404

Bakalash, S., Kessler, A., Mizrahi, T., Nussenblatt, R., & Schwartz, M. (2003). Antigenic specificity of immunoprotective therapeutic vaccination for glaucoma. *Investigative Ophthalmology & Visual Science* Vol.44, No.8, pp.3374-3381, ISSN 0146-0404

Baltmr, A., Duggan, J., Nizari, S., Salt, T.E., & Cordeiro, M.F. (2010). Neuroprotection in glaucoma - Is there a future role? *Experimental Eye Research* Vol.91, No.5, pp.554-566, ISSN 0014-4835

Beal, M.F. (2003). Bioenergetic approaches for neuroprotection in Parkinson's disease. *Annals of Neurology* Vol.53 No.Suppl 3, pp.S39-47; discussion S47-38, ISSN 0364-5134

Becker, B., Stamper, R.L., Asseff, C., & Podos, S.M. (1972). Effect of diphenylhydantoin on glaucomatous field loss: a preliminary report. *Transactions - American Academy of Ophthalmololgy and Otolaryngology* Vol.76, No.2, pp.412-422, ISSN 0002-7154

Bender, A., Auer, D.P., Merl, T., Reilmann, R., Saemann, P., Yassouridis, A., Bender, J., Weindl, A., Dose, M., Gasser, T., *et al.* (2005). Creatine supplementation lowers brain glutamate levels in Huntington's disease. *Journal of Neurology* Vol.252, No. 1, pp.36-41, ISSN 0340-5354

Berkelaar, M., Clarke, D.B., Wang, Y.C., Bray, G.M., & Aguayo, A.J. (1994). Axotomy results in delayed death and apoptosis of retinal ganglion cells in adult rats. *Journal of Neuroscience* Vol.14, No.7, pp.4368-4374, ISSN 1813-1948

Bosco, A., Inman, D.M., Steele, M.R., Wu, G., Soto, I., Marsh-Armstrong, N., Hubbard, W.C., Calkins, D.J., Horner, P.J., & Vetter, M.L. (2008). Reduced retina microglial activation and improved optic nerve integrity with minocycline treatment in the DBA/2J mouse model of glaucoma. *Investigative Ophthalmology & Visual Science* Vol.49, No.4, pp.1437-1446, ISSN 0146-0404

Brdiczka, D., & Wallimann, T. (1994). The importance of the outer mitochondrial compartment in regulation of energy metabolism. *Molecular and Cellular Biochemistry* Vol.133-134, pp.69-83, ISSN 0300-8177

Broderick, R., & Somlyo, A.P. (1987). Calcium and magnesium transport by in situ mitochondria: electron probe analysis of vascular smooth muscle. *Circulation Research* Vol.61, No.4, pp.523-530, ISSN 0009-7330

Casson, R.J. (2006). Possible role of excitotoxicity in the pathogenesis of glaucoma. *Clinical & Experimental Ophthalmology* Vol.34, No.1, pp.54-63, ISSN 1442-6404

Chen, H.S., & Lipton, S.A. (1997). Mechanism of memantine block of NMDA-activated channels in rat retinal ganglion cells: uncompetitive antagonism. The *Journal of Physiology* Vol.499 No.Pt 1, pp.27-46, ISSN 0022-3751

Cheng, L., Sapieha, P., Kittlerova, P., Hauswirth, W.W., & Di Polo, A. (2002). TrkB gene transfer protects retinal ganglion cells from axotomy-induced death in vivo. *The Journal of Neuroscience* Vol.22, No.10, pp.3977-3986, ISSN 0270-6474

Cheung, W., Guo, L., & Cordeiro, M.F. (2008). Neuroprotection in glaucoma: drug-based approaches. *Optometry and Vision Science* Vol.85, No.6, pp.406-416, ISSN 1040-5488

Cheung, Z.H., So, K.F., Lu, Q., Yip, H.K., Wu, W., Shan, J.J., Pang, P.K., & Chen, C.F. (2002). Enhanced survival and regeneration of axotomized retinal ganglion cells by a mixture of herbal extracts. *Journal of Neurotrauma* Vol.19, No.3, pp.369-378, ISSN 0897-7151

Chiu, K., Yeung, S.C., So, K.F., & Chang, R.C. (2010). Modulation of morphological changes of microglia and neuroprotection by monocyte chemoattractant protein-1 in experimental glaucoma. *Cellular & Moecular Immunology* Vol.7, No.1, pp.61-68, ISSN 1672-7681

Chung, H.S., Harris, A., Kristinsson, J.K., Ciulla, T.A., Kagemann, C., & Ritch, R. (1999). Ginkgo biloba extract increases ocular blood flow velocity. *Journal of Ocular Pharmacology and Therapeutics* Vol.15, No.3, pp.233-240, ISSN 1080-7683

Collaborative Normal-Tension Glaucoma Study Group. (1998a). Comparison of glaucomatous progression between untreated patients with normal-tension glaucoma and patients with therapeutically reduced intraocular pressures. *American Journal of Ophthalmology* Vol.126, No.4, pp.487-497, ISSN 0002-9394

Collaborative Normal-Tension Glaucoma Study Group. (1998b). The effectiveness of intraocular pressure reduction in the treatment of normal-tension glaucoma. *American Journal of Ophthalmology* Vol.126, No.4, pp. 498-505, ISSN 0002-9394

Crompton, M. (1999). The mitochondrial permeability transition pore and its role in cell death. *The Biochemical Journal Vol.341, No.Pt 2, pp.*233-249, ISSN 0264-6021

Crompton, M., Virji, S., Doyle, V., Johnson, N., & Ward, J.M. (1999). The mitochondrial permeability transition pore. *Biochemical Society Symposium* Vol.66, pp.167-179, ISSN 0067-8694

Danesh-Meyer, H.V., & Levin, L.A. (2009). Neuroprotection: extrapolating from neurologic diseases to the eye. *American Journal of Ophthalmology* Vol.148, No.2, pp.186-191 e182, ISSN 0002-9394

Danylkova, N.O., Alcala, S.R., Pomeranz, H.D., & McLoon, L.K. (2007). Neuroprotective effects of brimonidine treatment in a rodent model of ischemic optic neuropathy. *Experimental Eye Research* Vol.*84*, No.2, pp.293-301, ISSN 0014-4835

Di Polo, A., Aigner, L.J., Dunn, R.J., Bray, G.M., & Aguayo, A.J. (1998). Prolonged delivery of brain-derived neurotrophic factor by adenovirus-infected Muller cells temporarily rescues injured retinal ganglion cells. *Proceedings of the National Academy of Sciences of the United States of America* Vol.95, No.7, pp.3978-3983, ISSN 0027-8424

Dong, C.J., Guo, Y., Agey, P., Wheeler, L., & Hare, W.A. (2008). Alpha2 adrenergic modulation of NMDA receptor function as a major mechanism of RGC protection in experimental glaucoma and retinal excitotoxicity. *Investigative Ophthalmology & Visual Science Vol.49*, No.10, pp.4515-4522, ISSN 0146-0404

Dreyer, E.B., Zurakowski, D., Schumer, R.A., Podos, S.M., & Lipton, S.A. (1996). Elevated glutamate levels in the vitreous body of humans and monkeys with glaucoma. *Archives of Ophthalmology* Vol.114, No.3, pp.299-305, ISSN 0003-9950

Dubal, D.B., Zhu, H., Yu, J., Rau, S.W., Shughrue, P.J., Merchenthaler, I., Kindy, M.S., & Wise, P.M. (2001). Estrogen receptor alpha, not beta, is a critical link in estradiol-mediated protection against brain injury. *Proceedings of the National Academy of Sciences of the United States of America* Vol.98, No.4, pp.1952-1957, ISSN 0027-8424

Ettaiche, M., Fillacier, K., Widmann, C., Heurteaux, C., & Lazdunski, M. (1999). Riluzole improves functional recovery after ischemia in the rat retina. *Investigative Ophthalmology and Visual Science* Vol.40, No.3, pp.729-736, ISSN 0146-0404

Fang, J.H., Wang, X.H., Xu, Z.R., & Jiang, F.G. (2010). Neuroprotective effects of bis(7)-tacrine against glutamate-induced retinal ganglion cells damage. *BMC Neuroscience* Vol.11, pp.31, ISSN 1471-2202

Finkel, T., & Holbrook, N.J. (2000). Oxidants, oxidative stress and the biology of ageing. *Nature* Vol.408, No.6809, pp.239-247, ISSN 0028-0836

Fisher M., UMass/Memorial Health Care (1999). Recommendations for standards regarding preclinical neuroprotective and restorative drug development. *Stroke* Vol.30, No.12, pp.2752-2758, ISSN 0039-2499

Fisher M., MD, UMass/Memorial Health Care (2001). Recommendations for clinical trial evaluation of acute stroke therapies. *Stroke* Vol.32, No.7, pp.1598-1606, ISSN 0039-2499

Flammer, J., Haefliger, I.O., Orgul, S., & Resink, T. (1999). Vascular dysregulation: a principal risk factor for glaucomatous damage? *Journal of Glaucoma Vol. 8*, No.3, pp.212-219, ISSN 1057-0829

Flammer, J., Orgul, S., Costa, V.P., Orzalesi, N., Krieglstein, G.K., Serra, L.M., Renard, J.P., & Stefansson, E. (2002). The impact of ocular blood flow in glaucoma. *Progress in Retinal and Eye Research* Vol.21, No.4, pp.359-393, ISSN 1350-9462

Fontaine, V., Mohand-Said, S., Hanoteau, N., Fuchs, C., Pfizenmaier, K., & Eisel, U. (2002). Neurodegenerative and neuroprotective effects of tumor Necrosis factor (TNF) in retinal ischemia: opposite roles of TNF receptor 1 and TNF receptor 2. *The Journal of Neuroscience* Vol.22, No.7, pp.RC216, ISSN 0270-6474

Fu, Q.L., Hu, B., Wu, W., Pepinsky, R.B., Mi, S., & So, K.F. (2008a). Blocking LINGO-1 function promotes retinal ganglion cell survival following ocular hypertension and optic nerve transection. *Investigative Ophthalmology & Visual Science* Vol.49, No.3, pp.975-985, ISSN 0146-0404

Fu, Q.L., Wu, W., Wang, H., Li, X., Lee, V.W., & So, K.F. (2008b). Up-regulated endogenous erythropoietin/erythropoietin receptor system and exogenous erythropoietin rescue retinal ganglion cells after chronic ocular hypertension. *Cellular and Molecular Neurobiology* Vol.28, No.2, pp.317-329, ISSN 0272-4340

Gandolfi, S.A., Cimino, L., & Mora, P. (2003). Effect of brimonidine on intraocular pressure in normal tension glaucoma: a short term clinical trial. *European Journal of Ophthalmology* Vol.13, No.7, pp.611-615, ISSN 1120-6721

Greenfield, D.S., & Bagga, H. (2005). Clinical variables associated with glaucomatous injury in eyes with large optic disc cupping. *Ophthalmic Surgery, Lasers & Imaging* Vol.36, No.5, pp.401-409, ISSN 1542-8877

Grus, F.H., Joachim, S.C., Wuenschig, D., Rieck, J., & Pfeiffer, N. (2008). Autoimmunity and glaucoma. *Journal of Glaucoma* Vol.17, No.1, pp.79-84, ISSN 1057-0829

Guo, L., Moss, S.E., Alexander, R.A., Ali, R.R., Fitzke, F.W., & Cordeiro, M.F. (2005). Retinal ganglion cell apoptosis in glaucoma is related to intraocular pressure and IOP-induced effects on extracellular matrix. *Investigative Ophthalmology & Visual Science* Vol.46, No.1, pp.175-182, ISSN 0146-0404

Guo, L., Salt, T.E., Luong, V., Wood, N., Cheung, W., Maass, A., Ferrari, G., Russo-Marie, F., Sillito, A.M., Cheetham, M.E., *et al.* (2007). Targeting amyloid-beta in glaucoma treatment. *Proceedings of the National Academy of Sciences of the United States of America* Vol.104, No.33, pp.13444-13449, ISSN 0027-8424

Guo, L., Salt, T.E., Maass, A., Luong, V., Moss, S.E., Fitzke, F.W., & Cordeiro, M.F. (2006). Assessment of neuroprotective effects of glutamate modulation on glaucoma-related retinal ganglion cell apoptosis in vivo. *Investigative Ophthalmology & Visual Science* Vol.47, No.2, pp.626-633, ISSN 0146-0404

Gupta, N., Ang, L.C., Noel de Tilly, L., Bidaisee, L., & Yucel, Y.H. (2006). Human glaucoma and neural degeneration in intracranial optic nerve, lateral geniculate nucleus, and visual cortex. *The British Journal of Ophthalmology* Vol.90, No.6, pp.674-678, ISSN 0007-1161

Gupta, N., Fong, J., Ang, L.C., &Yucel, Y.H. (2008). Retinal tau pathology in human glaucomas. *Canadian Journal of Ophthalmology* Vol.43, No.1, pp.53-60, ISSN 0008-4182

Gupta, N., Greenberg, G., de Tilly, L.N., Gray, B., Polemidiotis, M., & Yucel, Y.H. (2009). Atrophy of the lateral geniculate nucleus in human glaucoma detected by magnetic resonance imaging. *The British Journal of Ophthalmology* Vol.93, No.1, pp.56-60, ISSN 0007-1161

Gupta, N., & Yucel, Y.H. (2001). Glaucoma and the brain. *Journal of Glaucoma* Vol.10, No.5 Suppl 1, pp.S28-29, ISSN 1057-0829

Hashizume, K., Mashima, Y., Fumayama, T., Ohtake, Y., Kimura, I., Yoshida, K., Ishikawa, K., Yasuda, N., Fujimaki, T., Asaoka, R., *et al.* (2005). Genetic polymorphisms in the angiotensin II receptor gene and their association with open-angle glaucoma in a Japanese population. *Investigative Ophthalmology & Visual Science* Vol.46, No.6, pp.1993-2001, ISSN 0146-0404

Hayreh, S.S., March, W., & Anderson, D.R. (1979). Pathogenesis of block of rapid orthograde axonal transport by elevated intraocular pressure. *Experimental Eye Research* Vol.28, No.5, pp.515-523, ISSN 0014-4835

Heijl, A., Leske, M.C., Bengtsson, B., Hyman, L., Bengtsson, B., & Hussein, M. (2002). Reduction of intraocular pressure and glaucoma progression: results from the Early Manifest Glaucoma Trial. *Archives of Ophthalmology* Vol.120, No.10, pp.1268-1279, ISSN 0003-9950

Hernandez, M., Urcola, J.H., & Vecino, E. (2008). Retinal ganglion cell neuroprotection in a rat model of glaucoma following brimonidine, latanoprost or combined treatments. *Experimental Eye Research 86*, 798-806, ISSN 0014-4835

Hirooka, K., Baba, T., Fujimura, T., & Shiraga, F. (2006). Prevention of visual field defect progression with angiotensin-converting enzyme inhibitor in eyes with normal-tension glaucoma. *American Journal of Ophthalmology* Vol.142, No.3, pp.523-525, ISSN 0002-9394

Hirooka, K., Tokuda, M., Miyamoto, O., Itano, T., Baba, T., & Shiraga, F. (2004). The Ginkgo biloba extract (EGb 761) provides a neuroprotective effect on retinal ganglion cells in a rat model of chronic glaucoma. *Current Eye Research* Vol.28, No.3, pp.153-157, ISSN0271-3683

Hoffman, G.E., Merchenthaler, I., & Zup, S.L. (2006). Neuroprotection by ovarian hormones in animal models of neurological disease. *Endocrine* Vol.29, No.2, pp.217-231, ISSN 1355-008X

Howell, G.R., Libby, R.T., Jakobs, T.C., Smith, R.S., Phalan, F.C., Barter, J.W., Barbay, J.M., Marchant, J.K., Mahesh, N., Porciatti, V., *et al.* (2007). Axons of retinal ganglion cells are insulted in the optic nerve early in DBA/2J glaucoma. *The Journal of Cell Biology* Vol.179, No.7, pp.1523-1537, ISSN 0021-9525

Husain, S., Liou, G.I., & Crosson, C.E. (2011). Opioid-Receptor-Activation: Suppression of Ischemia/Reperfusion-Induced Production of TNF-{alpha} in the Retina. *Investigative Ophthalmology & Visual Science,* Feb 4. [Epub ahead of print], ISSN 0146-0404

Ishii, Y., Kwong, J.M., & Caprioli, J. (2003). Retinal ganglion cell protection with geranylgeranylacetone, a heat shock protein inducer, in a rat glaucoma model. *Investigative Ophthalmology & Visual Science* Vol.44, No.5, pp.1982-1992, ISSN 0146-0404

Ishikawa, H., Takano, M., Matsumoto, N., Sawada, H., Ide, C., Mimura, O., & Dezawa, M. (2005). Effect of GDNF gene transfer into axotomized retinal ganglion cells using in vivo electroporation with a contact lens-type electrode. *Gene Therapy* Vol.12, No4. pp.289-298, ISSN 0969-7128

Izzotti, A., Bagnis, A., & Sacca, S.C. (2006). The role of oxidative stress in glaucoma. *Mutation Research* Vol.612, No.2, pp.105-114, ISSN 0027-5107

Ji, D., Li, G.Y., & Osborne, N.N. (2008). Nicotinamide attenuates retinal ischemia and light insults to neurones. *Neurochemistry International* Vol.52, No.4-5, pp.786-798, ISSN 0197-0186

Ji, J.Z., Elyaman, W., Yip, H.K., Lee, V.W., Yick, L.W., Hugon, J., & So, K.F. (2004). CNTF promotes survival of retinal ganglion cells after induction of ocular hypertension in rats: the possible involvement of STAT3 pathway. *The European Journal of Neuroscience* Vol.19, No.2, pp.265-272, ISSN 0953-816X

Johnson, E.C., Deppmeier, L.M., Wentzien, S.K., Hsu, I., & Morrison, J.C. (2000). Chronology of optic nerve head and retinal responses to elevated intraocular pressure. *Investigative Ophthalmology & Visual Science* Vol.41, No.2, pp.431-442, ISSN 0146-0404

Johnson, J.W., & Ascher, P. (1987). Glycine potentiates the NMDA response in cultured mouse brain neurons. *Nature* Vol.325, No.6104, pp.529-531, ISSN 0028-0836

Johnson, L.V., Leitner, W.P., Rivest, A.J., Staples, M.K., Radeke, M.J., & Anderson, D.H. (2002). The Alzheimer's A beta -peptide is deposited at sites of complement activation in pathologic deposits associated with aging and age-related macular degeneration. *Proceedings of the National Academy of Sciences of the United States of America* Vol.99, No.18, pp.11830-11835, ISSN 0027-8424

Ju, W.K., Kim, K.Y., Angert, M., Duong-Polk, K.X., Lindsey, J.D., Ellisman, M.H., & Weinreb, R.N. (2009). Memantine blocks mitochondrial OPA1 and cytochrome c release and subsequent apoptotic cell death in glaucomatous retina. *Investigative Ophthalmology & Visual Science* Vol.50, No.2, pp.707-716, ISSN 0146-0404

Ju, W.K., Kim, K.Y., Lindsey, J.D., Angert, M., Duong-Polk, K.X., Scott, R.T., Kim, J.J., Kukhmazov, I., Ellisman, M.H., Perkins, G.A., *et al.* (2008). Intraocular pressure elevation induces mitochondrial fission and triggers OPA1 release in glaucomatous optic nerve. *Investigative Ophthalmology & Visual Science* Vol.49, No.11, pp.4903-4911, ISSN 0146-0404

Kass, M.A., Heuer, D.K., Higginbotham, E.J., Johnson, C.A., Keltner, J.L., Miller, J.P., Parrish, R.K., 2nd, Wilson, M.R., & Gordon, M.O. (2002). The Ocular Hypertension Treatment Study: a randomized trial determines that topical ocular hypotensive medication delays or prevents the onset of primary open-angle glaucoma. *Archives of Ophthalmology* Vol.120, No.6, pp.701-713; discussion 829-730, ISSN 0003-9950

Khan, N., Huang, J.J., & Foster, C.S. (2006). Cancer associated retinopathy (CAR): An autoimmune-mediated paraneoplastic syndrome. *Seminars in Ophthalmology* Vol.21, No.3, pp.135-141, ISSN 0882-0538

Khoury, R., Cross, J.M., Girkin, C.A., Owsley, C., & McGwin, G., Jr. (2009). The association between self-reported glaucoma and ginkgo biloba use. *Journal of Glaucoma* Vol.18, No.7, pp.543-545, ISSN 1057-0829

Kipnis, J., Yoles, E., Porat, Z., Cohen, A., Mor, F., Sela, M., Cohen, I.R., & Schwartz, M. (2000). T cell immunity to copolymer 1 confers neuroprotection on the damaged optic nerve: possible therapy for optic neuropathies. *Proceedings of the National Academy of Sciences of the United States of America* Vol.97, No.13, pp.7446-7451, ISSN 0027-8424

Kitsos, G., Zikou, A.K., Bagli, E., Kosta, P., & Argyropoulou, M.I. (2009). Conventional MRI and magnetisation transfer imaging of the brain and optic pathway in primary open-angle glaucoma. *The British Journal of Radiology* Vol.82, No.983, pp.896-900, ISSN 0007-1285

Ko, M.L., Hu, D.N., Ritch, R., Sharma, S.C., & Chen, C.F. (2001). Patterns of retinal ganglion cell survival after brain-derived neurotrophic factor administration in hypertensive eyes of rats. *Neuroscience Letters* Vol.305, No.2, pp.139-142, ISSN 0167-6253

Kobayashi, K., Kobayashi, H., Ueda, M., & Honda, Y. (1998). Estrogen receptor expression in bovine and rat retinas. *Investigative Ophthalmology & Visual Science* Vol.39, No.11, pp.2105-2110, ISSN 0146-0404

Koeberle, P.D., & Ball, A.K. (2002). Neurturin enhances the survival of axotomized retinal ganglion cells in vivo: combined effects with glial cell line-derived neurotrophic factor and brain-derived neurotrophic factor. *Neuroscience* Vol.110, No.3, pp.555-567.

Kroemer, G., Galluzzi, L., & Brenner, C. (2007). Mitochondrial membrane permeabilization in cell death. *Physiological Reviews* Vol.87, No.1, pp.99-163, ISSN 0031-9333

Krupin, T., Liebmann, J.M., Greenfield, D.S., Rosenberg, L.F., Ritch, R., & Yang, J.W. (2005). The Low-pressure Glaucoma Treatment Study (LoGTS) study design and baseline characteristics of enrolled patients. *Ophthalmology* Vol.112, No.3, pp.376-385, ISSN 0161-6420

Kuehn, M.H., Kim, C.Y., Ostojic, J., Bellin, M., Alward, W.L., Stone, E.M., Sakaguchi, D.S., Grozdanic, S.D., & Kwon, Y.H. (2006). Retinal synthesis and deposition of complement components induced by ocular hypertension. *Experimental Eye Research* Vol.83, No.3, pp.620-628, ISSN 0014-4835

Lagreze, W.A., Knorle, R., Bach, M., & Feuerstein, T.J. (1998). Memantine is neuroprotective in a rat model of pressure-induced retinal ischemia. *Investigative Ophthalmology & Visual Science* Vol.39, No.6, pp.1063-1066, ISSN 0146-0404

Lai, R.K., Chun, T., Hasson, D., Lee, S., Mehrbod, F., & Wheeler, L. (2002). Alpha-2 adrenoceptor agonist protects retinal function after acute retinal ischemic injury in the rat. *Visual Neuroscience* Vol.19, No.2, pp.175-185, ISSN 0952-5238

Lambiase, A., Aloe, L., Centofanti, M., Parisi, V., Mantelli, F., Colafrancesco, V., Manni, G.L., Bucci, M.G., Bonini, S., & Levi-Montalcini, R. (2009). Experimental and clinical evidence of neuroprotection by nerve growth factor eye drops: Implications for glaucoma. *Proceedings of the National Academy of Sciences of the United States of America* Vol.106, 13469-13474, ISSN 0027-8424

Lensman, M., Korzhevskii, D.E., Mourovets, V.O., Kostkin, V.B., Izvarina, N., Perasso, L., Gandolfo, C., Otellin, V.A., Polenov, S.A., & Balestrino, M. (2006). Intracerebroventricular administration of creatine protects against damage by global cerebral ischemia in rat. *Brain Research* Vol.1114, No.1, pp.187-194, ISSN 0006-8993

Leske, M.C., Heijl, A., Hussein, M., Bengtsson, B., Hyman, L., & Komaroff, E. (2003). Factors for glaucoma progression and the effect of treatment: the early manifest glaucoma trial. *Archives of Ophthalmology* Vol.121, No.1, pp.48-56, ISSN 0003-9950

Levkovitch-Verbin, H., Harris-Cerruti, C., Groner, Y., Wheeler, L.A., Schwartz, M., a&Yoles, E. (2000). RGC death in mice after optic nerve crush injury: oxidative stress and neuroprotection. *Investigative Ophthalmology & Visual Science* Vol.41, No.13, pp.4169-4174, ISSN 0146-0404

Lipton, S.A. (1993). Prospects for clinically tolerated NMDA antagonists: open-channel blockers and alternative redox states of nitric oxide. *Trends in Neurosciences* Vol.16, No.12, pp.527-532, ISSN 0166-2236

Lipton, S.A., Choi, Y.B., Pan, Z.H., Lei, S.Z., Chen, H.S., Sucher, N.J., Loscalzo, J., Singel, D.J., & Stamler, J.S. (1993). A redox-based mechanism for the neuroprotective and neurodestructive effects of nitric oxide and related nitroso-compounds. *Nature* Vol.364, No.6438, pp.626-632, ISSN 0028-0836

Lipton, S.A., & Rosenberg, P.A. (1994). Excitatory amino acids as a final common pathway for neurologic disorders. *The New England Journal of Medicine* Vol.330, No.9, pp.613-622, ISSN 0028-4793

Mahadevan, S., & Park, Y. (2008). Multifaceted therapeutic benefits of Ginkgo biloba L.: chemistry, efficacy, safety, and uses. *Journal of Food Science* Vol.73, No.1, pp.R14-19, ISSN 0022-1147

Maier, K., Merkler, D., Gerber, J., Taheri, N., Kuhnert, A.V., Williams, S.K., Neusch, C., Bahr, M., & Diem, R. (2007). Multiple neuroprotective mechanisms of minocycline in autoimmune CNS inflammation. *Neurobiology of Disease* Vol.25, No.3, pp.514-525, ISSN 0969-9961

Mansour-Robaey, S., Clarke, D.B., Wang, Y.C., Bray, G.M., & Aguayo, A.J. (1994). Effects of ocular injury and administration of brain-derived neurotrophic factor on survival and regrowth of axotomized retinal ganglion cells. *Proceedings of the National*

Academy of Sciences of the United States of America Vol.91, No.5, pp.1632-1636, ISSN 0027-8424

Martin, D., Thompson, M.A., & Nadler, J.V. (1993). The neuroprotective agent riluzole inhibits release of glutamate and aspartate from slices of hippocampal area CA1. *European Journal of Pharmacology* Vol.250, No.3, pp.473-476, ISSN 0014-2999

Martin, K.R., Quigley, H.A., Zack, D.J., Levkovitch-Verbin, H., Kielczewski, J., Valenta, D., Baumrind, L., Pease, M.E., Klein, R.L., & Hauswirth, W.W. (2003). Gene therapy with brain-derived neurotrophic factor as a protection: retinal ganglion cells in a rat glaucoma model. *Investigative Ophthalmology & Visual Science* Vol.44, No.10, pp.4357-4365, ISSN 0146-0404

McKinnon, S.J., Lehman, D.M., Tahzib, N.G., Ransom, N.L., Reitsamer, H.A., Liston, P., LaCasse, E., Li, Q., Korneluk, R.G., & Hauswirth, W.W. (2002). Baculoviral IAP repeat-containing-4 protects optic nerve axons in a rat glaucoma model. *Molecular Therapy* Vol.5, No.6, pp.780-787, ISSN 1525-0016

Mosinger, J.L., Price, M.T., Bai, H.Y., Xiao, H., Wozniak, D.F., & Olney, J.W. (1991). Blockade of both NMDA and non-NMDA receptors is required for optimal protection against ischemic neuronal degeneration in the in vivo adult mammalian retina. *Experimental Neurology* Vol.113, No.1, pp.10-17, ISSN 0196-6383

Mosser, D.D., Caron, A.W., Bourget, L., Meriin, A.B., Sherman, M.Y., Morimoto, R.I., & Massie, B. (2000). The chaperone function of hsp70 is required for protection against stress-induced apoptosis. *Molecular and Cellular Biology* Vol.20, No.19, pp.7146-7159, ISSN 0270-7306

Mozaffarieh, M., Grieshaber, M.C., & Flammer, J. (2008). Oxygen and blood flow: players in the pathogenesis of glaucoma. *Molecular Vision* Vol.14, pp.224-233, ISSN 1090-0535

Nakajima, Y., Inokuchi, Y., Nishi, M., Shimazawa, M., Otsubo, K., & Hara, H. (2008). Coenzyme Q10 protects retinal cells against oxidative stress in vitro and in vivo. *Brain Research* Vol.1226, pp.226-233, ISSN 0006-8993

Nakazawa, T., Nakazawa, C., Matsubara, A., Noda, K., Hisatomi, T., She, H., Michaud, N., Hafezi-Moghadam, A., Miller, J.W., & Benowitz, L.I. (2006a). Tumor necrosis factor-alpha mediates oligodendrocyte death and delayed retinal ganglion cell loss in a mouse model of glaucoma. *The Journal of Neuroscience* Vol.26, No.49, pp.12633-12641, ISSN 0270-6474

Nakazawa, T., Takahashi, H., & Shimura, M. (2006b). Estrogen has a neuroprotective effect on axotomized RGCs through ERK signal transduction pathway. *Brain Research* Vol.1093, No.1, pp. 141-149, ISSN 0006-8993

Neufeld, A.H., & Liu, B. (2003). Comparison of the signal transduction pathways for the induction of gene expression of nitric oxide synthase-2 in response to two different stimuli. *Nitric Oxide* Vol.8, No.2, pp.95-102, ISSN 1089-8603

Nguyen, S.M., Alexejun, C.N., *and* Levin, L.A. (2003). Amplification of a reactive oxygen species signal in axotomized retinal ganglion cells. *Antioxiadants & Redox Signaling* Vol.5, No.5, pp.629-634, ISSN 1523-0864

Nikolskaya, T., Nikolsky, Y., Serebryiskaya, T., Zvereva, S., Sviridov, E., Dezso, Z., Rahkmatulin, E., Brennan, R.J., Yankovsky, N., Bhattacharya, S.K., *et al.* (2009). Network analysis of human glaucomatous optic nerve head astrocytes. *BMC Medical Genomics* Vol.2, pp.24, ISSN 1755-8794

Osborne, N.N. (2008). Pathogenesis of ganglion "cell death" in glaucoma and neuroprotection: focus on ganglion cell axonal mitochondria. *Progress in Brain Research* Vol.173, pp.339-352, ISSN 0079-6123

Osborne, N.N. (2009). Recent clinical findings with memantine should not mean that the idea of neuroprotection in glaucoma is abandoned. *Acta Ophthalmologica* Vol.87, No.4, pp.450-454, ISSN 1755-375X

Palmer, G.C. (2001). Neuroprotection by NMDA receptor antagonists in a variety of neuropathologies. *Current Drug Targets* Vol.2, No.3, pp.241-271, ISSN 1389-4501

Park, K.H., Cozier, F., Ong, O.C., & Caprioli, J. (2001). Induction of heat shock protein 72 protects retinal ganglion cells in a rat glaucoma model. *Investigative Ophthalmology & Visual Science* Vol.42, No.7, pp.1522-1530, ISSN 0146-0404

Pieper, A.A., Verma, A., Zhang, J., & Snyder, S.H. (1999). Poly (ADP-ribose) polymerase, nitric oxide and cell death. *Trends in Pharmacological Sciences* Vol.20, No.4, pp.171-181, ISSN 0165-6147

Pin, J.P., & Duvoisin, R. (1995). The metabotropic glutamate receptors: structure and functions. *Neuropharmacology* Vol.34, No.1, pp.1-26, ISBN 9780716745105

Prass, K., Royl, G., Lindauer, U., Freyer, D., Megow, D., Dirnagl, U., Stockler-Ipsiroglu, G., Wallimann, T., & Priller, J. (2007). Improved reperfusion and neuroprotection by creatine in a mouse model of stroke. *Journal of Cerebral Blood Flow and Metabolism* Vol.27, No.3, pp.452-459, ISSN 0271-678X

Quaranta, L., Bettelli, S., Uva, M.G., Semeraro, F., Turano, R., & Gandolfo, E. (2003). Effect of Ginkgo biloba extract on preexisting visual field damage in normal tension glaucoma. *Ophthalmology* Vol.110, No.2, pp.359-362; discussion 362-354, ISSN 0161-6420

Ray, K., and Mookherjee, S. (2009). Molecular complexity of primary open angle glaucoma: current concepts. *Journal of Genetics* Vol.88, No.4, pp.451-467, ISSN 0022-1333

Reisberg, B., Doody, R., Stoffler, A., Schmitt, F., Ferris, S., & Mobius, H.J. (2003). Memantine in moderate-to-severe Alzheimer's disease. *The New England Journal of Medicine* Vol.348, No.14, pp.1333-1341, ISSN 0028-4793

Rhone, M., & Basu, A. (2008). Phytochemicals and age-related eye diseases. *Nutrition Reviews* Vol.66, No.8, pp.465-472, ISSN 0029-6643

Rudzinski, M., Wong, T.P., & Saragovi, H.U. (2004). Changes in retinal expression of neurotrophins and neurotrophin receptors induced by ocular hypertension. *Journal of Neurobiology* Vol.58, No.3, pp.341-354, ISSN 0022-3034

Salt, T.E., & Cordeiro, M.F. (2006). Glutamate excitotoxicity in glaucoma: throwing the baby out with the bathwater? *Eye* (London, England) Vol.20, No.6, pp.730-731; author reply 731-732, ISSN 0950-222

Santel, A., & Frank, S. (2008). Shaping mitochondria: The complex posttranslational regulation of the mitochondrial fission protein DRP1. *IUBMB Life* Vol.60, No.7, pp.448-455, ISSN 1521-6543

Scheff, S.W., & Dhillon, H.S. (2004). Creatine-enhanced diet alters levels of lactate and free fatty acids after experimental brain injury. *Neurochemical Research* Vol.29, No.2, pp.469-479, ISSN 0364-3190

Schober, M.S., Chidlow, G., Wood, J.P., & Casson, R.J. (2008). Bioenergetic-based neuroprotection and glaucoma. *Clinical and Experimental Ophthalmology* Vol.36, No.4, pp.377-385, ISSN 1442-6404

Schori, H., Kipnis, J., Yoles, E., WoldeMussie, E., Ruiz, G., Wheeler, L.A., & Schwartz, M. (2001). Vaccination for protection of retinal ganglion cells against death from glutamate cytotoxicity and ocular hypertension: implications for glaucoma. *Proceedings of the National Academy of Sciences of the United States of America* Vol.98, No.6, pp.3398-3403, ISSN 0027-8424

Schwartz, M. (2001). T cell mediated neuroprotection is a physiological response to central nervous system insults. *Journal of Molecular Medicine* Vol.78, No.11, pp.594-597, ISSN 0946-2716

Seki, M., Soussou, W., Manabe, S., & Lipton, S.A. (2010). Protection of retinal ganglion cells by caspase substrate-binding peptide IQACRG from N-methyl-D-aspartate receptor-mediated excitotoxicity. *Investigative Ophthalmology & Visual Science* Vol.51, No.2, pp.1198-1207, ISSN 0146-0404

Shimazawa, M., Inokuchi, Y., Okuno, T., Nakajima, Y., Sakaguchi, G., Kato, A., Oku, H., Sugiyama, T., Kudo, T., Ikeda, T., *et al.* (2008). Reduced retinal function in amyloid precursor protein-over-expressing transgenic mice via attenuating glutamate-N-methyl-d-aspartate receptor signaling. *Journal of Neurochemistry* Vol.107, No.1, pp.279-290, ISSN 0022-3042

Sieving, P.A., Caruso, R.C., Tao, W., Coleman, H.R., Thompson, D.J., Fullmer, K.R., & Bush, R.A. (2006). Ciliary neurotrophic factor (CNTF) for human retinal degeneration: phase I trial of CNTF delivered by encapsulated cell intraocular implants. *Proceedings of the National Academy of Sciences of the United States of America* Vol.103, No.10, pp.3896-3901, ISSN 0027-8424

Siu, A.W., Ortiz, G.G., Benitez-King, G., To, C.H., & Reiter, R.J. (2004). Effects of melatonin on the nitric oxide treated retina. *The British Journal of Ophthalmology* Vol.88, No.8, pp.1078-1081, ISSN 0007-1161

Smith, J.R., & Rosenbaum, J.T. (2000). Management of immune-mediated uveitis. *BioDrugs Vol.13*, No.1, pp.9-20, ISSN 1173-8804

Sommer, A., Tielsch, J.M., Katz, J., Quigley, H.A., Gottsch, J.D., Javitt, J., & Singh, K. (1991). Relationship between intraocular pressure and primary open angle glaucoma among white and black Americans. The Baltimore Eye Survey. *Archives of Ophthalmology* Vol.109, No.8, pp.1090-1095, ISSN 0003-9950

Soti, C., Nagy, E., Giricz, Z., Vigh, L., Csermely, P., & Ferdinandy, P. (2005). Heat shock proteins as emerging therapeutic targets. *British Journal Pharmacology* Vol.146, No.6, pp.769-780, ISSN 0007-1188

Sribnick, E.A., Ray, S.K., Nowak, M.W., Li, L., & Banik, N.L. (2004). 17beta-estradiol attenuates glutamate-induced apoptosis and preserves electrophysiologic function in primary cortical neurons. *Journal of Neuroscience Research* Vol.76, No.5, pp.688-696, ISSN 0360-4012

Stasi, K., Nagel, D., Yang, X., Wang, R.F., Ren, L., Podos, S.M., Mittag, T., & Danias, J. (2006). Complement component 1Q (C1Q) upregulation in retina of murine, primate, and human glaucomatous eyes. *Investigative Ophthalmology & Visual Science* Vol.47, No.3, pp.1024-1029, ISSN 0146-0404

Straten, G., Schmeer, C., Kretz, A., Gerhardt, E., Kugler, S., Schulz, J.B., Gravel, C., Bahr, M., & Isenmann, S. (2002). Potential synergistic protection of retinal ganglion cells from axotomy-induced apoptosis by adenoviral administration of glial cell line-derived neurotrophic factor and X-chromosome-linked inhibitor of apoptosis. *Neurobiology of Disease* Vol.11, No.1, pp.123-133, ISSN 0969-9961

Swanson, K.I., Schlieve, C.R., Lieven, C.J., & Levin, L.A. (2005). Neuroprotective effect of sulfhydryl reduction in a rat optic nerve crush model. *Investigative Ophthalmology & Visual Science* Vol.46, No.10, pp.3737-3741, ISSN 0146-0404

Tang, Q., Hu, Y., & Cao, Y. (2006). Neuroprotective effect of melatonin on retinal ganglion cells in rats. *Journal of Huazhong University of Science and Technology Medical Sciences* Vol.26, No.2, pp.235-237, 253, ISSN 1672-0733

Tarnopolsky, M.A., & Beal, M.F. (2001). Potential for creatine and other therapies targeting cellular energy dysfunction in neurological disorders. *Annals of Neurology* Vol.49, No.5, pp.561-574, ISSN 0364-5134

Tatton, W.G., Chalmers-Redman, R.M., Sud, A., Podos, S.M., & Mittag, T.W. (2001). Maintaining mitochondrial membrane impermeability. an opportunity for new therapy in glaucoma? *Survey of Ophthalmology* Vol.45, No.Suppl 3, pp.S277-283; discussuin S295-276, ISSN 0039-6257

Tezel, G. (2006). Oxidative stress in glaucomatous neurodegeneration: mechanisms and consequences. *Progress in Retinal and Eye Research* Vol.25, No.5, pp.490-513, ISSN 1350-9462

Tezel, G., Chauhan, B.C., LeBlanc, R.P., & Wax, M.B. (2003). Immunohistochemical assessment of the glial mitogen-activated protein kinase activation in glaucoma. *Investigative Ophthalmology & Visual Science* Vol.44, No.7, pp.3025-3033, ISSN 0146-0404

Tezel, G., Hernandez, R., & Wax, M.B. (2000). Immunostaining of heat shock proteins in the retina and optic nerve head of normal and glaucomatous eyes. *Archives of Ophthalmology* Vol.118, No.4, pp.511-518, ISSN 0003-9950

Tezel, G., Li, L.Y., Patil, R.V., & Wax, M.B. (2001). TNF-alpha and TNF-alpha receptor-1 in the retina of normal and glaucomatous eyes. *Investigative Ophthalmology & Visual Science* Vol.42, No.8, pp.1787-1794, ISSN 0146-0404

Tezel, G., Seigel, G.M., & Wax, M.B. (1998). Autoantibodies to small heat shock proteins in glaucoma. *Investigative Ophthalmology & Visual Science* Vol.39, No.12, pp.2277-2287, ISSN 0146-0404

Tezel, G. & Wax, M.B. (2000a). Increased production of tumor necrosis factor-alpha by glial cells exposed to simulated ischemia or elevated hydrostatic pressure induces apoptosis in cocultured retinal ganglion cells. *The Journal of Neuroscience* Vol.20, No.23, pp.8693-8700, ISSN 0270-6474

Tezel, G., & Wax, M.B. (2000b). The mechanisms of hsp27 antibody-mediated apoptosis in retinal neuronal cells. *The Journal of Neuroscience* Vol.20, No.10, pp.3552-3562, ISSN 0270-6474

Tezel, G., & Wax, M.B. (2007). Glaucoma. *Chemical Immunology and Allergy* Vol.92, pp.221-227, ISSN 1660-2242

Tezel, G., & Yang, X. (2004). Caspase-independent component of retinal ganglion cell death, in vitro. *Investigative Ophthalmology & Visual Science* Vol.45, No.11, pp.4049-4059, ISSN 0146-0404

Tezel, G., Yang, X., & Cai, J. (2005). Proteomic identification of oxidatively modified retinal proteins in a chronic pressure-induced rat model of glaucoma. *Investigative Ophthalmology & Visual Science* Vol.46, No.9, pp.3177-3187, ISSN 0146-0404

Tezel, G., Yang, X., Luo, C., Peng, Y., Sun, S.L., & Sun, D. (2007). Mechanisms of immune system activation in glaucoma: oxidative stress-stimulated antigen presentation by the retina and optic nerve head glia. *Investigative Ophthalmology & Visual Science* Vol.48, No.2, pp.705-714, ISSN 0146-0404

Tezel, G., Yang, X., Yang, J., & Wax, M.B. (2004). Role of tumor necrosis factor receptor-1 in the death of retinal ganglion cells following optic nerve crush injury in mice. *Brain Research* Vol.996, No.2, pp.202-212, ISSN 0006-8993

Thiagarajan, G., Chandani, S., Harinarayana Rao, S., Samuni, A.M., Chandrasekaran, K., & Balasubramanian, D. (2002). Molecular and cellular assessment of ginkgo biloba extract as a possible ophthalmic drug. *Experimental Eye Research* Vol.75, No.4, pp.421-430, ISSN 0014-4835

Thoreson, W.B., & Witkovsky, P. (1999). Glutamate receptors and circuits in the vertebrate retina. *Progress in Retinal and Eye Research* Vol.18, No.6, pp.765-810, ISSN 1350-9462

Tulsawani, R., Kelly, L.S., Fatma, N., Chhunchha, B., Kubo, E., Kumar, A., & Singh, D.P. (2010). Neuroprotective effect of peroxiredoxin 6 against hypoxia-induced retinal ganglion cell damage. *BMC Neuroscience* Vol.11, pp.125, ISSN 1471-2202

van Adel, B.A., Arnold, J.M., Phipps, J., Doering, L.C., & Ball, A.K. (2005). Ciliary neurotrophic factor protects retinal ganglion cells from axotomy-induced apoptosis via modulation of retinal glia in vivo. *Journal of Neurobiology* Vol.63, No.3, pp.215-234, ISSN 0022-3034

Walland, M.J., Carassa, R.G., Goldberg, I., Grehn, F., Heuer, D.K., Khaw, P.T., Thomas, R., & Parikh, R. (2006). Failure of medical therapy despite normal intraocular pressure. *Clinical & Experimental Ophthalmology* Vol.34, No.9, pp.827-836, ISSN 1442-6404

Wallimann, T., & Hemmer, W. (1994). Creatine kinase in non-muscle tissues and cells. *Molecular and Cellular Biochemistry* Vol.133-134, pp.193-220, ISSN 0300-8177

Wang, W.H., McNatt, L.G., Pang, I.H., Hellberg, P.E., Fingert, J.H., McCartney, M.D., & Clark, A.F. (2008). Increased expression of serum amyloid A in glaucoma and its effect on intraocular pressure. *Investigative Ophthalmology & Visual Science* Vol.49, No.5, pp.1916-1923, ISSN 0146-0404

Ward, M.S., Khoobehi, A., Lavik, E.B., Langer, R., & Young, M.J. (2007). Neuroprotection of retinal ganglion cells in DBA/2J mice with GDNF-loaded biodegradable microspheres. *Journal of Pharmaceutical Sciences* Vol.96, No.3, pp.558-568, ISSN 0022-3549

Wax, M.B., Tezel, G., Yang, J., Peng, G., Patil, R.V., Agarwal, N., Sappington, R.M., & Calkins, D.J. (2008). Induced autoimmunity to heat shock proteins elicits glaucomatous loss of retinal ganglion cell neurons via activated T-cell-derived fas-ligand. *The Journal of Neuroscience* Vol.28, No.46, pp.12085-12096, ISSN 0270-6474

Wen, R., Cheng, T., Li, Y., Cao, W., & Steinberg, R.H. (1996). Alpha 2-adrenergic agonists induce basic fibroblast growth factor expression in photoreceptors in vivo and ameliorate light damage. *The Journal of Neuroscience* Vol.16, No.19, pp.5986-5992, ISSN 0270-6474

Wheeler, L.A., Gil, D.W., & WoldeMussie, E. (2001). Role of alpha-2 adrenergic receptors in neuroprotection and glaucoma. *Survey of Ophthalmology* Vol.45 No.Suppl 3, pp.S290-294; discussion S295-296, ISSN 0039-6257

Whitmore, A.V., Libby, R.T., & John, S.W. (2005). Glaucoma: thinking in new ways-a role for autonomous axonal self-destruction and other compartmentalised processes? *Progress in Retinal and Eye Research* Vol.24, No.6, pp.639-662, ISSN 1350-9462

Xu, C.J., Klunk, W.E., Kanfer, J.N., Xiong, Q., Miller, G., & Pettegrew, J.W. (1996). Phosphocreatine-dependent glutamate uptake by synaptic vesicles. A comparison with atp-dependent glutamate uptake. *The Journal of Biological Chemistry* Vol.271, No.123, pp.13435-13440, ISSN 0021-9258

Yan, Q., Wang, J., Matheson, C.R., & Urich, J.L. (1999). Glial cell line-derived neurotrophic factor (GDNF) promotes the survival of axotomized retinal ganglion cells in adult rats: comparison to and combination with brain-derived neurotrophic factor (BDNF). *Journal of Neurobiology* Vol.38, No.5, pp.382-390, ISSN 0022-3034

Yancheva, S., Ihl, R., Nikolova, G., Panayotov, P., Schlaefke, S., & Hoerr, R. (2009). Ginkgo biloba extract EGb 761(R), donepezil or both combined in the treatment of Alzheimer's disease with neuropsychiatric features: a randomised, double-blind, exploratory trial. *Aging & Mental Health* Vol.13, No.2, pp.183-190, ISSN 1360-7863

Yang, H., Hirooka, K., Fukuda, K., & Shiraga, F. (2009). Neuroprotective effects of angiotensin II type 1 receptor blocker in a rat model of chronic glaucoma. *Investigative Ophthalmology & Visual Science* Vol.50, No.12, pp.5800-5804, ISSN 0146-0404

Yang, J., Yang, P., Tezel, G., Patil, R.V., Hernandez, M.R., & Wax, M.B. (2001). Induction of HLA-DR expression in human lamina cribrosa astrocytes by cytokines and simulated ischemia. *Investigative Ophthalmology & Visual Science* Vol. 42, No.2, pp.365-371, ISSN 0146-0404

Yoneda, S., Tanaka, E., Goto, W., Ota, T., & Hara, H. (2003). Topiramate reduces excitotoxic and ischemic injury in the rat retina. *Brain Research* Vol.967, No.1-2, pp.257-266, ISSN 0006-8993

Yucel, Y.H., Gupta, N., Zhang, Q., Mizisin, A.P., Kalichman, M.W., & Weinreb, R.N. (2006). Memantine protects neurons from shrinkage in the lateral geniculate nucleus in experimental glaucoma. *Archives of Ophthalmology* Vol.124, No.2, pp.217-225, ISSN 0003-9950

Yucel, Y.H., Zhang, Q., Weinreb, R.N., Kaufman, P.L., & Gupta, N. (2001). Atrophy of relay neurons in magno- and parvocellular layers in the lateral geniculate nucleus in experimental glaucoma. *Investigative Ophthalmology & Visual Science* Vol.42, No.13. pp.3216-3222, ISSN 0146-0404

Zeevalk, G.D., & Nicklas, W.J. (1992). Evidence that the loss of the voltage-dependent Mg2+ block at the N-methyl-D-aspartate receptor underlies receptor activation during inhibition of neuronal metabolism. *Journal of Neurochemistry* Vol.59, No.4, pp.1211-1220, ISSN 0022-3042

Part 2

Optic Nerve Head and Nerve Fiber Layer

7

The Optic Nerve in Glaucoma

Ivan Marjanovic
University Eye clinic, Clinical Centre of Serbia
Belgrade

1. Introduction

To recognize and to assess glaucomatous changes at the optic nerve, it is important to know the characteristics of the normal optic disc. As in the other biological variables, the appearance of the optic disc varies widely among healthy individuals. This fact is complicate the recognition of the pathological changes.

'Optic Disc' is frequently used to describe the portion of the optic nerve clinically visible on examination. This, however, may be slightly inaccurate as 'disc' implies a flat, 2 dimensional structure without depth, when in fact the 'optic nerve head' is very much a 3 dimensional structure which should ideally be viewed stereoscopically.

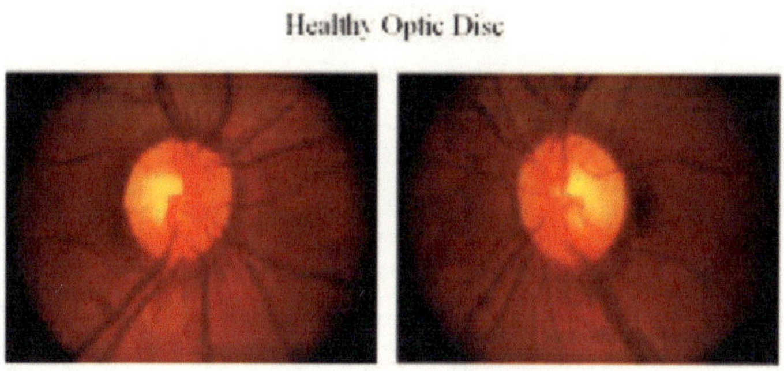

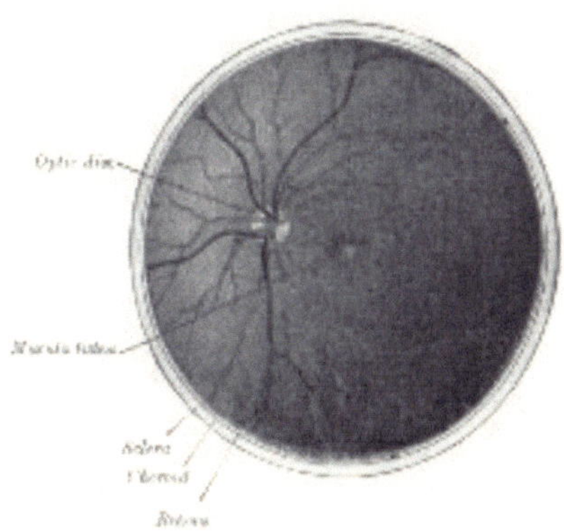

Fig. 1. Posterior part of the left eye. The veins are darker in appearance than the arteries.

The optic nerve itself is a cylindrical structure of approximately 50mm in length, between the retina and the optic chiasm. This can be divided into 4 main parts:

1. Intraocular (the optic nerve head)
2. Intraorbital (between globe and optic canal)
3. Intracanalicular (within the optic canal)
4. Intracranial (between optic canal and chiasm)

The optic nerve head, or disc, is defined as the distal portion of the optic nerve extending from the myelinated portion of nerve that begins just behind the sclera, to the retinal surface. Typically, it is slightly oval with the vertical diameter being about 9% greater than the horizontal. On average the vertical disc diameter is approximately 1500 micrometers, although this may be greater in a myopic eye and less in a hypermetropic eye.

This can also be divided into 4 component parts:

1. Superficial nerve fibre layer - contiguous with the nerve fibre layer of the retina
2. Prelaminar area - consists of nerve fibre bundles and astroglia, which form sheaths around each bundle
3. Laminar (Scleral) portion - contains a modification of sclera called the Lamina Cribrosa. This is made up of sheets of connective and elastic tissue, and contains fenestrations which give passage to the nerve fibre bundles and retinal blood vessels. It also serves to maintain intra-ocular pressure (IOP) against a gradient between the intra-ocular and extra-ocular spaces.
4. Retrolaminar portion - myelinated nerve fibres, circumscribed by leptomeninges of the CNS.[1]

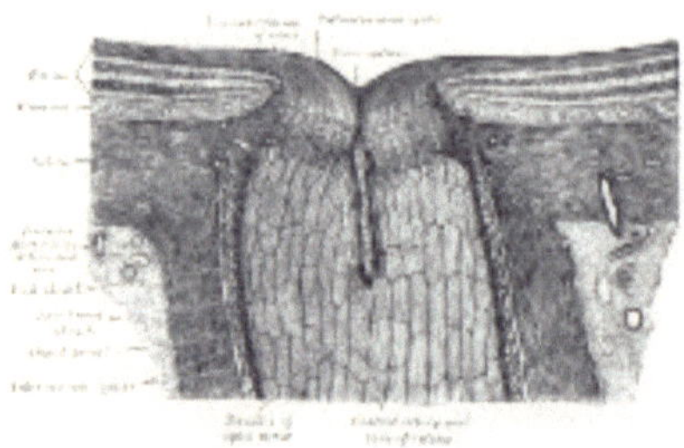

Fig. 2. The terminal portion of the optic nerve and its entrance into the eyeball, in horizontal section.

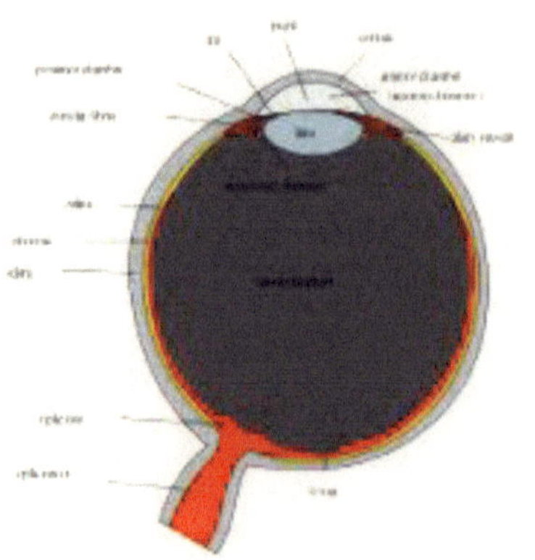

Fig. 3. Schematic diagram of the human eye, with the optical disc, or blind spot, at the bottom.

Optic Disc Basic Examination

When assessing a disc for glaucoma there are many subtle characteristics which should be examined. There are also various ways to examine the optic disc.
For an assessment of the optic disc, there is "the 3 Cs" rule- the cup, colour and contour.

The Contour

The borders of the optic disc should be clear and well defined. If not one becomes concerned that the disc may be swollen such as in the case of papilloedema - disc swelling secondary to raised intracranial pressure. Alternatively, the disc margins may appear blurred due to presence of optic disc drusen.

The Colour

Typically the optic disc looks like an orange-pink donut with a pale centre. The orange-pink appearance represents healthy, well perfused neuro-retinal tissue. There are many pathological reasons why a disc may lose this orange-pink colour and appear pale ie optic atrophy. These include advanced glaucoma, optic neuritis, arteritic or non-arteritic ischaemic optic neuropathy or a compressive lesion.
The causes of an optic neuropathy can be remembered by **NIGHT TIC**:
Neuritis
Ischaemic
Granulomatous
Hereditory
Traumatic
Toxic
Irradiation
Compression

The Cup

The disc has an orange-pink rim with a pale centre. This pale centre is devoid of neuroretinal tissue and is called the cup. The vertical size of this cup can be estimated in relation to the disc as a whole and presented as a "cup to disc ratio". A cup to disc ratio of 0.3 (i.e. the cup occupies 1/3 of the height of the entire disc) is generally considered normal, and an increased cup to disc ratio may indicate a decrease in the quantity of healthy neuro-retinal tissue and hence, glaucomatous change.

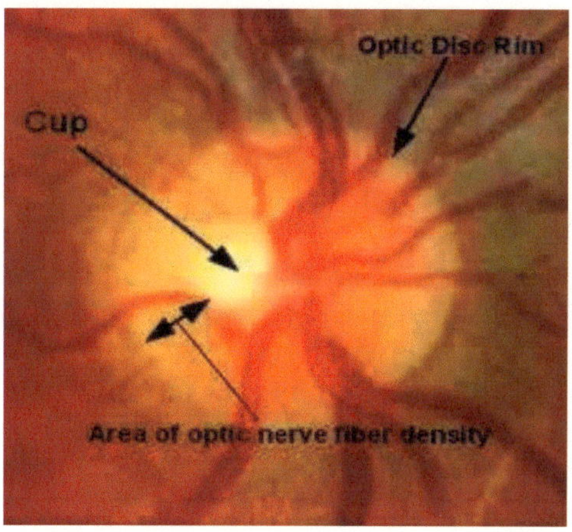

The optic disc (or optic disk optic nerve head, optic papilla or blind spot) is the location where ganglion cell axons exit the eye to form the optic nerve. There are no light sensitive rods or cones to respond to a light stimulus at this point thus it is also known as "the blind spot". A blind spot, also known as a scotoma, is an obscuration of the visual field. A particular blind spot known as the blind spot, or physiological blind spot, is the specific scotoma in the visual field that corresponds to the lack of light-detecting photoreceptor cells on the optic disc. Since there are no cells to detect light on the optic disc, a part of the field of vision is not perceived. The brain fills in with surrounding detail and with information from the other eye, so the blind spot is not normally perceived.[2]

2. The glaucomatous optic disc and glaucomatous cupping

Considering that the axons of the retinal ganglion cells are lost, changes occur in the structural appearance of the retinal nerve fiber layer and optic nerve head that often precede the development of visual field defects. The most important characteristics of the glaucomatous process are changes that occur in the optic nerve. Therefore, it is important for the ophthalmologist to be familiar with the characteristic signs of glaucoma in the optic disc.

The optic disc cupping has been recognized as an important characteristic of the glaucomatous process since the 19th Century. Quantification of the size of the cup and its relationship to the size of the optic disc, i.e the cup/disc (C/D) ratio, has been widely used in the differentiation of glaucomatous from normal eyes. Vertical elongation of the cup is a characteristic feature of glaucomatous optic neuropathy and the vertical C/D ratio is a simple indicator of neuroretinal rim loss that can be assessed in clinical practice without the use of sophisticated techniques or devices.[1]

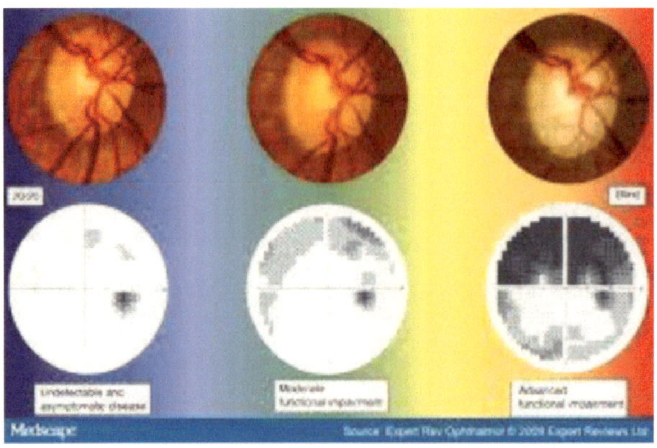

Fig. 4. Glaucomatous disc progression and corresponding VF defects.

The diagnosis of primary open angle glaucoma (POAG) is traditionally based on the triad of increased intraocular pressure(IOP),visual field changes and optic nerve head changes. It is well established that IOP is only a risk factor, albeit, the only risk factor that can be therapeutically manipulated. The fact that upto 50% of POAG patients can present with normal IOP[2] makes it imperative that the diagnosis of POAG be made independent of IOP increase. Occurance of arcuate nerve fibre bundle visual field defects has been taken as the sine qua non for the diagnosis of POAG. Studies by Quigley et al have shown that upto 40%

of the axons could be lost before a visual field defect develops on Goldmann perimetry and that 20% of axons are lost before a 5 db loss is detected on standard automated perimetry.[3] The current research efforts in the early "preperimetric glaucoma" diagnosis are aimed either at psychological tests or alterations in the optic nerve head morphology as assesed by scanning laser ophthalmoscope, digital image processing of optic nerve head images or optical coherence tomography.[4,5] While these advanced technologies are relevant in glaucoma diagnosis and research, they are not practical in routine clinical practice.
With some training it is possible to clinically evaluate the optic nerve head stereoscopically and detect early glaucomatous disc damage.

Features of glaucomatous disc damage

Cup-disc ratio

Cup to disc ratio greater than 0.5:1 is the most often reported sign of glaucomatous disc damage. In a given disc with a cup-disc ratio of more than 0.5:1, it is important to establish if the cup-disc ratio has been large from the onset (large physiological cup) or if it increased over a period of time. Increase in the cup-disc ratio (or enlargement of the cup) over a period of time is diagnostic of glaucomatous disc damage even in the absence of visual field defect. This definitive sign has practical limitation because one time diagnosis is not possible and followup over a period of time is neccesary. The physiological variability of the cup-disc ratio ocurs because of the large variation in the normal optic nerve head size.[1]
Though the normal optic nerve head size is reported to be 1.5 mm in diameter it can vary from 0.96 mm to 2.91 mm.[6] As a result, the physiological cup can be as small as 0.1:1 or as large as 0.8:1.

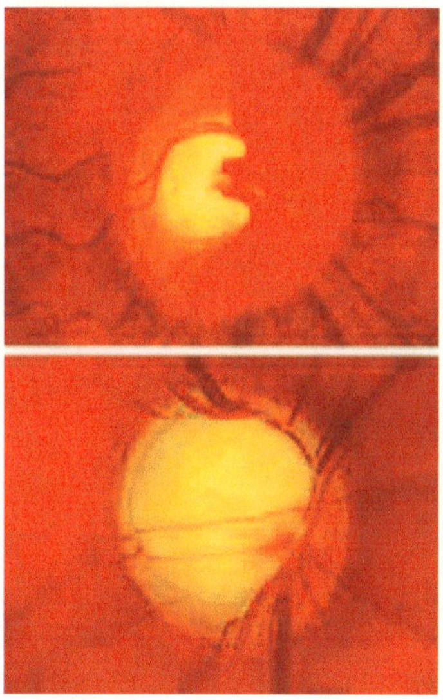

Fig. 5. Glaucomatous optic disc progression.

Neuroretinal Rim Evaluation

Loss of axons in glaucoma is reflected as abnormalities of the neuroretinal rim. Normally the rim is widest in the inferior temporal sector, followed by the superior temporal sector, the nasal and the temporal horizontal sector.[7] Since localised field defects restricted to one hemisphere are an early sign of glaucoma, stereoscopic examination of the neuroretinal rim in the superior and inferior poles comparing carefully their thickness, pallor and notching can aid in the diagnosis of very early glaucomatous damage.

Contour Cupping vs Colour Cupping

To asses the width of the neuroretinal rim, the edge of the cup has to be clearly delineated, the usual temptation is to equate the central pallor of the disc with cup, but atleast in some glaucomatous discs there is a discrepancy between the extent of central pallor (colour cup) and the site at which the vessels change their contour (contour cup). In the evaluation of glaucomatous disc damage it is the contour cup that is of relevance and not the colour cup.[1]

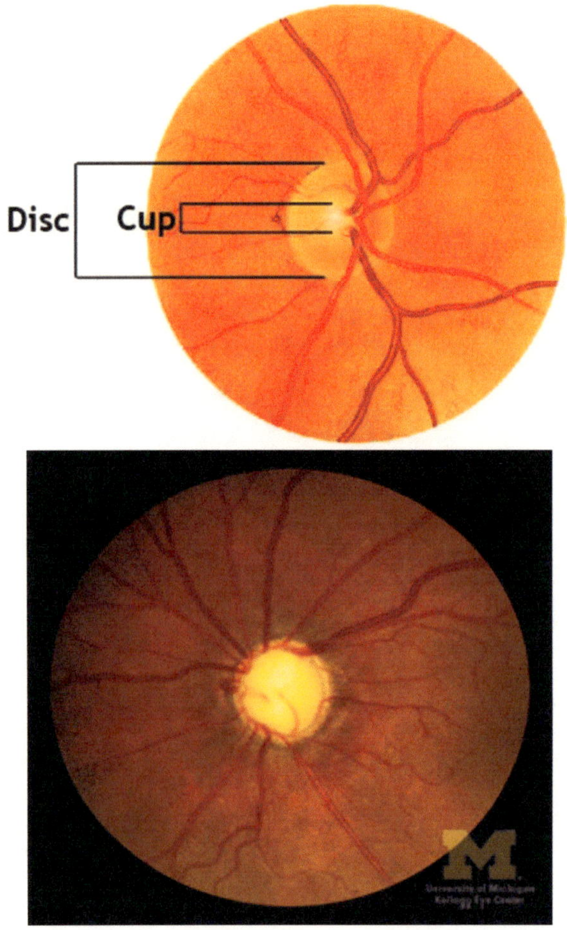

Fig. 6. Right: Cup/Disc ratio; Left: Glaucomatous cupping, change of colour and contour.

Myopic Changes vs Glaucoma

Myopic disc can cause difficulties in glaucomatous disc evaluation either because of the oblique entry resulting in tilted disc or because of the peripapillary changes. A myopic disc the glaucomatous damage is not obvious. The inferior peripapillary atrophy results in a wrong estimation of the extent of the cup as this is mistaken for a part of the disc.

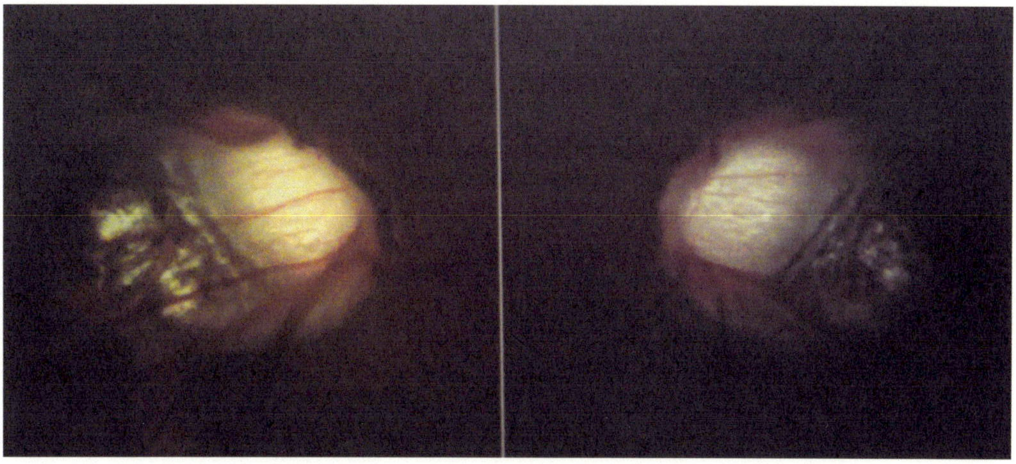

Fig. 7. Degenerative myopic changes of the optic disc.

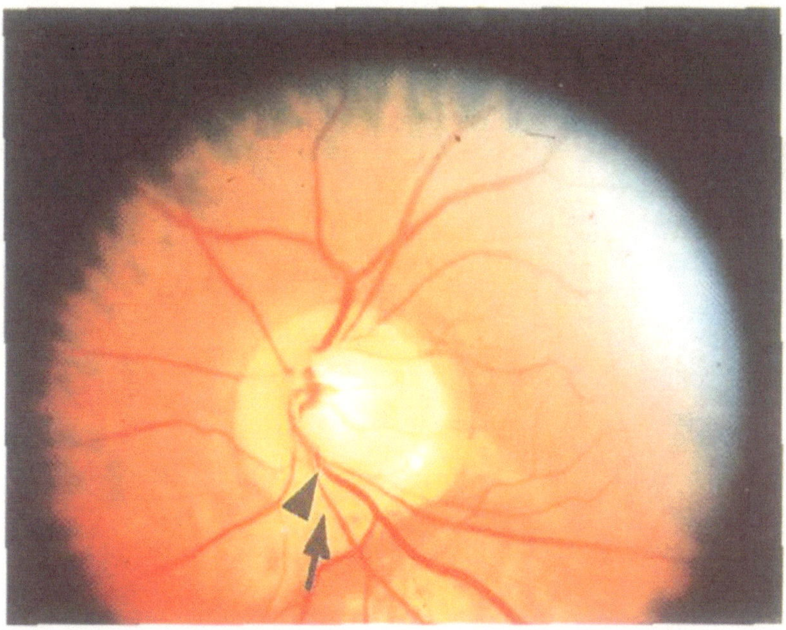

Fig. 8. A myopic disc with peripapillary atrophy(arrow) which can be confused as a part of the disc, resulting in missing of the inferior notch (arrowhead) which shows the edge of the disc where the vessel is changing contour.

Careful evaluation reveals the edge of the disc to be more central with a change in vessel contour at the edge of the disc revealing the inferior notch. The corresponding superior field defect.

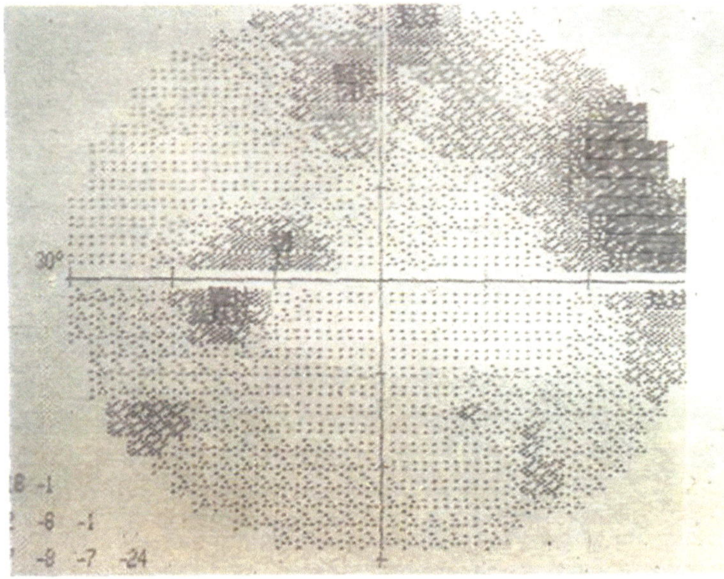

Fig. 9. Superior paracentral scotoma corresponding to the disc shown on previous photo.

Peripapillary Changes

Acquired peripapillary atrophy has been described to be secondary to glaucomatous disc damage. Some authorities feel such changes may predispose to glaucomatous damage.

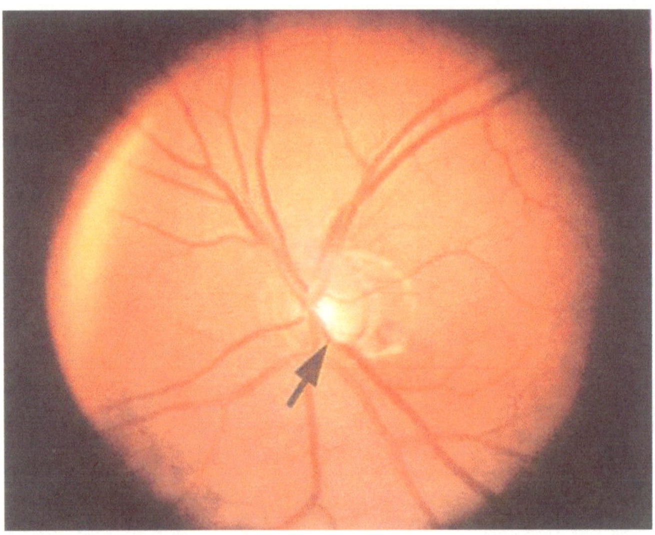

Fig. 10. Glaucomatous cupping in a small disc. Cup size is small but the inferior notch(arrow) indicated by the change in contour of the infero-temporal vessel is typical.

The zone closer to the optic nerve head with retinal pigment epithelial (RPE) and choroidal atrophy with sclera showing through is called zone- β. The more peripheral zone with only RPE atrophy is called zone- α. Since these changes could be seen in myopia also appearance of these changes de-novo or their occurrence in small discs or non myopic eyes is more suggestive of glaucomatous disc damage. A correlation between the location of disc haemorrhage and location of peripapillary atrophy has been reported. If this is so, peripapillary atrophy could be a more reliable and permanent marker for progression than disc hemorrhages.[8]

Nerve Fibre Layer (NFL) Changes

NFL atrophy is associated with a high risk for field loss. Localised defects are the easiest to detect and may be very specific to differentiate early glaucoma from normal eyes. While they occur in 10 to 20% of ocular hypertensive eyes they must be looked for in every glaucoma suspect as the high specificity is clinically useful in identifying patients with impending or established perimetric loss.

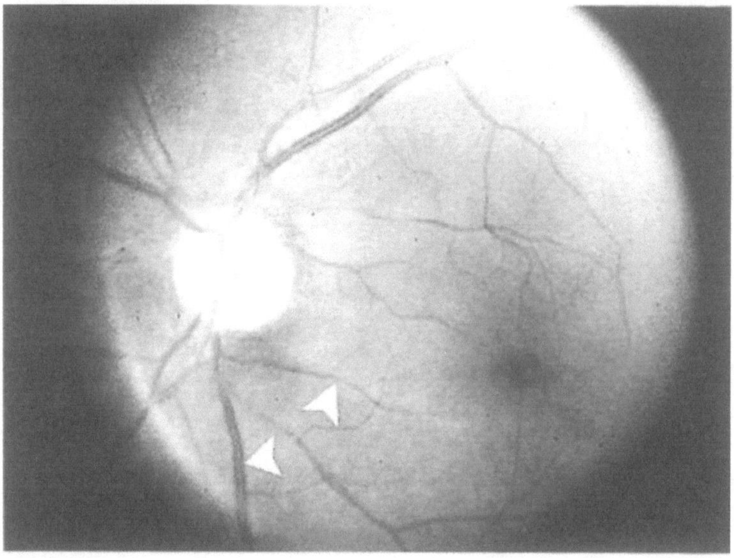

Fig. 11. Red free disc photo showing NFL loss in the inferior arcuate area (arrowheads).

Differential diagnosis

A large physiological cup. If one takes care to asses the neuroretinal rim carefully and measures the optic nerve head size, one can be reasonably sure of a large physiological cup in a large disc.

Congenital colobomas of the optic nerve head are some times easy to diagnose because of the morning glory appearance or other associated colobomas. Optic nerve pit and conus of the disc can some times cause diagnostic difficulties.

Pallor disproportionate to cupping, normal intraocular pressure or unusual history of onset, progression and age should arouse suspicion of a neurological cause for the disc changes and appropriate investigations should be carried out. Photo shows cupping and pallor secondary to pituitary tumour which was mistaken for glaucoma. Also the correspoding temporal hemianopia is shown.

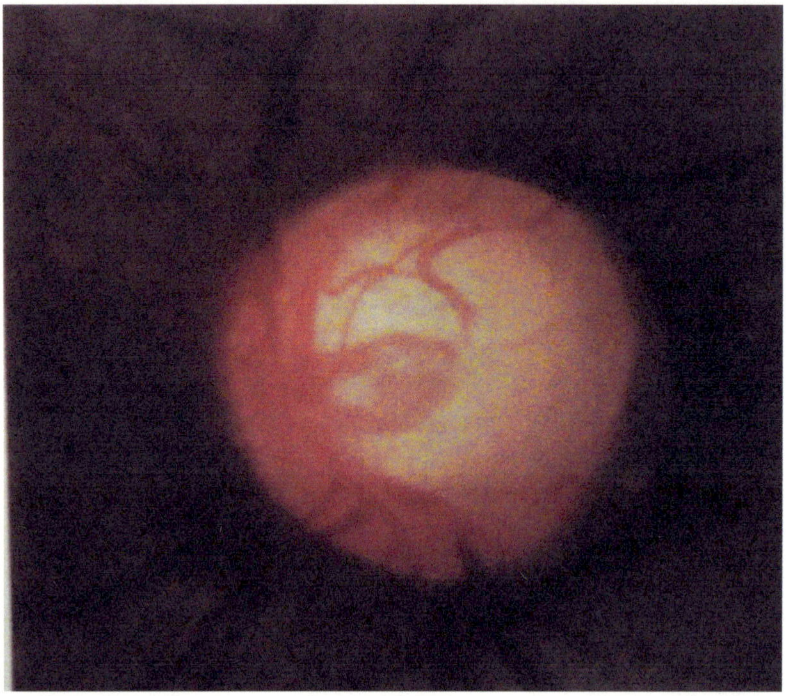

Fig. 12. A Large left optic disc.

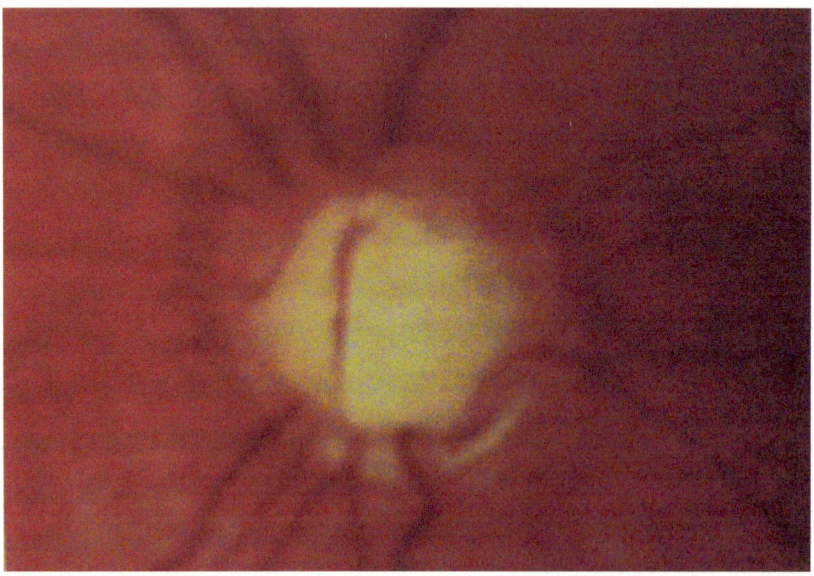

Fig. 13. An Optic disc coloboma.

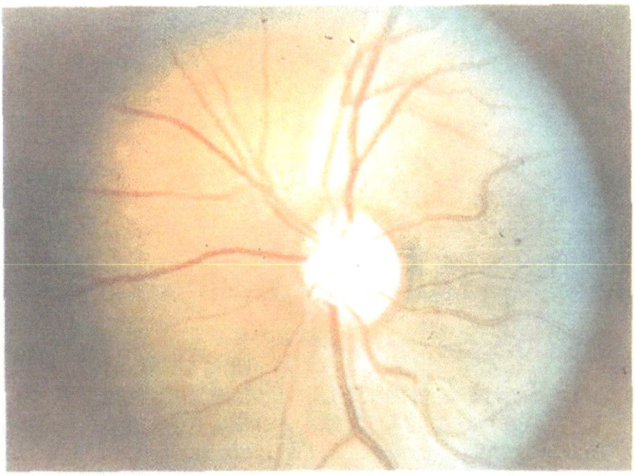

Fig. 14. Cupping of the optic disc and pallor secondary to pituitary tumor.

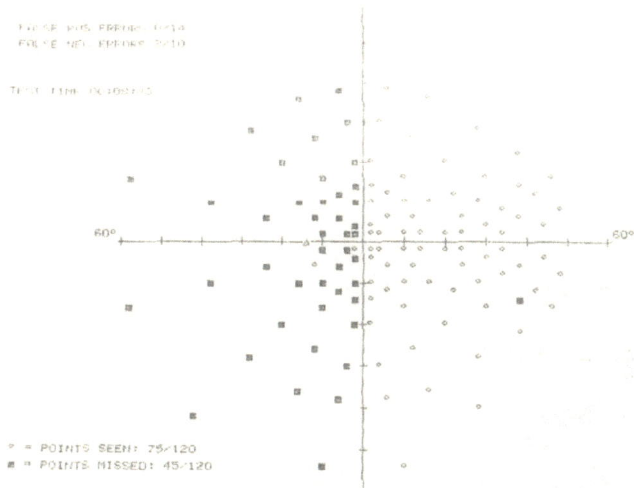

Fig. 15. Temporal hemianopsia corresponding to the disc changes shown in previous photo.

Evaluation tehniques

The most important points in clinical evaluation of the Optic nerve head are a stereoscopic view with magnification for proper evaluation of the neuroretinal rim changes and an estimation of the optic nerve head size.

Stereoscopic view of the optic nerve head is possible by indirect ophthalmoscopy, central part of goniolens, Hruby lens and Volk 90, 78 and 60 D lenses. Indirect ophthalmoscopy is inappropriate for assesement of the optic disc in glaucoma. I prefer the Volk lens systems. While the 78D lens provides a good balance between the field of view and magnification, the 60D lens can make measurement of optic nerve head size simple.

With one of these lenses and slitlamp with redfree light source, it is possible to asses the NFL abnormalities also, though specialised NFL photography systems are more sensitive. Use of direct ophthalmoscope in serious glaucomatous disc evaluation is to be discouraged.

Clinical estimation of optic nerve head size is possible with a Welsch Allen Ophthalmoscope or with Volk 60D lens. The smallest white round spot of the Welsch Allen ophthalmoscope usually illuminates a cone angle of 5° and casts a light of 1.5 mm in diameter on the retina.[9] This retinal spot size remains constant in phakic eyes with refractive errors between -5.00 D and + 4.00 D.

The location of the originating point of the light cone does not significantly affect the retinal spot size as long as it is ± 3mm from the anterior focal point of the patient's eye. Since 1.5 mm is the usual size of the optic nerve head, this can be used as a yard stick for measuring disc size. Simplistically, in eyes with large physiological cups due to large discs the area illuminated is less than the area occupied by the cup.

Disc diameter can be measured by adjusting the slitlamp beam height to the edges of the disc while viewing the disc with a 60 D lens.7 This measurement is roughly equal to the measurement obtained by planimetry of disc photos with Littmann's correction.

A similar measurement of the vertical and horizontal disc diameter can be obtained with other lenses by multiplying the measured value with the appropriate magnification factor: Goldmann contact lens (1.26) and Volk superfield lens (1.5).[7]

It is useful to get habituated to a routine pattern of examination of the disc and look sequentially for findings as follows:

1. Overall impression of the disc
2. Size and shape of the disc
3. Evaluation of the neuroretinal rim keeping in mind the variability of its thickness in various zones mentioned in the text and also look for notch and neuroretinal rim haemorrhage.
4. Peripappillary atrophy
5. Nerve fibre layer abnormalities
6. Vertical cup-disc ratio and asymmetry.

Stereoscopic evaluation of the optic nerve head with emphasis on changes of the neuro retinal rim and not estimation of cup-disc ratio will aid in early diagnosis of glaucoma.

3. Neuroretinal rim loss and retinal nerve fiber layer (RNFL) defects

Examination of the neuroretinal rim is therefore of fundamental importance for the identification of glaucomatous damage to the optic nerve, and its changes are closely related to those occurring in the optic disc cup.[1]

The neuroretinal rim is the intrapapillary equivalent of the retinal nerve fiber layer, and qualitative and quantitative changes in this structure reflect the nerve fiber loss that occurs in glaucoma.

Glaucoma is a progressive optic neuropathy that is accompanied by typical changes in the visual field.[2] Progressive neuroretinal rim thinning, increased excavation, and diffuse and localized loss of the retinal nerve fiber layer are all recognizable features of structural damage in the disease.[3] However, their precise relationship with functional deterioration in patients with glaucoma remains largely unclear.[4-8]

Regulatory agencies throughout the world generally have not approved structural assessment of the optic nerve as a primary end point in clinical trials of glaucoma drugs and devices.[9] The Food and Drug Administration has suggested the need to demonstrate that structural measures are predictive of clinically relevant functional outcomes in patients with glaucoma before they can reliably be used as end points in clinical trials. Currently acceptable end points according to the Food and Drug Administration include only intraocular pressure (IOP) and methods for assessment of visual function, such as standard automated perimetry (SAP). However, IOP is only a surrogate for clinically relevant outcomes in glaucoma and its relationship with disease progression is certainly imperfect.[10-12] Also, although assessment of visual function is critically important for all patients with glaucoma, there is evidence to suggest that many patients may show evidence of progressive optic disc damage before functional loss is detected by SAP. Both the Ocular Hypertension Treatment Study[13] and the European Glaucoma Prevention Study[14] demonstrated that a substantial proportion of patients with ocular hypertension who developed glaucoma showed a change first in optic disc photographs. However, despite being included as end points for glaucoma conversion in these studies, progressive optic disc damage has not yet been demonstrated to translate into worse clinically relevant outcomes for these patients.

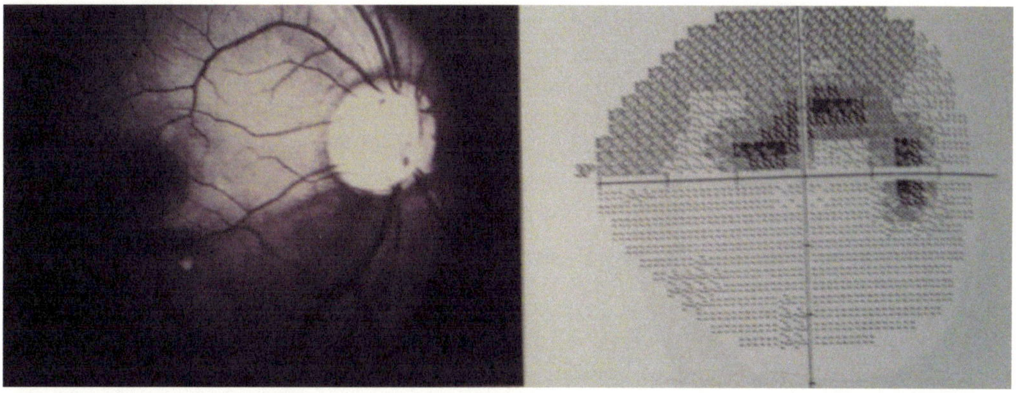

Fig. 16. NFL defect in glaucoma. Left: inferior NFL wedge defect; Right: corresponding superior visual field defect.

Previous investigations have shown that cross-sectional baseline structural measurements, either by expert assessment of stereophotographs or objective imaging methods, are predictive of future development of visual field loss in those with suspected glaucoma, suggesting a potential role for these measurements in early detection of disease.[15-21] However, measures of predictive ability reported in these studies have generally indicated a low accuracy of cross-sectional structural measures for predicting individual functional outcomes. This is likely due to the wide variation in the appearance of the optic nerve, which makes it difficult to identify early signs of disease at one time. Although detection of progressive optic disc change over time is likely to be a more specific indicator of the presence of structural damage from glaucoma and to correlate better with functional outcomes, the ability of progressive optic disc change in predicting functional outcomes in patients with glaucoma has not been elucidated. The purpose of this study was to evaluate the value of progressive optic disc damage detected by expert assessment of longitudinal stereophotographs in predicting future development of visual field loss in suspected glaucoma.

At times when pre-perimetric diagnosis of glaucoma is the goal, the search for the subtle signs of damage in the NFL is of utmost importance. Retinal nerve fiber layer defects have been shown to be among the earliest signs of glaucomatous damage, and they can indeed precede visual field defects.[22,23] They are especially helpful for early glaucoma diagnosis and in eyes with small optic disks. The localized wedge-shaped defect of the NFL is usually seen in association with notching of the neuroretinal rim, vertical enlargement of the cup, or following disk hemorrhages. Nevertheless, in early glaucoma, bundle defects in the NFL may not be associated with neuroretinal rim thinning because the initial damaged NFL is located in the deep retinal layers. Hence, typical wedge-shaped defects can be found in disks with normal appearance.[24-26] Since NFL defects are not present in normal eyes, they always indicate an abnormality. Although typically occurring in about 20% of all eyes with glaucoma, they are not pathognomonic and can also be found in other ocular diseases, such as optic disk drusen, ischemic retinopathies with cotton-wool spots, toxoplasmotic retinochoroidal scars, long-standing papilledema, or optic neuritis due to multiple sclerosis. The incidence is higher in normal-tension glaucoma than in the other forms, which makes the differential diagnosis somewhat difficult. Some authors have shown that NFL defects may be a common finding in diabetic patients with early diabetic retinopathy, and one of the risk factors is concomitant high blood pressure.[27] Retinal nerve fiber layer thickness has been found to decrease with the development of diabetic retinopathy and with impairment of metabolic regulation.[28] Cotton-wool spots are frequently a feature of systemic arteriolar disease, most commonly hypertension, diabetes, and collagen vascular disease; they represent infarcts at the nerve fiber layer. Cotton-wool spots have been described to be followed in some patients by localized NFL defects, with and without associated visual field defect.[29,30]

4. Peripapillary atrophy and optic disc haemorrhage

Glaucoma structural diagnosis has been focused on the optic disc and the peripapillary retinal nerve fiber layer (RNFL). Objective and quantitative assessment of the optic disc and the peripapillary RNFL is useful both in glaucoma diagnosis and monitoring of disease progression.[1-3]

Evaluation of the glaucoma optic neuropathy may be done by direct or indirect ophthalmoscopy of the optic nerve, optic nerve photography, or computerized imaging technologies. Clinical features of glaucomatous optic neuropathy include atrophy of the retinal nerve fiber layer, focal or diffuse narrowing of the neuroretinal rim, optic disc splinter haemorrhage (DH) and para papillary atrophy (PPA).[4-6]

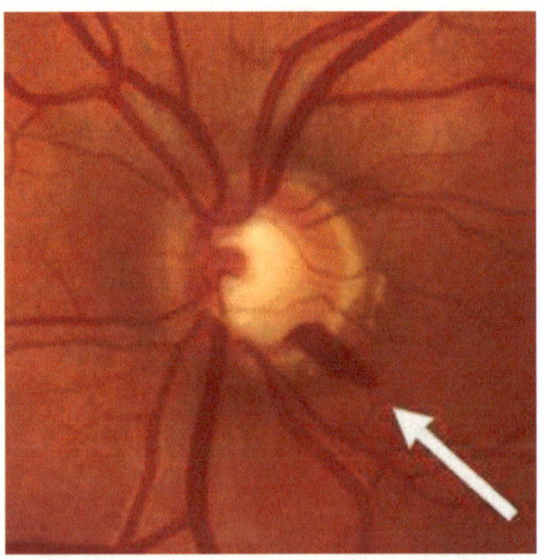

Fig. 17. Optic disc splinter haemorrhage (arrow).

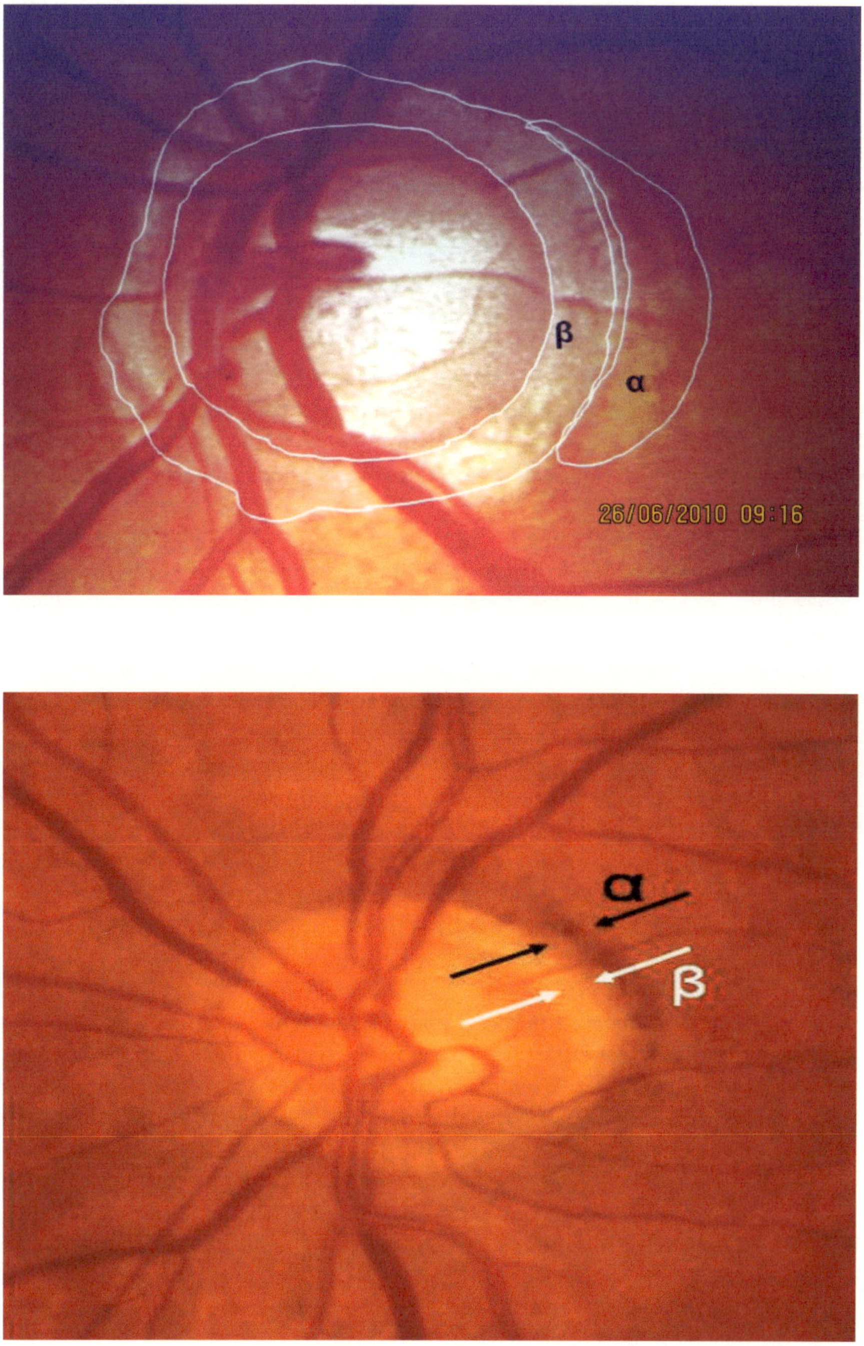

Fig. 18. α and β zones of peripapillar atrophy.

Para papillar atrophy (PPA) is a form of outer retinal atrophy that abuts the optic disc and can be divided into alpha(α) and beta(β) zones.[7-9] Because this atrophy most often lies adjacent to but does not completely surround the nerve, the term parapapillary may be preferable to peripapillary atrophy, though they are used interchangeably in the literature.

In βPPA the sclera and large choroidal vessels are visible, as the retinal pigment epithelium (RPE) and most of the photoreceptors are absent.[7,8] In α PPA, there is an irregular arrangement of RPE cells that can result clinically in both hypo- and hyperpigmentation. The α zone is more peripheral than the β zone when both are present.

However, there are no imaging devices to provide automated assessment of DH or PPA, which at the present time are assessed either by patient examination or by photographic interpretation. Interestingly, several studies addressing the topic have found that PPA and DH tend to occur together in eyes and, additionally, tend to occur in the same regions of the eye, leading to the possibility that PPA may be useful as an indicator of increased likelihood of prior, present, or future disc hemorrhage.[10-15] Because βPPA is present in 15%–20% of normal eyes, its presence is less specific for glaucoma than DH, which occurs only in 0.6% of healthy eyes.[14,16] Given that DH is transient, lasting weeks to months, and that PPA is stable and progressive, it maybe advantageous to rely on PPA parameters for glaucoma diagnosis and monitoring.[11,15]

αPPA and βPPA have been evaluated in glaucoma using quantitative analysis of optic nerve photographs (morphometry) typically by manually outlining and measuring the area of PPA using a slide projector, imaging processing software, or with confocal scanning laser ophthalmoscopy.[8-10,17-23] Both αPPA and βPPA are larger and occur more frequently in eyes with glaucoma than in normal eyes, though βPPA is more specific for glaucoma.[8,9,17,18] Using these morphometric techniques, PPA has been reported to be helpful in differentiating between normal and glaucomatous eyes.[8,9,17,18,24-27]

While many morphometric investigations of PPA in glaucomatous and normal eyes have reported significant differences between these 2 groups, there is a paucity of information on how clinical evaluation of PPA may guide the clinician in the diagnosis of open-angle glaucoma (OAG). Additionally, it is difficult clinically to estimate quantitative PPA parameters, such as area of PPA, due to its heterogenous shape. Despite this, in a clinical assessment using direct ophthalmoscopy alone, information including the PPA circumferential extent and amount of neuroretinal rim narrowing increased the sensitivity and specificity for detection of glaucomatous visual field loss.[4]

Disc hemorrhages seem to mean different things to different clinicians. Many see them as a sign of glaucomatous progression. Some consider disc hemorrhages by themselves to represent a diagnosis of normal-tension glaucoma. Others view the hemorrhages as an indication of inadequate therapy. The development of these hemorrhages often is followed by amplification in glaucoma therapy, either adding medications or performing surgery.

Hemorrhages occur in patients with glaucoma and ocular hypertension and, rarely, in seemingly normal eyes. True glaucomatous disc hemorrhages typically occur at the superior, superior-temporal, inferior, or inferior-temporal aspect of the disc. They typically are small and reside in the retinal nerve fiber layer (RNFL), and they are contiguous with the neuroretinal rim of the optic disc. They often occur in association with notching of the neuroretinal rim or RNFL defects.

Hemorrhages that do not fit this clinical pattern are more likely caused by vascular occlusion, posterior vitreous detachment, other optic neuropathy, or blood dyscrasia such as anemia. Disc hemorrhages typically recur and in the same location on the disc. The etiology and pathogenesis of these hemorrhages remains unknown. It has been theorized that they are the result of a microvascular occlusion of the disc blood supply.

Several well-known glaucoma studies have looked at the implication of optic disc hemorrhages and virtually all indicate that the presence of one in a patient with glaucoma is a risk factor for progression. These findings themselves are not without controversy, however. For example, in the Ocular Hypertension Treatment Study (OHTS), patients with ocular hypertension who developed a disc hemorrhage during the course of the study had a nearly four-fold increased risk of progression to glaucoma compared with those who did not. The increased risk of conversion to glaucoma was about 87% of eyes that demonstrated a disc hemorrhage. That hemorrhages easily can be missed on clinical examination.

The Collaborative Normal Tension Glaucoma Study (CNTGS) found disc hemorrhages in normal-tension glaucoma to indicate the greatest risk of progression of the disease. It also discovered that reduction of IOP did not affect the outcome. Lowering IOP in patients with normal-tension glaucoma manifesting a hemorrhage did nothing to halt disease progression.

In the Early Manifest Glaucoma Treatment (EMGT) Study, disc hemorrhages, likewise, were seen as a major risk factor for disease progression. As with the CNTGS, however, IOP reduction was seen to have little benefit in altering the course of disease in eyes demonstrating disc hemorrhages. Although the hemorrhages were predictive of progression, IOP-reducing treatment was unrelated to the presence or frequency of hemorrhages. These were equally common in both the treated and untreated groups of patients in this study.

The EMGT seems to suggest that disc hemorrhages cannot be considered an indication of insufficient IOP-lowering treatment and that glaucoma progression in eyes with disc hemorrhages cannot be totally halted by IOP reduction.

It should be noted that none of the major glaucoma studies considered the development of a hemorrhage to be a clinical study endpoint for glaucoma progression or conversion to glaucoma from ocular hypertension.

Disc hemorrhages themselves are not progression but are a significant risk factor for progression

5. Progression of the glaucomatous optic disc damage

Insight of progressive glaucomatous damage to the optic disc is one of the most important aspects of glaucoma management, yet it remains largely subjective and imprecise. Progressive change in the appearance of the optic disc or retinal nerve fiber layer (RNFL) often precedes the development of visual field defects in glaucoma. Because visual field defects on standard automated perimetry may only be detected after a substantial number of nerve fibers has been lost, assessment of the optic disc and RNFL is essential for monitoring the initial stages of the disease. Before the development of visual field defects, structural changes in the optic disc or RNFL may be the only evidence for the ophthalmologist that the glaucoma is progressing and treatment needs to be intensified. Even in the presence of visual field defects, progression of optic disc damage may occur without any detectable evidence of functional deterioration.

Disc Damage Likelihood Score (**DDLS**)

Glaucoma is defined as a process wherein there is progressive loss of retinal ganglion cells manifest clinically as loss of neuroretinal rim tissue from the optic nerve. In order to detect this, a clinician must have a method to identify these changes and distinguish them from normal. There is also a need for a system to document any change in optic nerve appearance with time in order to determine progression. The concept of cup:disc ratio(CDR) was developed by Armaly in 1967[1] as a standardised way of documenting disc appearance in order to address these issues. Whilst an enlarging cup:disc ratio is undoubtedly linked with glaucomatous loss, this system does not take into consideration the influence of optic disc size nor yet the focal changes seen in glaucomatous optic neuropathy. It is also well recognised that there is significant intra and inter observer error with this method.

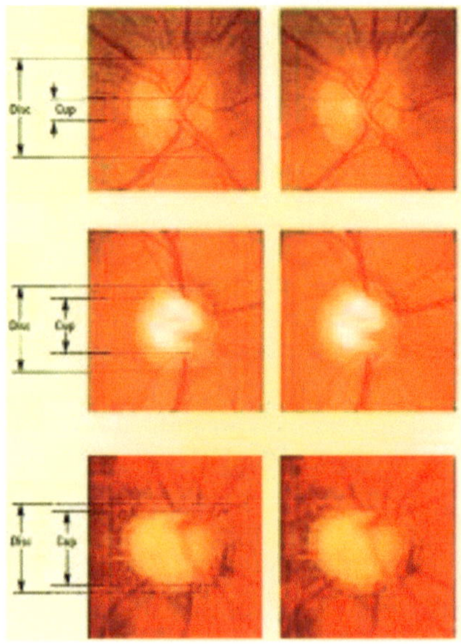

Fig. 19. Cup/Disc ratio progression in glaucoma.

The disc damage likelihood scale (DDLS) was devised by Spaeth et al in 2002 to incorporate the effect of disc size and focal rim width into a clinical grading scale.[2] It is highly reproducible and does correlate strongly with the degree of field loss.[3] The system categorises the disc as small (<1.5mm), medium(1.5-2.0mm) or large(>2.0mm). This ensures that the disc size is measured thereby reducing misclassification bias based on disc size. Disc size can be measured using a fundus lens at the slit-lamp. A slit beam is directed onto the disc and the graticule at the top used to reduce the height of the beam until it corresponds in size to the disc. The lens used will determine the correction factor. A 66D gives the exact measure from the graticule.[4]

Correction factors for the other lenses are -

Volk
60D-0.88
78D-1.2
90D-1.33
Nikon
60D-1.03
90D-1.63

The next stage is to measure the width of the thinnest part of the rim. This forces the examiner to evaluate the rim throughout its entire circumference in order to identify the area of greatest thinning. The measurement is expressed in rim:disc. Where there is no rim present at the thinnest point the value is 0. The circumferential extent of rim absence is then measured in degrees. Care must be taken when evaluating a sloping rim because a sloping rim is not an absent rim.

Whilst simply documenting a CDR is quick, in the main it is of little use in either the diagnosis or longitudinal monitoring of glaucoma. The DDLS not only forces the clinician to determine the size of the disc, which by itself already is alerting the observer to which discs are big and which are small but it also formalises the evaluation of the neuroretinal rim. Because each grade is assigned a numerical value the system can then be used in research settings to determine severity or degree of progression.

Optic nerve heads come in many shapes and forms. No method of classification will fit all of these different patterns and forms. The DDLS cannot be used to evaluate certain types of discs, such as those that are congenitally anomalous. Myopic discs may be difficult to grade. Probably one of the first mental steps one takes when considering the nature of the optic disc is, "Is this an anomalous disc? Is there any system that can be used to stage or characterize this disc?" There will be those situations which the answer to that question is, "No." It is unwise in such situations to use any of the standard systems, such as cup/disc ratio, HRT evaluations, OCT evaluations, or the DDLS.[4,5]

Another problem with the DDLS is that a disc may show progressive damage by having a continuing generalized narrowing of the neuroretinal rim, but not have an increase in the circumferential extent of rim absence. In such a situation the disc would unquestionably have become worse, but the DDLS score will not change. Fortunately this seems to be a rare occurrence.[5]

It takes some effort to learn it and initially a copy of the table should always be to hand. However, given practice and used accordingly the DDLS is an excellent tool for classifying and monitoring the optic nerve in glaucoma.

6. References

[1] Ahn JK, Kang JH, Park KH. Correlation between a disc hemorrhage and peripapillary atrophy in glaucoma patients with a unilateral disc hemorrhage. J Glaucoma. 2004;13(1):9–14.

[2] Alencar LM, Bowd C, Weinreb RN, Zangwill LM, Sample PA, Medeiros FA. Comparison of HRT-3 glaucoma probability score and subjective stereophotograph assessment for prediction of progression in glaucoma. Invest Ophthalmol Vis Sci. 2008;49(5):1898–1906.

[3] Anderson DR., Normal Tension Glaucoma Study Collaborative normal tension glaucoma study. Curr Opin Ophthalmol. 2003;14(2):86–90.

[4] Armaly M. Genetic determination of cup/disc ratio of the optic nerve. Arch Ophthalmol 1967;78:35-43

[5] Bayer A. Harasymowycz P. Henderer JD, et al. Validity of a new disc grading scale for estimating glaucomatous damage: correlation with visual field damage. Am J Ophthalmol 2002;133:758-763

[6] Bochmann F, Howell JP, Meier C, et al. The disc damage likelihood scale (DDLS): interobserver agreement of a new grading system to assess glaucomatous optic disc damage. Klin Monatsbl Bugenheilkd 2009;226:280-3.
[7] Budenz DL, Anderson DR, Feuer WJ, et al. Detection and prognostic significance of optic disc hemorrhages during the Ocular Hypertension Treatment Study. Ophthalmology. 2006;113(12):2137–2143.
[8] Chaum E, Drewry RD, Ware GT, Charles S. Nerve fiber bundle visual field defect resulting from a giant peripapillary cotton-wool spot. J Neuroophthalmol. 2001;21:276-7.
[9] Chihara E, Honda Y. Topographic changes in the optic disc in eyes with cotton-wool spots and primary open-angle glaucoma. Graefes Arch Clin Exp Ophthalmol. 1991;229:13-8
[10] Chihara E, Matsuoka T, Ogura Y and Matsumura M, Retinal nerve fiber layer defect as an early manifestation of diabetic retinopathy, Ophthalmology. 1993;100:1147-51
[11] Danesh-Meyer H, et al, Regional Correlation of Structure and Function in Glaucoma, Using the Disc Damage Likelihood Scale, Heidelberg Retina Tomograph, and Visual Fields, Ophthalmology 2006;113:603-611 © by the American Academy of Ophthalmology.
[12] Fingeret M, Medeiros FA, Susanna R, Jr, Weinreb RN. Five rules to evaluate the optic disc and retinal nerve fibre layer for glaucoma. Optometry. 2005 Nov;76(11):661–8.
[13] Gardiner SK, Johnson CA, Cioffi GA. Evaluation of the structure-function relationship in glaucoma. Invest Ophthalmol Vis Sci. 2005;46(10):3712–3717.
[14] Garway-Heath DF, Wollstein G, Hitchings RA. Aging changes of the optic nerve head in relation to open angle glaucoma. Br J Ophthalmol, 1998; 81:840-5.
[15] Geijssen HC,Greve EL. Disc haemorrhages and peripapillary atrophy. Invest Ophthalmol Vis Sci 32:1017, 1991.
[16] Gonzalez-Hernandez M, Pablo LE, Armas-Domingue K, Rodriguez de la Vega R, Ferreras A, Gonzalez de la Rosa M. Structure-function relationship depends on glaucoma severity. Br J Ophthalmol. 2009
[17] Gordon MO, Beiser JA, Brandt JD, et al. The Ocular Hypertension Treatment Study: baseline factors that predict the onset of primary open-angle glaucoma. Arch Ophthalmol. 2002;120(6):714–720. discussion 829-830.
[18] Gordon MO, Torri V, Miglior S, et al. Ocular Hypertension Treatment Study Group. European Glaucoma Prevention Study Group Validated prediction model for the development of primary open-angle glaucoma in individuals with ocular hypertension. Ophthalmology. 2007;114(1):10–19.
[19] Gross PG, Drance SM. Comparison of a simple ophthalmoscopic and planimetric measurement of glaucomatous neuroretinal rim areas. J Glaucoma 4:314-316, 1995.
[20] Harper R, Reeves B. The sensitivity and specificity of direct ophthalmoscopic optic disc assessment in screening for glaucoma: a multivariate analysis. Graefes Arch Clin Exp Ophthalmol. 2000;238(12):949–955.
[21] Harwerth RS, Carter-Dawson L, Smith EL, III, Crawford ML. Scaling the structure-function relationship for clinical perimetry. Acta Ophthalmol Scand. 2005;83(4):448–455.

[22] Hayakawa T, Sugiyama K, Tomita G, et al. Correlation of the peripapillary atrophy area with optic disc cupping and disc hemorrhage.J Glaucoma. 1998;7(5):306–311.
[23] Henderer JD, Liu C, Kesen M, et al. Reliability of the disc damage likelihood scale. Am J Ophthalmol 2003;135:44-8
[24] Johnson CA, Cioffi GA, Liebmann JR, Sample PA, Zangwill LM, Weinreb RN. The relationship between structural and functional alterations in glaucoma: a review. Semin Ophthalmol. 2000;15(4):221–233.
[25] Jonas JB, Budde WM, Panda-Jonas S. Ophthalmoscopic evaluation of the parapapillary region of the optic nerve head. Klin Oczna. 2004; 106 Suppl 1-2:279–289.
[26] Jonas JB, Naumann GO. Parapapillary chorioretinal atrophy in normal and glaucoma eyes. II. Correlations. Invest Ophthalmol Vis Sci.1989;30(5):919–926.
[27] Jonas JB, Nguyen XN, Gusek GC, Naumann GO. Parapapillary chorioretinal atrophy in normal and glaucoma eyes. I. Morphometric data.Invest Ophthalmol Vis Sci. 1989;30 (5):908–918.
[28] Jonas JB, Martus P, Budde WM. Inter-eye differences in chronic open-angle glaucoma patients with unilateral disc hemorrhages. Ophthalmology.2002;109(11):2078–2083.
[29] Jonas JB. Predictive factors of the optic nerve head for development or progression of glaucomatous visual field loss. Invest Ophthalmol Vis Sci. 2004;45(8):2613–2618.
[30] Jonas JB, Martus P, Budde WM, Jünemann A, Hayler J. Small neuroretinal rim and large parapapillary atrophy as predictive factors for progression of glaucomatous optic neuropathy. Ophthalmology. 2002;109(8):1561–1567.
[31] Jonas JB, Bergua A, Schmitz-Valckenberg P, Papastathopoulos KI, Budde WM. Ranking of optic disc variables for detection of glaucomatous optic nerve damage. Invest Ophthalmol Vis Sci. 2000;41(7):1764–1773.
[32] Jonas JB. Clinical implications of peripapillary atrophy in glaucoma. Curr Opin Ophthalmol. 2005;16(2):84–88.
[33] Jonas JB, Budde WM, Panda-Jonas S. Ophthalmoscopic evaluation of the optic nerve head. Surv Ophthalmol. 1999;43(4):293–320.
[34] Jonas JB, Dichtl A. Evaluation of the retinal nerve fiber layer. Surv Ophthalmol. 1996;40:369-78.
[35] Jonas JB, Fernandez MC, Sturmer J. Pattern of glaucomatous neuroretinal rim loss. Ophthalmology. 1993;100:63-8.
[36] Jonas JB, Schiro D. Localised wedge shaped defects of the retinal nerve fibre layer in glaucoma. Br J Ophthalmol. 1994;78:285-90.
[37] Jonas JB, Gusek GC, Naumann GOH. Optic disc, cup and neuroretinal rim size, configuration and correlations in normal eyes. Invest Ophthalmol Vis Sci 29:1151-1158, 1988.
[38] Jonas JB,Dichtl A. Advances in assessment of the optic disc changes in early glaucoma. Cur Opi Ophthalmol 6:61-66, 1995.
[39] Jonas JB, Budde WM, Panda-Jonas S. Ophthalmoscopic evaluation of the optic nerve head. Surv Ophthalmol. 1999;43(4):293–320.
[40] Kanamori A,Nagai-Kusuhara A,Escaño MF,et al. Comparison of confocal scanning laser ophthalmoscopy, scanning laser polarimetry and optical coherence tomography to

discriminate ocular hypertension and glaucoma at an early stage. Graefes Arch Clin Exp Ophthalmol 2006;244:58–68.

[41] Kass MA, Heuer DK, Higginbotham EJ, et al. The Ocular Hypertension Treatment Study: a randomized trial determines that topical ocular hypotensive medication delays or prevents the onset of primary open-angle glaucoma. Arch Ophthalmol. 2002;120(6):701-713. discussion 829-830.

[42] Kwon YH, Kim YI, Pereira MLM, et al. Rate of optic disc cup progression in treated primary open-angle glaucoma. J Glaucoma. 2003;12(5):409–416.

[43] Kubota T, Jonas JB, Naumann GO. Direct clinico-histological correlation of parapapillary chorioretinal atrophy. Br J Ophthalmol.1993;77(2):103–106.

[44] Lalezary M, Medeiros FA, Weinreb RN, et al. Baseline optical coherence tomography predicts the development of glaucomatous change in glaucoma suspects. Am J Ophthalmol. 2006;142(4):576–582.

[45] Law SK, Choe R, Caprioli J. Optic disk characteristics before the occurrence of disk hemorrhage in glaucoma patients. Am J Ophthalmol. 2001;132(3):411–413.

[46] Leibowitz HM, Kruger DE, Maunder LR, et al. The Framingham Eye Study monograph: An ophthalmological and epidemiological study of cataract, glaucoma, diabetic retinopathy, macular degeneration and visual acuity in general population. Surv Ophthalmol 24 (suppl):335 610, 1980.

[47] Lester M, Garway-Heath D, Lemij H. Optic Nerve Head and Retinal Nerve Fibre Analysis. European Glaucoma Society. 2005.

[48] Leung CK,Chan WM,Chong KK,et al. Comparative study of retinal nerve fiber layer measurement by Stratus OCT and GDx VCC. I: correlation analysis in glaucoma. Invest Ophthalmol Vis Sci 2005;46:3214–3220.

[49] Medeiros FA, Alencar LM, Zangwill LM, et al. The relationship between intraocular pressure and progressive retinal nerve fiber layer loss in glaucoma. Ophthalmology. 2009;116(6):1125.e1-3–1133.e1-3.

[50] Medeiros FA,Zangwill LM,Bowd C,Weinreb RN. Comparison of the GDx VCC scanning laser polarimeter, HRT II confocal scanning laser ophthalmoscope, and stratus OCT optical coherence tomograph for the detection of glaucoma. Arch Ophthalmol 2004;122:827–837.

[51] Medeiros FA, Weinreb RN, Sample PA, et al. Validation of a predictive model to estimate the risk of conversion from ocular hypertension to glaucoma. Arch Ophthalmol. 2005;123(10):1351–1360.

[52] Medeiros FA, Zangwill LM, Bowd C, Vasile C, Sample PA, Weinreb RN. Agreement between stereophotographic and confocal scanning laser ophthalmoscopy measurements of cup/disc ratio: effect on a predictive model for glaucoma development. J Glaucoma. 2007;16(2):209–214.

[53] Miglior S, Zeyen T, Pfeiffer N, Cunha-Vaz J, Torri V, Adamsons I., European Glaucoma Prevention Study (EGPS) Group Results of the European Glaucoma Prevention Study. Ophthalmology. 2005;112(3):366–375.

[54] Mohammadi K, Bowd C, Weinreb RN, Medeiros FA, Sample PA, Zangwill LM. Retinal nerve fiber layer thickness measurements with scanning laser polarimetry predict glaucomatous visual field loss. Am J Ophthalmol. 2004;138(4):592–601.

[55] Ozdek S, Lonneville YH, Onol M, Yetkin I, Hasanreisoglu B. Assessment of nerve fiber layer in diabetic patients with scanning laser polarimetry. Eye. 2002;16:761-5.
[56] Park KH, Park SJ, Lee YJ, Kim JY, Caprioli J. Ability of peripapillary atrophy parameters to differentiate normal-tension glaucoma from glaucomalike disk. J Glaucoma. 2001;10(2):95–101. Armaly M. Genetic determination of cup/disc ratio of the optic nerve. Arch Ophthalmol 1967;78:35 -43.
[57] Quigley HA, Dunkelbarger GR, Green WR. Retinal ganglion cell atrophy correlated with automated perimetry in human eyes with glaucoma. Am J Ophthalmol 107: 453-464, 1989.
[58] Racette L, Medeiros FA, Bowd C, Zangwill LM, Weinreb RN, Sample PA. The impact of the perimetric measurement scale, sample composition, and statistical method on the structure-function relationship in glaucoma. J Glaucoma. 2007;16(8):676–684.
[59] Radcliffe NM, Liebmann JM, Rozenbaum I, et al. Anatomic relationships between disc hemorrhage and parapapillary atrophy. Am JOphthalmol. 2008;146(5):735–740.
[60] Rockwood EJ, Anderson DR. Acquired peripapillary changes and progression in glaucoma. Graefes Arch Clin Exp Ophthalmol. 1988;226(6):510–515.
[61] Schuman JS, Hee MR, Puliafito CA. et al. Quantification of nerve fibre layer thickness in normal and glaucomatous eyes using optical coherence tomography. Arch Ophthalmol 113:586-596, 1995.
[62] Sommer A, Quigley HA, Robin AL, Miller NR, Katz J, Arkell S. Evaluation of nerve fiber layer assessment. Arch Ophthalmol. 1984;102:1766-71.
[63] Sommer A, Katz J, Quigley HA, Miller NR, Robin AL, Richter RC, et al. Clinically detectable nerve fiber atrophy precedes the onset of glaucomatous field loss. Arch Ophthalmol. 1991;109:77-83.
[64] Sugiyama K, Tomita G, Kawase K, et al. Disc hemorrhage and peripapillary atrophy in apparently healthy subjects. Acta Ophthalmol Scand. 1999;77(2):139–142.
[65] Theodossiades J, Murdoch I. What optic disc parameters are most accurately assessed using the direct ophthalmoscope? Eye (Lond).2001;15(Pt 3):283–287.
[66] Uchida H. Increasing peripapillary atrophy is associated with progressive glaucoma. Ophthalmology. 1998;105(8):1541–1545.
[67] Uhm KB, Lee DY, Kim JT, Hong C. Peripapillary atrophy in normal and primary open-angle glaucoma. Korean J Ophthalmol. 1998;12(1): 37–50.
[68] Weinreb RN, Khaw PT. Primary open-angle glaucoma. Lancet. 2004;363(9422):1711–1720.
[69] Weinreb RN, Kaufman PL. The glaucoma research community and FDA look to the future: a report from the NEI/FDA CDER Glaucoma Clinical Trial Design and Endpoints Symposium. Invest Ophthalmol Vis Sci. 2009;50(4):1497–1505.
[70] Weinreb RN. Diagnosing and monitoring glaucoma with confocal scanning laser ophthalmoscopy. J Glaucoma 4:225-227, 1995.
[71] Wilensky JT, Kolker AE. Peripapillary changes in glaucoma. Am J Ophthalmol. 1976;81(3):341–345.
[72] Xu L, Wang Y, Yang H, Jonas JB. Differences in parapapillary atrophy between glaucomatous and normal eyes: the Beijing Eye Study. Am J Ophthalmol. 2007;144(4):541–546.

[73] Zangwill LM, Weinreb RN, Beiser JA, et al. Baseline topographic optic disc measurements are associated with the development of primary open-angle glaucoma: the Confocal Scanning Laser Ophthalmoscopy Ancillary Study to the Ocular Hypertension Treatment Study. Arch Ophthalmol. 2005;123(9):1188–1197.

8

The use of Confocal Scanning Laser Tomography in the Evaluation of Progression in Glaucoma

Liamet Fernández Argones, Ibraín Piloto Díaz, Marerneda Domínguez Randulfe, Germán A. Álvarez Cisneros and Marcelino Río Torres
Cuban Institute of Ophthalmology, Havana, Cuba

1. Introduction

Monitoring of glaucomatous damage is critical in a modern glaucoma practice. Confocal scanning laser tomograph or Heidelberg Retina Tomograph (HRT) is one of the imaging techniques that allow clinicians to examine more patients and to obtain objectives measurements compared to the gold standard of optic disc stereo- photography.

It employs a diode laser with a wavelength of 670nm. In a confocal optical system light can only reach the photo detector if it is reflected from a narrow area surrounding the set focal plane. Light reflected outside of the focal plane is highly suppressed (Heidelberg Engineering, 2005).

A two- dimensional sector of the retina is scanned sequentially. The amount of reflected light at each point is measured using a light sensitive detector. To obtain a topography image (three- dimensional image), the height of the retinal surface is computed at each point (Heidelberg Engineering, 2005).

Analysis of glaucomatous progression is performed with the HRT operating software by quantitatively describing temporal changes of the optic nerve head topography. It is particularly important as glaucoma progression occurs slowly and changes often are subtle and missed easily. The HRT has the advantage that the new technology enables backward compatibility. So progression can be analysed since the introduction of the first HRT (HRT Classic).

2. Progression analysis

2.1 Basis for a confident progression analysis

During the progression analysis the follow- up exam and the baseline are compared. To ensure that differences between the images are for glaucomatous progression and not for imaging conditions, the image quality, the alignment and normalization procedures should be addressed.

The control label of good or better must be present in all the images (defined as a scan standard deviation less than 30 µm). It means that the three 15° scans used to generate a mean topographic image are uniform. For each pixel in the topography image, the standard deviation of the pixel height is calculated from the three scanned images and then averaged over the entire topography image (Heidelberg Engineering, 2005).

The image quality can be affected by age, incorrectly adjusted refraction, eye movement, dry eye, size of the pupil, media opacity or other physical characteristics of the eye. It is recommended to perform HRT scan before other diagnostic measures are taken. In dry eyes artificial tear fluid can be applied shortly before the examination while ointments, fluorescein, among others should be avoided. If the pupil diameter is smaller than 3 mm or if image quality is thought to be affected by media opacity, the pupil should be dilated with 0.5% tropicamide (Sihota et al., 2002; Heidelberg Engineering, 2005; Strouthidis & Garway-Heath, 2008; Fogagnolo et al., 2011). The good quality of images is determinant for the accuracy of the HRT progression analysis (figure 1).

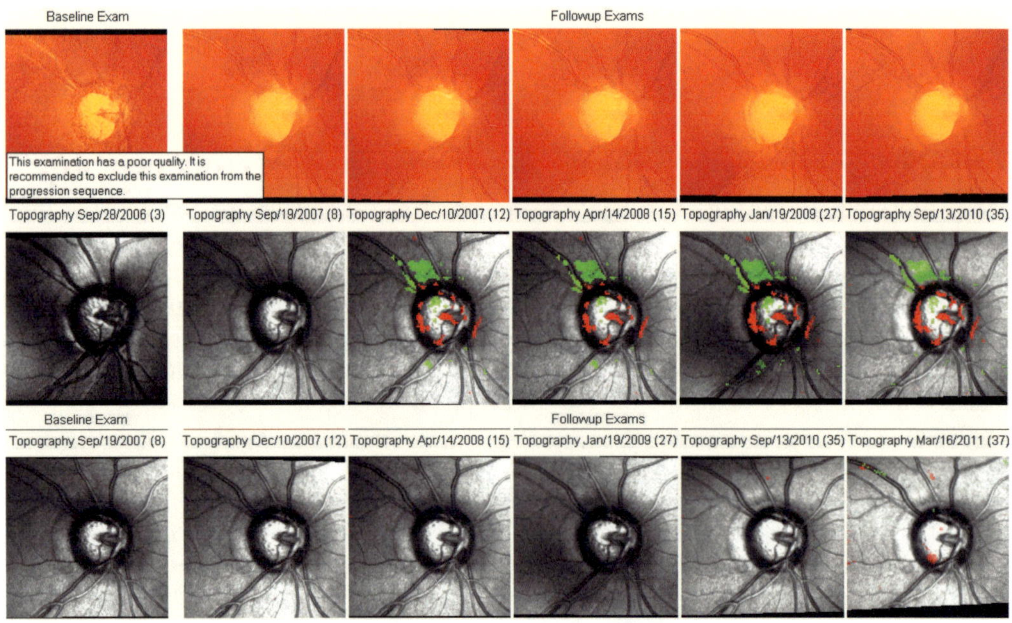

Fig. 1. This figure illustrates the importance of a good quality image in the progression analysis. The two superior rows show the difficulties in the evaluation of glaucomatous progression generated by a poor quality baseline. The inferior row shows the result when a poor quality image is excluded of the progression sequences.

The HRT has the ability to monitor quality control during follow- up image acquisition. There is a warning message which starts to blink if the current focus setting differs from the previous setting. There is also a blue frame which appears close to the line image margin, with a blue cross located in the center of the optic disc live image when the same retinal region as the baseline examination is adjusted (Heidelberg Engineering, 2005).

After the examination, a quickly view to the follow- up images may give information about the quality of the alignment. Black margins around the image appear when the optic nerve head is not centered (figure 2).

For the progression analysis based on stereometric parameters the demarcation of contour line is essential. It is manually located along the inner edge of the scleral (Elschnig´s) ring by the operator. The margin of the optic disc is used as a reference. The contour line can be

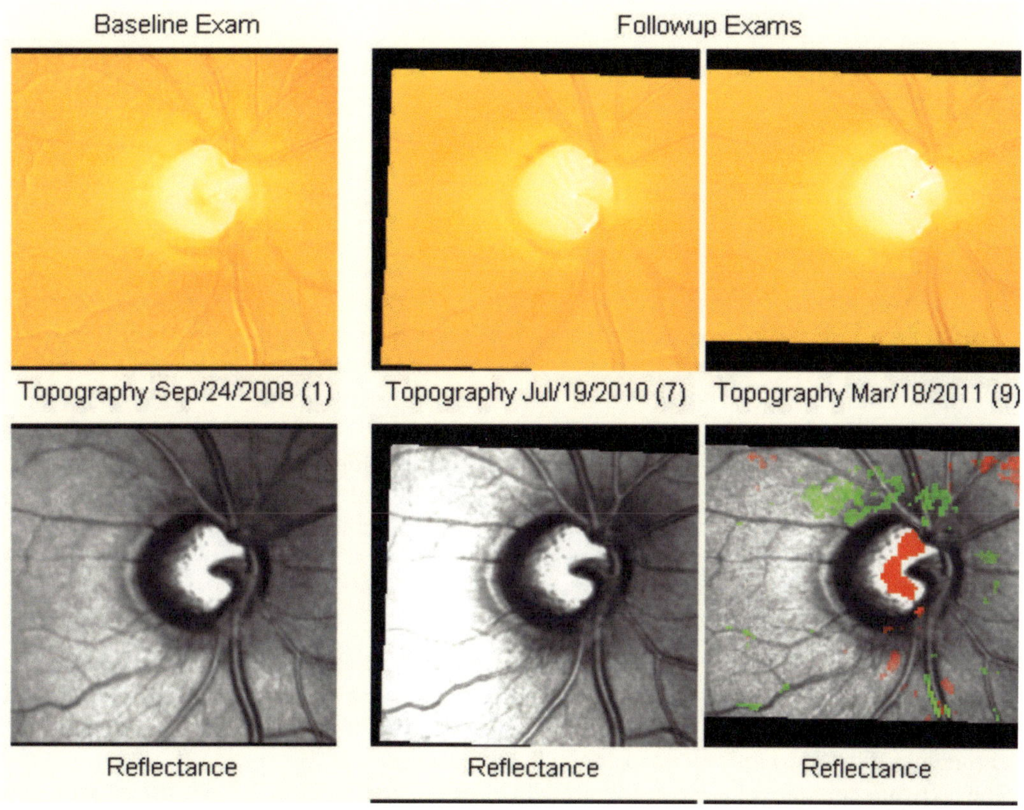

Fig. 2. Black margins around the images as a result of bad alignment during follow- up image acquisition. May be the image differences are due to different imaging conditions.

modified at any time later on. Every modification of the contour line in the baseline or follow-up examinations is transferred directly to all other examinations. Excluding a baseline examination results in the loss of the contour line. This will delete the stereometric parameter until a new contour line is drawn (Heidelberg Engineering, 2005).

The reference plane is parallel to the peripapillary retinal surface and located 50 µm below the retinal surface at the contour line and in the papillomacular bundle (350° - 356°). It is used to define structures above the plane as "rim" and below as "cup." In general, stereometric parameters are strongly influenced by the position of the reference plane. (Kamal et al., 2000; Tan et al., 2003a; Strouthidis et al., 2005a; Breusegem et al., 2008). It has been reported that the 320 Âµm plane, which is offset from the reference ring in the image periphery, is less likely to be affected by disease severity, resulting in more stable rim area measurements (Deleon et al., 2007).

Image acquisition- induced variability seemed larger than operator-induced variability (Miglior et al., 2002). Some factors such as image quality and the noise of HRT measurements, among others, influence the results (Owen et al., 2006; Bowd et al., 2009). It has been described that in some eyes, the optic nerve head is more elevated at the lower pressure (Harju et al., 2008; Vizzeri et al., 2011). On the other hand, it was found that intraocular pressure increases and decreases on the order of 5 mm Hg did not appear to have an effect on optic disc topography (Nicolela et al., 2006).

A follow- up examination is automatically normalized to its baseline examination. The six images are aligned and normalized to each other. It includes correction of displacement, rotation, tilt, magnification and prospective changes. It ensures that differences between the images that are due to different imaging conditions are eliminated and that baseline and follow- up examinations can be compared to detect glaucomatous progression. The Glaucoma Module 3.0 software uses an enhanced automatic alignment and normalization procedure, which is likely to improve progression analyses, both for assessment of surface height change by topographical change analysis, and serial analysis of stereometric parameters (Heidelberg Engineering, 2005; Strouthidis & Garway-Heath, 2008).

In rare cases, the automatic alignment procedure may not be able to precisely align the images. As a result, the contour line appears misplaced in the follow- up examination. To resolve this, a manual alignment procedure may be used (Heidelberg Engineering, 2005).

It is highly recommended to start a new progression analysis after any kind of invasive surgery, as this will modify the optic properties of the eye. The images before and after the surgery are not comparable to each other in most cases (Heidelberg Engineering, 2005).

When the baseline and the follow- up image are optimal to be compared, it is time to looking for glaucomatous progression by the Topographic Change Analysis and by the changes on Stereometric Parameters over time.

2.2 Topographic Change Analysis (TCA)

The most important method to detect glaucomatous progression is the TCA. It is a technique that compares the variability within a baseline examination to that between baseline and follow-up examinations. It is independent of the optic disc head contour line and it takes the chronologically oldest follow- up examinations as the baseline.

The software compares the "within variability" of all baseline and follow- up examination with the "pooled variability" of all baseline and follow- up examinations. If the pooled variability of all baseline and follow- up examinations is significantly increased, then there is a height change at the corresponding location. Super pixels with an error probability of less than 5% for rejecting the equal variances hypothesis indicate a significant change at the corresponding location (Heidelberg Engineering, 2005; Strouthidis & Garway-Heath, 2008) (figure 3).

A region of at least 20 super pixels with significant changes in surface height that are connected to each other is called a cluster. With the cluster analysis, it is possible to evaluate the temporal change of the size and the amount of change in a cluster of significant super pixels. For the computation of the cluster volume, all super pixels inside the cluster boundaries are considered, but only the significant super pixels inside the cluster boundaries contribute to the cluster area (Heidelberg Engineering, 2005; Strouthidis & Garway-Heath, 2008) (figure 3). The largest clustered super pixel area within the optic disc margin was the TCA parameter providing the best sensitivity/specificity tradeoff for the detection of glaucomatous progression. Authors suggested early progression detection using TCA (Bowd et al., 2009).

The TCA Cluster Change- Graph (figure 4) displays changes in cluster volume (red, right vertical axis) and cluster area (blue, left vertical axis) over time for all follow- up examinations compared to the baseline exam.

To successfully appreciate the follow- up information given by TCA it is necessary to know the following reproducibility rules: in the first follow- up exam no results is displayed, in the second follow- up exam only changes reproducible over both two follow- up exams are

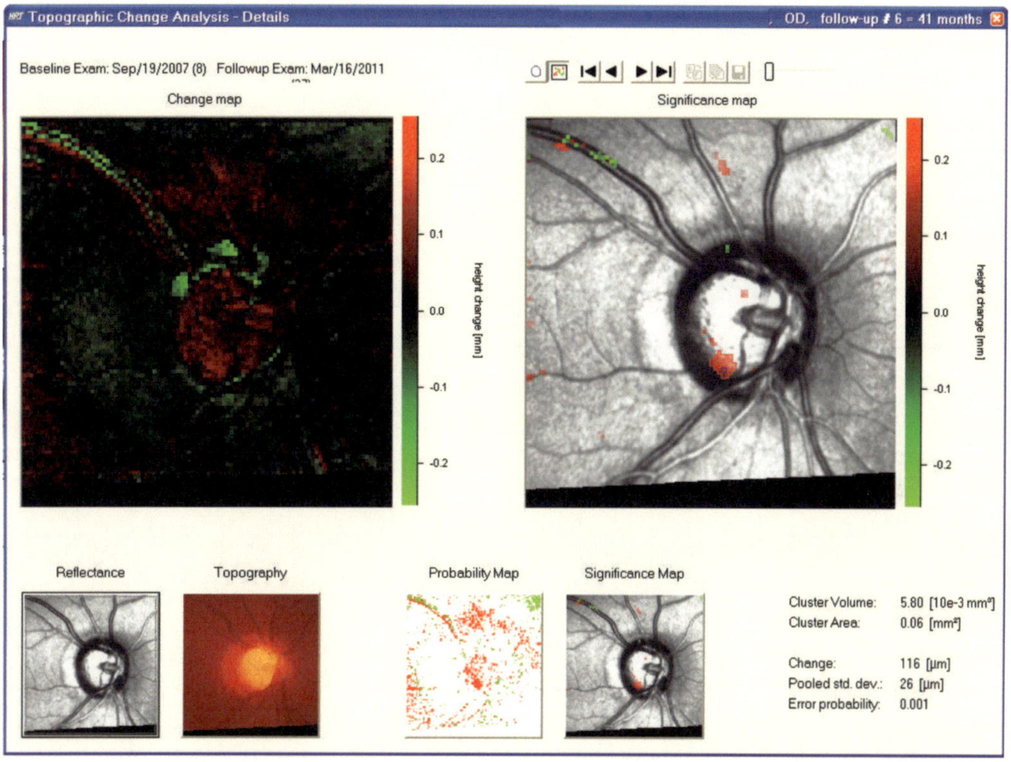

Fig. 3. Topographic Change Analysis- Details. It appears when double- click in an image of the progression sequence. It shows the cluster in the significance map (color red). The cluster volume and area are displayed on the right- inferior corner. The change of the local surface height in microns of the selected super pixel and the probability error of this change (corresponding to the current position of blue circle inside the cluster) are displayed below.

displayed, in the third follow- up exam only changes reproducible over all three follow- up exams are displayed, and in the further follow- up exam only changes reproducible in any three out of the last four follow- up exams are displayed (Heidelberg Engineering, 2005) (figure 4).

It has been suggested that significant TCA change may precede the visible progression by stereophotograph or by currently available visual field-based progression detection techniques (Chauhan et al., 2001; Budenz et al., 2006; Strouthidis & Garway-Heath, 2008; Bowd et al., 2009; Vizzeri et al., 2009; Asaoka et al., 2009). The TCA has demonstrated that it performs at least as well as either the individual or best combination of observer for detecting progressive glaucomatous disc changes of disc photographs (Chauhan et al., 2009). It has been considered that assessment of the HRT and stereophotography may be identifying different aspects of structural change. Some eyes progressing by TCA alone may have only areas of surface height change, which is less easily appreciated from photographs (Kourkoutas et al., 2007; Strouthidis & Garway-Heath, 2008). On the other hand, stereophotographic examination can assesses certain features of the optic disc, such as rim pale, splinter haemorrhages, Alfa and Beta-Zone parapapillary atrophy, among others; that are important to evaluate the individual risk for progression (Budenz et al., 2006; Teng et al., 2010) (figure 5).

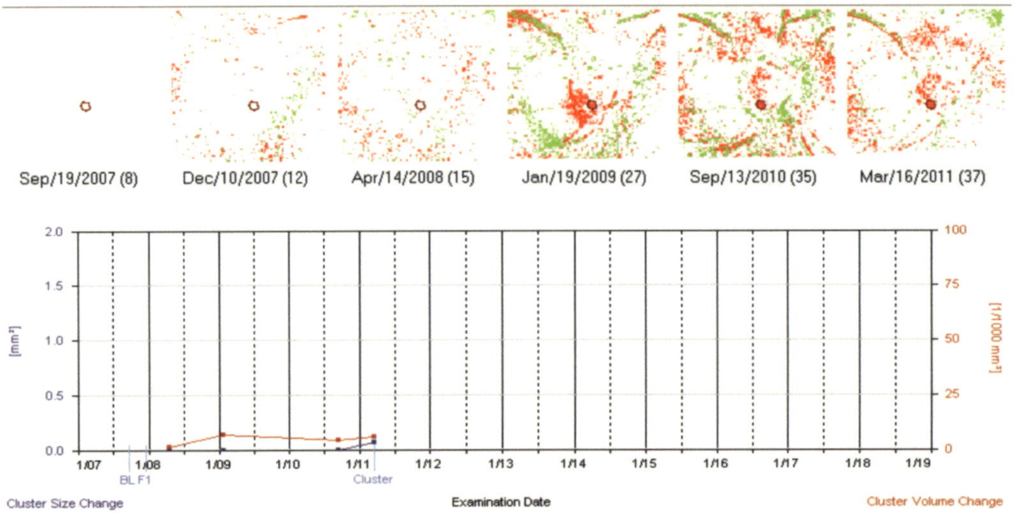

Fig. 4. Probability map and TCA Cluster Change- Graph. The TCA Cluster Change- Graph appears when double- click in a cluster area. Real progression of glaucomatous damage at the inferior- temporal cup is suspected in the right eye of the patient showed in figure 1. When there are more than four exams only significant changes reproducible in any three out of the last four follow-up are displayed (cluster delineated by a blue circle first appeared in the probability map in 2009 while it was first displayed in the significance map superimposed on the reflectance image in 2011).

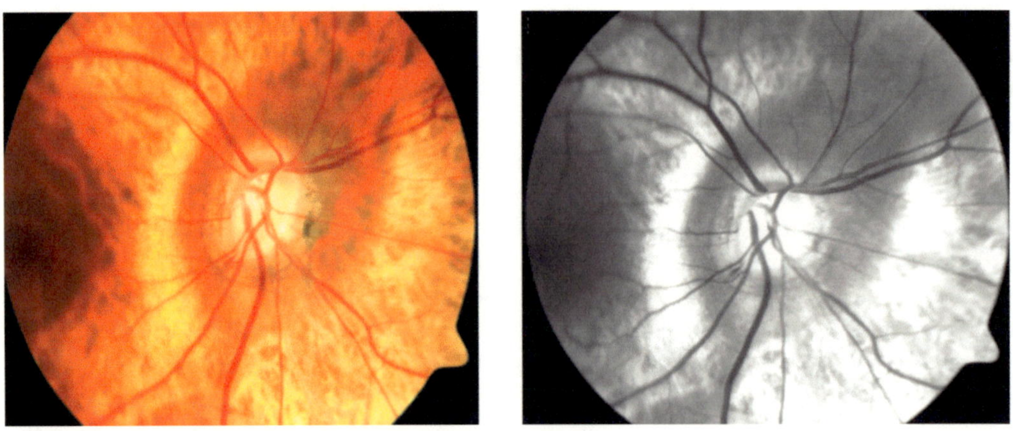

Fig. 5. Colour and red free photograph of the optic disc ad retinal nerve fiber layer in a glaucomatous patient. A splinter haemorrhage is present at the inferior optic disc margin.

Results suggested that ideal parameters for separating glaucomatous and healthy groups are small clusters (between 1% and 2% of disc areas), with shallow depth changes (20-50 µm) (Bowd et al., 2009). Using the same cluster size in small and in large optic disc may cause that the required change has to be relatively bigger in small disc. TCA may fail to identify progressive structural damage in case of large disc with narrow neuro- retinal rim or in the presence of advanced optic nerve head damage with little anatomic reserve (Martinez de la Casa et al., 2006; Hudson et al., 2007).

At present, TCA progression alone should not indicate a treatment change. HRT change must be evaluated in conjunction with other clinical features of deterioration before altering therapy (Kourkoutas et al., 2007).

2.3 Glaucomatous progression in stereometric parameters

The progressions of stereometric parameters can be assessed by monitoring the change in a particular stereometric parameter over time, the event analysis, the trend analysis and different algorithms that have been described.

The event analyses identify progression when a measurement exceeds a predetermined criterion for change (or an event); it is assumed that any change below the criterion represents measurement variability and that changes above the criterion represent true disease change.

The trend analysis examines the change of stereometric parameters over time, with each value being normalized by using the ratio of the difference between a given value and baseline to the difference between the average value in a normal eye and an eye with advanced glaucoma. It does not give a statistical analysis of the rate of change (Strouthidis & Garway-Heath, 2008).

It is recommended a minimum of 7-8 images to increase the accuracy in the detection of progression, although a downward tendency in three consecutively images is suggestive of change. Using the downward tendency of more that 0.05 (normalized parameter value) in three consecutively image, as the criterion of progression, the specificity is increased to more that 90% (Martinez de la Casa et al., 2006).

Two progression algorithms assessing rim area change have been described: a trend analysis based on linear regression of sector rim area over time (Strouthidis et al., 2006) and an event analysis based on defining the criteria for change according to sector rim area coefficient of repeatability (Fayers et al., 2007). For both algorithms authors concluded that poor agreement exists between HRT rim area progression and visual field progression and suggested that on a practical level, both structural and functional measures need to be monitored to have the best chance of identifying glaucomatous progression.

The greatest challenge in detecting progression is the ability to discriminate true change (disease process) from measurement variability.

A difference of 10% or more in the standard reference height compared with the baseline is considered excess variability. It has been identified that excess standard reference height variability (average 24%) does occur in a considerable proportion of follow-up HRT 3 scans (46% of all HRT 3 scans) and that more than half the variability in retinal nerve fiber layer, rim area, and rim volume could be attributed to variability in the standard reference height (Breusegem et al., 2008). Increased test-retest variability is associated with the degree of glaucomatous damage even after taking into account effects from age, visual acuity and lens media (Deleon et al., 2007).

The top five parameters considered by Heidelberg manufacturer are rim area, rim volume, cup shape measure, height variation contour and mean retinal nerve fiber layer (Heidelberg Engineering, 2005).

Rim area has been identified as a repeatable and reliable parameter in test–retest studies; it therefore represents a good marker for measuring disease progression (Kamal et al., 2000; Tan et al., 2003; Strouthidis et al., 2005a, 2005b; Artes et al., 2005; Jampel et al., 2006; Strouthidis & Garway-Heath, 2008). In a cohort study in ocular hypertensive and control subjects, the rim area event analysis had a higher detection rate of progression, at 95% specificity, than rim area trend analysis and the visual field progression criteria (Fayers et al., 2007). In a comparative study, the scanning laser polarimetry ability to discriminate eyes with progressing glaucoma by standard achromatic perimetry and/or stereophotographs from stable eyes was significantly greater for retinal nerve fiber layer thickness measured than for rim area measurements from HRT (Alencar et al., 2010).

Intertest differences in reference height and image quality had a strong relationship with intertest rim area differences and together they are responsible for 70% of the intertest variability of rim area measurements (Strouthidis et al., 2005a). The position of the reference plane with respect to the optic nerve head was considered the most frequent contributor to rim area variability (Tan et al., 2003b) and it has been demonstrated that the false positive progression can be reduce by increasing the quality follow- up image acquisition (Owen et al., 2006; Patterson et al., 2006; Bergin et al., 2008).

The detection of glaucomatous progression based on stereometric parameters, other than rim area, has been proposed. The best correlation with glaucomatous progression was found with the cup: disc area ratio (Saarela et al; 2010). In advanced glaucomatous damage the vertical cup: disc ratio may have a higher potential for detecting progression, where it maintains low test–retest variability (Deleon et al., 2007). In eyes with early glaucoma or suspected glaucoma, perimetry progression showed higher correlations with the cup area and the vertical cup: disc area. Those eyes with baseline Moorfields regression analysis changes were at a higher risk of having perimetry abnormalities and a faster progression (Garcia-Martin et al., 2010).

In a group of ocular hypertensive eyes converted to early glaucoma the parameters which changed most frequently were inferonasal cup volume (11% of discs), inferotemporal cup volume (8.5%), superotemporal cup area (7.3%) and global cup volume (6.7%) (Kamal et al., 2000). In a similar subject group, the optic disc parameters detect only a small amount of the converters, although the hit rate could be increased with the sectoral based analysis. The cup shape measure showed the highest rate (Philippin et al., 2006).

In a group of progressive optic neuropathy, a statistically significant change between baseline and follow-up examination was found for the following HRT parameters: cup shape measurement, classification index, the third moment in contour, cup/disc ratio, cup area, rim area, and area below reference while in the stable group no HRT parameters had changed significantly (Kalaboukhova et al., 2006).

The cup shape measure could be a preferred HRT3 parameter to determine glaucoma progression because it appeared to be independent of standard reference height, although considerable variability exists by other factors (Breusegem et al., 2008). It was the only parameter which provides a significant correlation with progression of the retinal nerve fiber layer defect, whereas the best combination of two parameters included the maximum cup depth and the linear cup: disc area ratio; and the best combination of three parameters included the maximum cup depth, the linear cup: disc area ratio and the horizontal cup: disc area ratio (Saarela & Airaksinen, 2008).

It has been proposed that despite good image quality, the change in the stereometric parameters did not have a high sensitivity and specificity for progression detected with photographs. So evaluation of glaucomatous progression in the optic nerve head should not rely solely on the stereometric parameters of the HRT (Saarela et al., 2010). At present, it is a general opinion that further refinement is required to eliminate some of the inherent variability of the stereometric parameter change analysis (Kamal et al., 2000; Philippin et al., 2006; Deleon et al., 2007; Breusegem et al., 2008; Alencar et al., 2010; Saarela et al., 2010).

It is important to highlight that age-dependent changes occur in optic nerve head topography detectable with the HRT. There were found significant changes indicating increased optic nerve head cupping in cup area, cup-to disc area ratio, rim area, mean cup depth and cup shape measure, after ten years of prospective follow- up in 36 healthy volunteers (Harju et al., 2010).

2.4 Progression analysis application (HRT 3)

The following patient is an African origin boy of 16 years old who was diagnosed of bilateral ocular hypertension in 2007. His grandfather received glaucoma filtration surgery in both eyes.

On clinical examination the average intraocular pressure measured by dynamic contour tonometer (Pascal tonometer) was 23.5mmHg (range 19.9-25.5) in the right eye and 23.7mmHg (range 20-27.7) in the left eye. The central corneal thickness was 642 and 630 for the respective eyes. The fundoscopic characteristics of both eyes are shown in figure 6. The visual field Octopus 101, 32 program, TOP strategy and Frequency- Doubling Technology (Humphrey Zeiss 710 FDT) were normal for both eyes.

The first step to analyze if glaucomatous progression occurred is the assessment of image quality in the baseline and the follow- up sequence. Those images with poor quality (more than 30µm) were excluded for the progression analysis in this patient.

The printed TCA and the trend analysis are displayed in figure 7 and 8 for the respective eyes. The TCA shows the significant height variation in different super- pixels within the disc margin (red colour) that do not form a cluster (both eyes).

The stereometric parameters were obtained after the contour line was delineated by an expert. The HRT computation revealed a disc area of 1.6mm^2 and 1.83mm^2 for respective eyes, so the disc size asymmetry may explain the slight asymmetry in cup appearance (figure 6).

The average reference height was 539.7µm and 516.5µm for the respective eyes. There was low variability between the baseline and the follow- up images in both eyes (average 1.6% and 2.1% respectively). The reference height can be obtained from the stereometric parameters window in each image analysis. The percentage of variability is then calculated.

Thanks to good quality images, proper alignment, and low variability in the standard reference plane, the trend analysis become reliable and can help to identify if real progression has occurred.

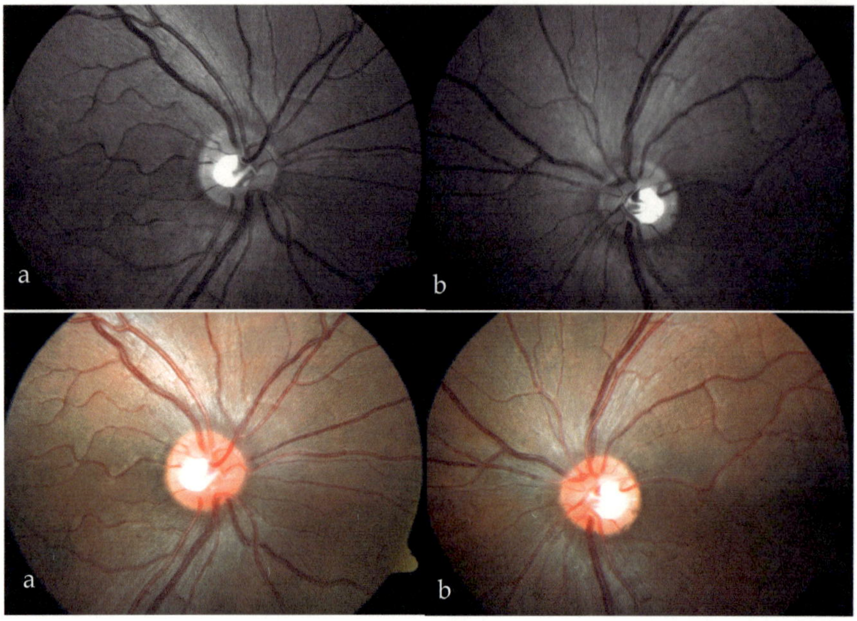

Fig. 6. Red- free and coloured photographs of the retinal nerve fiber layer and optic disc in the right eye (a) and in the left eye (b). As positive details the cup: disc area ratio and the vertical cup: disc diameter are both slightly increased in the left eye. The superior neuroretinal rim is larger than the inferior in both eyes.

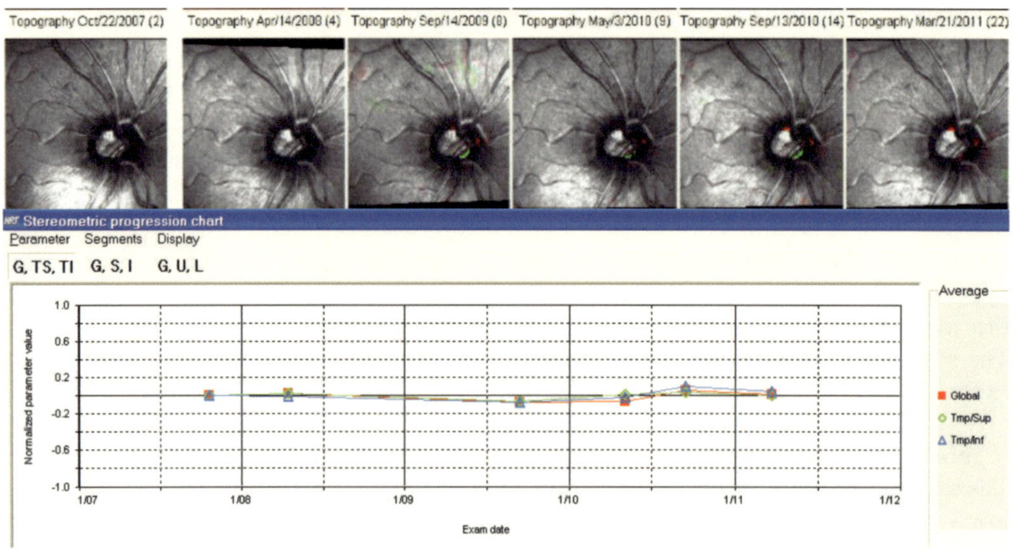

Fig. 7. Topographic Change Analysis and Trend Analysis of the right eye. The superior row shows the significance map superimposed on the reflectance image in the progression sequence. The inferior row shows the trend analysis. There were no significant changes on stereometric parameters over time.

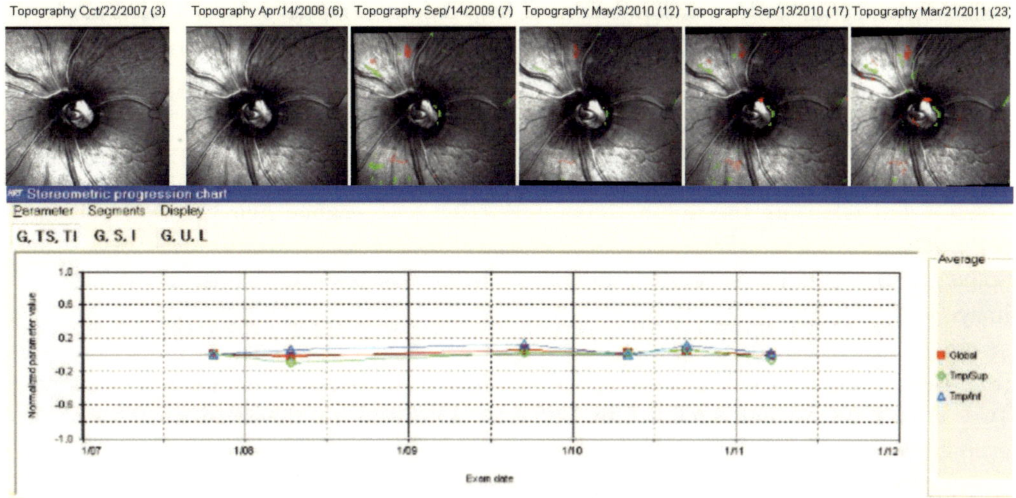

Fig. 8. Topographic Change Analysis and Trend Analysis of the left eye. The superior row illustrates a cluster in the superior retinal nerve fiber layer and significant height changes in super- pixels of the supero- temporal neuroretinal rim. There were no significant changes on stereometric parameters over time.

Progression analysis was also assessed following the changes on the main five stereometric parameters over time (figure 9). There was no variability in the four years follow- up.

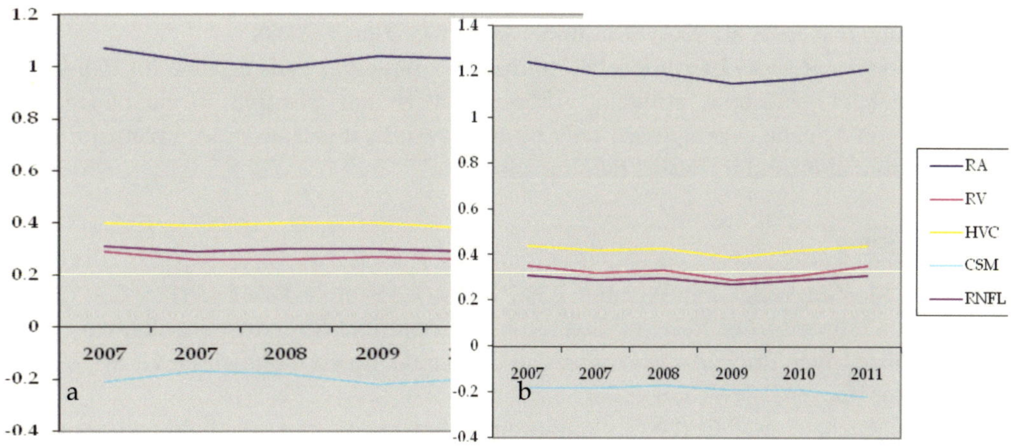

Fig. 9. Variability on the main five stereometric parameters over time in the right eye (a) and in the left eye (b). RA: rim area, RV: rim volume, HVC: height variation contour, CSM: cup shape measure, RNFL: retinal nerve fiber layer thickness.

In this patient longer follow- up is needed to identify if progression occurred by optic disc deterioration or visual fields abnormalities. Until now he receives early preventive treatment since he is considered at high risk of progression basis on his African origin, positive family history of glaucoma and long life expectance (Kass et al., 2010).

3. Conclusion

No consensus yet exists as to how best to integrate the new technology into clinical practice and what are the optimal operating criteria to enable their full potential to be realized.

Some authors prefer the TCA for progression analysis because it provides appropriate image alignment correction and considering guidelines for clinical versus statistical significant progress, whereas stereometric parameters measurements show big variability (Breusegem et al., 2008). Others consider that unlike rim area, the anatomical correlate of TCA is less easily understood. The HRT rim area may be observed both by clinical examination and by assessment of optic disc stereo-photographs (Asaoka et al., 2009). A recent study concluded that statistical methods for detecting structural changes in HRT images exhibit only moderate agreement with each other and have poor agreement with expert-assessed change in optic disc stereophotographs (O'Leary et al., 2010). For the most advantageous use of HRT it has been proposed the use of TCA as a tool for screening and the trend analysis as a confirmation of positive TCA cases. (Martinez de la Casa et al., 2006).

Different articles show evidence suggesting that there is poor agreement between structural and functional measurements of progression despite similar high levels of specificity and regardless of stage of disease. It has been suggested that it is the result of differences in measurement variability between the two methods in individual patients or different forms of presentation of the disease. It is not possible to be certain that there is an ordered structure–function relationship in glaucoma until the issue of test variability has been resolved fully (Fayers et al., 2007; Strouthidis & Garway-Heath, 2008).

The progression analysis by confocal scanning laser tomography is a powerful tool in the management of glaucoma patients. Although it is not possible to guarantee that glaucomatous damage is progressed only by HRT results, it is a strong complement to the clinical examination and the visual field function.

4. References

Alencar, L.M.; Zangwill, L.M.; Weinreb, L.N.; Bowd, C.; Sample, P.A. & Girkin, C.A. (2010). A Comparison of Rates of Change in Neuroretinal Rim Area and Retinal Nerve Fiber Layer Thickness in Progressive Glaucoma. Invest Ophthalmo. Vis Sci, Vol.51, No.7, pp. 3531-3539, ISSN: 1552-5783.

Artes, P.H. & Chauhan, B.C. (2005). Longitudinal changes in the visual field and optic disc in glaucoma. Prog Retin Eye Res, Vol.24, pp. 333-354, ISSN: 1350-9462.

Asaoka, R.; Strouthidis, N.G.; Kappou, V.; Gardiner, S.K. & Garway-Heath, D.F. (2009). HRT-3 Moorfields reference plane: effect on rim area repeatability and identification of progression. Br J Ophthalmol, Vol.93, pp. 1510-1513, ISSN: 1468-2079

Bergin, C.; Garway-Heath, D.F. & Crabb, D.P. (2008). Evaluating the effect of the new alignment algorithm for longitudinal series of Heidelberg retina tomography images. Acta Ophthalmologica. Vol.86, No.2, pp. 207-214, ISSN: 1755-3768.

Bowd, C.; Balasubramanian, M.; Weinreb, R.N.; Vizzeri, G.; Alencar, L.M.; et al. (2009). Performance of Confocal Scanning Laser Tomograph Topographic Change Analysis (TCA) for Assessing Glaucomatous Progression. Invest Ophthalmol Vis Sci, Vol.50, No.2, pp. 691-701, ISSN:1552-5783.

Breusegem, C.; Fieuws, S.; Stalmans, I. & Zeyen, T. (2008). Variability of the Standard Reference Height and Its Influence on the Stereometric Parameters of the Heidelberg Retina Tomograph 3. Invest Ophthalmol Vis Sci, Vol.49, No.11, pp. 4881-4885, ISSN: 1552-5783.

Budenz, D.L.; Anderson, D.R.; Feuer, W.J.; et al. (2006). Detection and prognostic significance of optic disc haemorraghes during the ocular hypertension treatment study. Ophthalmology, Vol.113, pp. 2137-2143, ISSN: 0161-6420.

Chauhan, B.C.; McCormick, B.A.; Nicolela, M.T. & Le Blanc, R.P. (2001). Optic Disc and Visual Field Changes in a Prospective Longitudinal Study of Patients with Glaucoma. Arch Ophthalmol, Vol.119, pp. 1492-1499, ISSN: 0003-9950.

Chauhan, B.C.; Hutchison, D.M.; Artes, P.H.; Caprioli, J.; Jonas, J.B.; LeBlanc, R.P. & Nicolela, M.T. (2009). Optic disc progression in glaucoma: comparison of confocal scanning laser tomography to optic disc photographs in a prospective study. Invest Ophthalmol Vis Sci, Vol.50, No.4, pp. 1682-1691, ISSN: 1552-5783.

Deleon, J.E.; Sakata, L.M.; Kakati, B.; McGwin, G. Jr.; Monheit, B.E.; Arthur, S.N. & Girkin, C.A. (2007). Effect of glaucomatous damage on repeatability of confocal scanning laser ophthalmoscope, scanning laser polarimetry, and optical coherence tomography. Invest Ophthalmol Vis Sci, Vol.48, No.3, pp. 1156-1163, ISSN: 1552-5783.

Fayers, T.; Strouthidis, N.G. & Garway-Heath, D.F. (2007). Monitoring glaucomatous progression using a novel Heidelberg retina tomograph event analysis. Ophthalmology, Vol.114, pp. 1973-1980, ISSN: 0161-6420.

Fogagnolo, P.; Romano, S.; Ranno, S.; Taibbi, G.; Pierrottet, C.; Ferreras, A.; Figus, M.;, Rossetti, L. & Orzalesi, N. (2011). Diagnostic assessment of normal and pale optic nerve heads by confocal scanning laser ophthalmoscope and stereophotography. J Glaucoma, Vol.20, No.1, pp. 10-4, ISSN: 1057-0829.

García-Martín, E.; Pablo, L.; Ferreras, A.; Idoipe, M.; Pérez, S. & Pueyo, V. (2010). Ability of Heidelberg Retina Tomograph III to predict progression in patients with early glaucoma or suspected primary open-angle glaucoma. Arch Soc Esp Oftalmol, Vol.85, No.4, pp. 138-143, ISSN: 0365-6691.

Harju, M.; Saari, J.; Kurvinen, L. & Vesti, E. (2008). Reversal of optic disc cupping in glaucoma. Br J Ophthalmol, Vol.92, No.7, pp. 901-905, ISSN: 1468-2079.

Harju, M.; Kurvinen, L.; Saari, J. & Vesti, E. (2010). Change in optic nerve head topography in healthy volunteers: an 11-year follow-up. Br J Ophthalmol ISSN: 1468-2079. doi:10.1136/bjo.2010.186213.

Heidelberg Retina Tomograph. (2005). Operating Instructions Software Version 3.0. Glaucoma Module, Heidelberg Engineering Gmgh, Alemania.

Hudson, C.J.; Kim, L.S.; Hancock, S.A.; et al. (2007). Some dissociating factors in the analysis of structural and functional progressive damage in open-angle glaucoma. Br J Ophthalmol, Vol.91, pp. 624-628, ISSN: 1468-2079.

Jampel, H.D.; Vitale, S.; Ding, Y.; Quigley, H.; Friedman, D.; Congdon, N. & Zeimer, R. (2006). Test-retest variability in structural and functional parameters of glaucoma damage in the glaucoma imaging longitudinal study. J Glaucoma, Vol.15, No.2, pp. 152-157, ISSN: 1057-0829 .

Kalaboukhova, L.; Fridhammar, V. & Lindblom, B. (2006). Glaucoma follow-up by the Heidelberg retina tomograph--new graphical analysis of optic disc topography changes. Graefes Arch Clin Exp Ophthalmol, Vol.244, No.6, pp. 654-662, ISSN: 0721-832X(prin version) 1435-702X(electronic version).

Kamal, D.S.; Garway-Heath, D.F.; Hitchings, R.A.; et al. (2000). Use of sequential Heidelberg retina tomograph images to identify changes at the optic disc in ocular hypertensive patients at risk of developing glaucoma. Br J Ophthalmol, Vol.84, pp. 993-998, ISSN: 1468-2079.

Kass, M.A.; Gordon, M.O.; Gao, F.; Heuer,, D.K.; Higginbotham, E.J.; et al; for the Ocular Hypertension Treatment Study Group. (2010). Delaying Treatment of Ocular Hypertension. *Arch Ophthalmol*, Vol.128 No.3, pp. :276-287. doi:10.1001/archophthalmol.2010.20

Kourkoutas, D.; Buys, Y.M.; Flanagan, J.G.; et al. (2007). Comparison of glaucoma progression evaluated with Heidelberg retina tomograph II versus optic nerve head stereophotographs. Can J Ophthalmol, Vol.42, pp. 82-88, ISSN: 1715-3360.

Martínez de la Casa, J.M.; García-Feijoó, J.; Vizzeri, G. & Bowd, C. (2006). Rentabilidad diagnóstica de los sistemas de análisis de progresión del tomógrafo retiniano de Heidelberg. Boletín de la Soc. Oftalmo. de Madrid - N.° 46, ISSN: 1132-3701.

Miglior, S.; Albé, E.; Guareschi, M.; Rossetti, L. & Orzalesi, N. (2002). Intraobserver and interobserver reproducibility in the evaluation of optic disc stereometric parameters by Heidelberg retina tomograph. Ophthalmology, Vol.109, No.6, pp. 1072-1077, ISSN: 0161-6420.

Nicolela, M.T.; Soares, A.S.; Carrillo, M.M.; et al. (2006). Effect of moderate intraocular pressure changes on topographic measurements with confocal scanning laser tomography in patients with glaucoma. Arch Ophthalmol, Vol.124, pp. 633-640, ISSN: 0003-9950.

O'Leary, N.; Crabb, D.P.; Mansberger, S.L.; Fortune, B.; Twa, M.D.; Lloyd, M.J.; Kotecha, A.; Garway-Heath, D.F.; Cioffi, G.A. & Johnson, C.A. (2010). Glaucomatous progression in series of stereoscopic photographs and Heidelberg retina tomograph images. Arch Ophthalmol. Vol.128, No.5, pp. 560-568, ISSN: 0003-9950.

Owen, V.M.; Strouthidis, N.G.; Garway-Heath, D.F. & Crabb, D.P. (2006). Measurement variability in Heidelberg retina tomograph imaging of neuroretinal rim area. Invest Ophthalmol Vis Sci, Vol.47, pp. 5322-5330, ISSN: 1552-5783.

Patterson, A.J.; Garway-Heath, D.F. & Crabb, D.P. (2006). Improving the repeatability of topographic height measurements in confocal scanning laser imaging using maximum-likelihood deconvolution. Invest Ophthalmol Vis Sci, Vol.47, pp. 4415-4421, ISSN: 1552-5783.

Philippin, H.; Unsoeld, A.; Maier, P.; Walter, S.; Bach, M. & Funk, J. (2006). Ten-year results: detection of long-term progressive optic disc changes with confocal laser tomography Graefes Arch Clin Exp Ophthalmol, Vol.244, No.4, pp. 460-464, ISSN: :0721-832X(prin version) 1435-702X(electronic version).

Saarela, V. & Airaksinen, P.J. (2008). Heidelberg retina tomograph parameters of the optic disc in eyes with progressive retinal nerve fibre layer defects. Acta Ophthalmol, Vol.86, No.6, pp. 603-608, ISSN: 1755-3768.

Saarela, V.; Falck, A.; Airaksinen, P.J. & Tuulonen, A. (2010). The sensitivity and specificity of Heidelberg Retina Tomograph parameters to glaucomatous progression in disc photographs. Br J Ophthalmol, Vol.94, pp. 68-73, ISSN: 1468-2079.

Sihota, R.; Gulati, V.; Agarwal, H.C.; Saxena, R.; Ajay, S. & Pandey, R.M. (2002). Variables Affecting Test-Retest Variability Of Heidelberg Retina Tomograph II Stereometric Parameters. J Glaucoma, Vol.11, No.4, pp. 321-328, ISSN: 1057-0829.

Strouthidis, N.G.; White, E.T; Owen, V.M.; et al. (2005a). Factors affecting the test-retest variability of Heidelberg retina tomograph and Heidelberg retina tomograph II measurements. Br J Ophthalmol, Vol.89, pp. 1427-1432, ISSN:1468-2079 ____.

Strouthidis, N.G.; White, E.T.; Owen, V.M.; et al. (2005b). Improving the repeatability of Heidelberg retina tomograph and Heidelberg retina tomograph II rim area measurements. Br J Ophthalmol, Vol.89, pp. 1433-1437, ISSN: 1468-2079_____.

Strouthidis, N.G.; Scott, A.; Peter, N.M. & Garway-Heath, D.F. (2006). Optic disc and visual field progression in ocular hypertensive subjects: detection rates, specificity, and agreement. Invest Ophthalmol Vis Sci. Vol.47, pp. 2904-2910, ISSN: 1552-5783_____.

Strouthidis, N.G. & Garway-Heath, D.F. (2008). New developments in Heidelberg retina tomograph for glaucoma. Current Opinion in Ophthalmology, Vol.19, No.2, pp. 141-148, ISSN: 1040-8738.

Tan, J.C.; Garway-Heath, D.F.; Fitzke, F.W. & Hitchings, R.A. (2003a). Reasons for rim area variability in scanning laser tomography. Invest Ophthalmol Vis Sci, Vol.44, pp. 1126-1131, ISSN: 1552-5783_____.

Tan, J.C.; Garway-Heath, D.F. & Hitchings, R.A. (2003b). Variability across the optic nerve head in scanning laser tomography. Br J Ophthalmol, Vol.87, pp. 557-559, ISSN: 1468-2079 .

Teng, C.C.; De Moraes, C.G.; Prata, T.S.; Tello, C.; Ritch, R.; Liebmann, M. (2010). Beta-Zone parapapillary atrophy and the velocity of glaucoma progression. Ophthalmology, Vol.117, No.5, pp. 909-915, ISSN: 0161-6420.

Vizzeri, G.; Weinreb, R.N.; Martinez de la Casa, J.M.; Alencar, L.M.; Bowd, C.; et al. (2009). Clinicians Agreement in Establishing Glaucomatous Progression Using the Heidelberg Retina Tomograph. Ophthalmology, Vol.116, No.1, pp. 14-24, ISSN: 0161-6420.

Vizzeri, G.; Kjaergaard, S.M.; Rao, H.L. & Zangwill, L.M. (2011). Role of imaging in glaucoma diagnosis and follow-up. Indian J Ophthalmol, Vol.59, pp. 59-68, ISSN: 0301-4738.

9

Nerve Fiber Layer Defects Imaging in Glaucoma

Kubena T., Kofronova M. And Cernosek P.
Glaucoma service
U zimniho stadionu 1759
Czech Republic

1. Introduction

Glaucoma is in the group of neurodegenerative diseases. A characteristic of this disease is glaucoma neuropathy which is caused by a loss of ganglion cells. In a healthy eye there is a vital optic nerve head and a thick layer of nerve fibres. With a glaucoma patient there are various stages of defects in nerve fibre layer. A subjective examination of the nerve fibre layer belongs in routine glaucoma examinations. It is beneficial for early glaucoma diagnostic. For documentation and follow-up examinations it is useful to make special adjusted red free photos to compare them with these baseline photos. This paper shows a step by step examination nerve fibre layer, its digital photo documentation, picture processing and archiving. Practical benefit of the adjusted red free photos of nerve fibre layer is highlighted in two interesting cases.

2. Nerve fibre layer defects and how to diagnose them

In a healthy eye the nerve fibre layer can be seen as silky and clear with fine strips in red free digital photos (Figure 1). The nerve fibre layer is thickest near to the optic nerve head, especially in the inferior part, slightly thinner is in the superior part. In the temporal part, which includes a maculopapillar bundle, nerve fibre layer is very silky, stripy but no perfectly clearly visible. In the nasal part it is difficult to detect the nerve fibre layer because in this area is naturally thin. In the temporal part of the macula a horizontal line connecting superior and inferior nerve fibre layers can be found. Some vessels are also very helpful in detecting nerve fibre layers. In a healthy eye vessels are overlapped of the nerve fibre layers like several veils.

In a routine ophthalmologic examination we used to provide a biomicroscopy with a Volk 65 or 90 dioptres lens. To detect the nerve fibre layer we use a red free light which reflects from nerve fibre layer and make visible its characteristic stripy structure. In location of a nerve fibre layer loss the red free light goes through the retina and is reflected from the retinal pigment epithelium. Such places are darker with loss of its characteristic stripping, widening from optic disc to periphery like a comet. Blood vessels are darker in the defects and vessels have sharp reflexes. Defect of nerve fiber layer bellow the optic disc (Fig 2a). corresponds with defect /scotoma/ in the upper part of visual field of the same eye (Fig 2b).

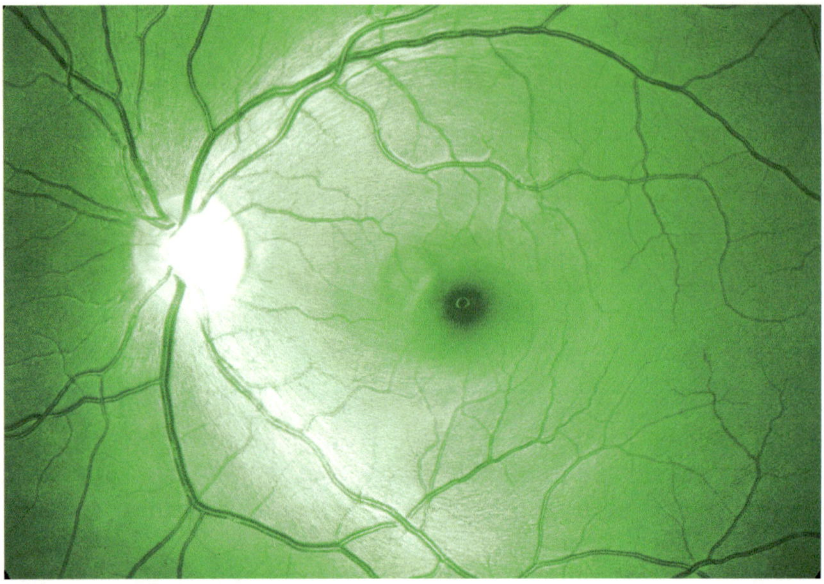

Fig. 1. Nerve fibre layer in healthy eye

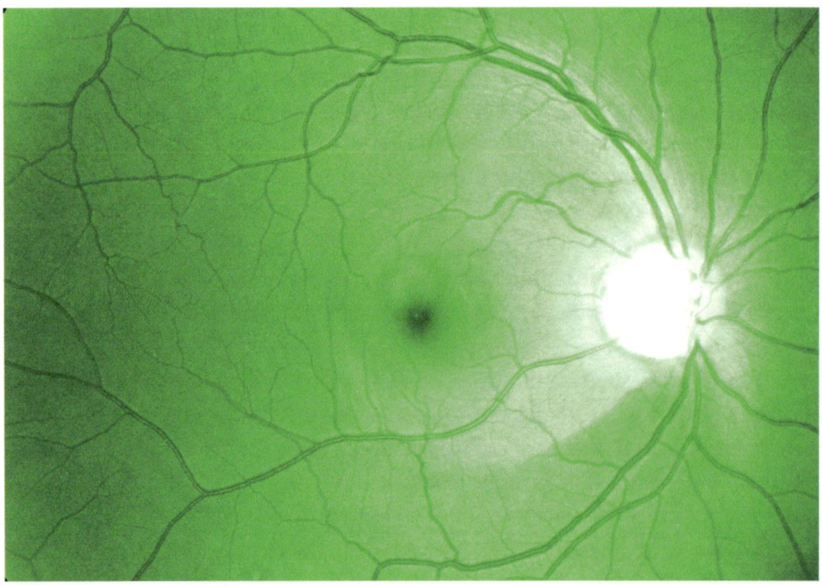

Fig. 2a. Nerve fibre layer defect bellow the optic disc

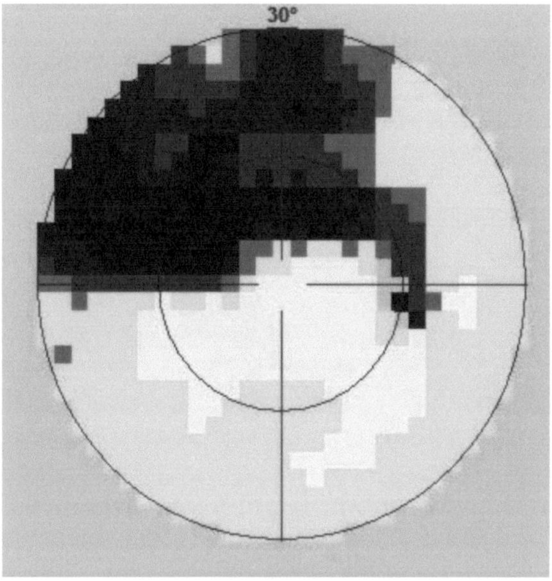

Fig. 2b. Defect /scotoma/ in the upper part of visual field

Small focal defects width of few retinal vessels do not cause visual field defects. This stage of glaucoma is called preperimetric stadium. For that reason the focal defects are very important and helpful in the diagnosis of early stage of glaucoma (Fig 3).

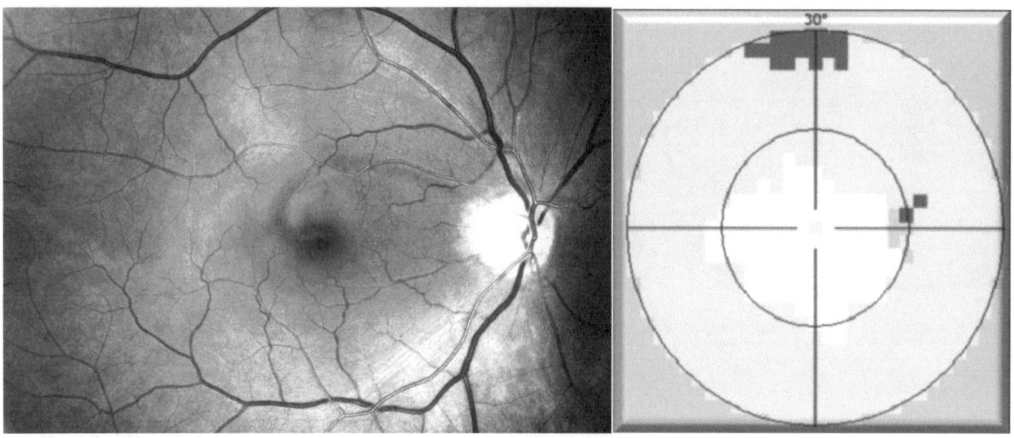

Fig. 3. Focal defect in nerve fibre layer in upper part of maculopapillar bundle with normal visual field of the same eye.

With glaucoma progression nerve fibre layer defects getting darker and enlarge from strip to wedge form. Than first visual field defects begin to appear. This stage of glaucoma is called perimetric stadium. Visual field defects usually begin in the nasal area of the visual field close horizontal line and are known as a Ronne´s nasal step (Fig 4). The wedge defect of the nerve fibre layer between 12 to 2 clock corresponds with her visual field defect bellow nasal horizontal line. The focal defect of her nerve fibre layer in 5 clock has not induce a visual field scotoma yet.

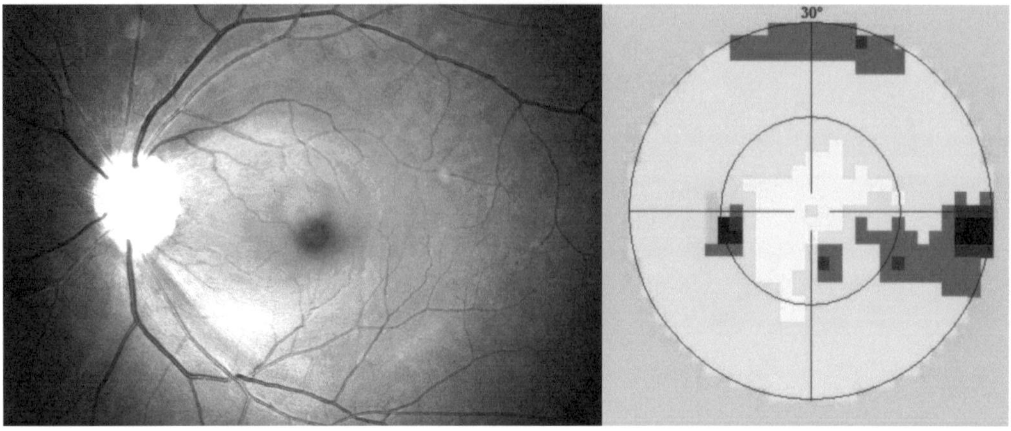

Fig. 4. Wedge defect in 12-2 clock correspond with lower Ronne´s nasal step of the visual field the same eye. Focal defect in 5 clock with normal upper part of visual field.

With glaucoma progression nerve fibre layer defects enlarge and visual field defects expand to paracentral part and lasts in blind spot area. Wedge defects well correspond with visual field defects (Fig 5).

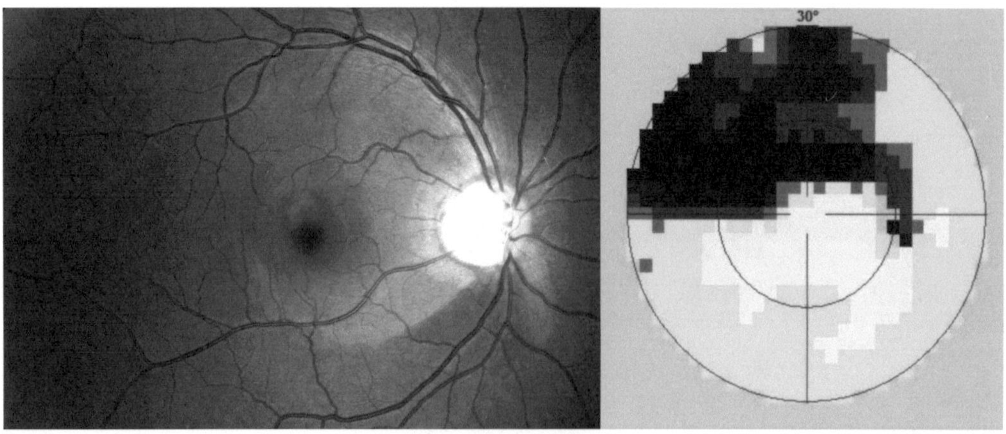

Fig. 5. Wedge defect of nerve fibre layer in lower part of retina and scotoma in upper part of the visual field of the same eye.

Diffuse thinning or diffuse atrophy of the nerve fiber layer can be seen in advanced glaucoma. It is usually difficult to detect on one eye, but when we compare both eyes together, glaucoma atrophy is usually asymmetric and is easily recognized.

3. Nerve fibre layer defecst and how to image them

Fundus camera Canon CF-60UV with digital camera Canon EOS 20D for digital picture performing is used. The camera setting of the visual field is 60 degrees and the excitation filter for fluorescein angiography with maximal transmission on wave length 480 nm is used. Flash intensity is performed to F2 level. Camera setting: Lens shutter time is 1/80, ISO 400 and picture quality L /3504x2669 pixels/ - type JPG. Personal computer with operating system Windows XP is connected with a digital camera by the way of a USB connector. Program EOS Viewer Utility is running. This program is attached to a digital camera CD. In this program we create a new folder for each patient with his or her ID, in which we save the pictures.

3.1 Performing of the digital picture

The examination is performed is at least in 5 mm pupil dilation. The patient is looking with his/her examination eye to the camera objective so in the centre of the picture is the central part of the retina. The next step is performing the correct approximation of the fundus camera close to the examination eye, focusing and pressing the shutter of the camera. The performed picture is taken within 1 second and is translate from the camera to the computer so we can examine the picture on the screen.

If the picture is too dark or too light, intensity of the flash is slightly changed and photo is repeated. Usually 3 to 5 pictures are taken from each eye. In full screen program EOS Viewer Utility the best picture is choose and other pictures are deleted.

3.2 Computer graphics adjustment in program Photoshop CS2

Original picture is adjusted in the following steps:

a. Downloading of the original picture to the program Photoshop - File/Open (Fig.6, 7)
b. Adjustment of the picture histogram - Image/ Adjustment / Levels - shift of the right, eventually left scroll bar close to the center. (Fig.8, 9)
c. Picture conversion to the monochromatic light- Image / Mode / Gray scale (Fig.10, 11)
d. Adjustment of the contrast- Image / Adjustment / brightness and contrast (Fig. 12)
e. Storing of the adjusted image (Fig. 13)

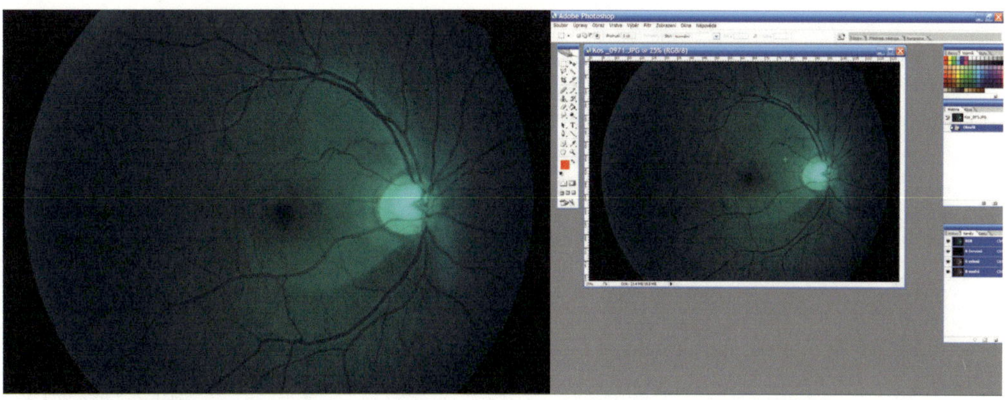

Fig. 6. and 7. Original picture and it s downloading to program Photoshop

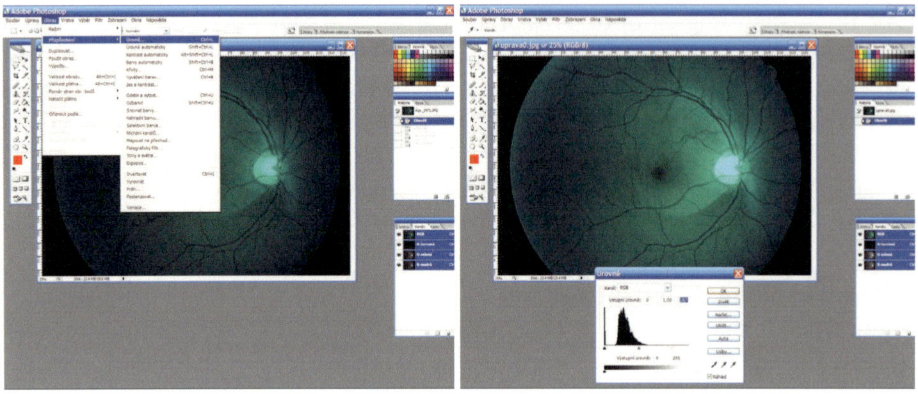

Fig. 8. 9. Histogram picture adjustment

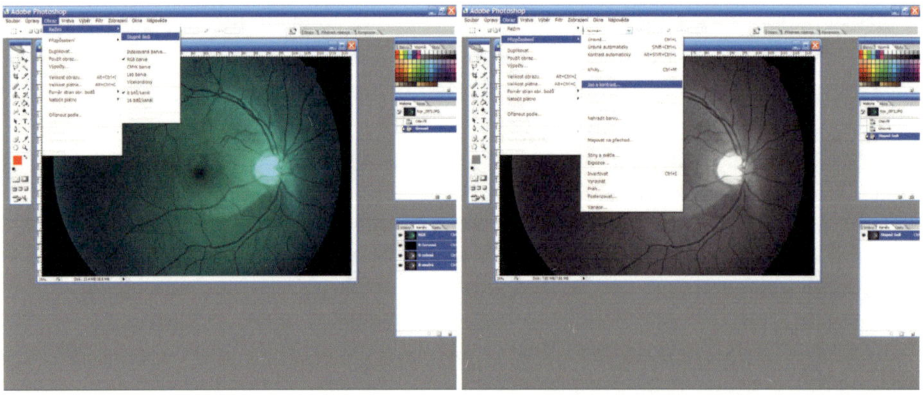

Fig. 10. 11. Picture conversion to monochromatic light

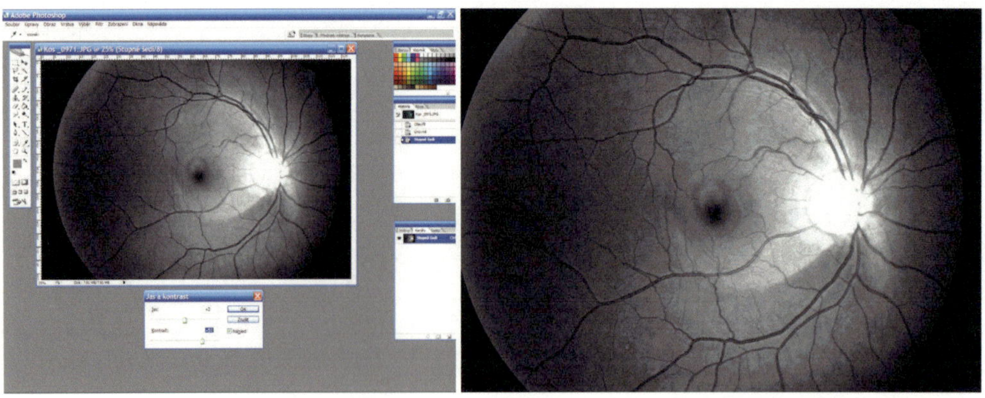

Fig. 12. 13. Brightness, contrast adjustment and picture storage.

4. Cases

4.1 Case 1

We would like to present 43 years old man under treatment for pigmentary glaucoma since year 2000. Even before year 2000 there was the visual field scotoma in upper part on the right eye corresponding with nerve fiber layer defect (Fig. 14), left eye optic nerve and visual field were normal. Prostaglandins were select as a first local antiglaucoma therapy. Although intraocular pressure was about 11,0/12,0 mm Hg, in April 2005 we found peripapillary hemorrhage in No 7 on the right eye, on September 2005 there was evident widening of the wedge nerve fiber layer defect in lower part of right eye, scotoma on the upper part of the right eye was getting deeper and wider. Focal defects on upper part of retina on the right eye and on the left eye are also visible. These small defects didn't cause visual field yet. We added local beta blockers to treatment. One year later, in 2006, Intraocular pressure was 16,5/15, 0 mm Hg. On the both eyes nerve fiber layer defects were similar, also the visual field defects was still on the right eye only, on the left eye was normal visual field. After next 3 years, in 2009, the right eye nerve fiber layer defect and scotoma were still the same extent, but on the left eye we have found peripapillary hemorrhage and the focal nerve fiber layer defect was getting wider (Fig. 15) and scotoma in the upper part of the visual field of the left eye have appeared. We indicated penetrating trabeculectomy on both eyes, et present are the values of intraocular pressure are about 10,0 mm Hg on both eye without local therapy.

In this case we tried to demonstrate how the focal nerve fiber defects (without visual field defects) can enlarge to wedge defects of nerve fiber layer corresponding with visual field defects. (Fig.16,17). Very useful are also peripapillary hemorrhages as indicator of the glaucoma progression.

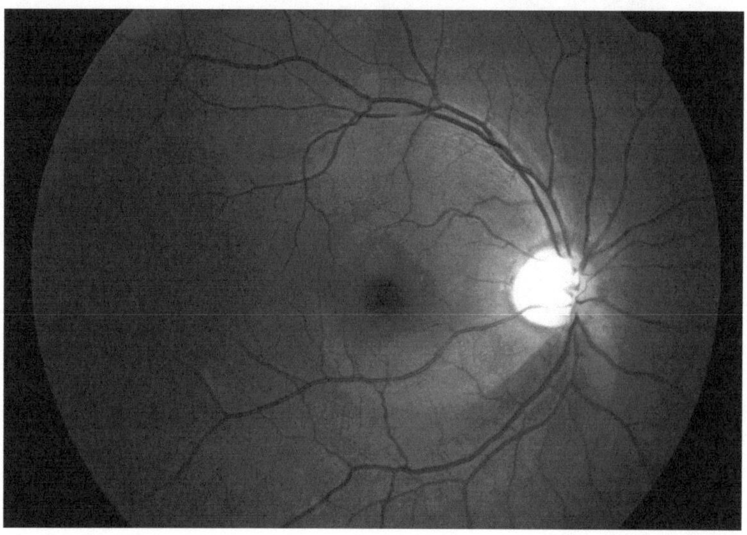

Fig. 14. Right eye: Bellow the optic disc wedge defect corresponding with visual field defect on the upper part.

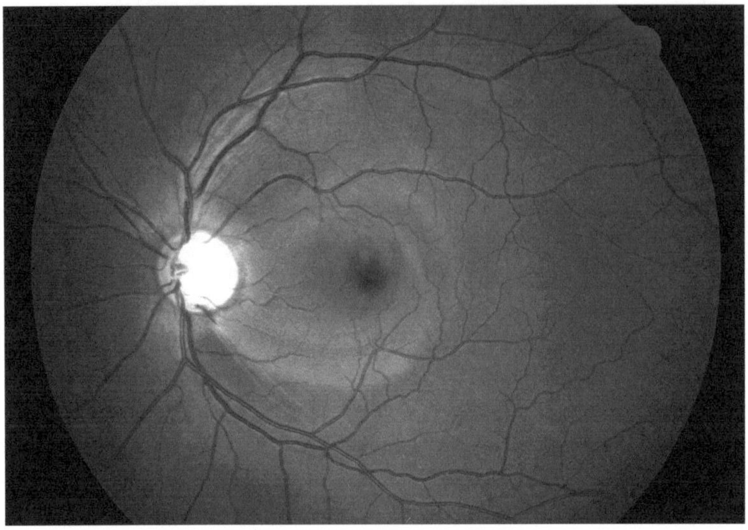

Fig. 15. Left eye: Optic disc splinter hemorrhage on 5 clock. Bellow the optic disc wedge defect

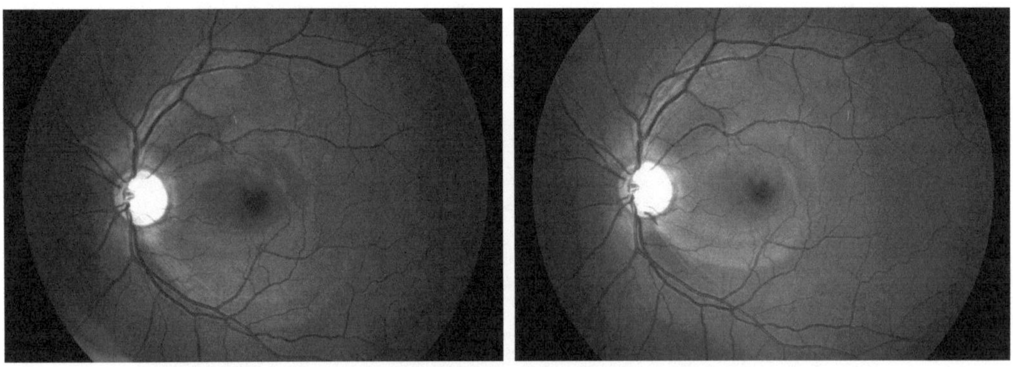

Fig. 16. 17. Left eye: widening of nerve fibre layer defect in lower part of retina in 5 clock position on optic nerve head, which is attending peripapillary hemorrhage. On the left picture (2005) there are only few focal nerve fibre layer defects, on the right picture (2009) peripapillary hemorrhage, wedge defect on the lower part of retina and identical focal defects on the upper part.

4.2 Case 2

47 years old man was sending to our service for reasons non proliferative diabetic retinopathy. This man undergo treatment hypertension (blood pressure 150/80 mm Hg) and diabetes mellitus - insulin.

On retinas of both eyes we have found optic nerve head with normal cupping, vessels with hypertonic changes - narrowing of arteries, dilatation of veins and cross signs. In both retinas was seen dot like hemorrhages. In red free light there were numerous focal nerve fibre layer defects (Fig. 18).

We speculated that nerve fibre layer defects are in consequences with multifocal micro infarcts of optic nerve head in praetrombotic status.

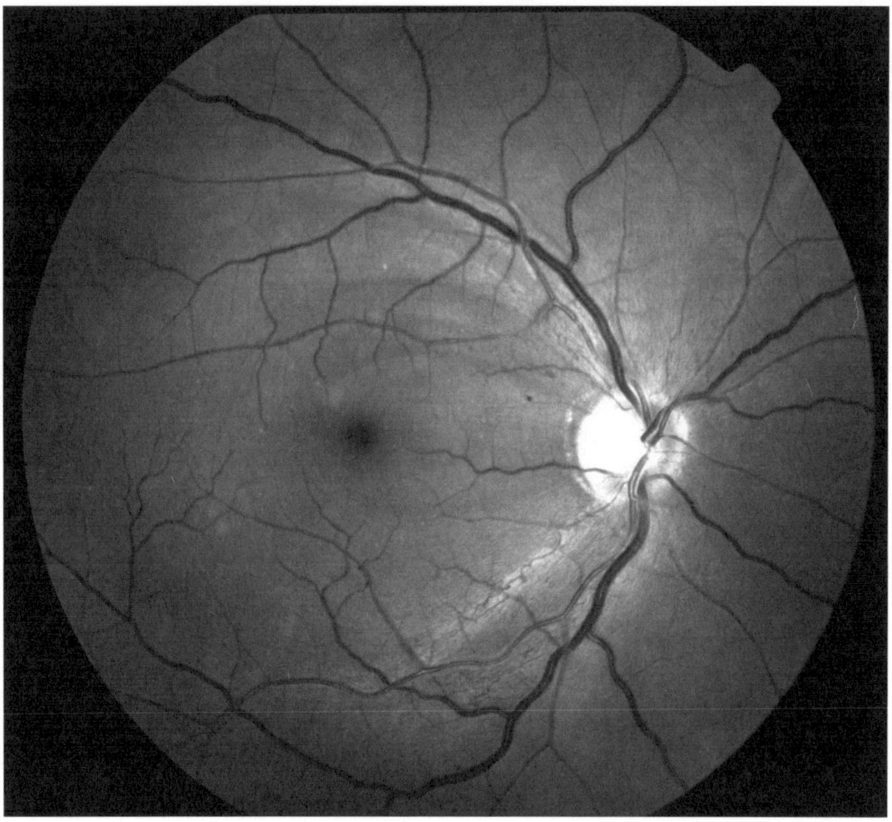

Fig. 18. Dilated veins, cross signs and numerous focal defects of nerve fibre layer

5. Discussion

Nerve fiber layer was firstly described by Vogt in 1913 (Vogt et all., 1913) Half an century later Berhrendt a Wilson (Behrendt et all., 1965) during photo of the retina found, that nerve fiber layer is not visible in the red light, but better visible on the green and blue light. This phenomenon they elucidated by the fact, that blue light does not penetrate through nerve fiber layer, but it is reflected back to the camera in contrast to places with damaged nerve fiber layer and light is absorbed by pigment epithelium of the retina. This is the principle of the contrast between normal and damage areas. Delori and Gradoudas (Delori et all., 1976) founded that best wave length of the light for photography of nerve fiber layer are these from 475 to 520 nm. Rohrschneider (Rohrschneider et all., 1995) recommend for patients with slightly pigmented retinas is useful green-blue filter 470-490 nm, for others green filters 520-540 nm. 15 Airaxinen (Airaxinen et all., 1984) refers about easy detection of nerve fiber layer wide-angle camera with blue monochromatic interference filter.

Nerve fiber layer defects was firstly described by Hoyt (Hoyt et all., 1973). In our national Czech literature published about nerve fiber layer and it s imaging Kurz (Kurz et all., 1956), Kraus (Kraus et all., 1996), Lestak (Lestak et al., 2000).

On our department we found good results with exiting filter for fluorescein angiography with maximal permeability on wave length 480 nm. (Kubena et all., 2008) This filter is usually constant component of the funduscamera. Film frame of the camera we used 60°, which is useful compare with the 30° visual field test. Nerve fiber layer visibility on native pictures is markedly worse in comparison with subjective examination. That is why we tried to find method of the adjustment of pictures so picture quality was nearly equal to our subjective feeling during biomicroscopy examination. We described method picture adjustment in Photoshop program to achieve this effect.

With compared 30 eyes adjusted photographs of nerve fiber layer pictures with results of Heidelberg Retina Tomography, Laser Polarimetry and Optic Coherence Tomography on each eye. Nerve fiber layer defect were comparable on each method, but in case of thin, early defects adjusted photography was superior other methods.

Benefit of nerve fiber layer digital pictures is there are familiar for ophthalmologists, wide-range field and good sensitivity for very thin and early defects.

Disadvantage of the wide-ranged digital pictures is necessity to dilate pupils in taking photos, subjectively evaluation of pictures only, which requires experience of the physicist and impossibility to compare pictures with normative data with sophisticated computer programs.

6. Conclusion

Nerve fiber layer and its defects is beneficial to document with digital red free mydriatic fundus camera. Usual fundus camera with exciting filter for fluorescein angiography can be used. Consecutive adjustment digital pictures in Photoshop CS2 improve visibility of nerve fiber layer. The nerve fiber layer defects in this adjustment photos are comparable with this defects detected by recent image methods. Early recognition of focal defects of retinal nerve fiber layer is useful for diagnosis preperimetric stage of glaucoma, its treatment and follow up.

7. References

Airaksinen, PJ., Drance, SM., Douglas, GR. et al.: Diffuse and localized nerve fiber loss in glaucoma. Am J Ophthalmol., 98, 1984, 566 p.

Airaksinen, PJ., Drance, SM., Douglas, GR. et al.: Visual field and retina nerve fiber layer comparisons in glaucoma, Arch Ophthalmol., 103, 1985, 205 p.

Airaksinen, PJ., Nieminen, H., Mustonen, E.: Retina nerve fiber layer photography with a wide-angle fundus kamera, Acta Ophthalmol (Copenh) 60, 1982: 362 p.

Airaksinen, PJ., Tuulonen, A.: Retinal nerve fiber layer evaluation. In Varma, R., Spaeth, GL. (Ed): The optic nerve in glaucoma, Philadelphia, JB Lippincott, 1993, 277-289 p.

Behrendt, T., Wilson, LA.: Spectral reflectance photography of the retina. Am J Ophthalmol 59, 1965.: 1079 p.

Behrendt, T., Duane, TD.: Investigation of fundus oculi with spectral reflectance photography. I. Depth and integrity of fundal structures, Arch Ophghalmol., 75, 1966, 375 p.

Delori, FC., Gradoudas, ES.: Examination of the ocular fundus with monochromatic light. Ann. Ophthalmol., 8, 1976, 703 p.

Hoyt, WF., Frisen, L., Newman, NM.: Funduscopy of nerve fiber layer defects in glaucoma, Incest Ophthalmol., 12, 1973: 814 p.

Kraus, H., Bartosova, L., Hycl, J.: Evaluation of Retinal Nerve Fiber Layer in Glaucoma. I. Introduction and Method. Ces. a slov. Oftal., 52, 1996, 4: 207-209.

Kraus, H., Bartosova, L., Hycl, J.: Evaluation of Retinal Nerve Fiber Layer in Glaucoma. II. Retinal Nerve Fiber Layer Examination and Development of Visual Field Defects in a Prospective Study. Ces. a slov. Oftal., 56, 2000, 3: 149-153.

Kraus, H., Konigsdorfer, E., Ciganek, L.: Nerve fiber bundle defects of the retina and alteration of computer perimetry in initial stages of glaucoma simplex. Cs. Oftal., 41, 1985, 5: 294-298.

Kubena, T., Klimesova, K., Kofronova M., Cernosek P.: Subjective Examination of the Nerve Fiber layer of the Retina and its Evaluation in Healthy eye and in Glaucoma. Ces. a slov. Oftal., 64, 2008, 1: 3-7.

Kubena, T., Klimesova, K., Kofronova M., Cernosek P.: Digital images of the Retinal Nerve Fiber Layer in Healthy Eye and in Glaucoma. Ces. a slov. Oftal., 65, 2009, 1: 3-7.

Kurz, J.: Oftamlo-neurologicka diagnostika, Praha, Statni zdravotnicke nakladatelstvi, 1956, 765.

Lestak J., Pitrova S., Peskova H.: Diagnostika glaukomu vysetrenim vrstvy nervových vlaken. Ces. a slov. Oftal., 56, 2000, 6: 394-400.

Rohrschneider, K., Kruse, F.E., Durk, R.O.: Possibilities for imaging the retina nerve fiber layer sign the SLO. Ophthalmologe, 92, 1995, s 515/520.

Vogt A: Demonstration eines von Rot befreiten Ophthalmoskopierlichtes. Ber. Dtsch. Ophthalm. Ges. Heidelberg 39, 1913: 416.

Vogt A: Die Nervenfaserstreifung der menschlichen Netzhaut mit besonderer Berucksichtigung der Differential-Diagnose gegenuber Pathologischen streifenformigen reflexen (preretinalen Faltelungen), Klin Monatsbl Augenheilkd., 58, 1917: 399.

Vogt A: Die Nervenfaserzeichnung der menschlichen Netzhaut im rotfreien Licht. Klin Monatsbl Augenheilkd., 66, 1921: 718.

10

Optic Neuropathy Mimicking Normal Tension Glaucoma Associated with Internal Carotid Artery Hypoplasia

Kyoko Shidara and Masato Wakakura
Inouye Eye Hospital/ Tokyo
Japan

1. Introduction

Most cases of ischemic optic neuropathy are of sudden onset without any prior indication of visual field loss. In contrast, a gradual loss of the visual field is observed in normal-tension glaucoma (NTG). We here present a case in which we initially diagnosed NTG but upon further examination it was evident that ICA hypoplasia was present.

Horowitz et el. previously reported an uncommon case of anterior ischemic optic neuropathy that was associated with hypoplasia of the interanal carotid aretry (ICA) (Horowitz et al., 2001) . Here, we report on a curious case in which clinical expression mimicked NTG, but upon further examination there was considered have been an ischemic event due to ICA hypoplasia that was responsible for the noted visual field change.

2. Case report

In 2006, a 41-year-old female visited an ophthalmologist for the purpose of purchasing contact lenses. During the contact lens examination the patient was found to have excavation of the right optic disc. In the past, she had not been aware of any visual dysfunction, including visual blurring, visual field loss or transient monocular blindness. After being diagnosed as having glaucoma treatment was immediately begun. However, the ophthalmologist in charge of the treatment considered her visual field to be atypical and that her disc morphology was not compatible with the observed field defect as is the case in glaucoma.

Therefore, in February of 2007, 1 year after her original examination, she was referred to our hospital. Upon initial presentation at our clinic, her visual acuity (VA) was 20/20 OU. She had a right relative afferent pupillary defect (RAPD) and her intraocular pressures (IOP) were 12 mmHg OD and 10 mmHg OS. Biomicroscopic examination showed normal findings in both eyes. Fundoscopy revealed large disc excavation in her right eye with an almost normal left eye, and there was chorioretinal atrophy in both eyes (Fig. 1). Goldmann perimetry indicated there was a multidirectional, irregular defect at the temporal and nasal quadrants of her right eye (Fig. 2).

Irregular depression at nasal and inferior quadrant of right eye and normal field of left eye on Goldman perimetry.

Over a 3.5-year period, there was no further significant progress noted for this multidirectional and irregular visual field defect. Fluorescein angiography (FA) showed neither leakage nor hyperfluorescence. The retinal nerve fiber layer thickness, as measured by optic coherence tomography (OCT), showed diffuse thinning in her right eye. Borderline results were found for the Moorfields Classification, which used the Heidelberg retina tomography (HRT).

Since she had a RAPD and her visual field and optic disc findings were not typical of glaucoma, we performed magnetic resonance imaging (MRI) and magnetic resonance angiography (MRA) of her head. MRA revealed there was approximately a 50% stenosis of the ophthalmic portion of the right internal carotid artery (ICA) (Fig. 3).

MRA showing approximately 50% stenosis of the right ICA of ophthalmic portion and slight narrowing of the right anterior cerebral artery on brain MRA.

However, there were no abnormality of the right anterior cerebral artery. Three-dimensional computed tomography (3D-CT) indicated that there was a partial stenosis of the right cervical ICA, which was strongly suggestive of hypoplasia (Fig. 4).

A part of hypoplasia and stenosis of the right cervical ICA on 3D-CT.

Color Doppler imaging (CDI) was performed in order to determine the functional characteristics of the internal carotid artery stenosis. As shown in Figure 5, CDI showed a downstream reversed diastolic flow in the right ophthalmic artery. In normal waveforms, there is an initial sharp rise with a small notch noted on the down slope of the peak.

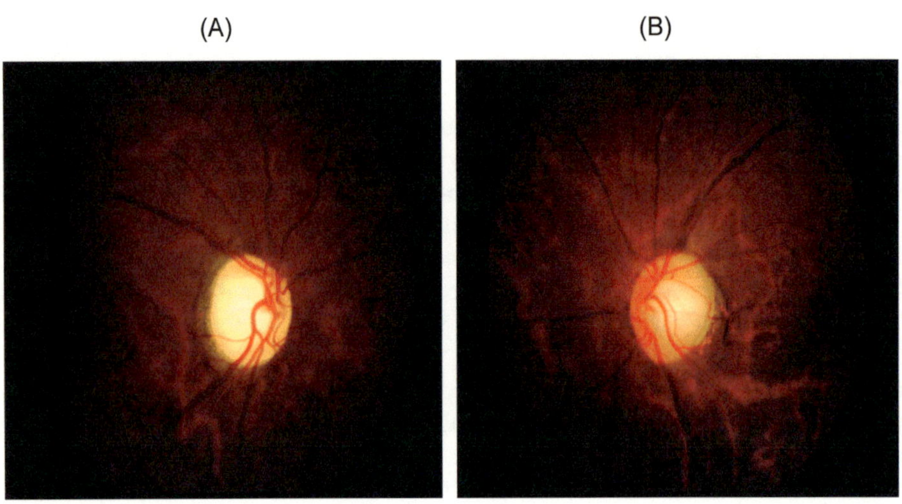

Fig. 1. Fundes photograph
A: right eye B: left eye. Note large cupping in the right eye and almost normal in the left eye.

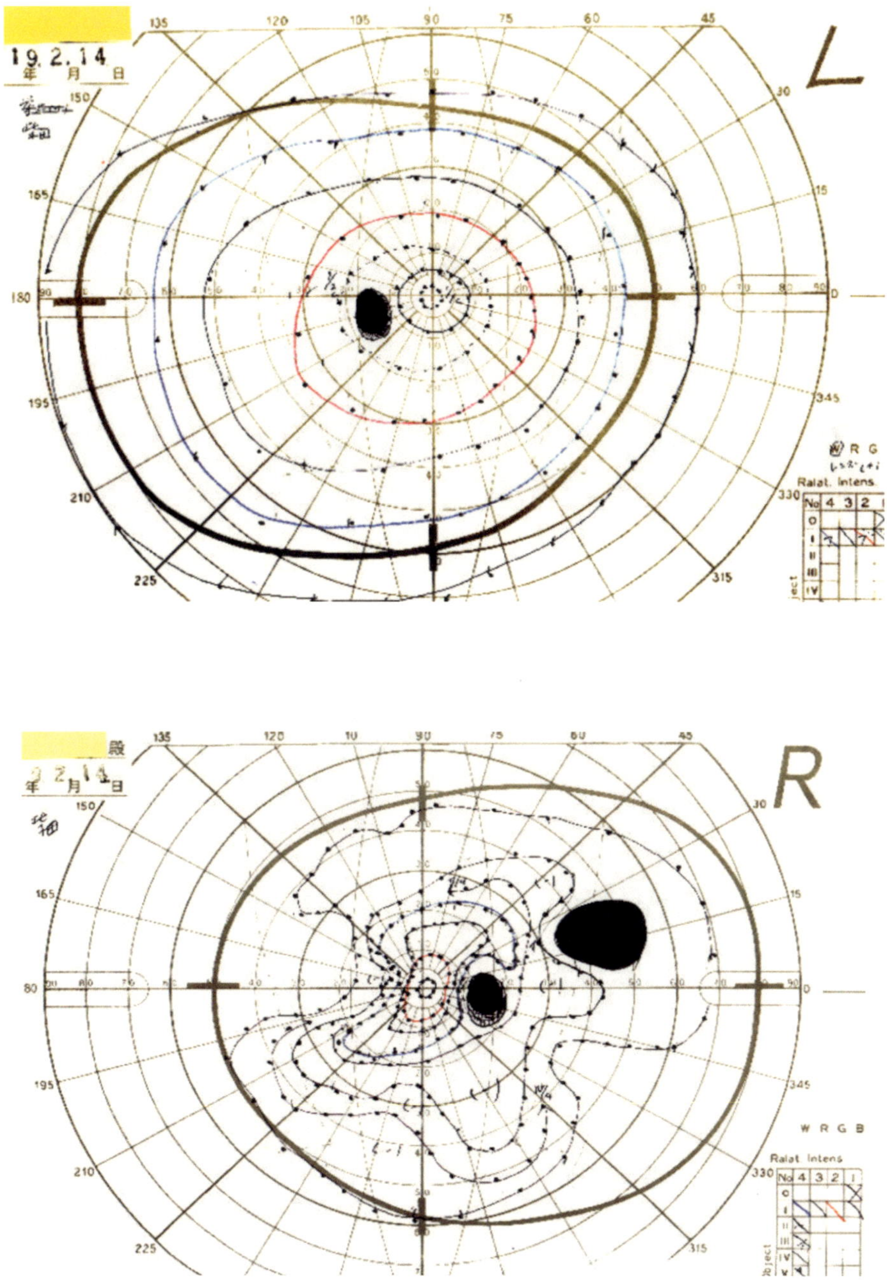

Fig. 2. Goldman perimetry.

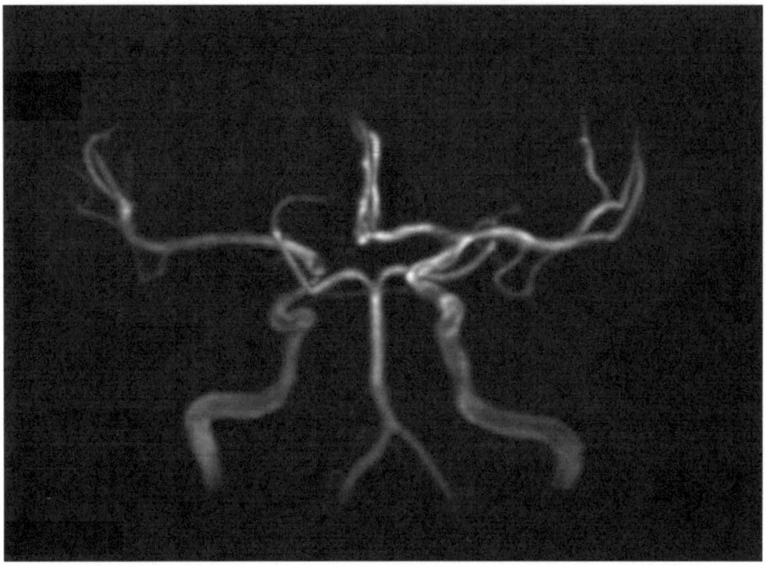

Fig. 3. MRA

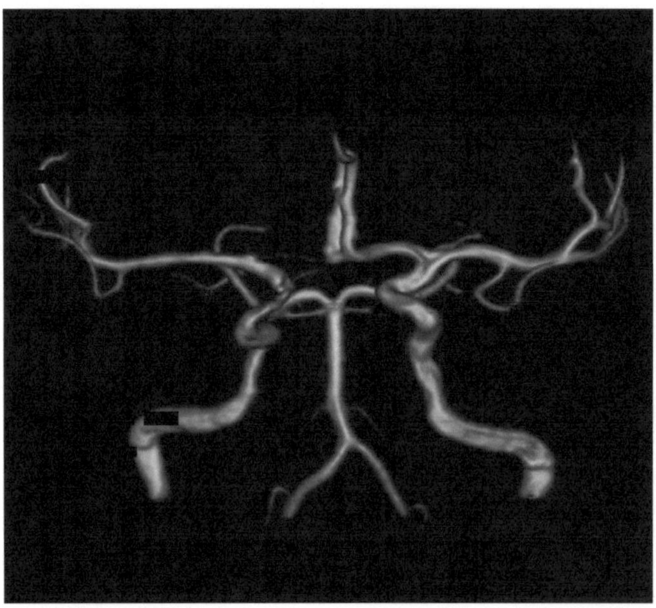

Fig. 4. 3D-CT

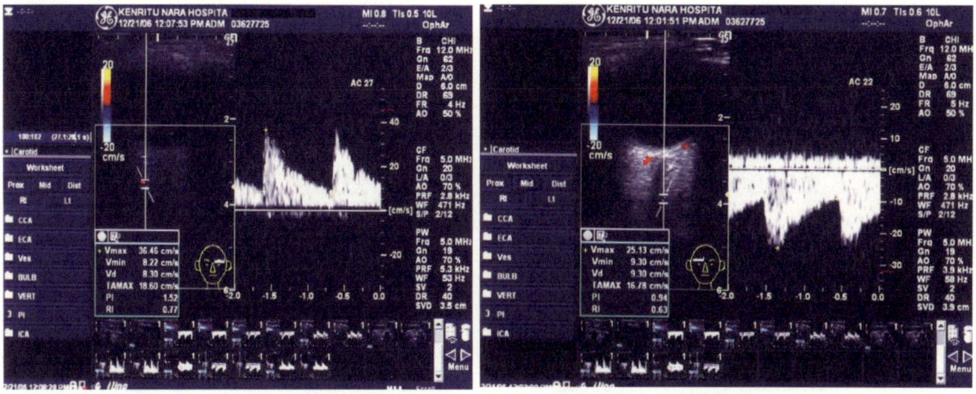

Left eye Right eye

Fig. 5. Orbital CDI.

Note downstream of the right ophthalmic artery and normal upstream of the left ophthalmic artery on orbital CDI.

In the current case, there was an atypical pattern with a slow rising wave that lacked the notch found in the normal waveform. There was a normal typical flow in the left ophthalmic artery. These findings indicated that there was regurgitation of the right ophthalmic artery. This can be explained by a significant stenosis of the right ICA leading to a reverse flow in the right ophthalmic artery (Fujioka S et al., 2003).

To assess the optic disc change, we repeatedly conducted HRT during the year that followed. No significant changes were observed.

We also examined the patient using a Humphrey Field Analyzer (program 30-2 SITA standard test). The patient is currently being seen every 3 months. At the present time, she has completed 3.5 years of follow-up and there has been neither progression of the visual field defect nor any change in the disc appearance (Fig. 6).

3. Discussion

It has been previously reported that ocular ischemic phenomena can result from disease of the cervical ICA: for example amaurosis fugax (AF), acute retinal artery obstruction, branch retinal artery obstruction (BRAO), ischemic optic neuropathy and the ocular ischemic syndrome where the entire globe shows evidence of poor perfusion. There are also case reports of normal tension glaucoma associated with chronic reduction of retrobulbar blood flow(Costa VP et al.,1998).

In the current case, the initial diagnosis was thought to be NTG, however the atypical disc and visual field defects were against this diagnosis. MRA and 3-D CT examinations suggested that there was hypoplasia of the right cervical ICA and orbital CDI of the right ophthalmic artery indicated reversed diastolic. These results suggested that the presumed ischemic optic neuropathy was associated with stenosis and hypoplasia of the right cervical ICA(Kawaguchi S et al., 1999).

Although the finding in the carotid artery could be incidental and unrelated to the optic cupping in this case, in our opinion the carotid artery abnormalities could have been

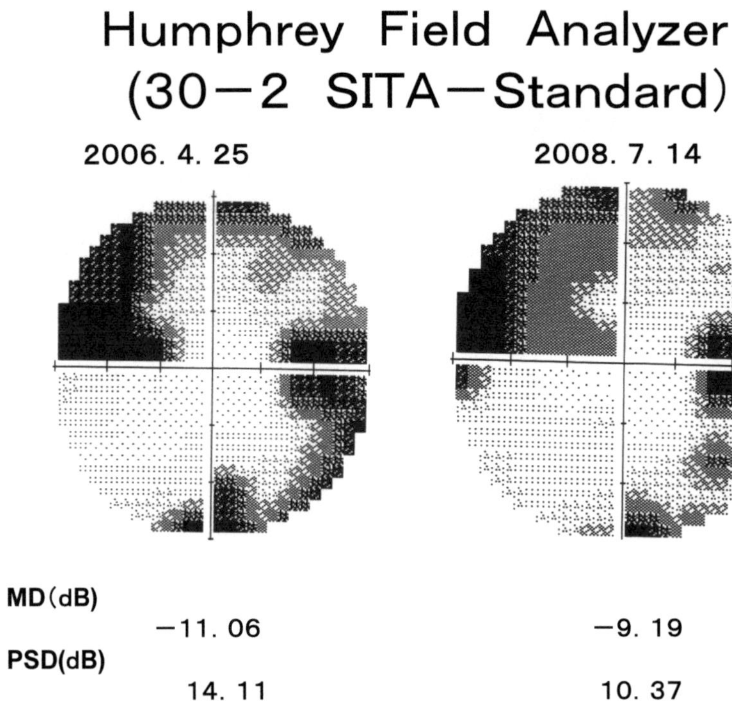

Fig. 6. Humphrey Field Analyzer (30-2 SITA standard test).
Humphrey Field Analyzer (30-2 SITA standard test) initially show decreased sensitivity at each quadrant and MD and PSD revealed no significant changes during 3.5 year.

associated with ischemia of the nerve head at some time. There may be several other possibilities that could explain the ischemic ocular neuropathy including, the accumulation of subclinical ischemic events on the optic nerve, which is referred to as chronic progressive ischemic optic neuropathy (Knox DL et al.,1971), hypoperfusion of the ophthalmic artery (Burghaus L et al.,2007), ischemic optic neuropathy in childhood(Chutorian AM et al,.2002), and conventional anterior or posterior ischemic optic neuropathy that was not noticed by the patient.

Of these optic neuropathy-related ischemic events, only anterior optic neuropathy has been reported to be associated with ICA hypoplasia. It is common knowledge that there is a sudden onset for ischemic events. In the present case, however, for at least 3.5 years there has been neither significant progression of the disc morphology nor any visual field defect. Within this context, there are two possibilities that might explain our observations. One is that there is a very slow progressive ischemic syndrome that is present. This type of ischemic optic neuropathy has been reported as chronic progressive ischemic optic neuropathy, although at the current time there is still much dispute with regard to this entity (Lessell S et al., 1999).

Another possibility is that this type of ischemic optic neuropathy occurs during infancy. Since the patient did not have any subjective symptoms and the current clinical stage of the optic neuropathy appears to be non-active, it very well could be that the patient may simply have had no previous awareness of the initial ischemic event.

Thus, based upon the ICA congenital anomaly, we speculate that the ischemic optic neuropathy could even have occurred during infancy. An ischemic event of this type in the optic nerve could result in a slight enlargement of cupping (Saito H et al., 2008), as well as a non-progressive change in the visual field.

In the ocular ischemic syndrome there are reports that the flow dynamics of the ophthalmic artery can spontaneously improve (Ward JB et al., 1995). In the current case, CDI documented that the right ophthalmic artery exhibited a reversed flow, indicating that there was the normal flow, indicating that there was the normal collateral pathway from the external carotid artery to the right ophthalmic artery. It is our belief that this collateral pathway provided indispensable circulation.

Hypoplasia of the ICA is rare : less than 100 cases having been reported (Horowitz et al., 2001). Although this condition rarely occurs, the possibility that hypoplasia of the ICA could be the associated with an ischemic ocular syndrome that mimics NTG needs to be taken into consideration when diagnosing such patients.

There is no report of the same or a similar case like our report in the literature, but the neurovascular contact of ICA or the anterior cerebral artery has been described in the literature. Compression of the optic nerve by a fusiform enlagement of the internal carotid artery is originally described in Japanese (Miyake Y et al.,1978).

Subsequently, Uchino et al reported a 71-yaer old woman who had a unilateral visual field defect due to optic nerve compression by sclerotic internal carotid artery. This case underwent decompression surgery and then, the visual field was improved(.Uchino M et al.,1999). According to a retrospective neuroimaging study for reasons unrelated to loss of vision, optic neuropathy, or carotid artery disorders, the frequency of the artery relationship included contact one or both optic nerves in 70 (70%) of 100 patients. The anatomic compression of the optic nerve depended upon the diameter of the carotid artery (Jacobson DM., 1997).

Although uncommon, intracranial compression of the optic nerve by the carotid artery should be always considered when seeing unknown optic neuropathy(Jacobson DM.,1999).

Compression of the optic nerve seems to also occure by megadolichoectatic ophthalmic artery (Gire J.,2010).

The compression may be induced not by anterior cerebral artery (Nishioka T.,1995), but they also suggested the progressive optic neuropathie s due to compression by the plolapsing gyrus rectus (Nishioka T.,2004).

Longstanding compression of the intracranial optic nerve may produce a nerve fiber bundle pattern of visual field loss and excavation of the optic disc, two signs consistent with glaucoma. However most patients with these two signs had other features atypical of glaucoma, including pallor of the neuroretinal rim and impairment of visual acuity and color vision. The presence of such signs should alert one the possibility that a patient with visual field loss and excavation of the optic disc may be harboring a compression lesion, not suffering from glaucoma(Jacobson DM.,1999).

It is necessary to assess a condition of intracranial using thin-slice MRI or angiography, whenever the patients has a optic neuropathy of an unknown etiology or the case having a visual field changes like a glaucoma, but does not agree with clinical findings.

4. References

Burghaus L et al(2007).. Acute loss of vision with hypoplasia of the contralateral carotid artery. *J Stroke Cerebrovasc Dis* ,2007,16,43-44.

Chutorian AM et al(2002).Anterior ischemic optic neuropathy in children. *Pediatr Neurol* ,2002,26,358-364.

Costa VP et el.(1998) Collateral blood supply through the ophthalmic artery. A steal phenomenon analyzed by color Doppler imaging. *Ophthalmology,* 1998,105,689-693.

Fujioka S.(2003). Use of orbital color Doppler imaging for detecting internal carotid artery stenosis in patients with amaurosis fugax. *Jpn J Ophthalmol* ,2003,47,276-280.

Gire J et al(2010). Optic Nerve Compression by an Intraorbitctatic Megadolichoectatic Ophtalmic Artery. *Orbit.* 2010,29,60-62.

Horowitz J et al.(2001). Internal carotid artery hypoplasia presenting as anterior ischemic optic neuropathy. *Am J Ophthalmol,* 2001,131,673-674.

Jacobson DM et al,(1997). Optic nerve contact and compression by the carotid artery in asymptomatic patients. *AJO* ,1997,123,677-683.

Jacobson DM.(1999).Symptomatic compression of the optic nerve by the carotid artery. *Ophthalmology.*1999, 106,1994-2004.

Kawaguchi S et al,(1999). Effects of bypass on ocular ischemic syndrome caused by reversed flow in the ophthalmic artery. *The Lancet,* 1999,354,2052-2053.

Knox DL et al,(1971).Slowly progressive ischemic optic neuropathy. A clinicopathologic case report. *Trans Am Acad Ophthalmol Otolaryngol* 1971,75,1065-1068.

Lessell S.(1999). Nonarteritic anterior ischemic optic neuropathy. *Arch Ophthalmol* 1999,117,386-388.

Miyake Y et al,(1978).A case of compression of the optic nerve by a fusiform enlargement of the internal carotid artery. *Rinsho Shinkeiganka.* ,1978,18,608-613.

Nishioka T et al(1995).Progressive blurring of vision in both eyes. *The Lancet.*1995,346,1402.

Nishioka T et al,(2000). Plolapsing gyrus rectus as a cause of progressive optic neuropathy. *Neoro Med Chir.* 2000,40,301-309.

Saito H et al,(2008).Optic disc and peripapillary morphology in unilateral nonarteritic anterior ischemic optic neuropathy and age- and refraction- matched normals. *Ophthalmology,* 2008, 115,1585-1590.

Uchino M et al,(1999). Unilateral visual field defect due to optic nerve compression by sclerotic internal carotid artery.*Nouge,*1999, 27,189-194.

Ward JB et al,(1995).. Reversible abnormalities in the ophthalmic arteries detected by color Doppler imaging. *Ophthalmology* 1995,102,1606-1610.

11

Optic Nerve Head Blood Flow in Glaucoma

Tetsuya Sugiyama, Maho Shibata, Shota Kojima and Tsunehiko Ikeda
Osaka Medical College
Japan

1. Introduction

These days it is commonly accepted that multiple factors are involved in the etiology of glaucoma. Although many studies have demonstrated that the major risk factor for glaucoma is an increase in intraocular pressure (IOP), some studies, including epidemiologic studies, have suggested an association between glaucoma, especially primary open-angle glaucoma (POAG) and normal-tension glaucoma (NTG), and vascular factors. In this chapter, previous studies regarding the implications of optic nerve head (ONH) blood flow in glaucoma will be reviewed, and then our recent studies will be presented.

Some population-based prevalence surveys demonstrated that lower perfusion pressure (blood pressure - intraocular pressure), especially diastolic perfusion pressure, was strongly associated with an increased prevalence of POAG or NTG in the US, Europe and Asia (Tielsch et al, 1995; Bonomi et al, 2000; Leske et al, 2002; Hulseman et al, 2007). These reports suggest that POAG including NTG is associated with alterations in factors related to ocular blood flow. There is also sufficient evidence that optic disc hemorrhage is an important risk factor for glaucoma progression (Daugeliene et al, 1999; Leske et al, 2003; Bengtsson et al, 2008; Prata et al, 2010). Additionally, increasing peripapillary atrophy, which might be related with hypoperfusion to the ONH, was reportedly associated with progressive glaucoma (Araie et al, 1994; Uchida et al, 1998; Daugeliene et al, 1999), and it has been reported that non-use of calcium channel blockers was significantly associated with the progression of visual field loss in NTG (Daugeliene et al, 1999).

Clinically usable methods for the measurement of ONH blood flow include fluorescein fundus angiography, scanning laser Doppler flowmetry, and laser speckle flowgraphy. Fluorescein fundus angiography has multiple limitations in quantitatively evaluating ONH blood flow (Hayreh, 1997). Above all, once the dense capillary network in the surface nerve fiber layer of the ONH fills completely with fluorescein-stained blood, underlying ciliary vessels are masked so that no information can be obtained about the circulation in the deeper capillaries. Laser Doppler flowmetry is predominantly sensitive to blood flow changes in the superficial layers of the ONH and gives very little information about the prelaminar and deeper regions of the ONH (Petrig et al, 1999). Laser speckle flowgraphy (LSFG) can detect capillary blood flow in the ONH, probably around the laminar region, and is suitable for monitoring the time-course of its change (Sugiyama et al, 2010). LSFG was develped to facilitate the non-contact analysis of ocular blood flow utilizing the laser speckle phenomenon (Tamaki et al, 1995). Originally, normalized blur and square blur rate had been used as indexes of blood velocity, but later they were experimentally shown to be well correlated with blood flow rate. In the recent version of LSFG, a new parameter, mean blur rate (MBR), which is

theoretically proportional to the square blur rate, is also commonly used as an idex of blood flow rate (Konishi, 2002). There have been many reports demonstrating the effects of various treatments on the ONH blood flow in humans using LSFG (Sugiyama et al, 2010).
Some investigators have reported that ONH blood flow is autoregulated in normal eyes, but not in patients with POAG. Several reports have suggested a larger diurnal fluctuation of parameters for ocular blood flow including ONH blood flow in patients with POAG or NTG (Claridge & Smith, 1994; Chung et al, 1999; Okuno T et al, 2004; Pemp et al, 2009). There has also been some evidence that endothelin (ET)-1 and nitric oxide may play roles in the dysregulation of ocular blood flow in glaucoma (Yorio et al, 2002; Flammer et al, 2007; Polak et al, 2007; Nicolela, 2008; Venkataraman et al, 2010).
There have been some studies on the effects of anti-glaucoma medication on ONH blood flow. The effects of prostaglandin (PG) derivatives, beta-blockers, and carbonic anhydrase inhibitors (CAIs) on ONH blood flow are summarized below. Regarding latanoprost, a representative PG derivative, some reports showed that it increased ONH blood flow, but others reported that it had no significant effect on ONH blood flow in healthy subjects or in glaucoma patients (Seong et al, 1999; Ishii et al, 2001; Gherghel et al, 2008; Sugiyama et al, 2009). Unoprostone, another PG derivative, reportedly increased ONH blood flow in healthy subjects (Tamaki et al, 2001; Makimoto et al, 2002). There has been no report regarding the effects of travoprost, bimatoprost or tafluprost on ONH blood flow in humans as far as we know. It is reported that timolol either had no significant effect on or decreased ONH blood flow in humans (Yoshida et al, 1991; Tamaki et al, 1997a, 1997b; Netland et al, 1999; Haefliger et al, 1999; Lübeck et al, 2001). In contrast, carteolol, betaxolol and nipradilol reportedly increased ONH blood flow in humans (Tamaki et al, 1997a, 1997b; Tamaki et al, 1999; Mizuno et al, 2002). It was reported that dorzolamide, a topical CAI, had no significant effect on ONH blood flow in healthy subjects but increased ONH blood flow in glaucoma patients (Pillunat et al, 1999; Fuchsjäger-Mayrl et al, 2005; Rolle et al, 2008). To the best of our knowledge, there have been few reports on the effect of brinzolamide, another topical CAI, on ONH blood flow in humans (Iester et al, 2004).

2. Clinical studies of ONH blood flow in glaucoma

2.1 Association of ONH blood flow with stages of glaucoma (Clinical study 1)

The correlation between the stages of the visual field defect and the impairment of ONH blood flow was investigated in a retrospective study involving glaucoma patients. The subjects included 18 eyes of 13 patients with preperimetric glaucoma, 54 eyes of 31 patients with POAG and 39 eyes of 21 age-matched normal control subjects. POAG was defined as showing the following criteria in two consecutive examinations by Humphrey Field Analyzer (HFA, Carl Zeiss Meditec, Dublin, CA) using Program 30-2, SITA standard strategy: 1) Outside normal limits by the glaucoma hemi-field test; 2) Pattern standard deviation with P values < 5%; 3) Cluster of 3 or more points in the pattern deviation plot in the abnormal hemifield with P values < 5% and one of which has a P value < 1%. POAG patients were divided into the initial, middle or advanced stage as classified by Anderson & Pattela (1999). Preperimetric glaucoma is defined as showing no abnormality in the HFA examination in spite of having glaucomatous optic neuropathy detected by the examination of the ocular fundus. The exclusion criteria for all patients were: best corrected visual acuity less than 10/20, myopia more than -6D, age less than 40 years old, history of ocular disease other than glaucoma and mild cataract, history of serious systemic disease such as hypertension or diabetes, and poor fixation for the measurement of the blood flow or visual field.

MBR value, an index of ONH blood flow, was measured on the same day or within 3 months after the HFA examination was done. In this study, 8 divisions of sectoral tissue blood flow in the ONH rim were analyzed using LSFG Analyzer (ver. 3) and Layer Viewer (Softcare, Fukuoka, Japan). The edge of ONH cupping was determined using Heidelberg Retina Tomograph 2 (Heidelberg Engineering, Heidelberg, Germany). The ratio of the MBR value of each sector was calculated and compared between groups.

As a result, less blood flow was observed at the superior and inferior sectors of the ONH rim in patients with preperimetric glaucoma compared to normal control subjects (Fig. 1). In contrast, the blood flow became reduced at the temporal sectors as POAG progressed in comparison to patients with preperimetric glaucoma (Fig. 2).

2.2 ONH blood flow and progression of glaucoma (Clinical study 2)

In order to verify the correlation between ONH blood flow and the progression of the visual field defect, a 3-year prospective study was performed in 12 patients with NTG. The inclusion criteria were: 1) Both eyes had a glaucomatous visual field defect with HFA mean deviation (MD) of -20 dB or more and IOP of 20 mmHg or less before treatment for glaucoma; and 2) The difference between the MD values of both eyes was 5 dB or less at the beginning of this study. The exclusion criteria were the same as in Clinical Study 1. During the study, all of the patients were treated with anti-glaucoma eye drops in both eyes in the same manner. HFA was examined every 6 months to calculate the MD slope. At the same time, the MBR value was measured at each temporal sector using LSFG. The difference of the MD slopes obtained from the right and left eyes, defined as ΔMDS, and the ratio of the MBR values or IOPs obtained from the right eye to those from the left eye, defined as relative MBR or relative IOP, were calculated and averaged throughout the study.

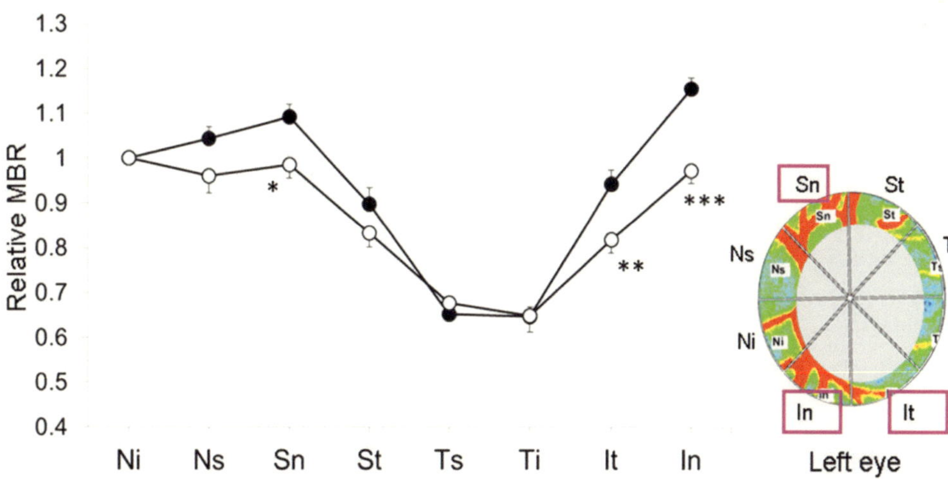

Fig. 1. Ratios of the MBR (mean blue rate) values of each sector of the ONH (optic nerve head) rim in patients with preperimetric glaucoma (open circles, n=18) and normal control subjects (closed circles, n=39). Data are expressed as mean ± SEM. Asterisks indicate significant differences between the two groups (unpaired t-test, *$p < 0.05$, **$p < 0.01$, ***$p < 0.001$).

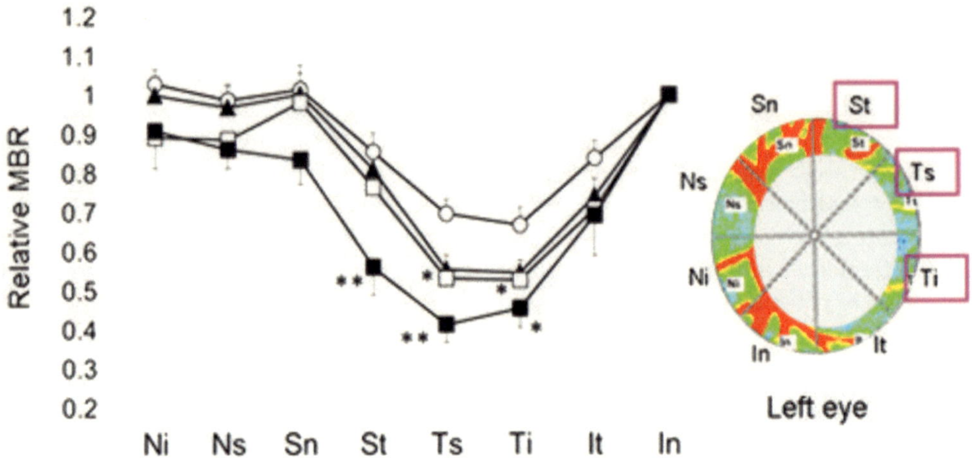

Fig. 2. Ratios of the MBR values of each sector of the ONH rim in patients with preperimetric glaucoma (open circles, n=18), initial POAG (closed triangles, n=26), middle POAG (open squares, n=21), and advanced POAG (closed squares, n=7). Data are expressed as mean ± SEM. Asterisks indicate significant differences when compared with the preperimetric glaucoma group (unpaired t-test, *p < 0.05, **p< 0.01).

The mean±SD of their ages at the start of this study was 63.7±10.6 years, male-to-female ratio was 4:8. Both the MD (dB) and MBR values were not different between both eyes at the initial level (right eyes:-4.48 ± 6.24 and 9.16 ± 3.35, left eyes: -5.32 ± 5.93 and 10.67 ± 4.16, respectively). In addition, throughout the study the mean IOP (mmHg) was not different between both eyes (right eyes: 12.1 ± 1.8, left eyes: 12.1 ± 1.9). There was a significant correlation between relative MBR and ΔMDS (Fig. 3). However, there was no correlation between relative IOP and ΔMDS (Fig. 4).

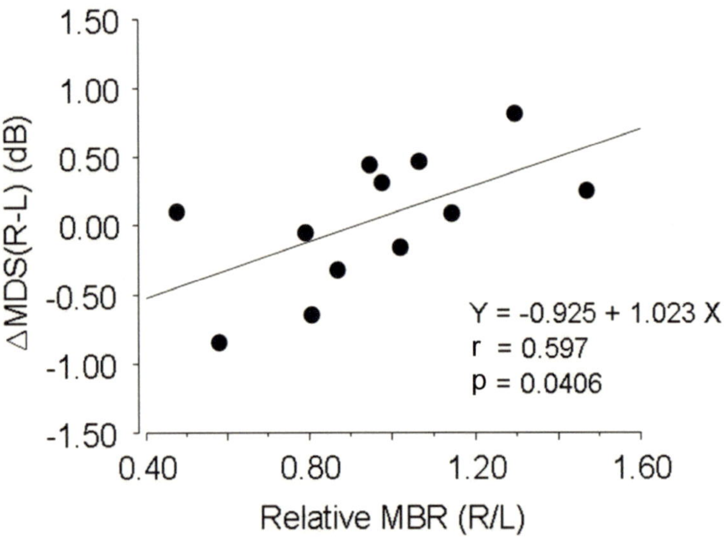

Fig. 3. The relationship between the relative MBRs and the differences of MD slopes, obtained from both eyes in 12 NTG patients.

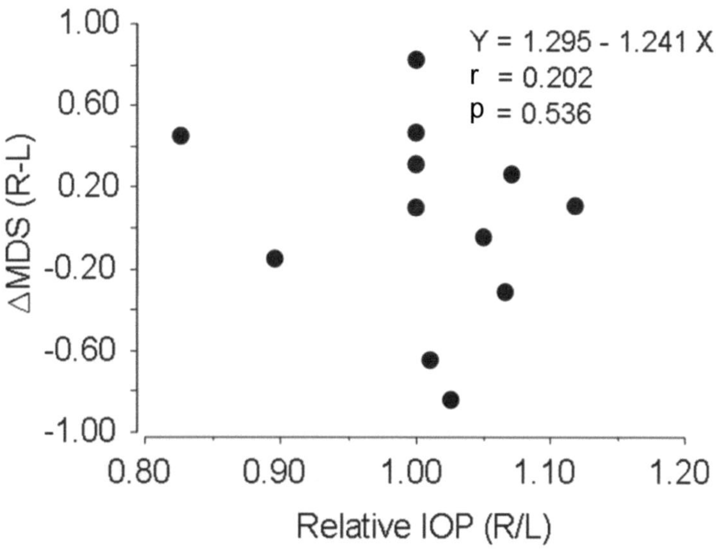

Fig. 4. The relationship between the relative IOP (intraocular pressure) and the differences of MD slopes, obtained from both eyes in 12 NTG patients.

2.3 Changes in ONH blood flow induced by PG derivatives (Clinical study 3)

The effect of tafluprost, a novel prostaglandin analogue, on the ONH blood flow was investigated in a randomized comparative study involving 24 patients with POAG. The IOPs of the subjects were 25 mmHg or less without any treatment for glaucoma. They were in the initial or middle stages of glaucoma according to Anderson & Patella (1999). They had no serious ocular or systemic diseases except for glaucoma as well as no present or past history of smoking. They were not on any systemic medications that could alter the ocular blood flow, such as calcium channel blockers or beta blockers. After random assignment, the tafluprost and latanoprost treatment groups included 11 patients and 13 patients, respectively. There were no significant differences between the subjects' ages, gender ratios or pretreatment IOPs. The IOP, blood flow in the rim of ONH, and blood pressure were measured before and 1, 3, and 6 months after treatment. ONH blood flow was measured as the MBR value using LSFG. Ocular perfusion pressure (OPP) was calculated as 2/3 of the mean blood pressure minus the IOP. The analyzed eyes were selected at random.

As a result, the IOP decreased significantly at 1, 3, and 6 months compared to the levels measured at the start of tafluprost or latanoprost treatment. Both groups had almost the same degree of IOP reduction (Fig. 5). Blood flow in the rim of ONH, except on the nasal side, increased significantly compared with the initial levels in the tafluprost-treated group, but not in the latanoprost-treated group (Fig. 6). OPP did not change significantly in either group (data not shown).

2.4 Changes in ONH blood flow induced by beta blockers (Clinical study 4)

We have already reported the effects of combined therapy with latanoprost and beta blockers on the ONH blood flow in NTG patients. In the present study, the effects of combined therapy with latanoprost and long-acting ophthalmic solutions of beta blockers

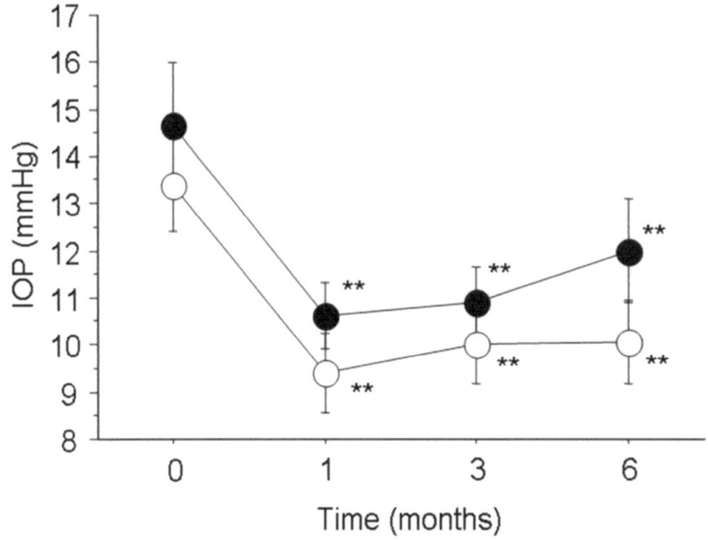

Fig. 5. IOP changes induced by tafluprost (closed circles, n=11) and latanoprost (open circles, n=13) in POAG patients. Data are expressed as mean ± SEM. Asterisks indicate significant differences when compared with initial levels (paired t-test, **p< 0.01).

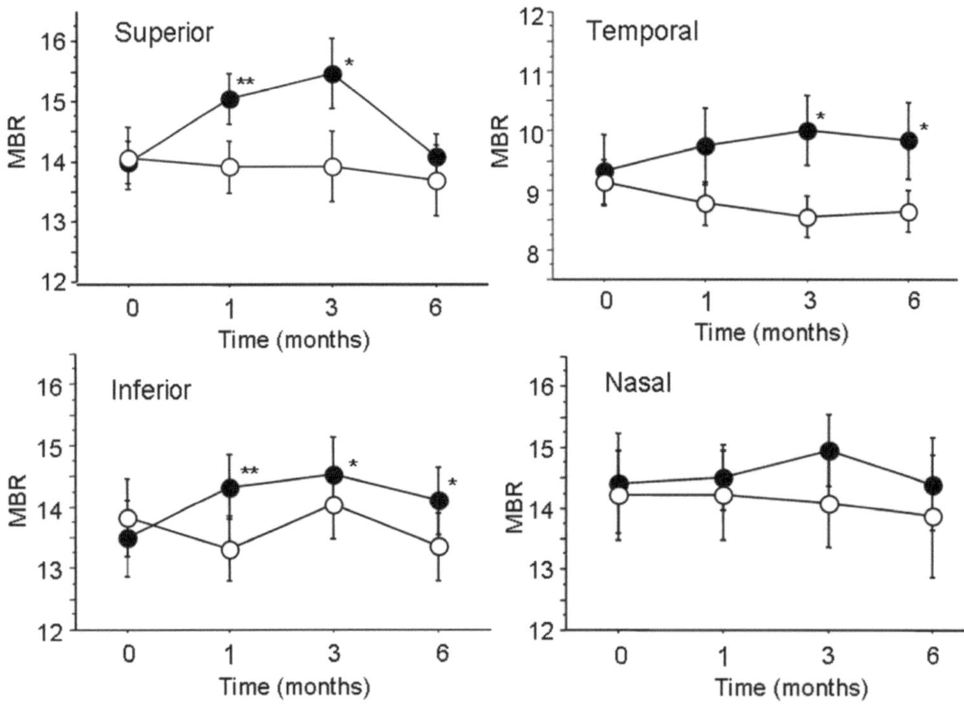

Fig. 6. MBR changes induced by tafluprost (closed circles, n=11) and latanoprost (open circles, n=13) in superior, inferior, temporal and nasal sectors of the ONH rim in POAG patients. Data are expressed as mean ± SEM. Asterisks indicate significant differences when compared with initial levels (paired t-test, *p < 0.05, **p< 0.01).

on the ONH blood flow were investigated in a crossover study involving 10 patients with POAG. They had been receiving treatment with latanoprost for 4 weeks or more. Patients with serious ocular or systemic diseases and those who were smokers were excluded from the study. The mean±SD of their ages and IOPs at the start of this study were 59.3±13.3 years and 15.7±1.4 mmHg, respectively, and the male-to-female ratio was 4:6. One of the long-acting ophthalmic solutions of beta blockers, Timoptol-XE (timolol) and Mikelan-LA (carteolol), was prescribed for these patients for 2 months each. Since the order of the beta blockers was decided randomly, the Timoptol-XE-preceding group included 5 patients, and the Mikelan-LA-preceding group included 5 patients. The IOP, blood flow in the rim of ONH, and blood pressure were measured before and at 2 and 4 months after treatment. ONH blood flow was measured as a MBR value using LSFG. OPP was calculated as mentioned above. The analyzed eyes were selected at random.

The results of the current study showed that IOP decreased significantly at 2 months after combined therapy with a beta blocker (either Timoptol-XE or Mikelan-LA) compared to the levels before the combined therapy. There was no significant difference between the IOP reductions induced by the two beta blockers (Fig. 7). Blood flow in the rim of ONH, except on the nasal side, was significantly higher with the coadministration of Mikelan-LA, but not with that of Timoptol-XE, compared to the administration of latanoprost alone (Fig. 8). OPP did not change significantly after the combined therapy with either beta blocker (data not shown).

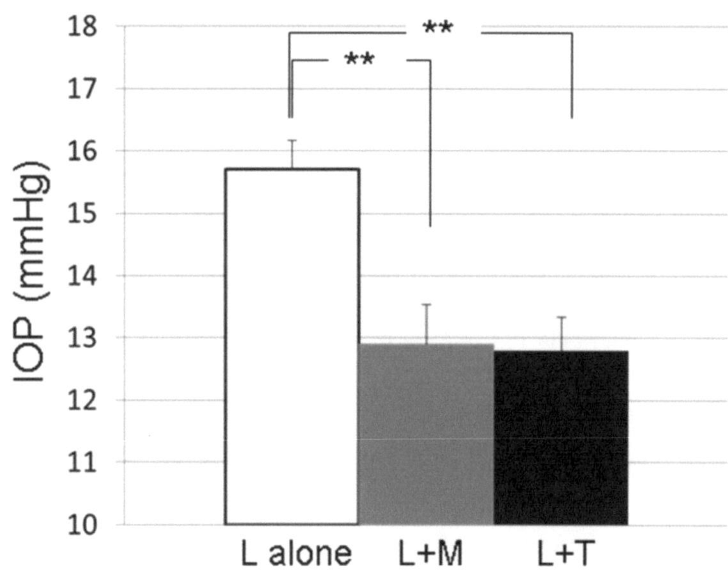

Fig. 7. IOP before and 2 months after the combined therapies with latanoprost (L) and a long-acting beta blocker (M: Mikelan-LA, T:Timoptol-XE) in 10 POAG patients. Data are expressed as mean ± SEM. Asterisks indicate significant differences between the bracketed groups (Dunnett's test, **$p < 0.01$).

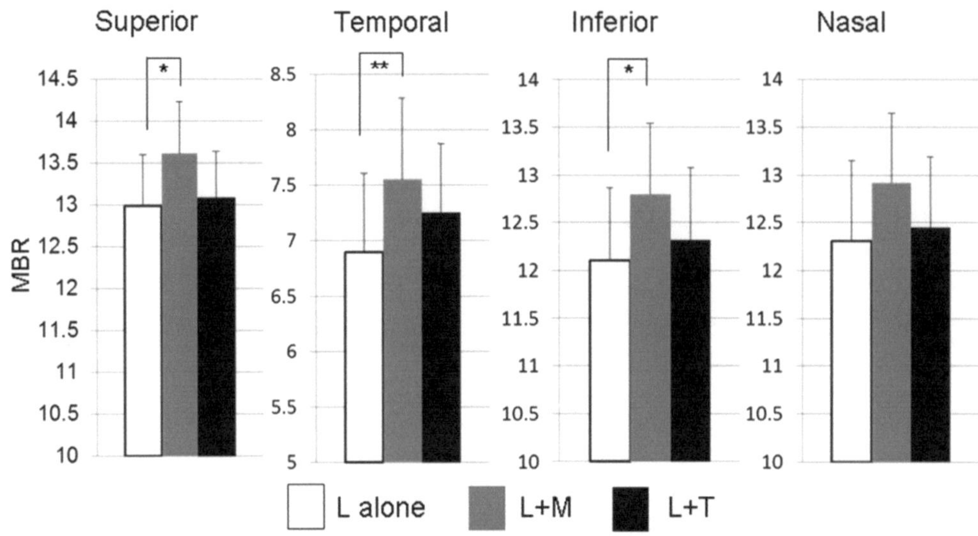

Fig. 8. MBR in superior, inferior, temporal and nasal sectors of the ONH rim before and 2 months after the combined therapies with latanoprost (L) and a long-acting beta blocker (M: Mikelan-LA, T:Timoptol-XE) in 10 POAG patients. Data are expressed as mean ± SEM. Asterisks indicate significant differences between the bracketed groups (Dunnett's test, *$p < 0.05$, **$p < 0.01$).

2.5 Discussions of clinical studies 1-4

Clinical study 1, a retrospective study, revealed that the blood flow was reduced in some sectors of the ONH rim even in preperimetric glaucoma. In addition, it was reduced in the other sectors in accordance with the progression of POAG. Clinical study 2, a prospective study, showed that the less blood flow there was in the ONH rim, the more the visual field defect progressed in NTG. Although it has been controversial whether the reduced ocular blood flow is only a result of the progression of optic neuropathy, our results show that reduced ONH blood flow is surely an important risk factor in the progression of open-angle glaucoma. Therefore, maintaining the ONH blood flow might be an effective therapy for POAG including NTG. Prospective clinical studies should be performed to verify the effects of agents that increase the ONH blood flow in POAG, even though such studies may be costly and time-consuming.

There are several methods for increasing the ocular blood flow. Anti-glaucoma eye drops usually reduce IOP, and OPP is then increased. Generally speaking, the following equation is valid:

Ocular blood flow $\propto$ OPP/Vascular resistance

If vascular resistance does not vary significantly, ocular blood flow is directly proportional to OPP. Therefore, anti-glaucoma eye drops might increase ocular blood flow including ONH blood flow. Glaucoma surgeries might have similar effects on ocular blood flow through the reduction of IOP. On the other hand, there are some medications that can reduce vascular resistance, including calcium channel blockers (Koseki et al, 2008; Mayama & Araie, 2011), ROCK inhibitors (Sugiyama et al, 2011), statins (Ozkiris, 2007; Nagaoka et al, 2007), ET-1 antagonists (Resch et al, 2009; Rosenthal & Fromm, 2011) and others. These kinds of medications might increase ocular blood flow if OPP is not changed significantly. There have also been several reports that stellate ganglion block might increase ocular blood flow mainly by reducing vascular resistance (Nagahara et al, 2001; Yu et al, 2003).

As mentioned above, reduction in IOP might lead to an increased OPP, which might result in enhancement of ocular blood flow. But Clinical studies 3 and 4, described in the present report, demonstrated that there might be a difference in the effect of anti-glaucoma medications on the ONH blood flow even though they have similar effects in terms of IOP reduction. In our study the difference was verified in the cases of some PG derivatives and beta blockers, but the difference also might be applied to other cases. These differences in the effects on the ONH blood flow, not only on the IOP, might be an important factor in the selection of anti-glaucoma medications for each glaucoma patient in the future. In addition, since there might be inter-individual differences in the effects of the same medications on the ONH blood flow, monitoring the changes in the ONH blood flow during the treatment for glaucoma would be helpful. For that purpose, more precise and easily usable instruments for measuring the ONH blood flow are needed in the near future.

3. Conclusion

The results of our clinical studies indicated that reduced ONH blood flow is an important risk factor for the progression of open-angle glaucoma including NTG, and that there might be a difference in the effect of anti-glaucoma medications on the ONH blood flow even though they have similar effects on IOP reduction. In conclusion, monitoring the changes in the ONH blood flow would be helpful in the treatment of glaucoma.

4. References

Anderson, D.R. & Pattela, V.M. (1999). In: *Automatic Static Perimetry* (2nd edition), pp.121-190, Mosby, St. Louis.

Araie, M., Sekine, M., Suzuki, Y. & Koseki, N. (1994). Factors contributing to the progression of visual field damage in eyes with normal-tension glaucoma. *Ophthalmology* 101, 8, pp.1440-1444.

Araie, M. & Mayama, C. (2011). Use of calcium channel blockers for glaucoma. *Prog Retin Eye Res* 30, 1, pp.54-71.

Bengtsson, B., Leske, M.C., Yang, Z. & Heijl, A.; EMGT Group. (2008). Disc hemorrhages and treatment in the early manifest glaucoma trial. *Ophthalmology* 115, 11, pp.2044-2048.

Bonomi, L., Marchini, G., Marraffa, M., Bernardi, P., Morbio, R. & Varotto, A. (2000). Vascular risk factors for primary open angle glaucoma: the Egna-Neumarkt Study. *Ophthalmology* 107, 7, pp.1287-1293.

Chung, H.S., Harris, A., Evans, D.W., Kagemann, L., Garzozi, H.J. & Martin, B. (1999). Vascular aspects in the pathophysiology of glaucomatous optic neuropathy. *Surv Ophthalmol* 43, Suppl 1, pp.S43-S50.

Claridge, K.G. & Smith, S.E. (1994). Diurnal variation in pulsatile ocular blood flow in normal and glaucomatous eyes. *Surv Ophthalmol* 38, Suppl, pp.S198-S205.

Daugeliene, L., Yamamoto, T. & Kitazawa, Y. (1999). Risk factors for visual field damage progression in normal-tension glaucoma eyes. *Graefes Arch Clin Exp Ophthalmol* 237, 2, pp.105-108.

Flammer, J. & Mozaffarieh, M. (2007). What is the present pathogenetic concept of glaucomatous optic neuropathy? *Surv Ophthalmol* 52, Suppl 2, pp.S162-S173.

Fuchsjäger-Mayrl, G., Wally, B., Rainer, G., Buehl, W., Aggermann, T., Kolodjaschna, J., Weigert, G., Polska, E., Eichler, H.G., Vass, C. & Schmetterer, L. (2005). Effect of dorzolamide and timolol on ocular blood flow in patients with primary open angle glaucoma and ocular hypertension. *Br J Ophthalmol* 89, 10, pp.1293-1297.

Gherghel, D., Hosking, S.L., Cunliffe, I.A. & Armstrong, R.A. (2008). First-line therapy with latanoprost 0.005% results in improved ocular circulation in newly diagnosed primary open-angle glaucoma patients: a prospective, 6-month, open-label study. *Eye* (Lond) 22, 3, pp.363-369.

Haefliger, I.O., Lietz, A., Griesser, S.M., Ulrich, A., Schötzau, A., Hendrickson, P. & Flammer J. (1999). Modulation of Heidelberg Retinal Flowmeter parameter flow at the papilla of healthy subjects: effect of carbogen, oxygen, high intraocular pressure, and beta-blockers. *Surv Ophthalmol* 43, Suppl 1, pp.S59-S65.

Hayreh, S. S. (1997) Evaluation of optic nerve head circulation: Review of the methods used. *J Glaucoma* 6, 5, pp.319–330.

Hulsman, C.A., Vingerling, J.R., Hofman, A., Witteman, J.C. & de Jong, P.T. (2007). Blood pressure, arterial stiffness, and open-angle glaucoma: the Rotterdam study. *Arch Ophthalmol* 125, 6, pp.805-812.

Iester, M., Altieri, M., Michelson, G., Vittone, P., Traverso, C.E. & Calabria, G. (2004). Retinal peripapillary blood flow before and after topical brinzolamide. *Ophthalmologica* 218, 6, pp.390-396.

Ishii, K., Tomidokoro, A., Nagahara, M., Tamaki, Y., Kanno, M., Fukaya, Y. & Araie, M. (2001). Effects of topical latanoprost on optic nerve head circulation in rabbits, monkeys, and humans. *Invest Ophthalmol Vis Sci* 42, 12, pp.2957-2963.

Konishi, N., Tokimoto, Y., Kohra, K. & Fujii, H. (2002). New laser speckle flowgraphy system using CCD camera. *Opt Rev* 9, pp.163–169.

Koseki, N., Araie, M., Tomidokoro, A., Nagahara, M., Hasegawa, T., Tamaki, Y. & Yamamoto, S. (2008). A placebo-controlled 3-year study of a calcium blocker on visual field and ocular circulation in glaucoma with low-normal pressure. *Ophthalmology* 115, 11, pp.2049-2057.

Leske, M.C., Wu, S.Y., Nemesure, B. & Hennis, A. (2002). Incident open-angle glaucoma and blood pressure. *Arch Ophthalmol* 120, 7, pp.954-959.

Leske, M.C., Heijl, A., Hussein, M., Bengtsson, B., Hyman, L. & Komaroff, E. (2003). Early Manifest Glaucoma Trial Group. Factors for glaucoma progression and the effect of treatment: the early manifest glaucoma trial. *Arch Ophthalmol* 121, 1, pp.48-56.

Lübeck, P., Orgül, S., Gugleta, K., Gherghel, D., Gekkieva, M. & Flammer J. (2001). Effect of timolol on anterior optic nerve blood flow in patients with primary open-angle glaucoma as assessed by the Heidelberg retina flowmeter. *J Glaucoma*. 10, 1, pp.13-17.

Makimoto, Y., Sugiyama, T., Kojima, S. & Azuma, I. (2002). Long-term effect of topically applied isopropyl unoprostone on microcirculation in the human ocular fundus. *Jpn J Ophthalmol* 46, 1, pp.31-35.

Mizuno, K., Koide, T., Saito, N., Fujii, M., Nagahara, M., Tomidokoro, A., Tamaki, Y. & Araie M. (2002). Topical nipradilol: effects on optic nerve head circulation in

humans and periocular distribution in monkeys. *Invest Ophthalmol Vis Sci* 43, 10, pp.3243-3250.
Nagahara, M., Tamaki, Y., Araie, M. & Umeyama, T. (2001). The acute effects of stellate ganglion block on circulation in human ocular fundus. *Acta Ophthalmol Scand* 79, 1, pp.45-48.
Nagaoka, T., Hein, T.W., Yoshida, A. & Kuo, L. (2007). Simvastatin elicits dilation of isolated porcine retinal arterioles: role of nitric oxide and mevalonate-rho kinase pathways. *Invest Ophthalmol Vis Sci* 48, 2, pp.825-832.
Netland, P.A., Schwartz, B., Feke, G.T., Takamoto, T., Konno, S. & Goger, D.G. (1999). Diversity of response of optic nerve head circulation to timolol maleate in gel-forming solution. *J Glaucoma* 8, 3, pp.164-71.
Nicolela, M.T.(2008). Clinical clues of vascular dysregulation and its association with glaucoma. Can J Ophthalmol 43, 3, pp.337-341.
Okuno, T., Sugiyama, T., Kojima, S., Nakajima, M. & Ikeda, T. (2004). Diurnal variation in microcirculation of ocular fundus and visual field change in normal-tension glaucoma. *Eye (Lond)* 18, 7, pp.697-702.
Ozkiris, A., Erkiliç, K., Koç, A. & Mistik, S. (2007). Effect of atorvastatin on ocular blood flow velocities in patients with diabetic retinopathy. *Br J Ophthalmol* 91, 1, pp.69-73.
Pemp, B., Georgopoulos, M., Vass, C., Fuchsjäger-Mayrl, G., Luksch, A., Rainer, G. & Schmetterer, L. (2009). Diurnal fluctuation of ocular blood flow parameters in patients with primary open-angle glaucoma and healthy subjects. *Br J Ophthalmol* 93, 4, pp.486-491.
Petrig, B. L., Riva, C. E. & Hayreh, S. S. (1999). Laser Doppler flowmetry and optic nerve head blood flow. *Am J Ophthalmol* 127, 4, pp.413–425.
Pillunat, L.E., Böhm, A.G., Köller, A.U., Schmidt, K.G., Klemm, M., Richard, G. (1999). Effect of topical dorzolamide on optic nerve head blood flow. *Graefes Arch Clin Exp Ophthalmol* 237, 6, pp.495-500.
Polak, K., Luksch, A., Berisha, F., Fuchsjaeger-Mayrl, G., Dallinger, S. & Schmetterer, L. (2007). Altered nitric oxide system in patients with open-angle glaucoma. *Arch Ophthalmol* 125, 4, pp.494-498.
Prata, T.S., De Moraes, C.G., Teng, C.C., Tello, C., Ritch, R. & Liebmann, J.M. (2010). Factors affecting rates of visual field progression in glaucoma patients with optic disc hemorrhage. *Ophthalmology* 117, 1, pp.24-29.
Resch, H., Karl, K., Weigert, G., Wolzt, M., Hommer, A., Schmetterer, L. & Garhöfer, G. (2009). Effect of dual endothelin receptor blockade on ocular blood flow in patients with glaucoma and healthy subjects. *Invest Ophthalmol Vis Sci* 50, 1, pp.358-363.
Rolle, T., Tofani, F., Brogliatti, B. & Grignolo, F.M. (2008). The effects of dorzolamide 2% and dorzolamide/timolol fixed combination on retinal and optic nerve head blood flow in primary open-angle glaucoma patients. *Eye (Lond)* 22, 9, pp.1172-1179.
Rosenthal, R. & Fromm, M. (2011). Endothelin antagonism as an active principle for glaucoma therapy. *Br J Pharmacol* 162, 4, pp.806-816.
Seong, G.J., Lee, H.K. & Hong, Y.J. (1999). Effects of 0.005% latanoprost on optic nerve head and peripapillary retinal blood flow. *Ophthalmologica* 213, 6, pp.355-359.
Sugiyama, T., Kojima, S., Ishida, O. & Ikeda, T. (2009). Changes in optic nerve head blood flow induced by the combined therapy of latanoprost and beta blockers. *Acta Ophthalmol* 87, 7, pp.797-800.

Sugiyama, T., Araie, M., Riva, C.E., Schmetterer, L. & Orgul, S. (2010). Use of laser speckle flowgraphy in ocular blood flow research. *Acta Ophthalmol* 88, 7, pp.723-729.

Sugiyama, T., Shibata, M., Kajiura, S., Okuno, T., Tonari, M., Oku, H. & Ikeda, T. (2011). Effects of fasudil, a Rho-associated protein kinase inhibitor, on optic nerve head blood flow in rabbits. *Invest Ophthalmol Vis Sci* 52, 1, pp.64-69.

Tamaki, Y., Araie, M., Kawamoto, E., Eguchi, S. & Fujii, H. (1995). Non-contact, two-dimensional measurement of tissue circulation in choroid and optic nerve head using laser speckle phenomenon. *Exp Eye Res* 60, 4, pp.373-383.

Tamaki, Y., Araie, M., Tomita, K., Nagahara, M. & Tomidokoro, A. (1997). Effect of topical beta-blockers on tissue blood flow in the human optic nerve head. *Curr Eye Res* 16, 11, pp.1102-10.

Tamaki, Y., Araie, M., Tomita, K., Tomidokoro, A. & Nagahara, M. (1997). Effects of topical adrenergic agents on tissue circulation in rabbit and human optic nerve head evaluated with laser speckle tissue circulation analyzer. *Surv Ophthalmol* 42, Suppl 1, pp.S52-S63.

Tamaki, Y., Araie, M., Tomita, K. & Nagahara, M. (1999). Effect of topical betaxolol on tissue circulation in the human optic nerve head. *J Ocul Pharmacol Ther* 15, 4, pp.313-321.

Tamaki, Y., Araie, M., Tomita, K., Nagahara, M., Sandoh, S. & Tomidokoro, A. (2001). Effect of topical unoprostone on circulation of human optic nerve head and retina. J Ocul Pharmacol Ther 17, 6, 517-527.

Tielsch, J.M., Katz, J., Sommer, A., Quigley, H.A & Javitt, J.C. (1995). Hypertension, perfusion pressure, and primary open-angle glaucoma. A population-based assessment. *Arch Ophthalmol* 113, 2, pp. 216-221.

Uchida, H., Ugurlu, S. & Caprioli, J. (1998). Increasing peripapillary atrophy is associated with progressive glaucoma. *Ophthalmology* 105, 8, pp.1541-1545.

Venkataraman, S.T., Flanagan, J.G. & Hudson, C. (2010). Vascular reactivity of optic nerve head and retinal blood vessels in glaucoma--a review. *Microcirculation* 17, 7, pp.568-581.

Yorio, T., Krishnamoorthy, R. & Prasanna, G. (2002). Endothelin: is it a contributor to glaucoma pathophysiology? *J Glaucoma* 11, 3, pp.259-270.

Yoshida, A., Feke, G.T., Ogasawara, H., Goger, D.G., Murray, D.L. & McMeel, J.W. (1991). Effect of timolol on human retinal, choroidal and optic nerve head circulation. *Ophthalmic Res* 23, 3, pp.162-170.

Yu, H.G., Chung, H., Yoon, T.G., Yum, K.W. & Kim, H.J. (2003). Stellate ganglion block increases blood flow into the optic nerve head and the peripapillary retina in human. *Auton Neurosci* 109, 1-2, pp.53-57.

Part 3

New Possibilities and Genetics

12

Measurement of Anterior Chamber Angle with Optical Coherence Tomography

De Orta-Arellano F, Muñoz-Rodriguez P and Salinas-Gallegos JL
Diagnóstico Visual de Guadalajara
México

1. Introduction

Evaluation of the width of the anterior chamber angle and its inlet during the ophthalmic examination is essential in determining the susceptibility of the angle to closure (Kalev-Landoy et al 2007, Leung et al 2007, Leung et al 2008, Radhakrishnan et al 2005).
There are factors that have been recognized as affecting the anterior chamber angle width include age, race/ethnicity, iris color, eye dominance, corneal curvature and refraction, and illumination open or narrow angles may become closed in dark lighting conditions, which can lead to the diagnosis of angle-closure glaucoma being missed (Liu L 2008).
Since the clinical introduction of the slitlamp into ophthalmology by Vogt, the dimensions of the anterior segment of the eye have usually been estimated by slit-lamp-supported biomicroscopy of the eye (Xu L 2008).
Although gonioscopy is the gold standard for anterior chamber angle assessment (Baikoff G 2004, Kalev-Landoy et al 2007, Leung et al 2007, Radhakrishnan et al 2005), its inevitable need for minimal illumination to visualize the angle, the uncertainty of the change in angle configuration when a goniolens is in direct contact on the cornea, and the dependence on individual skill and experience for interpretation of the angle configuration, serve to limit its role in providing precise angle assessment. Reliable measurement of the anterior chamber angle was not possible until ultrasound biomicroscopy (UBM) became available (Kalev-Landoy et al 2007, Leung et al 2007). With UBM, detailed spatial relationships of the anterior chamber angle iridocorneoscleral junction can be visualized and quantified.

1.1 UBM and Anterior Segment-Optical Coherence Tomography (AS-OCT)

Optical coherence tomography has several advantages over the other techniques for objective assessment of the anterior chamber angle (Dada et al 2007).
UBM is a close contact immersion technique (Kalev-Landoy et al 2007, Leung et al 2007 Radhakrishnan et al 2005), There is a risk of infection or corneal abrasion due to the contact nature of the examination (Dada et al 2007, Radhakrishnan et al 2005). Inadvertent corneal indentation can cause artifactitious widening of the angle (Baikoff G 2004, Dada et al 2007, Leung et al 2007). By the time the image is captured, it may be difficult to judge the exact globe position and the precise clock-hour location at which the scan was aligned (Leung et al 2007). Ultrasound biomicroscopy is performed with the patient supine, positioning that theoretically causes the iris diaphragm to fall back. This deepens the anterior chamber and opens the angle (Dada et al 2007).

In UBM, there is no fixed reference point and the angle region measured is located subjectively as nasal, temporal, superior, inferior, and so forth, not in exact degrees of an arc. With UBM, only 1 quadrant can be imaged at a time. With AS-OCT, 4 quadrants can be scanned at once. The UBM procedure is more time consuming and requires a highly skilled operator to obtain high-quality precision images (Dada et al 2007, Radhakrishnan et al 2005). As a result, intra- and interobserver reproducibilities for angle measurements have been generally poor (Leung et al 2007).

Anterior Segment Optical Coherence Tomography (AS-OCT) is a non-contact, non-invasive light-based imaging modality of diagnostic technique (Dacosta et al 2008 Spectral Domain, Dacosta et al 2008 Indian J Ophthalmol, Dada, T et al. 2008, Leung et al 2007, Leung et al 2008, Sakata LM, Sunita et al) that provides image resolution higher than that of UBM (axial resolution of 18 µm in Visante OCT versus 50 µm in UBM) of the anterior segment in cross section (Dacosta et al 2008 Spectral Domain, Dada, T et al. 2008, Leung et al 2007, Leung et al 2008, Sunita et al) in vivo. Fig. 1 (Boyd S et al). Furthermore the use of wide-field scanning optics (16 mm) and deep axial scan range (8 mm) permit the AS-OCT to image the entire anterior chamber in a single frame. After acquisition, the scanned images are processed by a customized "dewarping" software, which compensates for the index of refraction transition at the air-tear interface and the different group indices in air, cornea, and aqueous to correct the images physical dimensions (Sakata LM). It allows for an objective assessment of the anterior chamber (AC) angle and is easy to use after minimal training. These characteristics compare favorably to the current gold standard, gonioscopy, which requires highly trained personnel, is subjective, and involves placing a lens on the eye of the patient (Sunita et al).

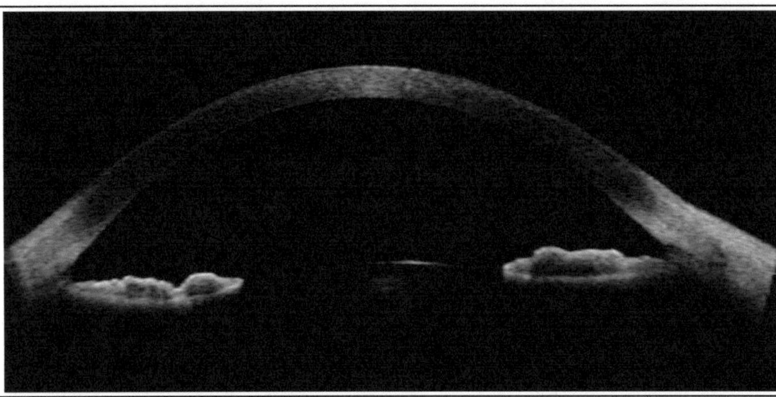

Fig. 1. OCT image of the anterior chamber

The working principle of OCT is similar to ultrasound (Dacosta et al 2008 Spectral Domain, Leung et al 2008, Dada et al 2007), which uses echoes to locate structures within the body. The speed of light being almost a million times faster than sound allows measurement of structures with a resolution of ≤10 microns as compared to 100 microns scale for ultrasound. (Dacosta et al 2008 Spectral Domain). OCT demonstrated excellent interobserver and intersession reproducibility for AC depth measurements and good to excellent interobserver and intersession reproducibility for angle parameters in the nasal and temporal quadrants. (Sunita et al).

With OCT, the user can view multiple cross-sectional image of the anterior chamber angle. As it use an infrared light, pupil doesn't close by providing a more natural image of angle structures without modifying their anatomy. Measurement software can be used to calculate the depth of the angle in degrees (Boyd S et al), or in mm (Angle Opening Distance, AOD) and mm^2 (Trabecular Iris Space Area, TISA) Fig 2.

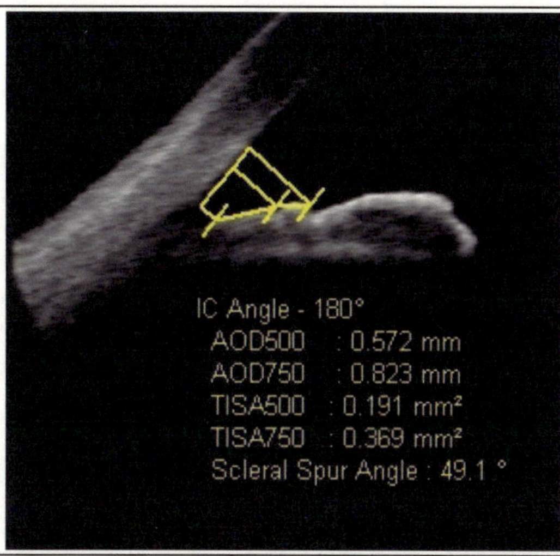

Fig. 2. Measurement of quantitative angle parameters using Visante OCT. Illustrated are angle opening distance (AOD), trabecular-iris space area (TISA) 500 or 750 µm from scleral spur.

Age and refractive error were found to be associated with anterior chamber angle measurement; one may argue that some adjustment would be required since the objective of the study was to provide population normative data (Xu L 2008).

2. Optical coherence tomography

Anterior segment optical coherence tomography is described as an attractive technique for optical biopsy because it can image tissue microstructure in situ, yielding micron- scale image resolution without the need to excise a specimen and process tissue processing. Optical coherence tomography has several advantages over the other techniques for objective assessment of the anterior chamber angle. Anterior segment optical coherence tomography can perform measurements without a coupling medium as it uses light energy (Dada et al 2007).
Optical Coherence tomography is based on the principle of Michelson interferometry. (Dacosta et al 2008 Spectral Domain, Dada T et al 2008). Broad bandwidth infrared light (of 1310 nm) first reported by Radhakrishnan et al using a system developed by Izatt's group Dada et al 2007 generated by using a superluminescent diode projected on the tissue (Boyd S et al, Dacosta et al, Leung et al 2007, Leung et al 2008, Sunita et al). 1310 nm wavelength of light is strongly absorbed by water in the ocular media and, therefore, only 10%of the light incident on the cornea reaches the retina (Radhakrishnan et al). The light is then broken into combination of reflected light from the sample arm and light from the reference arm gives rise to an interference pattern. By scanning the mirror in the reference arm, a reflectivity profile of the sample can be obtained. This reflectivity profile, called an A-scan contains information about the spatial dimension and location of structures within the item of interest. A cross-sectional tomography (B-Scan) may be achieved by laterally combining a series of these axial depth scan (A-scan) (Dacosta et al 2008 Spectral Domain). Images generated are easy to interpret (Dacosta et al 2008 Spectral Domain, Dada T et al 2008).

With standard software, the lateral resolution of AS-OCT is 60 mm and the axial resolution is 18 mm compared with 50 mm and 25 mm, respectively, with UBM. With high-resolution corneal software, axial resolution of AS-OCT can reach 8 mm. With the Visante AS-OCT, anterior segment scans up to 6.0 mm deep and 16.0 mm wide can be performed (data by Carl Zeiss Meditec). Important landmarks such as the scleral spur are more distinct in AS OCT images. With AS-OCT, one can also examine the posterior capsule of the lens, which is not possible with UBM (Dada et al 2007).

The AS-OCT image represents the differential backscattering contrast between different tissue types on a micron scale. It is a gray scale or false color 2-dimensional representation of backscattered light intensity in a cross-sectional plane (Dada et al 2007). It gives almost same details as that of UBM, with an additional advantage of being non-contact. This provides a detailed view of cornea, angle and angle recess, sclera and scleral spur; iris and its rood, ciliary body and ciliary body band and the limbus Fig 3. Sclera and the scleral spur are seen as highly reflective structures and ciliary body is seen as a hyporeflective structure. It allows a direct measure the anterior chamber angle.

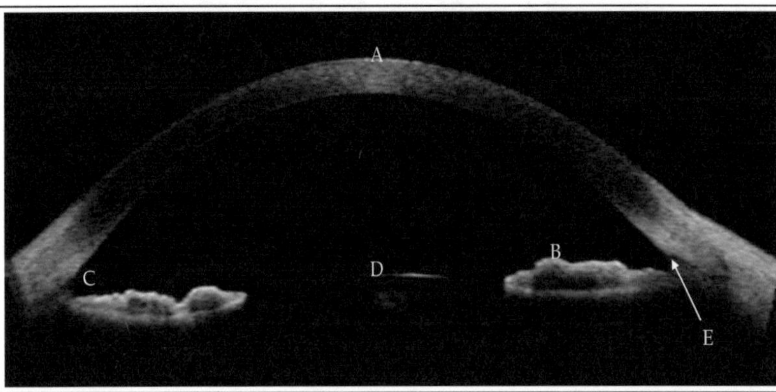

Fig. 3. Anterior segment OCT image. Illustrated (A) cornea, (B) iris, (C) anterior chamber angle, (D) lens and (E) scleral spur.

The imaging information provided by anterior segment OCT equates well with the UBM findings, biggest advantage of OCT over UBM is that the former being non-invasive and non contact (Dada, T et al 2008, Leung et al 2007, Leung et al 2008) it can be used in the imaging of the angle in immediate postoperative period and also in eyes with anterior segment trauma. Nozaki et al reported the anterior segment OCT findings after non-penetrating deep sclerectomy. They showed that OCT is capable of providing information regarding the status of bleb, trabeculo-Descemet's membrane, and bleb height (Dada, T et al).

Reliable documentation of the angle dimensions is also dependent on precise localization of the scleral spur (Leung et al 2008). The scleral spur in anterior segment imaging is marked by a prominent inner extension of the sclera (its thickest part) and represents an anatomical landmark for the trabecular meshwork, which is located approximately 250 to 500 μm anterior to the scleral spur along the angle wall (Sakata LM).

Previous UBM studies failed to attain repeatable measurements of the angle. The study by Urbak et al., who used the same UBM images for measurement, the intraobserver coefficient of variation for AOD was up to 16.97%, with significant differences ($P < 0.001$) found between observers. Measurement reproducibility was affected by subjective interpretation of visualized anatomic landmarks, which is directly related to image resolution (Leung et al 2008).

2.1 Image acquisition

In a retrospective observational study, the anterior chamber angle was measured using anterior segment images of OCT in 130 eyes of 72 patients. All subjects underwent an ophthalmic examination including visual acuity, slit-lamp biomicroscopy, autokeratorefractometry with KR-8000 (Topcon).

Exclusion criteria in our group of patients were history of glaucoma, trauma, ocular disease, previous ocular surgery including laser trabeculoplasty, laser iridotomy, laser photocoagulation, pterygium surgery, refractive surgery.

Scans were acquired with internal fixation target under dark conditions with angle protocol, which gives enhanced anterior segment single scan and global pachymetry map. This analysis detects corneal tissue, iris, lens anterior surface, anterior chamber. Angle measurements can be determined by manual detection of scleral spur. The inbuilt algorithm measures angle in both side of anterior chamber giving AOD 500, AOD 750, TISA 500, TISA 750. To perform AS OCT imaging in a non-accommodated state, the subjects refractive correction was used to adjust the internal fixation target for the patients distance correction.

All scans were taken by a single examiner. Scans were centered on the pupil and taken along the horizontal meridian (nasal - temporal angles at 0 to 180 degrees).

We analyzed the nasal and temporal angles, because they are more accessible than the superior and inferior angles. Lid manipulation is always necessary for superior and inferior angle imaging and may lead to inadvertent change in angle configuration.

3. Results

3.1 Mesurement obtainted of anterior chamber angle in myopic eyes

Measures were obtained from 52 eyes of 26 patients with mean of myopic refraction of -2.23 D (range - 0.75 to - 3.75) Fig. 4 and cylinder less than - 2.75 D obtained from Autokeratorefractometer KR-8000 (Topcon): 11 men, 15 women. Mean of age 28 years (range 18 to 67 years old). The mean of AOD 500 measured was 0.636 mm (SD 0.202), AOD 750: 0.912 mm (SD 0.274), TISA 500 0.217 mm^2 (SD 0.071), TISA 750: 0.412 mm^2 (SD 0.131).

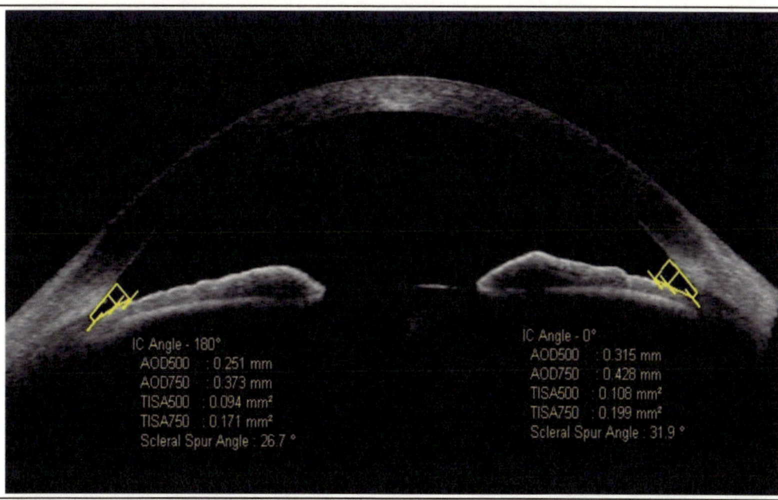

Fig. 4. Measurement of anterior chamber angle in myopic patient (- 2.50 = - 0.50 x 20°)

3.2 Mesurement obtainted of anterior chamber angle in hypermetropic eyes

Measures were obtained from 43 eyes of 24 patients with mean of refraction + 1.60 D (+ 0.25 to + 9.25 D): 10 men, 14 women. Mean of age 45 years (range 21 to 75 years). The mean of AOD 500 measured was 0.372 mm (SD 0.167), AOD 750: 0.528 mm (SD 0.210), TISA 500 0.131 mm^2 (SD 0.062), TISA 750: 0.243 mm^2 (SD 0.105).

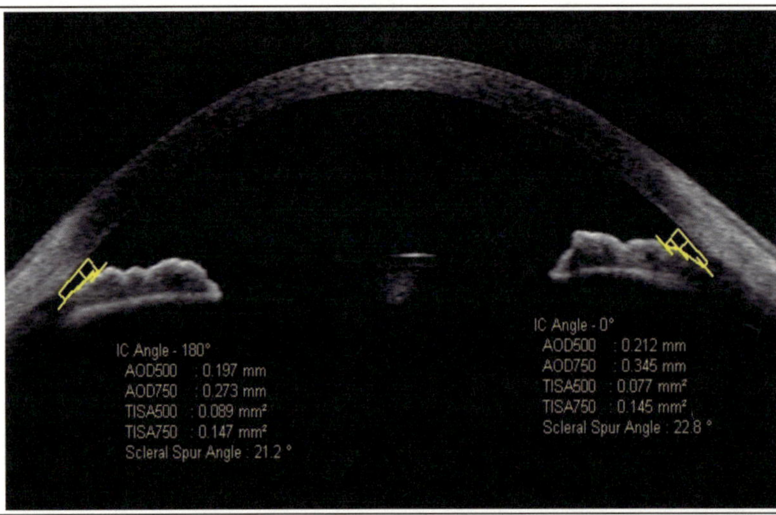

Fig. 5. Measurement of anterior chamber angle in hypermetropic patient (+ 6.00 = - 1.25 x 130°)

3.3 Mesurement obtainted of anterior chamber angle in high myopic eyes

Measures were obtained from 20 eyes of 11 patients with mean of refraction of - 6.61 (- 4.00 to - 10.50 D) cylinder less than - 2.75 D: 6 men, 5 women. Aged 26 years old (from 18 to 49 years). The AOD 500 measured was 0.845 mm (SD 0.398), AOD 750: 1.181 mm (SD 0.510) , TISA 500 0.286 mm^2 (SD 0.134) , TISA 750: 0.555 mm^2 (SD 0.282).

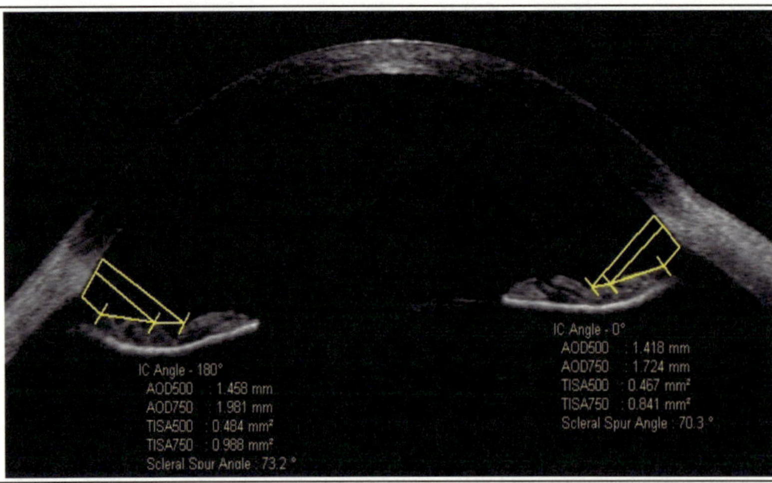

Fig. 6. Measurement of anterior chamber angle in high myopia patient (- 9.00 = - 0.50 x 100°).

3.4 Mesurement obtainted of anterior chamber angle in high astigmatic eyes

Measures were obtained from 15 eyes of 11 patients: 5 men, 6 women. Aged 25 years (from 17 to 33 years) with cylinder refraction - 5.32 (- 4.00 to - 7.00), spherical refraction - 2.23 (-0.25 to -3.75). The AOD 500 measured was 0.660 mm (SD 0.270), AOD 750: 0.910 mm (SD 0.357), TISA 500 0.220 mm^2 (SD 0.096), TISA 750: 0.415 mm^2 (SD 0.172).

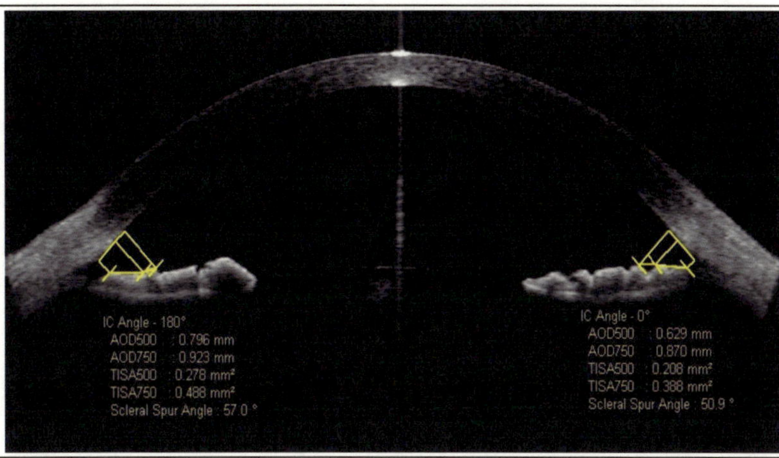

Fig. 7. Measurement of anterior chamber angle in astigmatic patient (+ 0.25 = - 5.00 x 180°)

	AOD 500 mm	AOD 750 mm	TISA 500 mm^2	TISA 750 mm^2
Hypermetropia	0.372	0.528	0.131	0.243
Myopia	0.636	0.912	0.217	0.412
High Astigmatism	0.660	0.910	0.220	0.415
High Myopia	0.845	1.181	0.286	0.555

Table 1. Difference of the media of anterior chamber angle measures between groups. AOD (Angle open distance), TISA (trabecular iris space area).

4. Conclusion

On routine gonioscopy, the angle structures may not be identified in eyes with a steep iris configuration and a narrow angle. A steep approach to the angle makes examination difficult in such cases. OCT Visante is one technique for objective estimation of angle measures even in difficult eyes. It is important to make angular measurements in greater groups of population to determine the normal variation of the angular values of AOD and TISA to compare it with glaucoma angles and to determine the angular values of risk for angular closing.

5. References

Baikoff G, Lutun E, Ferraz C, Wei J (2004) Static and dynamic of the Anterior Segment with Optical Coherence Tomography. *J Cataract Refract Surg* (Sept 2004) Vol. 30 No.9 pp. 1843-50.

Boyd S., Brancato R., Straatsma B. (2009) *Tomografía de Coherencia Óptica. Atlas y texto.* Jaypee-Highlights. ISBN 978-9962-678-05-2, Panamá, Panamá.

Dacosta S, Fernandes G, Rajendran B, Janakiraman P (2008) Assessment of anterior segment parameters under photopic and scotopic conditions in Indian eyes using anterior segment optical coherence tomography *Indian J Ophthalmol* (Febrary 2008) ; Vol 56 No. 1. pp. 17-22.

Dacosta S., Rajendran B., Janakiraman (2008). *Spectral Domain OCT.* 1a ed. Mc Graw Hill, ISBN 978-81-8448-311-6. New Delhi, India.

Dada T, Sihota R, Gadia R, Aggarwal A, Mandal S, Gupta V (2007) Comparison of anterior segment optical coherence tomography and ultrasound biomicroscopy for assessment of the anterior segment J Cataract Refract Surg (May 2007); Vol. 33 pp 837–840.

Dada,T., Sony P.,Sihota R. (2008). Clinical Utility of OCT in Glaucoma, In: *Techniques in Glaucoma Diagnosis and Treatment* , Garg, A., Mortensen JN., Marchini G., Mehta KR., Khalil AK., Melamed S., Bovet JJ., Carassa R., Dada T., Mehta C. (116-127). Mc Graw Hill, ISBN-13: 978-0-07-160195-5, New Delhi, India.

Kalev-Landoy M, Day AC, Cordeiro MF & Migdal C (2007). Optical coherence tomography in anterior segment imaging. *Acta Ophthalmol Scand.* Vol. 85, No.4 (June 2007) pp 427–430.

Leung CK, Cheung CY, Li H, Dorairaj S, Yiu CK, Wong AL, Liebmann J, Ritch R, Weinreb R & Lam DS (2007) Dynamic Analysis of Dark–Light Changes of the Anterior Chamber Angle with Anterior Segment OCT *Invest Ophthalmol Vis Sci.*, Vol. 48, No. 9 (September 2007) pp. 4116–4122

Leung CK, Li H, Weinreb RN, Liu J, Cheung CY, Lai RY, Pang CP & Lam DS (2008) Anterior Chamber Angle Measurement with Anterior Segment Optical Coherence Tomography: A Comparison between Slit Lamp OCT and Visante OCT *Invest Ophthalmol Vis Sci* Vol. 49 , No. 8, (August 2008) pp. 3469-74.

Liu L (2008) Anatomical Changes of the Anterior Chamber Angle With Anterior-Segment Optical Coherence Tomography *Arch Ophthalmol.* (Dec 2008) Vol. 126 No. 12. pp.1682-1686

Radhakrishnan S, Goldsmith J, Huang D, Westphal V, Dueker DK, Rollins AM, Izatt JA, Smith SD (2005) Comparison of optical coherence tomography and ultrasound biomicroscopy for detection of narrow anterior chamber angles *Arch Ophthalmol* (Aug 2005) Vol 123 No. 8. pp. 1053-9.

Sakata LM, Lavanya R, Friedman DS, Aung HT, Seah SK, Foster PJ & Aung T. (2008). Assessment of the scleral spur in anterior segment optical coherence tomography images. *Arch Ophthalmol.*Vol. 126 No. 2. pp 181-5.

Sunita Radhakrishnan, Jovina See, Scott D. Smith, Winifred P. Nolan, Zheng Ce,David S. Friedman, David Huang, Yan Li, Tin Aung, & Paul T. K. Chew (2007). Reproducibility of Anterior Chamber Angle Measurements Obtained with Anterior Segment Optical Coherence Tomography, *Invest Ophthalmol Vis Sci.* Vol.48, No. 8. (August 2007): pp. 3683–3688.

Xu L, Cao WF, Wang YX, Chen CX & Jonas JB (2008). Anterior Chamber Depth and Chamber Angle and Their Associations with Ocular and General Parameters: The Beijing Eye Study. *Am J Ophthalmol. Vol.* 145 no. 5 (May 2008) pp. 929-36

13

Association of TNF-α and TNF-β Gene Polymorphisms with Primary Open Angle and Primary Angle Closure Glaucoma

Najwa Mohammed Al- Dabbagh[1], Nourah Al-Dohayan[1], Abdulrahman Al-Asmari[2], Misbahul Arfin[2] and Mohammad Tariq[2]
[1]Department of Ophthalmology, [2]Research Center, Riyadh Military Hospital, Riyadh, Saudi Arabia

1. Introduction

Glaucoma is a complex disease that comprises a group of heterogeneous optic neuropathies characterized by a progressive degeneration of the optic nerve head and visual field defects. It starts with unnoticeable blind spots at the edges of field vision progressing to the tunnel vision and finally leading to blindness (Quigley & Broman, 2006). The disease process is insidious, and the central vision is usually not lost until the disease is advanced, a significant proportion of individuals remain either undiagnosed or undertreated. The most common forms of glaucoma are age-related, generally beginning in midlife and progressing slowly but relentlessly as the age advances (A.T.G.S.R.S.G., 2009). If detected early enough, disease progression can be slowed with drug and/or surgical treatment, emphasizing the importance of identifying the disease in its earliest stages.

Glaucoma is broadly classified into primary and secondary glaucoma based on their etiology and aqueous humor dynamics (Shields, 2005). Based on anatomy of the anterior chamber (gonioscopy), primary glaucomas are further classified as primary open angle glaucoma (POAG) and primary angle closure glaucoma (PACG). Depending on the time of onset, glaucoma is also termed as infantile, juvenile and adult type. Rarely glaucoma may be found in babies at birth this form of glaucoma called congenital glaucoma. Secondary glaucomas are characterized by the involvement of predisposing ocular or systemic diseases such as uveitis, trauma, or diabetes thereby resulting in an alteration of aqueous humor dynamics. Pseudoexfoliation glaucoma (XFG) and pigmentary glaucoma (PG) are the most frequently reported type of secondary glaucoma (Shields, 2005).

Glaucoma affects 70 million people and is the second leading cause of blindness worldwide. It is estimated that by the year 2020, this number would rise to around 79.6 million (Quigley & Broman, 2006). The prevalence of glaucoma varies widely across the different ethnic groups (He et al., 2006; Wong et al., 2006; Sakata et al., 2007; Cedrone et al., 2008; Vijaya et al., 2008a; 2008b; Pekmezci et al., 2009) and is significantly higher in blacks (4.7%) as compared to in the white (1.3%) population (Kwon et al., 2009). Primary open angle glaucoma is the predominant disease among whites and Africans (Tielsch et al., 1991; Klein et al., 1992; Rotchford & Johnson, 2002; Rotchford et al., 2003; Varma et al., 2004; Friedman et al., 2006; Sakata et al., 2007) while PACG is a major form of glaucoma in Asians (Hu et al.,

1989; Jacob et al., 1998; Foster & Johnson, 2001; Casson et al., 2007). Epidemiological studies reveal that the prevalence of POAG around the world varies by about 2 orders of magnitude with the lowest estimates found among Eskimos (0.06%) residing in Alaska (Arkell et al., 1987) and the highest prevalence among African-derived people living in the Caribbean (7.1– 8.8%) (Mason et al., 1989; Leske et al., 1994). PACG is leading cause of the most of the bilateral glaucoma related blindness in Singapore, China, and India. It has been estimated that PACG blinds more people than POAG worldwide (Dandona et al., 2000; Foster et al., 2000). According to a recent study glaucoma is the major cause of blindness in Saudi Arabia. The prevalence of both POAG and PACG is higher in western region of Saudi Arabia as compared to other Asian countries (Eid et al., 2009). To date no national study has been undertaken to determine the exact prevalence of glaucoma in this country.

Elevated intraocular pressure (IOP) is a major risk factor in glaucoma which is supported by the fact that experimentally induced elevation of IOP leads to glaucoma in animals (Levkovitch-Verbin et al., 2002). The etiology of raised IOP and resulting glaucoma is not fully understood. Fluid formed by the ciliary body (aqueous humor) is removed by the trabecular outflow pathways, which includes the trabecular meshwork, the juxtacanalicular connective tissue, the endothelial lining of Schlemm's canal, and the collecting channels and the aqueous veins (A.T.G.S.R.S.G., 2009). The IOP is dependent on the rate of fluid removal, which under normal conditions matches the rate of formation. In most patients with glaucoma, the rate of fluid removal declines so that it no longer keeps pace with the rate of formation resulting in the increased IOP. The increase in IOP has been associated with genetic factors, age and oxidative stress (Tschumper & Johnson, 1990; Leske et al., 1995; Green et al., 2007). Although elevation of intraocular pressure (IOP) is often related to the optic nerve damage in glaucoma, factors other than IOP are likely to play a role in the pathogenesis of glaucomatous optic neuropathy, particularly in individuals with normal tension glaucoma (NTG).

The loss of retinal ganglion cells (RGC) is the typical pathology in glaucoma. Progressive loss of optic nerve axons and RGCs result in characteristic optic nerve atrophy and visual field defects in glaucoma patients. A number of hypotheses have been put forward that describe the sequence of events responsible for triggering ganglion cell degeneration in glaucoma. These include compromised blood flow of the optic nerve, mechanical compression due to raised IOP, loss of neurotrophic factors, autoimmune mechanisms, nitric oxide-induced injuries to the optic nerve and glutamate excitotoxicity (Mozaffarieh et al., 2008). A combination of these factors may be involved in causing glaucomatous RGC loss. Animal models also confirmed that acute IOP elevation causes blockage of brain-derived neurotrophic factor (BDNF) transport and may contribute to neuronal death (Pease et al., 2000). On the other hand the mechanisms involved in the pathophysiology and development of PACG are rather complicated and involve the anatomy of the angle, and the spatial and structural relationships between the lens and the anatomy of the angle, the iris, and the lens. Most mechanisms for PACG impute to the increasing lens thickness during aging in a relatively small eye and a shallow anterior chamber. Acute PACG has been attributed to morphometeric characteristics of the eye. Human sclera undergoes active remodeling during the development of myopia. Biochemical assays from highly myopic eyes show markedly reduced amounts of biochemical markers for collagen and glycosaminoglycans, when compared with the similar sclera of emmetropic eyes. This remodeling process occurs in concert with an increase in the production and enhanced activation of collagen degrading enzymes, particularly matrix metalloproteases (MMPs) (McBrien & Gentle, 2001). The net effect of these changes is a loss of scleral tissue at the posterior pole of the eye.

Growing evidence obtained from clinical and experimental studies strongly suggests the involvement of the immune system in glaucoma (Helpern & Grosskreutz, 2002; Wax & Tezel, 2002; Tezel & Wax, 2000; 2003). Paradoxically the role of immune system in Glaucoma has been described as either neuroprotective or neurodestructive. A balance between beneficial immunity and harmful neurodegeneration may ultimately determine the fate of RGCs in response to various stresses in glaucomatous eye (Tezel & Wax 2007). T-cell-mediated immune response may initially be beneficial to limit neurodegeneration (Schwartz & Kipnis, 2001, 2002; Kipnis et al., 2002). However, a failure to properly control aberrant, stress-induced immune response likely converts the protective immunity to an autoimmune neurodegenerative process that can facilitate the progression of neurodegeneration in some, if not all, glaucoma patients (Tezel & Wax, 2007). Expansion and secondary recruitment of circulating T cells through an antigen mediated process is supported by the evidence of abnormal T-cell subsets (Yang et al., 2001a) and increased production of serum autoantibodies to different optic nerve and retina antigens in many glaucoma patients (Tezel et al., 1998, 1999; Wax et al., 1998a, 1998b; Yang et al., 2001b) Furthermore, initial *in vivo* studies support the feasibility of eliciting an experimental autoimmune model of glaucomatous neurodegeneration in which RGCs progressively die in specific antigen-immunized animals by exhibiting a pattern of neuronal damage similar to that of human glaucoma (Wax &Tezel, 2009). As the role of the immune system in glaucoma is one of the surveillance, in which signal pathways of the immune system regulate cell death in response to conditions that stress retinal neurons in glaucoma. Recent studies have focused on immunological changes occurring in glaucoma pathogenesis and possible preventive therapies based along those lines have been proposed. The major targets of interest are cytokines, as these inflammatory mediators play an important role in the pathogenesis of glaucoma and may regulate RGC survival or death (Tezel & Wax, 2004).

The role of tumor necrosis factor (TNF), an important proinflammatory cytokine is a subject of interest in glaucoma studies. Both TNF-α, produced mainly by monocytes and activated macrophages and TNF-β, produced mainly by activated T-cells, play important immunoregulatory roles in various diseases. TNF-α is up regulated in several neurodegenerative disorders including optic nerve microglia and astrocytes in glaucoma (Yuan & Neufeld, 2000; 2001). It has been suggested that cell death mediated by TNF-α is a contributing factor in the progression of neurodegeneration in glaucoma (Tezel et al., 2001). TNF-α plays a critical role in optic neuropathy by initiating the inflammatory pathways through the induction of NOS-2 in astrocytes (Yuan & Neufeld, 2000). It has been observed that ischemic or pressure-loaded glial cells produce TNF-α which results in oligodendrocytes death and the apoptosis of RGC leading to glaucomatous neurodegeneration (Tezel & Wax, 2000). Furthermore, TNF-α directly induces apoptosis through TNF-α receptor-I (TNFRI) also known as death receptor which is mainly localized on the retinal ganglion cells (Tezel et al., 2001). The substantial role of TNF-α/TNFRI in the pathogenesis of glaucoma has also been supported by experimental study on mouse model of glaucoma in which induction of ocular hypertension resulted in a rapid up regulation of TNF-α followed by loss of optic nerve oligodendrocytes (Nakazawa et al., 2006). Moreover, intravitreal TNF-α injection in normal mice mimicked glaucoma like RGCs degeneration whereas anti-TNF-α neutralizing antibody or deleting the TNF-α gene blocked the deleterious effects of ocular hypertension (Nakazawa et al., 2006). Tezel et al. (2004) also reported that unilateral optic nerve crush injury in mice resulted in significantly less glial activation, TNF-α production and retinal ganglion cell death in *TNFRI* -knockout mice. In fact, histopathologic studies have also shown increased immunostaining for TNF-α and TNFRI in the glaucomatous optic nerve head as compared to age-matched control samples (Yan et al., 2000; Yuan & Neufeld, 2000). Interestingly, a new antiglaucoma drug (GLC756) significantly suppressed LPS-induced TNF-α production (Laengle et al., 2006a, 2006b). These observations further confirm the hypothesis of an involvement of the TNF-α /TNFRI signaling pathway in the pathogenesis of glaucoma.

The genes for TNF-α (OMIM 191160) and TNF-β also known as lymphotoxin-α (LT-α, MIM 153440), located within the MHC III region of chromosome 6, shows close linkage to the HLA class I (*HLA-B*) and class II (*HLA-DR*) genes. Studies on monozygotic twins and their first-degree relatives, using *ex vivo* endotoxin stimulated whole blood samples, have provided evidence that 60% of variation in the production capacity of TNF-α appears to be genetically determined (Westendorp et al., 1997). Several polymorphisms within the promoter region of *TNF*-α and the intron 1 polymorphism of TNF–β, in particular, have been associated with altered levels of circulating TNF-α (Sharma et al., 2006; 2008).

With regard to PACG a number of lines of evidence have suggested that both genetic and environmental factors contribute to the development of PACG (Lowe, 1972). There are various published studies that suggested a genetic basis of the PACG (Aung et al., 2008a; 2008b). PACG, as a common complex disease, has become an important target for association studies in recent years. Genetic heterogeneity is illustrated by the several loci in many glaucoma causing genes identified to date. Single nucleotide polymorphisms in several genes such as matrix metalloproteases-9 (MMP-9), Cytochrome P450 1B1 (CYP1B1), membrane-type frizzled-related protein (MFRP) , methylenetetrahydrofolate reductase gene (MTHFR), myocilin (MYOC), calcitonin receptor-like gene (CALRL), endothelial nitric oxide synthase (eNOS), heat shock protein 70 (HSP70), retinal homeobox gene (CHX10), have been associated with PACG (Wang et al., 2006; Chakrabarti et al., 2007; Michael et al., 2008; 2009, Aung et al., 2008; Dai et al., 2008; Cong et al., 2009; Cao et al., 2009, Ayub et al., 2010). However, ethnic variations exist in the association between these polymorphisms and PACG, and many cases such association has not been replicated in subsequent research (Wang et al., 2006; Aung et al., 2008a). Moreover, the biological significance of the some associated single nucleotide polymorphisms (SNPs) in the development of PACG is still unknown (Michael et al., 2008). PACG has been reported to be associated with genes related to regulation of axial length and structural remodeling of connective tissues, such as *MFRP*, *MMP-9*, and *MTHFR* genes (Michael et al., 2008; Wang et al., 2006; Aung et al., 2008a; 2008 b; Wang et al., 2008). It has also been reported that TNF-α is capable of inducing both increased synthesis and activity of matrix metalloproteinases (MMPs) (Rajavashisth et al., 1999; Siwik et al., 2000; Uchida et al., 2000) therefore the polymorphism in TNF genes might be associated with regulation of axial length and structural remodeling of connective tissues and ultimately to the development of PACG.

Several polymorphisms have been reported in the promoter region of TNF-α gene. One of the best described single nucleotide polymorphisms (SNPs) is located at nucleotide position -308 within the TNF-α promoter region (rs1800629) and affects a consensus sequence for a binding site of transcription factor AP-2 (Abraham & Kroeger, 1999). TNF-α promoter polymorphism leads to a less common allele-A (allele 2) which has been associated with increased TNF-α production in vitro (Braun et al., 1996; Wilson et al., 1994) and higher rate of TNF-α transcription than wild type GG genotype (Wilson et al., 1997; Jeong et al., 2004). This polymorphism has been linked to increased susceptibility to several chronic metabolic degenerative, inflammatory and autoimmune diseases (Cuenca et al., 2001). It has also been reported to be involved in increased susceptibility to different eye diseases including diabetic retinopathy and glaucoma (Limb et al., 1999; Yoshioka et al., 2006; Huang et al., 2009). TNF-α ıs involved in T-cell dependent B-cell responses, T-cell proliferation, natural killer (NK)-cell activity and dendritic cell maturation. The previously published data indicate that the host's ability to produce TNF-α may play an important role in vulnerability to glaucoma.

Of interest, G/A polymorphism at nucleotide position -308 within the human TNF-α promoter region is associated with elevated TNF levels, disease susceptibility, and poor prognosis in several diseases (Messer et al., 1991; Wilson et al., 1992; Galbraith & Pendey, 1995; Patino-Garcia et al., 2000). Adenine at position -308 makes the TNF-α promoter a much more powerful transcription activator than guanine (Messer et al., 1991). The TNF-α is up regulated in several neurodegenerative disorders including multiple sclerosis, Parkinson's disease, Alzheimer's disease (Shohami et al., 1999; Yan et al., 2000; Liu et al., 2006) and in optic nerve microglia and astrocytes in glaucoma patients (Yuan & Neufeld, 2000; 2001]. Increased TNF-α level have been associated with a poor prognosis after trauma in the brain (Munoz-Fernandez & Fresno, 1998; Ertel et al., 1995), whereas a decrease in TNF-α is known to reduce nerve damage. In a rat cerebral ischemic model, exogenous TNF-α was found to exacerbate focal ischemic injuries, whereas blocking endogenous TNF-α was neuroprotective (Shohami et al., 1996).

TNF-β resembles to TNF-α in terms of several biological activities including apoptosis and gives rise to a similar pro-inflammatory response and has been shown to play a critical role in pathogenesis of many diseases. TNF-β gene polymorphism at nucleotide position 252 within first intron (A252G) (rs909253) affects a phorbol ester-responsive element. The presence of G at this position defines the mutant allele known as TNF-β * 1 (allele-1) which is less frequent allele in white subjects and is associated with higher TNF-α and TNF-β production (Messer et al., 1991; Abraham et al., 1993). Association of TNF-β +252 A/G polymorphism has been reported with various autoimmune disorders including Gravis' disease (Kula et al., 2001) idiopathic membranous glomerulonephritis, IgA nephropathy, insulin dependent diabetes mellitus (Medcraft et al., 1993) , myasthenia gravis (Zelano et al., 1998), asthma diathesis (Albuquerque et al., 1998), SLE with nephritis(Lu et al., 2005), systemic sclerosis (Pandey &Takeuchi, 1999), plaque psoriasis (Vasku et al., 2000), rheumatoid arthritis (Takeuchi et al., 2005), myocardial infarction in patients with rheumatoid arthritis (Panoulas et al., 2008), and type 1 diabetes (Boraska et al., 2009). Recently TNF-β +252 A/G polymorphism is reported to be associated with both susceptibility to and mortality from sepsis (Watanabe et al., 2010; Tiancha et al., 2011).

A few studies have been undertaken to determine the association of TNF-α polymorphisms and glaucoma in different part of the world (Limb et al., 1999; Yoshioka et al., 2006; Huang et al., 2009). The results of these studies on association of TNF-α polymorphism with POAG are inconsistent. These differences in findings have been attributed to variation in sample size, ethnicity and method of diagnosis (Lin et al., 2003; Mossbock et al., 2006; Tekeli et al., 2008; Razeghinejad et al., 2009). To date there is no report available on the association between TNF-β polymorphism and glaucoma. The joint analysis of polymorphism at TNF-α and TNF-β given that both are involved in the expression of TNF-α and in a suggested mechanism for autoimmune diseases, will provide further insight into the pathogenesis of glaucoma and help in developing effective therapeutic agents. Therefore the present study was undertaken to determine the possible association of TNF-α-308 and TNF-β +252 gene polymorphisms with POAG and PACG in Saudi population.

2. Methods

2.1 Subjects

The present study was undertaken to evaluate the association of TNF-α and TNF-β alleles and genotypes in Saudi primary glaucoma patients. A total of 200 unrelated Saudi patients with Primary Glaucoma [primary open angle glaucoma (POAG) and primary angle closure glaucoma (PACG)] were recruited from ophthalmology clinic of the Riyadh Military Hospital (RMH), Saudi Arabia. The patient group consisted of 94 males and 106 females, with age at diagnosis ranging from 25 to 78 years (mean ± SD: 58 ± 14.4). The control group consisted of 200 unrelated subjects, 100 males and 100 females, ages ranging from 25 to 68 years (mean ± SD: 55 ± 11.6). The diagnosis of primary glaucoma was based on comprehensive clinical examination as mentioned below.

2.2 Preliminary examination

The preliminary examination was performed in ophthalmology clinic of RMH. Detailed demographic data and medical history were recorded for each case and control subject. The preliminary examination included oblique flashlight test, anterior segment evaluation by slit lamp, Goldmann applanation tonometry, and direct fundoscopy (all examinations performed by resident/consultant ophthalmologists). The optic disc was examined after each pupil was dilated with 2 drops of tropicamide, unless contraindicated by the presence of a shallow anterior chamber depth at the slit lamp examination. The vertical cup-disc ratio (VCDR) was estimated for each eye. The rim border was determined based on the course of the blood vessels and the gradation of color, shadows, and texture (Spaeth, 1993). A suspect appearance of the optic disc (glaucomatous-appearing optic disc; GAOD) was defined in eyes with VCDR ≥ 0.6, asymmetry of the VCDR between the two eyes ≥ 0.2, focal thinning of the neuroretinal rim, localized or diffuse retinal nerve fiber layer defect, and/or optic disc hemorrhage. A glaucoma specialist confirmed the presence of a GAOD in the participants. Fundus photography, automated perimetry, and gonioscopy were not part of the preliminary examination protocol.

2.3 Detailed examination

Patients with GAOD status and/or intraocular pressure (IOP) measurements > 21 mm Hg at the screening underwent a definitive examination. At first each subject underwent a comprehensive ophthalmic examination, including review of medical history, best corrected visual acuity(BCVA) (using Snellen distance vision chart), retinoscopy and subjective refraction (when visual acuity < 20/30), slit lamp biomicroscopy, IOP measurement (using Goldmann applanation tonometry), standard automated perimetry tests, gonioscopy (using Sussman four-mirror lens), and fundoscopy examination. Gonioscopy was performed by a consultant (glaucoma specialist). Indentation gonioscopy with four-mirror Posner lens was performed in eyes with an anatomically narrow angle. The angle was graded according to the Scheie scheme (Scheie, 1957) and the peripheral iris contour, degree of pigmentation, presence of peripheral anterior synechiae, and other angle abnormalities were recorded. When the gonioscopy showed no contraindications, dilated direct fundoscopy and slit lamp

biomicroscopy of the optic disc (using a 78-D lens) were performed. The VCDR was determined independently in a masked fashion by two glaucoma specialists and cases of disagreement were resolved by consensus between the two graders during the definite examination visit. There was a good agreement between the two graders in determining VCDR (0.7 or more). The presence of any notching, optic disc hemorrhages, or nerve fiber layer defects was documented. Initially, most of the standard automated perimetry tests were performed with the Octopus 101 perimeter (Haag-Strreit Octopus, Switzerland). In an attempt to avoid the influence of learning effect in visual field (VF) results, these VF examinations were not considered for assessing visual function status.
The patients were further subjected to a second VF examination using a Humphrey visual field perimeter (Humphrey Visual Field Analyzer; Carl Zeiss Meditec, Inc., Dublin, CA), with the 24-2 full-threshold or SITA (Swedish interactive threshold algorithm) standard strategy. The visual function status was determined based on this single VF test, and only reliable VF examinations were considered for analysis. An abnormal VF examination was determined by the presence of one of the following criteria: (1) glaucoma hemifield test (GHT) result outside normal limits and (2) the presence of a cluster of ≥ 3 contiguous points in the pattern deviation (PD) probability plot with $P < 5\%$ or worse (within the same hemifield) (Foster et al., 2002). A reliable visual field test was defined as an examination with less than 33% of fixation losses, false positive and false negative. The glaucoma specialist verified whether the VF defects were consistent with glaucoma.

2.4 Criteria for glaucoma diagnosis

Glaucoma was diagnosed according to the International Society of Geographical and Epidemiologic Ophthalmology (ISGEO) classification, which uses three levels of evidence (Foster et al 2002). Briefly, in category 1, diagnosis was based on structural and functional evidence. It required CDR or CDR asymmetry ≥ 97.5th percentile for the normal population or a neuroretinal rim width reduced to ≥ 0.1 CDR (between 11- and 1-o'clock or 5- and 7-o'clock) with a definite VF defect consistent with glaucoma using the Swedish interactive threshold algorithm 30-2. Category 2 was based on advanced structural damage with unproved field loss. This included those subjects in whom VFs could not be determined or were unreliable, with CDR or CDR asymmetry ≥ 99.5th percentile for the normal population. Lastly, category 3 consisted of persons with an IOP ≥ 99.5th percentile for the normal population, whose optic discs could not be examined because of media opacities.

2.5 Glaucoma classification

Participants who fulfilled any of the three categories of evidence mentioned earlier were classified as having POAG or PACG
POAG: Anterior chamber angles open and appearing normal by gonioscopy, typical features of glaucomatous optic disc as defined earlier, and visual field defects corresponding to the optic disc changes.
PACG: At least two of the criteria mentioned: glaucomatous optic disc damage or glaucomatous visual field defects in combination with anterior chamber angle partly or totally closed, appositional angle closure or synechiae in angle, absence of signs of secondary angle closure (e.g., uveitis, lens related glaucoma, microspherophakia, evidence of neovascularization in the angle and associated retinal ischemia or congenital angle anomalies). Patients with signs of intracranial disease that would cause optic nerve atrophy

in x-ray, computerized tomography or magnetic resonance imaging were excluded. An anatomically narrow-angle eye should have pigmented trabecular meshwork not visible in ≥ 270° of the iridocorneal angle (as assessed by nonindentation gonioscopy) and/or the presence of peripheral anterior synechiae not explained by other causes but a primary angle-closure process.

2.6 Sample collection

Venous blood was collected from the patients (POAG, PACG) and controls and stored at - 20°C before extraction of DNA. The study protocol was approved by the Ethics Committee of the Hospital.

2.7 Genotyping

2.7.1 PCR amplification

Genomic DNA was extracted from the peripheral blood of patients and controls using QIAamp[R] DNA mini kit (Qiagen CA, USA). TNF-α and TNF-β genes were amplified using amplification refractory mutation systems (ARMS)-PCR methodology (Perry et al., 1999) to detect any polymorphism involved at position -308 of TNF-α and +252 in Interon1 of TNF-β gene respectively. The set of primers used to amplify target DNA in the promoter region of TNF-α and TNF-β genes are summarized in Table 1.

Locus	Generic (antisense) primer	Sense primers
TNF-α (G308A)	5′-TCT CGG TTT CTT CTC CAT CG-3′	5′-ATA GGT TTT GAG GGG CAT GG-3′ 5′-AAT AGG TTT TGA GGG GCA TGA-3′
TNF-β (A252G)	5′-AGA TCG ACA GAG AAG GGG ACA-3′	5′-CAT TCT CTG TTT CTG CCA TGG-3′ 5′-CAT TCT CTG TTT CTG CCA TGA-3′

Table 1. Showing sets of primers used to amplify the TNF-α and TNF-β to detect polymorphism

PCR amplification was carried out using Ready to Go PCR Beads (Amersham Biosciences, USA). Reaction consisted of 10 temperature cycles of denaturation for 15 s at 94 °C, annealing for 50 s at 65 °C and extension for 40 s at 72 °C. Then 25 cycles of denaturation for 20s at 94 °C, annealing for 50 s at 59 °C, extension for 50s at 72 °C. Final extension was performed at 72 °C for 7 m. A positive control was included in the PCR assay by amplification of the human growth hormone (HGH) gene. The amplified product for various samples were separated on the 1.5 % agarose gel, stained with ethidium bromide and photographed.

2.7.2 Statistical analysis

The differences in allele/ genotype frequencies between patients and controls were analyzed by the Fisher's exact test. *P* values less than 0.05 were considered significant. The strength of the association of disease with respect to a particular allele/genotype is expressed by odd ratio interpreted as *relative risk* (RR) following the Woolf's method as out lined by Schallreuter et al. (1993). It is calculated only for those Alleles/ genotypes which are increased or decreased in patients as compared to control group. The RR in this study has been calculated for all the subjects.

$$RR = (a) \times (d) \, / \, (b) \times (c) \quad \text{where,}$$

(a) = number of patients with expression of allele or genotype
(b) = number of patients without expression of allele or genotype
(c) = number of controls with expression of allele or genotype
(d) = number of controls without expression of allele or genotype
Etiologic Fraction (EF): The EF indicates the hypothetical genetic component of the disease. The values between 0 and 1 are of significance. EF is calculated for positive association only where RR> 1 (Savejgaard et al., 1983).

$$EF= (RR-1) f / RR, \text{ where } f= a/a+c$$

Preventive Fraction (PF): The PF indicates the hypothetical protective effect of one specific allele/ genotype for the disease. PF is calculated for negative association only where RR< 1 (Savejgaard et al., 1983). Values < 1.0 indicate the protective effect of the allele/genotype against the manifestation of disease.

$$PF= (1-RR) f / RR (1-f) +f, \text{ where } f= a/a+c$$

3. Results

In this case control study TNF-α and TNF-β genes were amplified to determine the allele and genotype frequencies in equal number of patients (200) and unrelated matched controls (200). The patient group consisted of POAG (135) and PACG (65) cases. The molecular analysis of the blood specimen of the patients and controls was performed in the same laboratory and at the same time. The investigator was blind to the phenotype of the subjects at the time of molecular analysis. Later on the results were separated for patient and control groups and analyzed for the determination of the frequencies of genotypes and alleles. Allelic frequencies and genotype distributions of both TNF-α and TNF-β gene polymorphisms differ between primary glaucoma (including both POAG and PACG cases) and control subjects (Tables 2-9).
The results of the genotypes and alleles distribution of TNF-α (-308) polymorphism in primary glaucoma (including total POAG and PACG cases) are summarized in Table 2. The frequency of GA (-308) genotype was significantly higher (*P*=0.02) while the frequency of GG (-308) genotype was lower in total primary glaucoma patients as compared to controls (*P*=0.01).

Genotype/ Allele	**Glaucoma (N=200)**		**Control (N=200)**		***P*-value**	**RR**	**EF*/PF**
	N	%	N	%			
GG	85	42.5	110	55	0.01‡	0.60	0.23
GA	100	50.0	76	38	0.02‡	1.63	0.22*
AA	15	7.5	14	7	0.85	1.08	0.04*
G-allele (TNF-α 1-allele)	270	67.5	296	74	0.04‡	0.73	0.15
A-allele (TNF-α 2-allele)	130	32.5	104	26	0.04‡	1.37	0.15*

N, number of subjects; RR, relative risk; EF, etiological fraction; PF, preventive fraction;
‡, statistically significant

Table 2. Genotype and allele frequencies of (G-308A) TNF-α variants in primary glaucoma patients and matched controls

No significant difference was noticed in distribution of AA genotype among the patients and controls (*P*=0.85). Frequency of allele A was found to be significantly increased in glaucoma patient while that of allele G was higher in control group (*P*=0.04).The higher frequencies of genotype GA and allele A in primary glaucoma patients as compared to controls indicated that the genotype GA and allele A are susceptible to the primary glaucoma (RR=1.63, EF=0.22 and RR=1.37, EF=0.15 respectively). The genotype GG and allele G being higher in controls indicating their protective nature for primary glaucoma (RR=0.60, PF=0.23 and RR=0.73, PF=0.15 respectively).

The results of TNF-α -308 polymorphism for total primary glaucoma cases were then stratified into POAG and PACG groups. The distribution of alleles and genotypes of TNF-α (-308) polymorphism in POAG are shown in Table 3.

Genotype/ Allele	**Open Angle Glaucoma (N=135)**		**Control (N =200)**		***P*-value**	**RR**	**EF*/PF**
	N	%	N	%			
GG	59	43.7	110	55	0.04‡	0.64	0.16
GA	68	50.4	76	38	0.03‡	1.66	019*
AA	8	5.9	14	7	0.82	0.84	0.06
G-allele (TNFα 1- allele)	186	68.9	296	74	0.16	0.83	0.07
A-allele (TNFα 2 -allele)	84	31.1	104	26	0.16	1.21	0.07*

N, number of subjects; RR, relative risk; EF, etiological fraction; PF, preventive fraction; ‡, statistically significant

Table 3. Genotype and allele frequencies of (G-308A) TNF-α variants in open angle glaucoma patients and controls

The frequency of genotype GA was significantly higher in POAG patients (*P*=0.03) while the frequency of GG was lower in POAG as compared to controls (*P*=0.04). The frequency of allele A was higher whereas the frequency of allele G was lower in PAOG patients as compared to control. However, the differences were not statistically significant for both alleles (*P*=0.16). The higher frequency of GA genotype in POAG indicated that the genotype GA of TNF-α -308 polymorphism might be susceptible to POAG (RR=1.66, EF=0.19) while the increased frequency of genotype GG in controls as compared to POAG patients indicated that genotype GG is resistant to POAG (RR=0.64,PF=0.16).

The frequencies of alleles and genotypes of TNF-α (-308) polymorphism in PACG is given in Table 4. The frequency of genotype GG was significantly lower in PACG as compared to controls (*P*=0.04). Although the frequency of genotype GA and AA was higher in PACG, the difference was not statistically significant (*P*=0.11 and *P*=0.42 respectively). The frequency of allele A was significantly increased in PACG as compared to controls (0.04) indicating that the allele A might be susceptible to the PACG (*RR*=1.56, EP= 0.11) while allele G might be protective (RR=0.64, PF=0.11) in Saudi patients with PACG. Similarly the lower frequency of genotype GG in PACG as compared to controls indicated that GG is protective for PACG (RR=0.55, PF=0.14).

Comparison of the distribution frequency of genotypes and alleles of TNF-α (-308) polymorphism between the POAG and PACG type of glaucoma is summarized in Table 5. The results of the genotype and allele distribution in the two types of glaucoma (POAG and PACG) show similar pattern without insignificant differences.

Genotype/ Allele	Angle closure glaucoma (N=65)		Control (N=200)		P-value	RR	EF*/PF
	N	%	N	%			
GG	26	40	110	55	0.04‡	0.55	0.14
GA	32	49.2	76	38	0.11	1.58	0.11*
AA	7	10.8	14	7	0.42	1.60	0.12*
G-allele (TNFα 1-allele)	84	64.6	296	74	0.04‡	0.64	0.11
A-allele (TNFα 2-allele)	46	35.4	104	26	0.04‡	1.56	0.11*

N, number of subjects; RR, relative risk; EF, etiological fraction; PF, preventive fraction;
‡, statistically significant

Table 4. Genotype and allele frequencies of (G-308A) TNF-α variants in angle closure glaucoma patients and controls

Genotype/Allele	Open angle glaucoma (135) N (%)	Angle closure glaucoma (65) N (%)	*P*-value
GG	59 (43.7)	26 (40)	0.76
GA	68 (50.4)	32 (49.2)	0.88
AA	8 (5.9)	4 (10.8)	0.25
G-allele (TNFα 1-allele	186 (68.9)	84 (64.6)	0.42
A-allele (TNFα 2-allele)	84 (31.1)	46 (35.4)	0.42

Table 5. Comparison of genotype/ allele frequencies of TNF-α (G308A) polymorphism between POAG and PACG

Our studies on TNF-β gene polymorphism at position +252 of intron1 showed that the frequency of GG was significantly higher in primary glaucoma (including total POAG and PACG cases) as compared to controls (*P*=0.001) while the frequency of GA genotype was significantly lower in glaucoma patients (*P*=0.001). Allele-G was predominantly distributed in glaucoma patients (*P*=0.001) whereas frequency of allele A was significantly higher in control group (*P*= 0.011). Though there was difference in the distribution of AA genotype among the primary glaucoma and control, the difference was not statistically significant (*P*=0.25) (Table 6).

Genotype/Allele	Glaucoma (N=200)		Control (N=200)		*P*-value	RR	EF*/PF
	N	%	N	%			
GG	69	34.50	28	14	0.001‡	3.235	0.491*
GA	99	49.50	148	74	0.001‡	0.344	0.432
AA	32	16.00	24	12	0.253	1.396	0.161*
G-allele (TNFβ 1-allele)	237	59.25	204	51	0.011‡	1.396	0.152*
A-allele (TNFβ 2-allele)	163	40.75	196	49	0.011‡	0.715	0.152

N, number of subjects; RR, relative risk; EF, etiological fraction; PF, preventive fraction;
‡, statistically significant

Table 6. Genotype and allele frequencies of TNF-β (LTα)- interon1 +252 variants in primary glaucoma patients and matched controls

The increased frequencies of genotype GG and allele G of TNF-β (LTα) - interon1 +252 polymorphism in patients group indicated that genotype GG/allele G is susceptible to the primary glaucoma (RR=3.235, EF=0.491and RR=1.396, EF=0.152 respectively) whereas the decreased frequencies of the genotype GA and allele A in glaucoma patients showed their resistant/ refractory nature (RR=0.344, PF=0.432 and RR=0.715, PF=0.52 respectively).

On stratification of results for two types of glaucoma (POAG and PACG), the distribution of genotypes and allele of TNF-β (LTα) - interon1 +252 polymorphism retained almost the same pattern in POAG and PACG as was in the results for the total primary glaucoma group (Tables 7, 8). The frequency of genotype GG and allele G were higher in POAG as compared to controls (*P*=0.001 and *P*=0.05 respectively) while the frequencies of genotype GA and allele A were higher in controls (*P*=0.001 and *P*=0.05 respectively).

The increased frequencies of genotype GG (RR=3.28, EF=0.435) and allele G (RR=1.376, EF=0.119) in POAG as compared to controls (Table 7) indicated that genotype GG and allele G are susceptible to the POAG in Saudis. The reduced frequencies of genotype GA (RR=0.326, PF= 0.386) and allele A (RR= 0.726, PF=0.119) in the POAG patients as compared to controls showed that genotype GA and allele A of TNF-β intron1+252 polymorphism are resistant for POAG.

Genotype/ Allele	**Open angle glaucoma (N=135)**		**Control (N=200)**		***P*-value**	**RR**	**EF*/PF**
	NO.	%	NO.	%			
GG	47	34.81	28	14	0.001‡	3.280	0.435*
GA	65	48.15	148	74	0.001‡	0.326	0.386
AA	23	17.04	24	12	0.20	1.506	0.164*
G-allele (TNFβ 1-allele)	159	58.89	204	51	0.05‡	1.376	0.119*
A-allele (TNFβ 2-allele)	111	41.11	196	49	0.05‡	0.726	0.119

N, number of subjects; RR, Relative risk; EF, etiological fraction; PF, preventive fraction;
‡, statistically significant

Table 7. Genotype and allele frequencies of TNF-β (LTα) - interon1+252 variants in Open angle glaucoma patients and matched controls

The distribution of genotypes and alleles of TNF-β intron1+252 polymorphism is shown in Table 8. The frequency of genotype GG was higher in PACG as compared to controls (*P*=0.001) while the frequencies of genotype GA was higher in controls (*P*=0.001). The higher frequencies of genotype GG in PACG as compared to controls indicated that genotype GG is susceptible to the disease (RR=3.142, EF=0.299) while genotype GA might be refractory for PACG as the frequency of GA was higher in controls RR=0.385, PF=0.229). The frequency of allele G was also higher in PACG and that of allele A was lower in PACG as compared to controls however, the difference in the frequency distribution of allele A and G was not significant in PACG (P=0.08).

Comparison of the distribution frequency of genotypes and alleles of TNF- β (LT-α) interon 1+252 polymorphism between the POAG and PACG is summarized in Table 9. The results clearly indicated that the genotype and allele distribution in the two types of glaucoma (POAG and PACG) have similar pattern with minor insignificant differences.

Genotype/Allele	Angle closure glaucoma (N=65)		Control (N=200)		*P*-value	RR	EF*/PF
	NO.	%	NO.	%			
GG	22	33.85	28	14	0.001‡	3.142	0.299*
GA	34	52.30	148	74	0.001‡	0.385	0.229
AA	9	13.85	24	12	0.67	1.078	0.041*
G-allele (TNFβ 1-allele)	78	60.00	204	51	0.08	1.441	0.084*
A-allele (TNFβ 2-allele)	52	40.00	196	49	0.08	0.693	0.084

N, number of subjects; RR, Relative risk; EF, etiological fraction; PF, preventive fraction;
‡, statistically significant

Table 8. Genotype and allele frequencies of TNF- β (LT-α) interon1+252 variants in angle closure glaucoma patients and matched controls

Genotype/Allele	Open angle glaucoma (135) N (%)	Angle closure glaucoma (65) N (%)	*P*-value
GG	47 (34.81)	22 (33.85)	1.00
GA	65 (48.15)	34 (52.30)	0.65
AA	23 (17.04)	9 (13.85)	0.68
G-allele (TNFβ 1-allele)	159 (58.89)	78 (60.00)	0.45
A-allele (TNFβ 2-allele)	111 (41.11)	52 (40.00)	0.45

Table 9. Comparison of genotype/ allele frequencies of TNF- β (G252 A) polymorphism in POAG and PACG

The comparison between the associations of TNF-α 308 polymorphism in glaucoma patients in various ethnic populations is given in Table 10. The distribution trend shows ethnic variations. TNF -α (-308) polymorphism is strongly associated with POAG in Saudis, Chinese and Iranian but not in Caucasians and Japanese.

4. Discussion

As early as 1873, Dooremal for the first time observed that the eye is one of the immune privileged region of the body which was later described by Streilein (1999). Multiple factors have been suggested to contribute to the immune privilege of the eye (Niederkorn, 2006) such as the blood- aqueous- barrier and the fact that eyes do not have a lymph drainage system. Aqueous humor is for example, capable of suppressing cytokine production by activated T-lymphcytes (Mochizuki et al., 2000).

The anterior chamber of the eye has an active immunomodulation (Streilein, 2003). It has also been suggested that autoimmune damage to the optic nerve may occur directly by autoantibodies or indirectly by a "mimicked" autoimmune response to a sensitizing antigen, which in turn injures retinal ganglion cells (Wax, 2000). In a study by Joachim et al. (2007) IgG antibody levels were found to be significantly higher in the aqueous humor of patients with POAG and PEXG as compared to controls, suggesting the role of multiple immune factors in glaucoma.

Study	Ethnicity	No. of Patients	Glaucoma	TNF -α (308) polymorphism
Present study	Saudis	200	Primary glaucoma (POAG +PACG)	Associated with TNF -α-308 GA
Lin et al., 2003	Chinese	60	POAG	Associated with TNF -α-308 AA
Fan et al., 2010	Chinese	405	POAG	Associated with TNF -α-308G
Razeghinejad et al., 2009	Iranian	223	POAG	Associated with TNF -α-308A
Funayama et al., 2004	Japanese	194	POAG	No association
Mossbock et al., 2006	Caucasia n	114	POAG	No association

Table 10. Association of TNF-α 308 polymorphism in glaucoma patients in various ethnic populations

Growing evidence obtained from clinical and experimental studies over the past decade strongly suggests the role of immune system in the pathogenesis of various types of glaucoma. It has been observed that immune mediators are not usually the primary causative agents but play a critical role in the progression of the disease (Funayama et al., 2004; Joachim et al., 2007). In addition, it has been reported that components of the immune system involved in the pathogenesis of glaucoma are also involved in neurodegeneration following brain injury. In such cases inflammation occurs in response to glutamate, reactive oxygen species (ROS), nitric oxide (NO), and cytokines including tumor necrosis factor-α (TNF-α), which are released from activated microglia or macrophages (Schwartz, 2007). As glaucoma is a disease of old age and involves optic nerve neuropathy, it has been proposed that both genetic as well as epigenetic factors are involved in the progression of the disease. Such factors cause a decrease in the cellular viability and self renewal capacity, which results in the generation of dysfunctional microglia. Such age-related attrition may contribute to the development of neurodegenerative diseases by diminishing glial neurosupportive functions. Secondary degeneration by the immune components leads to the neurodegenerative injury in glaucoma (Levkovitch-Verbin et al., 2003).

TNF-α is considered to be a neuroprotective component of the immune system, because it activates the ubiquitous transcription factor NF-κB through binding to the high affinity TNF receptors (TNF-R2), which in turn mediates the expression of a wide range of genes essential for neuronal survival. Contrary to its neuroprotective role, TNF-α can also serve as a neurodegenerative factor when it binds to the low affinity death receptors TNF-R1 and activates the mitochondria mediated apoptotic pathway (Lilienbaum & Israel, 2003; Marchetti et al., 2004, Tezel & Yang, 2005). Thus a delicate balance between the two pathways determines the survival of the cell, and any shift in equilibrium might have deleterious effects. An increased expression of TNF-α can shift the balance toward TNF-R1 signaling, as seen in glaucoma, and thus promote retinal ganglion cell death.

In the present study we found a strong association of GA genotype of TNF-α (-308) polymorphism with primary glaucoma, suggesting its role in the pathogenesis of the glaucoma. The results of our study showing the association between TNF-α-308 polymorphism and glaucoma are in agreement with some of the published data on Asian populations. A recent study from Iran showed that inheritance of high producer TNF -α-308 A allele is susceptibility factor for development of POAG (Razeghinejad et al., 2009). A highly significant association of POAG and TNF -α-308 AA genotype has also been observed in the Chinese population (Lin et al., 2003). These investigators suggested that the close association between TNF-α 308 A/AA and POAG could be used as genetic marker for the disease mapping and identifying subjects susceptible to glaucoma. On the other hand in another study from China the frequency of allele G of TNF-α 308 was higher in patient group than controls and it was suggested that variants in TNF were risk factors for POAG in the Chinese population (Fan et al., 2010). The variations in association of TNF-α(-308) polymorphism with POAG (Table 10) could be due to racial differences, sample size, poorly characterized controls and clinical heterogeneity between different samples. Khan et al. (2009) found a close association between TNF-α 308 polymorphism and pseudoexfoliation glaucoma (PEXG, a type of secondary glaucoma) in Pakistani population. These findings clearly suggest that transcriptional regulation of TNF-α is essential to circumvent the deleterious effects of over expression by transcriptional up regulation. The results of this study clearly suggest that excessive production of TNF-α associated with the G-308A polymorphism may have an important role in the development of glaucoma and may act as a genetic susceptibility factor driven by a high TNF-α expression, which would subsequently lead to immune responses causing the onset and /or progression of the disease. This hypothesis is further supported by the findings of several earlier investigators showing upregulation of the expression of TNF-α and TNF-α receptor-1 in the retina and optic nerve head in glaucomatous eyes (Yan et al., 2000; Tezel et al., 2001; Yuan & Neufeld, 2000). Agarwal et al. (2000) reported that the G to A transition at position −308 results in a six- to sevenfold increase in transcription of TNF-α as compared to normal basal level. Similarly Abraham & Kroeger (1999) demonstrated the functionality of TNF-α-308 polymorphism in the reporter gene assays with a significant up regulation of up to five fold in the constructs of TNF1 (G-allele) and TNF2 (A-allele). A recent study by Sawada et al. (2010) demonstrated that TNF-α levels were significantly elevated in the aqueous humor of glaucoma patients as compared to controls.

Contrary to our findings on Saudi population, studies on Japanese and Austrian Caucasian populations showed no association between TNF-α polymorphism G-308A and primary glaucoma (Funayama et al., 2004; Mossbock et al., 2009). These differences may be attributed to the variation in ethnicity, sample size, poorly characterized controls and clinical heterogeneity of the patients. However, Funayama et al. (2004) noticed a definite interaction between polymorphism in Optineurin (OPTN) and TNF-α genes that would increase the risk for glaucoma in Japanese which indirectly suggest the participation of immune mechanism in glaucoma. The variation in Japanese population to some extent may be attributed to the fact that G-308 A polymorphism is very rare in this population (Allen, 1999).

The role of immune system in glaucoma is further substantiated by the fact that TNF-α mediated activation of matrix metalloproteinases (MMPs) in aqueous humor of the eye results into optic neuropathies. Several *in vitro* studies have shown that TNF-α is capable of inducing both increased synthesis and activity of MMPs (Rajavashisth et al., 1999; Siwik et al., 2000; Uchida et al., 2000). The MMPs are a family of zinc-dependent endopeptidases that have been reported to cause the degradation of the extracellular matrix (ECM) (Stamenkovic, 2003) and involved in wide range of normal and pathological conditions. Uncontrolled activation of MMPs is counterbalanced by specific tissue inhibitors of metalloproteinases (TIMPs), and a delicate balance of MMPs and TIMPs is required for physiologic ECM turnover. An impaired balance between MMPs and TIMPs may thus contribute to the development of glaucoma (Schlötzer-Schrehardt et al., 2003; Määttä et al., 2005). The higher frequency of Allele-A in our patients clearly suggest increased secretion of TNF-α which lead to increased synthesis and activity of MMPs. Increased expression of MMPs has been associated with structural remodeling of connective tissues of eye which might lead to the development of PACG (Papp et al., 2006). Further studies are warranted to confirm the role of MMPs in TNF-α mediated genesis of glaucoma and other eye diseases.

In our study the GG genotypes of TNF-β (+252) polymorphism were significantly over-represented in glaucoma patients as compared to the controls (P= 0.001) while GA genotype was significantly higher in controls as compared to glaucoma patients (P=0.001) indicating that GG, genotypes at +252 were susceptible to glaucoma (RR=3.235, EF=0.491), whereas GA was found to be refractory (RR=0.344, PF=0.432). Similarly the higher frequency of allele-G of TNF-β (+252) polymorphisms in patients (P=0.011) indicated that Allele G is associated with glaucoma. TNF-β (+252) polymorphism has earlier been reported to be associated with a number of autoimmune diseases (Albuquerque et al., 1998; Zelano et al., 1998; Pandey et al., 1999; Vasku et al., 2000; Kula et al., 2001; Lu et al., 2005; Takeuchi et al., 2005; Panoulas et al., 2008; Boraska et al., 2009; Watanabe et al., 2010; Tiancha et al., 2011) however, this is the first report on the association between TNF-β polymorphism and glaucoma. The presence of allele G at +252 position defines the mutant allele also known as TNF-β* 1 (allele-1) is reported to be associated with higher TNF-α and TNF-β production (Messer et al., 1991; Abraham et al., 1993). Therefore the higher frequencies of allele G and genotype GG of TNF-β (+252) along with increased genotype GA of TNF-α (308) polymorphism might act in tandem to increase TNF- α secretion in ocular tissue of the patients that might lead to the development of glaucoma.

Several studies have shown the relationships between increased TNF-α levels and several ocular diseases including retinopathy (Doganay et al., 2002; Zorena et al., 2007). Sugita et al. (2007) detected significantly elevated levels of TNF-α and TNF-α receptors in the ocular fluid of patients with active uveitis. In an animal model of high intraocular pressure, elevation of TNF-α precedes the loss of retinal ganglion cells and oligodendrocytes. In addition, retinal cell degeneration has been observed by administering of TNF-α even without the elevated intraocular pressure (Nakazawa et al., 2006). TNF-α contributes to this process by adversely affecting oligodendrocytes (Butt & Jenkins, 1994) which increases the susceptibility of axons to excitotoxicity in the optic nerve head and retinal ganglion cell death (Coleman, 2005). It has been observed that both mRNA and protein levels of TNF-α or TNF-α receptor-1 (TNF-R1) are raised in the retina of glaucomatous eyes as compared to normal eyes, and therefore it was suggested that cell death mediated by TNF-α is a contributing factor in the neurodegeneration in glaucoma (Tezel et al., 2001). Using animal models, Nakazawa et al. (2006) showed that ocular hypertension or increased intraocular pressure induces TNF-α upregulation in the retina, which in turn leads to RGC degeneration. It has also been observed that anti-TNF- α antibodies can prevent death of RGCs suggesting that reducing the expression of TNF- α would be beneficial in treating glaucoma.

5. Conclusion

This study clearly showed that the TNF-α (-308) and TNF-β (+252) polymorphisms are significantly associated with the susceptibility to primary glaucoma (POAG and PACG) in

Saudis and could be used as a genetic marker for disease mapping. To the best of our knowledge this is the first study showing an association of TNF-β (+252) polymorphism with POAG and PACG. Immune hypotheses of glaucoma go very well with the findings of this study performed on the polymorphisms of TNF-α and of TNF-β genes. These cytokines might play a crucial role in the signaling glaucomatous neurodegeneration. The TNF-α (G-308A) and TNF-β (A+252G) polymorphisms alter and modulate the production of cytokines such as TNF–α which is consistently proposed to be involved in the RGC degeneration. Moreover, TNF has been found to be associated with the regulation of glial cells and stimulation of the synthesis and secretion of nerve growth factors (NGF).Therefore understanding the role of gene polymorphism like TNF-α (-308) and TNF-β (+252) in various ethnic populations could be helpful in predicting the predisposition to glaucoma and might help in developing novel therapeutic strategies for the management of this disease.

6. References

Abraham, L.J. & Kroeger, K.M. (1999). Impact of the –308 TNF promoter polymorphism on the transcriptional regulation of the TNF gene: relevance to disease. *Journal of Leukocyte Biology*, 66, 562-566, *ISSN* 0741-5400

Abraham, L.J., French, M.A.H. & Dawkins, R.L. (1993). Polymorphic MHC ancestral haplotypes affect the activity of tumour necrosis factor-alpha. *Clinical & Experimental Immunology*, 92, 14-18, *ISSN* 0009-9104

Agarwal, P., Oldenburg, M.C., Czarneski, J.E., Morse, R.M., Hameed, M.R., Cohen, S. & Fernandes, H. (2000). Comparison study for identifying promoter allelic polymorphism in interleukin 10 and tumor necrosis factor alpha genes. *Diagnostic Molecular Pathology*, 9, 158-164, *ISSN* 1052-9551

Albuquerque, R.V., Hayden, C.M., Palmer, L.J., Laing, I.A., Rye, P.J., Gibson, N.A., Burton, P.R., Goldblatt, J., Lesouef, P.N. (1998).Association of polymorphism within the tumour necrosis factor (TNF) genes and childhood asthma. *Clinical and Experimental Allergy*, 28, 578-584, ISSN 0954-7894

Allen, R.D. (1999). Polymorphism of the human TNF- α promoter random variation or functional diversity? *Molecular Immunology*, 36, 1017-1027, *ISSN* 0161-5890

Appropriateness of Treating Glaucoma Suspects RAND Study Group. (2009). For which glaucoma suspects is it appropriate to initiate treatment? *Journal of Ophthalmology*, 116, 710-716, *ISSN* 2090-0058

Arkell, S.M., Lightman, D.A., Sommer, A., Taylor, H.R., Korshin, O.M. & Tielsch J.M. (1987). The revalence of glaucoma among Eskimos of northwest Alaska. *Archives of Ophthalmology*, 105, 482-485, *ISSN* 0003-9950

Aung, T., Lim, M.C., Wong, T.T., Thalamuthu, A., Yong, V.H., Venkataraman,D., Venkataraman, A., Chew, P.T., Vithana, E.N. (2008a). Molecular analysis of CHX10 and MFRP in Chinese subjects with primary angle closure glaucoma and short axial length eyes. *Molecular Vision*, 14, 1313-1318, *ISSN* 1090-0535

Aung, T., Victor, H.K., Lim, M.C., Venkataraman, D., Toh, J.Y., Chew, P.T. &Vithana, E.N. (2008b). Lack of association between the rs2664538Polymorphism in the MMP-9

Gene and Primary angle Closure Glaucoma in Singaporean Subjects. *Journal of Glaucoma,* 17, 257-258, *ISSN* 1057-0829

Ayub, H., Khan, M.I., Micheal, S., Akhtar, F., Ajmal, M., Shafique, S., Ali, S.H.B., Den Hollander, A.I., Ahmed ,A., Qamar, R. (2010). Association of eNOS and HSP70 gene polymorphism with glaucoma in Pakistani cohorts. *Molecular Vision* , 16, 18-25, *ISSN* 1090-0535

Boraska, V., Zeggini, E., Groves, C.J., Rayner, N.W., Skrabic, V., Diakite, M., Rockett, K.A., Kwiatkowski, D., McCarthy, M.I. & Zemunik, T. (2009). Family based analysis of tumor necrosis factor and lymphotoxin-alpha Tag polymorphism with type 1 diabetes in the population of South Croatia. *Human Immunology,* 70, 159-9, *ISSN* 0198-8859

Braun, N., Michel, U., Ernst, B.P., Metzner, R., Bitsch, A., Weber, F. & Riechmann, P. (1996). Gene polymorphism at position -308 of the tumor-necrosis-factor-alpha (TNF-alpha) in multiple sclerosis and its influence on the regulation of TNF-alpha production. *Neuroscience Letters,* 215, 75-78, *ISSN 0304-3940*

Butt, A.M. & Jenkins, H.G. (1994). Morphological changes in oligodendrocytes in the intact mouse optic nerve following intravitreal injection of tumor necrosis factor. *Journal of Neuroimmunology,* 51,27–33, *ISSN* 0165-5728

Cao, D., Lu, X., Guo X., Cong, Y., Huang, J. & Mao, Z. (2009). Investigation of the association between CALCRL polymorphisms and primary angle closure glaucoma. *Molecular Vision,* 15, 2202-2208, *ISSN* 1090-0535

Casson, R.J., Newland, H.S., Muecke, J., McGrovern, S., Abraham, L., Shein, W.K., Selva, D. & Aung T. (2007). Prevalence of glaucoma in rural Myanmar: the Meiktila Eye study. *British Journal of Ophthalmology,* 91, 710-714, *ISSN* 1468-2079

Cedrone, C., Mancino, R., Cerulli, A., Cesareo, M. & Nucci, C. (2008). Epidemiology of primary glaucoma : prevalence, incidence, and blinding effects. *Progress in Brain Research,* 173, 3-14, *ISSN* 0079-6123

Chakrabarti, S., Devi, K.R., Komatireddy, S., Kaur, K., Parikh, R.S., Mandal, A.K., Chandrasekhar, G. & Thomas, R. (2007). Glaucoma-Associated CYP1B1 mutations share similar haplotypes backgrounds in POAG and PACG phenotypes. *Investigative Ophthalmology &Visual Science,* 48, 5439-5444, *ISSN* 0146-0404

Coleman, M. (2005). Axon degeneration mechanisms: commonality amid diversity. *Nature Reviews Neuroscience,* 6, 889–898, *ISSN* 1471-003X.

Cong, Y., Guo, X., Liu, X., Cao, D., Jia, X., Xiao, X., Li, S., Fang, S. & Zhang, Q.(2009). Association of the single nucleotide polymorphisms in the extracellular matrix metalloprotease- 9 gene with PACG in southern China. *MolecularVision,* 15,1412-1417, *ISSN* 1090-0535

Cuenca, J., Perez, C., Aguirre, A., Schiattino, I. & Aguillon, J.C. (2001). Genetic polymorphism at position –308 in the promoter region of the tumor necrosis factor (TNF): implications of its allelic distribution on susceptibility or resistance to diseases in the Chilean population. *Biological Research,* 34, 237-241, *ISSN* 0716-97.

Dai, X., Nie, S., Ke, T., Liu, J., Wang, Q. & Liu, M.(2008).Two variants in MYOC and CYP1B1 genes in a Chinese family with primary angle closure glaucoma. *Zhonghua Yi Xue Yi Chaun Xue Za Zhi,* 25, 493-496, *ISSN* 1003-9406

Dandona, L., Dandona, R., Srinivas, M., Mandal, P., John, R.K., McCarty, C.A., et al. (2000). Open angle glaucoma in an urban population in southern India, the Andhra Pradesh eye disease study. *Ophthalmology*, 107, 1702-1709, *ISSN* 2090-004X

Doganay, S., Evereklioglu, C. Er, H., Türköz, Y, Sevinç , A., Mehmet, N. & Savli, H. (2002). Comparison of serum NO, TNF-α, IL-1 , sIL-2R, IL-6 and IL-8 levels with grades of retinopathy in patients with diabetes mellitus. *Eye*, 16,163–170, *ISSN* 0950-222X

Eid, T.M., El –Harwary, I. & El- Menawy, W. (2009). Prevalence of glaucoma types and legal blindness from glaucoma in the Western region of Saudi Arabia: a hospital based study. *International Ophthalmology*, 29, 477-483, ISSN 0165-5701.

Ertel, W., Keel, M., Bonaccio, M., Steckholzer, U., Gallati, H., Kenney, J.S. & Trentz,O(1995). Release of anti-inflammatory mediators after mechanical trauma correlates with severity of injury and clinical outcome. *Journal of Trauma*, 39, 879–887, *ISSN* 0022-5282

Fan, B.J., Liu, K., Wang, D.Y., Tham, C.C., Tam, P.O., Lam, D.S. & Pang, C.P. (2010). Association of polymorphisms of tumor necrosis factor and tumor protein p53 with primary open-angle glaucoma. *Investigative Ophthalmology & Visual Science*, 51, 4110-4116, *ISSN* 0146-0404

Foster, P.J. & Johnson, G.J. (2001). Glaucoma in China: how big is the problem? *British Journal of Ophthalmology*, 85, 1277-1282, *ISSN* 0007-1161

Foster, P.J., Oen, F.T., Machin, D., Ng, T.P., Devereux, J.G., Johnson, G.J., Khaw, P.T. & Seah, S.K. (2000). The prevalence of glaucoma in Chinese residents of Singapore: a cross-sectional population survey of the Tanjong Pagar district. *Archives of Ophthalmology*, 118, 1105-1111, *ISSN* 0003-9950

Foster, P.J., Buhrmann, R., Quigley, H.A. & Johnson, G.J. (2002). The definition and classification of glaucoma in prevalence surveys. *British Journal of Ophthalmology*, 86, 238-242, *ISSN* 0007-1161

Friedman, D.S., Jampel, H.D., Munoz, B. & West, S.K. (2006).The prevalence of open angle glaucoma among blacks and whites 73 years and older: the Salisbury eye evaluation glaucoma study. *Archives of Ophthalmology*, 124, 1625-1630, *ISSN* 0003-9950

Funayama, T., Ishikawa, K., Ohtake, Y., Tanino, T., Kurosaka, D., Kimura, I., et al. (2004).Variants in optineurin gene and their association with tumor necrosis factor-alpha polymorphisms in Japanese patients with glaucoma. *Investigative Ophthalmology & Visual Science*, 45, 4359-4367, *ISSN* 0146-0404

Galbratith, G.M. & Pendey, J.P. (1995). Tumor necrosis factor alpha (TNF-alpha) gene polymorphism in alopecia areata. *Human Genetics*, 96, 433-436, *ISSN* 0340-6717

Green, C.M., Kearns, L.S., Wu, J., Barbour, J.M., Wilkinson, R.M., Ring, M.A., et al. (2007). How significant is a family history of glaucoma? Experience from the glaucoma inheritance study in Tasmania. *Clinical & Experimental Ophthalmology*, 35, 793 -799, *ISSN* 2155-9570

Halpern, D.L. & Grosskreutz, C.L. (2002). Glaucomatous optic neuropathy: mechanisms of disease. *Ophthalmology Clinics of North America*, 15, 61-68, *ISSN* 0896-1549

He, M., Foster, P.J., Huang, W., Zheng, Y., Freidman, D.S, Lee, P.S. & Khaw, P.T. (2006). Prevalence and Clinical characteristics of Glaucoma in Adult Chinese: A population based study in Liwan District, Guangzhou. *Investigative Ophthalmology & Visual Science,* 47, 2782-2788, ISSN 0146-0404

Hu, Z., Zhao, Z.L. & Dong, F.T. (1989). An epidemiological investigation of glaucoma in Beijing and Shun Yi county. *Chinese Journal of Ophthalmology,* 25, 115-118, *ISSN* 0412-4081

Huang, P., Zhang, S.S. & Zhang, C. (2009). The two sides of cytokine signaling and glaucomatous optic neuropathy. *Journal of Ocular Biology, Diseases, and Informatics,* 2, 78-83, ISSN 1936-8437

Jacob, A., Thomas, R., Koshi, S.P., Braganza, A. & Muliyil, J. (1998). Prevalence of primary glaucoma in an urban south Indian population. *Indian Journal of Ophthalmology,* 46, 81-86, *ISSN* 0301-4738

Jeong, P., Kim, E.J., Kim, E.G., Byun, S.S., Kim, C.S. & Kim, W.J. (2004). Association of bladder tumors and GA genotype of –308 nucleotide in tumor necrosis factor-alpha promoter with greater tumor necrosis factor-alpha expression. *Urology,* 64, 1052-1056, *ISSN* 1677-5538

Joachim, S.C., Wuenschig, D., Pfeiffer, N. & Grus, F.H. (2007). IgG antibody patterns in aqueous humor of patients with primary open angle glaucoma and psuedoexfoliation glaucoma. *Moleuclar Vision,* 13, 1573-1579, *ISSN* 1090-0535

Khan, M.I., Michael, S., Akhtar, F., Naveed, A., Ahmed, A. & Qamar, R. (2009). Association of ABO blood groups with glaucoma in the Pakistani population. *Canadian Journal* of *Ophthalmology,* 44, 582-586, *ISSN* 1715-3360

Kipnis, J., Mizrahi, T., Hauben, E., Shaked, I., Shevach, E., Schwartz, M. (2002). Neuroprotective autoimmunity: naturally occurring CD4+ CD25+ regulatory T cells suppress the ability to withstand injury to the central nervous system. *Proceedings of the National Academy of Sciences,* 99, 15620–15625, ISSN 0027-8424

Klein, B.E., Klein, R., Sponsel, W.E., Frank ,T., Cantor, L.B., Martone, J. & Menage, M.J. (1992). Prevalence of glaucoma. The Beaver Dam Eye study. *Journal of Ophthalmology,* 99, 1499-1504, *ISSN* 2090-004X

Kula, D., Jurecka-Tuleja, B., Gubala, E., Krawczyk, A., Szpak, S., Jarzab, M. (2001). Association of polymorphism of LT alpha and TNF genes with Graves disease. *Folia Histochem Cytobiol,* 39 Suppl 2: 77-8, *ISSN* 0258-851X

Kwon, Y.H., Fingert, J.H., Kuehn, M.H. & Alward, W.L. (2009). Primary open angle glaucoma. *New England Journal of Medicine,* 360, 1113-1124, *ISSN* 0028-4793

Laengle, U.W., Markstein, R., Pralet, D., Seewald, W. & Roman, D. (2006a). Effect of GLC756, a novel mixed dopamine D1 receptor antagonist and dopamine D2 receptor agonist, on TNF-alpha release in vitro from activated rat mast cells. *Experimental Eye Research,* 83, 1335-1339, *ISSN* 0014-4835

Laengle, U.W., Trendelenburg, A.U., Markstein, R., Nogues, V., Provencher-Bollinger, A. & Roman, D. (2006b). GLC756 decreases TNF-alpha via an alpha2 and beta2 adrenoceptor related mechanism. *Experimental Eye Research,* 83, 1246-1251, *ISSN* 0014-4835

Leske, C., Connell, M., Wu, Y., Hyman, G. & Schachat, A.P. (1995). Risk factors for open-angle glaucoma. The Barbados Eye Study. *Archives of Ophthalmology,* 113, 918-924, *ISSN* 0003-9950.

Leske, M.C., Connell, A.M., Schachat, A.P.& Hyman, L. (1994). The Barbados Eye Study. Prevalence of Open Angle Glaucoma. *Archives of Ophthalmology,*112, 821-829, *ISSN* 0003-9950

Levkovitch-Verbin, H., Quigley, H. A., Martin K.R., Valenta ,D., Baumrind, L.A. & Pease, M.E. (2002). Translimbal laser photocoagulation to the trabecular meshwork as a model of glaucoma in rats. *Investigative Ophthalmology & Visual Science,* 43, 402-410, *ISSN* 0146-0404

Levkovitch-Verbin, H., Quigley, H.A., Martin, K.R., Zack, D.J., Pease, M.E. & Valenta, D.F. (2003). A model to study differences between primary and secondary degeneration of retinal ganglion cells in rats by partial optic nerve transaction. *Investigative Ophthalmology & Visual Science*, 44, 3388-3393, *ISSN* 0146-0404

Lilienbaum, A. & Israel, A. (2003). From calcium to NF-kappa B signaling pathways in neurons. *Molecular and Cellular Biology,* 23, 2680-2698. *ISSN*: 1098-5549

Limb, G.A., Soomro, H., Janikoun, S., Hollifield, R.D.& Shilling J. (1999). Evidence for control of tumour necrosis factor –alpha(TNF-alpha) activity by TNF receptors in patients with proliferative diabetic retinopathy. *Clinical and Experimental Immunology,* 115, 409-414, *ISSN* 0009-9104

Lin, H.J., Tsai, F.J., Chen, W.C., Shi, Y.R., Hsu, Y. & Tsai, S.W. (2003). Association of tumor necrosis factor alpha -308 gene polymorphism with primary open-angle glaucoma in Chinese. *Eye,* 17, 31-34, ISSN 0950-222X

Liu, B. (2006). Modulation of microglial pro-inflammatory and neurotoxic activity for the treatment of Parkinson's disease. *The American Association of Pharmaceutical Scientists Journal,* 8, 606-621, *ISSN* 1550-7416

Lowe, R.F. (1972). Primary angle-closure glaucoma. Inheritance and environment. *British Journal of Ophthalmology,* 56, 13-20, *ISSN* 0007-1161

Lu, L.Y., Cheng, H.H., Sung, P.K., Tai, M.H., Yeh, J.J., Chen, A. (2005). Tumor necrosis factor –beta +252A polymorphism is associated with systemic lupus erythematosus in Taiwan. *Journal of the Formosan Medical Association,* 104, 563-570, *ISSN* 0929-6646

Määttä, M., Tervahartiala, T., Harju, M., Airaksinen, J., Autio-Harmainen, H. & Sorsa, T. (2005). Matrix metalloproteinases and their tissue inhibitors in aqueous humor of patients with primary open-angle glaucoma, exfoliation syndrome, and exfoliation glaucoma. *Journal of Glaucoma,* 14, 64-69, *ISSN* 1057-0829

Marchetti, L., Klein, M., Schlett, K., Pfizenmaier, K. & Eisel, U.L. (2004). Tumor necrosis factor (TNF)-mediated neuroprotection against glutamate-induced excitotoxicity is enhanced by N-Methyl-D-aspartate receptor activation: Essential role of a TNF receptor 2-mediated phosphatidylinositol 3-kinase-dependent NF-kappa B pathway. *Journal of Biological Chemistry,* 279, 32869-32881, ISSN 0021-9258

Mason, R.P., Kosoko, O., Wilson, M.R., et al. (1989). National survey of the prevalence and risk factors of glaucoma in St. Lucia, West Indies. Part I. Prevalence findings. *Ophthalmology,* 96, 1363–1368, *ISSN* 2090-004X

McBrien ,N.A. & Gentle, A. (2001). Timp -2 regulation of MMP-2 activity during visually guided remodeling of the tree shrew sclera in lens-induced myopia. *Investigative Ophthalmology & Visual,* 42 Suppl: 314, *ISSN*: 0146-040

Medcraft, J., Hitman, G.A., Sachs, J.A., Whichelow, C.E., Raafat, I. & Moore, R.H. (1993). Autoimmune renal disease and tumour necrosis factor beta gene polymorphism. *Clinical Nephrology,* 40, 63-68, *ISSN* 0301-0430

Messer, G., Spengler, U., Jung, M.C., Honold, G., Biomer, K., Pape, G.R., et al. (1991). Polymorphic structure of the tumor necrosis factor (TNF) locus: an Ncol Polymorphism in the first intron of the human TNF-beta gene correlates with a variant amino acid in position 26 and a reduced level of TNF-beta production. *Journal of Experimental Medicine,* 173, 209-219, *ISSN*:1540-9538

Micheal, S., Qamar, R., Akhtar, F., Khan, W.A. & Ahmed, A. (2008). C677T polymorphism in the methylene tetrahydrofolate reductase gene is associated with primary closed angle glaucoma. *Molecular Vision,* 14, 661-5, *ISSN* 1090-0535

Micheal, S., Qamar, R., Akhtar ,F., Khan, M.I, Khan, W.A. & Ahmed, A. (2009).MTHFR gene C677T and A1298C polymorphisms and homocystein levels in primary open angle and primary closed angle glaucoma. *Molecular Vision,* 15, 2268-2278, *ISSN* 1090-0535

Mochizuki, M., Sugita, S., Ishikawa, N. & Wantanabe, T.(2000). Immunoregulation by aqueous humor. *Cornea,* 19, S24-5, *ISSN*: 0277-3740

Mossbock, G., Weger, M., Moray, M., Renner, W., Haller-Schober, E.M., Mattes, D., Schmut, O., Wegscheider, B. & El-Shabrawi, Y. (2006). TNF-promoter polymorphisms and primary open-angle glaucoma. *Eye,* 20, 1040-1043, ISSN 0950-222X

Mozaffarieh, M., Greishaber, M.C. & Flammer, J. (2008). Oxygen and blood flow: Players in the pathogenesis of glaucoma. *Molecular Vision,* 14, 224-233, *ISSN* 1090-0535

Munoz-Fernandez, M.A., Fresno, M. (1998). The role of tumor necrosis factor, interleukin 6, interferon- and inducible nitric oxide synthase in the development and pathology of the nervous system. *Progress in Neurobiology,*56, 307–340, *ISSN* 0301-0082

Nakazawa, T., Nakazawa, C., Matsubara, A., Noda, K., Hisatomi, T., She, H., Michaud, N., Hafezi-Moghadam, A., Miller, J.W. & Benowitz, L.I. (2006). Tumor necrosis factor-alpha mediates oligodendrocyte death and delayed retinal ganglion cell loss in a mouse model of glaucoma. *Journal of Neuroscience,* 26, 12633-12641, *ISSN* 0270-6474.

Niederkorn, J.Y. (2006). See no evil, hear no evil, do no evil: the lessons of immune privilege. *Nature Immunology,* 7, 354-359, ISSN 1529- 2908

Pandey, J.P. & Takeuchi, F. (1999). TNF- alpha and TNF-beta gene polymorphism in systemic sclerosis. *Human Immunology,* 60, 1128-1130, ISSN 0198-8859

Panoulas, V.F., Nikas, S.N., Smith, J.P.,Douglas, K.M., Nightingale, P.,Milionis, H.J., Treharne, G.J., Toms, T.E., Kita, M.D., Kitas, G.D. (2008). Lymphotoxin 252A>G polymorphism is common and associates with myocardial infarction in patients with Rheumatoid Arthritis. *Annals of the Rheumatic Diseases,* 67, 1550-1556, ISSN 0003-4967

Papp, A.M., Nyilas, R., Szepesi, Z., Lorinez, M.L., Lorinez, M.L., Takacs, E., Abraham , I., Szilagyi, N., et al. (2007). Visible light induces matrix metalloprotinase-9 expression in rat eye. *Journal of Neurochemistry* ,103, 2224-2233, ISSN 0022-3042

Patino-Gracia, A., Sotillo- Pineiro, E., Modesto, C. & Sierrasesumaga, L. (2000). Analysis of the human tumour necrosis factor-alpha(TNF α) gene promoter polymorphisms in children with bone cancer, *Journal of Medical Genetics*, 37, 789-792, ISSN 0148-7299

Pease, M.E., Mc Kinnon, S.J., Quigley, H.A., Kerrigan-Baumrind, L.A. & Zack, D.J. (2000). Obstructed axonal transport of BDNF and its receptor TrkB in experimental glaucoma. *Investigative Ophthalmology & Visual Science*, 41, 764-774, *ISSN* 0146-0404

Pekmezci, M., Vo, B., Lim, A.K., Hirabayashi, D.R., Tanaka, G.H., Weinreb, R.N. & Lin, S.C. (2009). The characteristics of Glaucoma in Japanese Americans. *Archives of Ophthalmology* , 127, 167-171, *ISSN* 0003-9950

Perrey, C., Turney, S., Pravica, V., Howell, W.M. & Hutchinson, I.V. (1999). ARMS-PCR methodologies to determine IL-10, TNF-α, TNF-β and TGF-β1 gene polymorphisms. *Transplant Immunology*, 7, 127-128, *ISSN* 0966-3274

Quigley, H.A. & Broman, A.T. (2006). The number of people with glaucoma worldwide in 2010 and 2020. *British Journal of Ophthalmology*, 90, 262-267, *ISSN* 1468-2079.

Rajavashisth, T.B., Liao, J.K., Galis, Z.S., Tripathi, S., Laufs, U., Tripathi, J., Cahi, N.N., Xu, X.P., Jovinge, S., Shah, P.K. & Libby, P. (1999). Inflammatory cytokines and oxidized low density liproteins increase endothelial cell expression of membrane type 1-matrix metalloproteinase. *Journal of Biological Chemistry*, 274, 11924-11929, *ISSN 0021-9258*

Razeghinejad, M.R., Rahat, F. & Kamali-Sarvestani, E. (2009). Association of TNFA –308 G/A and TNFRI +36 A/G gene polymorphisms with glaucoma. *Ophthalmic Research*, 42, 118-124, *ISSN* 0030-3747

Rotchford, A.P., Kirwan, J.F., Muller, M.A., Johnson, G.J. & Roux P. (2003). Temba glaucoma study: a population – based cross- sectional survey in urban South Africa. *Journal of Ophthalmology*, 110, 376-382, *ISSN* 2090-004X

Rotchford, A.P. & Johnson, G.J. (2002). Glaucoma in Zulus: a population -based cross sectional survey in a rural district in South Africa. *Archives of Ophthalmology*, 120, 471-478, *ISSN* 0003-9950

Sakata, K., Sakata, L.M., Sakata, V.M., Santini, C., Hopker, L.M., Bernardes,R., Yabumoto, C. & Moreira, A.T. (2007). Prevalence of Glaucoma in a South Brazilian Population: Projeto Glaucoma. *Investigative Ophthalmology & Visual Science*, 48, 4974-4979, *ISSN* 0146-0404

Savejgaard, A., Platz, P. & Ryder, L.P. (1983). HLA and disease-1982: a survey. *Immunological Reviews*, 70:193-218, *ISSN* 0105-2896

Sawada, H., Fukuchi, T., Tanaka, T. & Abe, H. (2010). Tumor necrosis factor-alpha concentrations in the aqueous humor of patients with glaucoma. *Investigative Ophthalmology & Visual Science*, 51, 903-906, *ISSN* 0146-0404

Schallreuter, K.U., Levenig, C., Kuhnl, P., Loliger, C., Hohl-Tehari, M. & Berger, J. (1993). Histocompatability antigens in vitiligo: Hamburg study on 102 patients from Northern Germany. *Dermatology*, 187, 186-192, *ISSN* 1167-1122

Scheie, H.G. (1957). Width and pigmentation of the angle of the anterior chamber, a system of grading by gonioscopy. *Archives of Ophthalmology American Medical Association*, 58, 510-512, *ISSN* 0096-6339

Schlötzer-Schrehardt, U., Lommatzsch, J., Kuchle, M., Konstas, A.G. & Naumann, G.O. (2003). Matrix metalloproteinases and their inhibitors in aqueous humor of patients with pseudoexfoliation syndrome/glaucoma and primary open-angle glaucoma. *Investigative Ophthalmology & Visual Science,* 44, 1117-1125, *ISSN* 0146-0404

Schwart, M. & Kipnis, J. (2002). Autoimmunity on alert: naturally occurring regulatory CD4(+) CD25(+) T cells as part of the evolutionary compromise between a "need " and a "risk ". *Trends in Immunology* , 23, 530–534, *ISSN* 1471-4906

Schwartz, M. & Kipnis, J. (2001). Protective autoimmunity: regulation and prospects for vaccination after brain and spinal cord injuries. *Trends in Molecular Medicine,* 7, 252–258, *ISSN* 1471-4914

Schwartz, M. (2007). Modulating the immune system: a vaccine for glaucoma. *Canadian Journal* of *Ophthalmology*, 42, 439-441, *ISSN* 1715-3360.

Sharma, S., Ghosh, B. & Sharma, S.K. (2008). Association of TNF polymorphisms with sarcoidosis, its prognosis and tumour necrosis factor(TNF)-alpha levels in Asian Indians. *Clinical & Experimental Immunology,* 151,251-259, *ISSN* 0009-9104

Sharma, S., Sharma, A., Kumar, S., Sharma, S.K. & Ghosh, B. (2006). Association of TNF haplotypes with asthma, serum IgE levels, and correlation with serum TNF-alpha levels. *American Journal of Respiratory Cell and Molecular Biology,* 35, 488-495, *ISSN* 1040-0605

Shields, M.B. (2005). *Shields' Textbook of Glaucoma.* 4th ed. Lippincott Williams and Wilkins publishers, ISBN 13: 978-1-60831-630-4 New York, USA

Shohami, E., Bass, R., Wallach, D., Yamin, A. & Gallily, R. (1996). Inhibition of tumor necrosis factor alpha (TNF-α) activity in rat brain is associated with cerebroprotection after closed head injury. *Journal of Cerebral Blood Flow & Metabolism,* 16, 378–384, *ISSN* 0271-678X

Shohami, E., Ginis, I. & Hallenbeck, J.M. (1999). Dual role of tumor necrosis factor alpha in brain injury. *Cytokine & Growth Factor,* 10, 119-130, *ISSN* 1359- 6101

Siwik, D.A., Chang, D.L. & Colucci, W.S. (2000). Interleukin-1 beta and tumor necrosis factor-alpha decrease collagen synthesis and increase matrix metalloproteinase activity in cardiac fibroblasts in vitro. *Circulation Research,* 86, 1259-1265, *ISSN*: 0009-7330

Spaeth, G.I. (1993). *Direct Ophthalmoscopy,* In: Varma, R., Spaeth, G.I., Parker, K.W., eds. The optic Nerve in Glaucoma, JB Lippincott Co, ISBN 0-397-51069-1, 127-135, Philadelphia, USA

Stamenkovic, I.(2003). Extracellular matrix remodeling: the role of matrix metalloproteinases. *Journal of Pathology,* 200, 448-464, *ISSN* 0022-3417

Sterilein, J.W. (2003). Ocular immune privilege: The eye takes a dim but practical view of immunity and inflammation. *J Leukocyte Biology,* 74, 179-85, *ISSN* 0741-5400

Streilein, J.W. (1999). Immunoregulatory mechanisms of the eye. *Progress in Retinal and Eye Research,* 18, 357-370, *ISSN* 1350-9462

Sugita, S., Takase, H., Taguchi, C. & Mochizuki, M. (2007). The role of soluble TNF receptors for TNF-alpha in uveitis. *Investigative Ophthalmology & Visual Science,* 48, 3246-3252, *ISSN* 0146-0404

Takeuchi, F., Nabeta, H., Hong ,G.H., Kawasugi, K., Mori, M., Matsuta, K.,Kuwata, S., Murayama, T., Nakano, K. (2005).The genetic contribution of the TNFa11 microsatellite allele and the TNFb +252*2 allele in Japanese RA. *Clinical & Experimental Rheumatology,* 23, 494-498, *ISSN* 0392-856X

Tekeli, O., Turacli, M.E., Egin, Y., Akar, N. & Elhan, A.H. (2008). Tumor necrosis factor alpha-308 gene polymorphism and psuedoexfoliation glaucoma. *Molecular Vision,* 14, 1815-1818, *ISSN* 1090-0535

Tezel , G. & Wax, M.B. (2007). Glaucoma . *Chemical Immunology and Allergy,* 92, 221-227, ISSN: 1660-2242

Tezel, G.& Wax, M.B. (2004). The immune system and glaucoma. *Current Opinion in Ophthalmology* ,15, 80–84, *ISSN* 1040-8738

Tezel, G. & Wax, M.B. (2003). Glial modulation of retinal ganglion cell death in glaucoma. *Journal of Glaucoma,* 12, 63–68, *ISSN* 1057-0829

Tezel, G. & Yang, X. (2005). Comparative gene array analysis of TNF-alpha-induced MAPK and NF-kappaB signaling pathways between retinal ganglion cells and glial cells. *Experimental Eye Research,* 81, 207-217, *ISSN* 0014-4835

Tezel, G. & Wax, M.B. (2000a). The mechanisms of hsp27 antibody-mediated apoptosis in retinal neuronal cells. *Journal of Neuroscience,* 20, 3552–3562, *ISSN* 0270-6474

Tezel, G.& Wax, M.B. (2000b). Increased production of tumor necrosis factor-alpha by glial cells exposed to simulated ischemia or elevated hydrostatic pressure induces apoptosis in cocultured retinal ganglion cells. *Journal of Neuroscience,* 20, 8693–8700, *ISSN* 0270-6474

Tezel, G., Edward, D. P. & Wax M.B.(1999). Serum autoantibodies to optic nerve head glycosaminoglycans in patients with glaucoma. *Archives of Ophthalmology,* 117, 917–924, *ISSN* 0003-9950

Tezel, G., Li, L.Y., Patil, R.V. & Wax, M.B. (2001). TNF-alpha and TNF-alpha receptor-1 in the retina of normal and glaucomatous eyes. *Investigative Ophthalmology & Visual Science* , 42, 1787-1794, *ISSN* 0146-0404

Tezel, G., Seigel, G.M. & Wax, M.B. (1998). Autoantibodies to small heat shock proteins in glaucoma. *Investigative Ophthalmology & Visual Science,* 39, 2277–2287, *ISSN* 0146-0404

Tezel, G., Yang, X., Yang, J. & Wax, M.B. (2004). Role of tumor necrosis factor receptor-1 in the death of retinal ganglion cells following optic nerve crush injury in mice. *Brain Research,* 996, 202–212, *ISSN*: 0006-8993

Tiancha, H., Huiqin, W., Jiyong, J., Jingfen, J. & Wei, C. (2011). Association between lymphotoxin-? intron +252 polymorphism and sepsis: Ameta analysis. *Scandinavian Journal of Infectious Diseases,* 1-12, *ISSN* 0036-5548

Tielsh, J.M., Sommer, A., Katz, J., Royall ,R.M., Quigley, H.A. & Javitt, J. (1991). Racial variation in prevalence of primary open angle glaucoma. *Journal of the American Medical Association,*266, 369-374, ISSN 0098-7484

Tschumper, R.C. & Johnson, D.H. (1990). Trabecular meshwork cellularity: Differences between fellow eyes. *Investigative Ophthalmology & Visual Science* , 31, 1327-1331, *ISSN* 0146-0404

Uchida, M., Shima, M., Shimoaka, T., Fujieda, A., Obara, K., Suzuki, H., Nagai, Y., Ikeda, T., Yamato, H. & Kawaguchi, H. (2000). Regulation of matrix metalloproteinases (MMPs) and tissue inhibitors of metalloproteinases (TIMPs) by bone resorptive factors in osteoblastic cells. *Journal of Cellular Physiology* ,185, 207-214, *ISSN* 0021-9541

Varma, R., Ying-Lai, M., Francis, B.A., Nguyen, B.B., Deneen, J., Wilson, M.R., Azen, S.P. & Los Angeles Latino Eye study group . (2004). Prevalence of open angle glaucoma and Ocular hypertension in Latinos: the Los Angeles Latino eye study. *Journal of Ophthalmology,* 111, 1439-1448, *ISSN* 2090-004X

Vasku, V., Vasku, A., Izakovicova Holla, L., Tschoplova, S., Kankova K, Benakova, N., Semradova, V. (2000). Polymorphism in inflammation genes (angiotensinogen, TAP1 and TNF-beta) in Psoriasis. *Archives of Dermatological Research,* 292, 531-534, *ISSN* 0340-3696

Vijaya, L., George, R., Arvind, H., Baskaran, M., Ramesh, V., Raju, P., Kumaramanickavel, G. & McCarty, C. (2008a). Prevalence of primary angle- closure disease in an urban South Indian population and comparison with a rular population. The Chennai glaucoma study. *Journal of Ophthalmology,* 115, 655-660, *ISSN* 2090-004X

Vijaya, L., George, R., Baskaran, M. , Arvind, H., Raju, P., Ramesh, V., Raju, P., Kumaramanickavel, G., & McCarty, C. (2008b). Prevalence of primary open angle glaucoma in an Urban South Indian population and comparison with a rural population. The Chennai glaucoma study. *Journal of Ophthalmology,* 115, 655-660, *ISSN* 2090-004X

Wang, I.J., Chiang, T.H., Shih, Y.F., Lu, S.C., Lin, L.L., Shieh, J.W., Wang, T.H., Samples, J.R. & Hung PT.(2006). The association of single nucleotide polymorphisms in the MMP-9 genes with susceptibility to acute primary angle closure glaucoma in Taiwanese patients. *Molecular Vision,* 12, 1223-1232, *ISSN* 1090-0535

Wantanabe, E., Buchman, T.G., Hirasawa, H., Zehnbauer, B.A. (2010). Association between lymphotoxin–α (tumor necrosis factor-β) intron polymorphism and predisposition to serve sepsis is modified by gender and age. *Critical Care Medicine,* 38,181-193, *ISSN* 0090-3493

Wax, M.B. & Tezel, G. (2002). Neurobiology of glaucomatous optic neuropathy: diverse cellular events in neurodegeneration and neuroprotection. *Molecular Neurobiology,* 26, 45–55, *ISSN* 0893-7648

Wax, M.B. (2000). Is there a role for the immune system in glaucomatous optic neuropathy? *Current Opinion in Ophthalmology,* 11, 145-150, *ISSN* 1040-8738

Wax, M.B. & Tezel, G. (2009). Immunoregulation of retinal ganglion cell fate in glaucoma. *Experimental Eye Research,* 88,825–830, *ISSN* 0014-4835

Wax, M.B., Barrett, D.A. & Pestronk, A. (1994). Increased incidence of paraproteinemia and autoantibodies in patients with normal pressure glaucoma. *American Journal of Ophthalmology,* 117, 561–568, *ISSN* 0002-9394

Wax, M.B., Tezel, G.& Edward, P.D. (1998a). Clinical and ocular histopathological findings in a patient with normal-pressure glaucoma. *Archives of Ophthalmology,* 116, 993–1001, *ISSN* 0003-9950

Wax, M.B., Tezel, G., Saito, I., Gupta , R.S., Harley, J.B., Li, Z. & Romano, C. (1998b). Anti-Ro/SS-A positivity and heat shock protein antibodies in patients with normal-pressure glaucoma. *American Journal of Ophthalmology,* 125,145–157, *ISSN* 0002-9394

Wax, M.B., Yang, J. & Tezel, G. (2001). Serum autoantibodies in patients with glaucoma. *Journal of Glaucoma,* 10, S22–24, *ISSN* 1057-0829

Westendrop, R. G., Langermans, J.A., Huizinga, T.W., Elouali, A.H., Verweij, C.L., Boomsma, D.I. & Vandenbroucke, J.P. (1997). Genetic influence on cytokine production and fatal meningococcal disease. *Lancet,* 349, 170-173, *ISSN 0140-6736*

Wilson, A.G., Di Giovine, F.S., Blakemore, A.I.F. & Duff, G.W. (1992). Single base polymorphism in the human tumor necrosis factor alpha (TNF-α) gene detectable by Nco1 restriction of PCR product. *Human Molecular Genetics,* 1, 353, *ISSN* 0964-6906

Wilson, A.G., Gordon, C., di Giovine, F.S., de Vries, N., van de Putte, L.B., Emery, P. & Duff, G.W. (1994). A genetic association between systemic lupus erythematosus and tumor necrosis factor alpha. *European Journal of Immunology,* 24, 191-195, *ISSN* 0014-2980

Wilson, A.G., Symons, J.A., McDowell, T.L., McDevitt, H.O. & Duff, G.W. (1997). Effects of a polymorphism in the human tumor necrosis factor alpha promoter on transcriptional activation. *Proceedings of the National Academy of Sciences of the United States of America* ,94, 3195-3099, *ISSN-0027-8424*

Wong, T.Y., Loon, S.C., Saw, S.M. (2006).The epidemiology of age related eye diseases in Asia. *British Journal of Ophthalmology,* 90, 506-511, *ISSN* 0007-1161

Yan, X., Tezel, G., Wax, M.B. & Edward, P. (2000). Matrix metalloproteinases and tumor necrosis factor alpha in glaucomatous optic nerve head. *Archives of Ophthalmology,* 118, 666–673, *ISSN* 0003-9950

Yang, J., Patil, R.V., Yu H., Gordon, M. & Wax, M.B. (2001a). T cell subsets and sIL-2R/IL-2 levels in patients with glaucoma. *American Journal of Ophthalmology,* 131, 421–426, *ISSN* 0002-9394

Yang, J., Tezel, G., Patil, R.V., Romano, C. & Wax, M.B. (2001b). Serum autoantibody against glutathione S-transferase in patients with glaucoma. *Investigative Ophthalmology & Visual Science,* 42, 1273–1276, *ISSN* 0146-0404

Yoshioka, K., Yoshida, T., Takakura, Y., Umekawa, T., Kogure, A., Toda, H. & Yoshikawa, T. (2006). Relationship between polymorphisms 804C/A and 252A/G of lymphotoxin-alpha gene and –308G/A of tumor necrosis factor alpha gene and diabetic retinopathy in Japanese patients with type 2 diabetes mellitus. *Metabolism,* 55, 1406-1410, ISSN 0026-0494

Yuan, L. & Neufeld, A.H. (2000). Tumor necrosis factor-alpha: a potentially neurodestructive cytokine produced by glia in the human glaucomatous optic nerve head. *Glia,* 32, 41-50, *ISSN* 1098-1136

Yuan, L. & Neufeld, A.H. (2001). Activated microglia in the human glaucomatous optic nerve head. *Journal of Neuroscience Research,* 64, 523-532, *ISSN* 0360-4012

Zelano, G., Lino, M.M., Evoli, A., Settesoldi, D., Batocchi,A.P., Torrente, I. & Tonali, P.A. (1998).Tumor necrosis factor beta gene polymorphism in myasthenia Gravis. *European Journal of Immunogenetics,* 25, 403-408, *ISSN* 0960 -7420

Zorena, K., Mysliwska, J., Mysliwec, M., Balcerska, A., Hak, L., Lipowski, P., & Raczynska K. (2007). Serum TNF-alpha level predicts non-proliferative diabetic retinopathy in children. *Mediators of Inflammation,* (92196), 1-5, ISSN 0962-9351

14

Immune Modulation in Glaucoma – Can Manipulation of Microglial Activation Help?

Kin Chiu, Kwok-Fai So and Raymond Chuen-Chung Chang
The University of Hong Kong, Hong Kong SAR
China

1. Introduction

A large body of experimental results from clinical and experimental studies has strongly suggested an aberrant activity of the immune system in glaucoma. The roles of the innate immune responses in glaucoma are unclear and have been controversial about the concept of neuroprotection or neurodestruction. Protective immunity has been suggested occurring as a homeostatic response to injury, which can prevent disease progression. Neurodegeneration of retinal ganglion cells (RGCs) may be the consequence from a failure of proper controls for the initial immune response right after injury in some glaucoma patients. Long-term tissue stress in glaucomatous eyes appears to be important for the balance between neuroprotective and neurodestructive immunity. The onset, progression, and termination of retinal specific immune responses are predominantly regulated by the interaction among the RGCs and different glia (astrocytes, Müller cells and microglia) in the glaucomatous eyes. As immunocompetent cell in the central nervous system (CNS), microglia have diverse phenotypes and produce beneficial or destructive factors depending on the microenvironments they encounter. In response to injury, activated microglia have been shown to trigger neuronal death by producing high levels of cytotoxic factors such as nitric oxide, superoxide and tumor necrosis factor-α (TNF-α). However, increasing lines of evidence have shown that microglia can elicit protective effects by releasing trophic and anti-inflammatory factors. To transform microglia into neuroprotective or neurodestructive depends on the disease state or the type of stimulus to trigger them into "classically activated" proinflammatory (M1) or "alternatively activated" anti-inflammatory (M2) cells (Polazzi and Monti, 2010). *In vitro* study have shown that it is possible to manipulate the activation state of microglia so that their activation can be beneficial, i.e., protecting rather than destroying neurons (Polazzi et al., 2001; 2009). However, it is difficult to achieve this goal *in vivo*, especially in chronic neurodegenerative model. Our studies focus on modulating the retinal microglial cells by application of chemokine, monocyte-chemoattractive protein-1 (MCP-1/CCL2) into the posterior chamber to provide direct circumstance for attracting microglia to the retina. Furthermore, we also try to evaluate whether modulation of microglia in the retina can be achieved by the anti-aging Chinese medicine wolfberry. In this review, we will demonstrate how basic science research can be further developed and translated into pharmacological interventions through modulating the activation of microglia to prevent RGC loss in experimental glaucoma. This kind of approach can be one of therapeutic interventions for glaucoma patients in future.

2. Immunoregulation determines the fate of RGC in glaucoma

Glaucoma is an aging-associated neurodegenerative disease. In 2002, statistics gathered by WHO shows that glaucoma is the second leading cause of blindness worldwide, after cataract (Resnikoff et al., 2004). Glaucoma accounts for 12.3% of 37 million people affected by blindness, and 82% of which were 50 years or older. The number of glaucoma will increase to 79.6 million and the resulting blindness will increase to 11.1 million by 2020 (Quigley and Broman, 2006). Glaucoma results in irreversible loss of retinal ganglion cells (RGCs) and their axons, thus it is even a greater challenge than cataract for public health system. Therefore, investigation on potential neuroprotective agents is critical to prevent this blind leading visual impairment.

Glaucoma is defined as a group of optic neuropathies characterized by the irreversible loss of RGCs and their axons, accompanied by the excavation and degeneration of the optic nerve head (ONH) (Quigley, 1996). Elevated intraocular pressure (IOP)-related factors play an important role in initiation and progression of glaucoma. The glaucomatous neurodegeneration may be mediated via a combination of IOP-dependent compressive effects of the cribriform plates in the lamina cribosa on the axons of the RGCs, pressure-induced tissue ischemia, and various local cellular responses. The fate of RGCs may involve two or more cell stressors with additive or even synergistic effects. Increasing lines of evidence obtained from clinical and experimental studies strongly suggests diverse roles of the immune system in glaucoma as beneficial or destructive (Tezel, *2010,* doi:10.1016/j.exer.2010.07.009). It is now commonly recognized that there is an increased risks of failure in immune regulation under glaucomatous stress conditions (Schwartz and Ziv, 2008; Wax and Tezel, 2009).

2.1 Autoimmune neurodegeneration in glaucoma

Autoimmune neurodegeneration results from a failure to properly rectify an aberrant and stress-induced immune response. Neuronal antigens can initiate immune responses by recruiting cytotoxic T cells. This occurs primarily in low tension glaucoma patients as evident by abnormal T cell subsets (Yang et al., 2001a).

Humoral immune response is also involved in the onset and the progression of neurodegeneration in some glaucoma patients. There is an increased prevalence of monoclonal gammopathy (Wax et al., 1994), elevated serum titers of auto-antibodies to optic nerve head glycosaminoglycans (Tezel et al., 1999), auto-antibodies to retinal antigen such as rhodopsin (Romano et al., 1995), small heat shock protein (Tezel et al., 1998; Tezel et al., 2004), glutathione S-transferase (Yang et al., 2001b), gamma-enolase (Maruyama et al., 2000) and phosphatidylserine (Kremmer et al., 2001). Immunoglobulin has also been detected in the glaucomatous retina (Wax et al., 1998a). Heat shock protein antibodies (e.g. hsp60, hsp27, and α-crystallins) have direct pathological potential to facilitate apoptotic RGC death *in vitro* and *ex vivo* (Tezel et al., 1998; Tezel and Wax, 1999, 2000). In addition, clinical findings show that serum titers of auto-antibodies to heat shock proteins were independent of the severity of glaucomatous damage (Wax et al., 2001). Antibody-mediated neuronal damage may occur indirectly by molecular mimicry of self-antigen from pathogen (Romano et al., 1995; Wax et al., 1998b; Romano et al., 1999). This is supported by the finding of elevated auto-antibodies to bacterial heat shock proteins, including hsp60 (Wax et al., 1998b), and the increased expressions of HLA-DR/CD8 circulating T cells in low tension glaucoma patients (Yang et al., 2001a). In addition, significant alterations of serum Th1 and

Th2 cytokines are detected, suggesting abbreant immune responses of glaucomatous neuropathy (Huang et al., 2010).

2.2 Neuroprotective immune response – involvement of retinal microglia

Protective immunity has been suggested to occur as a homeostatic response to injury with the intent of preventing disease progression (Schwartz, 2007). The most important sites for immune modulation in glaucoma are retina and the optic nerve, which are thought to have an actively regulated immune privilege mechanism (Forrester, 2009). As the major immunocompetent cells in the CNS, the principal function of microglia is the quick response to the presence of pathogens and to CNS damage. In both human glaucomatous eye samples and animal models, the involvement of microglia in glaucoma has been reported (Schwartz et al., 2006). In human glaucomatous ocular specimens, microglia in the ONH and the parapapillary chorioretinal region of the ONH are activated and redistributed (Neufeld, 1999). In rat glaucoma model induced by cauterization, microglia in retinas exposed to chronic ocular hypertension appear as early as three days and last for about two months after IOP elevation (Wang et al., 2000; Naskar et al., 2002). Whether these retinal microglia play a protective or cytotoxic role in glaucoma deserve further investigation.

The balance between beneficial and deleterious immune responses is a critical issue for the treatment of neurodegenerative diseases. The use of immune-modulation drugs which are able to shift the immune response towards neuroprotection will be an effective therapeutic approach. As an FDA-approved drug for multiple sclerosis, glatiramer acetate (GA), also known as Copolymer-1 (Cop-1), was used as a treatment for autoimmune diseases and as a therapeutic vaccine for neurodegenerative diseases (Polazzi and Monti, 2010). GA is a synthetic oligopeptide of four naturally occurring amino acids, its activity derives from its ability to serve as a "universal antigen' that weakly activates a wide spectrum of self-reactive T-cells (Kipnis and Schwartz, 2002). T-cell-based vaccination with GA resulted in decreased plaque formation, reduction of excitotoxicity and induction of neurogenesis in Alzheimer's disease (AD) mouse model (Butovsky et al., 2006a; 2006b). This GA vaccination caused a phenotype switch in brain microglia to dendritic-like morphology, with the ability to produce insulin-like growth factor 1 (IGF-1) that counteracted the adverse Aβ-induced effects (Butovsky et al., 2006a; 2006b; 2007). Vaccination with GA significantly reduces loss of RGCs in rodent models of optic nerve crush injury, intraocular glutamate toxicity, glaucoma and macular degeneration (Schori et al., 2001). These results suggest that GA induced recruitment of dendritic-like microglia from bone marrow might contribute significantly to the anti-neurodegenerative effect. Vaccination has the impact on the entire body, how about using other immune-modulation drugs locally? Our laboratory has investigated the modulation of retinal microglia in a rat glaucoma model through intravitreous application of chemokine, monocyte chemoattractant protein-1 (MCP-1) (Chiu et al., 2010a). Furthermore, we also tested the involvement of retinal microglial cells in this glaucoma model which oral application of herbal medicine wolfberry polysaccharides have proved to be neuroprotective (Chan et al., 2007; Chiu et al., 2009). Our data showed that when the retinal microglia was tune to a neuroprotective state, named as police-state, there was a positive correlation with an increase in RGC survival under ocular hypertension (Chang et al., 2009).

3. Diverse activation of retinal microglia associated with divergent effects on retinal ganglion cell survival under chronic ocular hypertension (COH)

In the normal mature brain, microglia typically exist in a resting state that is highly ramified. In contrast to their non-moving cell body, processes of the "resting" microglia display high mobility, especially extension and retraction (Davalos et al., 2005). The brain microglia perform tissue surveillance and can patrol the entire neural parenchyma every few hours (Nimmerjahn et al., 2005). Use of Z-stack mode by multiphoton to scan different layers of retina from the nerve fiber layer to the outer segment on whole mounted retina allows us to observe the morphology of the resting state microglia. Similar to other reports in the brain, the resting microglia in the normal rat retina are highly ramified shape with small nuclei and long thin processes and was located in the inner retina with almost no overlapping of processes (diameter: ~50 μm, scattered throughout the retinal ganglion cell layer and the inner plexiform layer). They may also play a surveillance role in the retina (Chang et al., 2009; Chiu et al., 2009).

Upon activation, microglia emerged from a resting state and underwent morphological transformation from ramified to different activated forms, such as dendritic or amoeboid. Microglia constitute a family of cells with diverse phenotypes, some are beneficial and others are detrimental to surrounding cells (Schwartz et al., 2006). Like macrophages, microglia can exhibit different activated phenotypes: "classically activated" proinflammatory (M1) or "alternatively activated" anti-inflammatory (M2) (Benoit et al., 2008; Geissmann et al., 2008; Kigerl et al., 2009; Polazzi and Monti, 2010).

Although it has been shown that it is possible to manipulate the activation state of microglia *in vitro* so that their activation can be beneficial - protecting rather than destroying neurons (Polazzi et al., 2001; 2009). It is difficult to achieve this goal *in vivo*, especially in chronic neurodegenerative model. Our group managed to use a chronic ocular hypertension (COH) model to mimic glaucoma in rats. We tested differential activation of microglia in the retina under COH and their co-relationship with RGC survival in this chronic neurodegenerative model.

Adult female Sprague-Dawley (SD) rats (250-280 g) were grouped and used. Ocular hypertension (OH) was induced in the right eye of each animal using laser photocoagulation according to our previous publications (Chan et al., 2007; Chiu et al., 2007; Chiu et al., 2009; Chiu et al., 2010a; Chiu et al., 2010b). Schematic diagram (Fig. 1) shows the front and back view of laser photocoagulation applied (indicated as red spots) to the limbal veins (front veiw) and the three episcleral veins (two at the superior and one at the inferior quadrant, back view). After two weeks of laser photocoagulation, the limbal veins were replaced by scar tissue and could not be seen in the limbal area except the nasal 90 degrees where no laser photocoagulation was applied. The corneas of the OH eyes were healthy and transparent, with no neovascularization existed. The OH eyes were free of infection, cataract, intraocular bleeding or retinal detachment.

Photocoagulation using the argon laser increased the IOP of the right eyes (OH eyes) from the baseline around 15 mmHg to 22 mmHg for up to one month. There was significant loss of RGCs in the experimental eyes starting at 2 weeks after the first laser treatment. The density of RGCs was decreased from 2,241 to 1,964/mm^2 (#P = 0.002), this loss was only about 17% of total RGC in normal retina at one month after the first laser (Luo et al., 2009). Since ocular hypertension is not an acute injury causing massive neuronal death, microglia in the glaucomatous retina were not activated as they were in the optic nerve axotomy model. The microglia detected in the inner retina of the OH eyes were in resting state under elevated IOP (Luo et al., 2009). The morphology of iba-1 positive microglia in the cross retinal sections was similar with the ramified one in the Naskar et al. (2002) study. The resting state morphology of microglia was also supported by Lam et al. (2003) in which they could not detect the phagocytic microglia in glaucomatous retina by using ED1 immunohistochemical staining. The microglial responses in this laser photocoagulation-induced COH model are similar to the situation in human glaucomatous retina where activated microglia are detected in the ONH and the parapapillary chorioretinal region of the ONH, where this region is not considered to be retina. Therefore, this model provides a good opportunity for us to investigate different morphologies of microglia modulated by different factors.

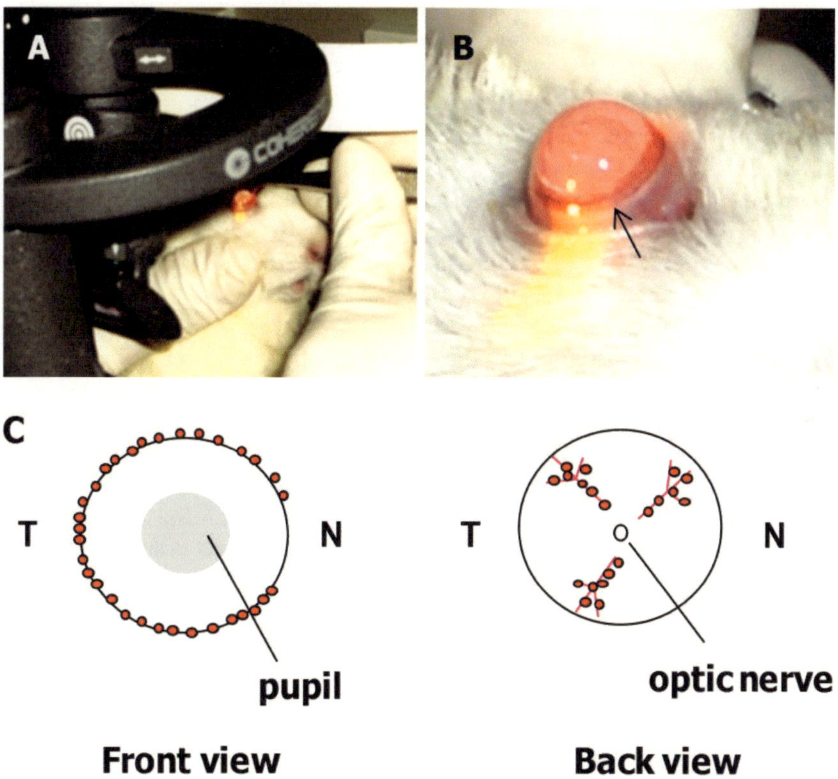

Fig. 1. **Photograph shows argon laser photocoagulation on the rat limbal and episcleral veins.** Right eye of the rat was photocoagulated by argon laser (A). Limbal veins of the eye (arrow) are indicated under slit-lamp (B). Schematic diagram (C) shows front view (observe from the corneal side) and back view (observe from the optic nerve side) of laser photocoagulation applied (indicated as red spots) to the limbal veins and three episcleral veins (two at the superior and one at the inferior quadrant). T: temporal; N: nasal.

3.1 Classical activation of retinal microglia is detrimental to RGC under COH

Conventional stimulation of microglia/macrophages by classical pathogens such as bacterial endotoxin lipopolysaccharide (LPS) or zymogen can be neurodestructive, because massive production of free-radicals triggered by these stimuli can induce both apoptosis and necrosis of neurons. Activated microglia have been considered to be endogenous malefactors in the CNS because they play important roles in neurological diseases such as Alzheimer's disease and amyotrophic lateral sclerosis (Sargsyan, et al., 2005). In response to injury, activated microglia have been shown to induce neuronal death by releasing excess cytotoxic factors such as superoxide (Lee, et al., 1993; Block, et al., 2007), nitric oxide (NO) and tumor necrosis factor-α (TNF-α) (Chang, et al., 2000a; 2000b; Colton and Gilbert, 1987). This kind of stimulation can eventually result in activation-induced cell death depleting the pool of these innate immune cells in the CNS. This is similar to the stimulation of LPS applied to the macrophages *in vitro*. LPS promotes the differentiation of "classically activated" M1 macrophages. These M1 macrophages secrete high levels of pro-inflammatory cytokines, release oxidative metabolites such as superoxide radicals (O^{2-}) and NO, and reduce production of neurotrophic factor (Benoit et al., 2008; Geissmann et al., 2008; Kigerl et al., 2009; Polazzi and Monti, 2010). Therefore, conventional stimulation of microglia/macrophages not only produces cytotoxic pro-inflammatory factors, but also depletes the pool of the innate immune cells to elicit possible neuroprotective effects.

In this COH model, a single intravitreous injection of 50 μg of LPS or MCP-1 1000 ng greatly alerted microglia to transform themselves from a resting state to a fully activated state in the glaucomatous eye up to four weeks under ocular hypertension (Chiu et al., 2010). The immunoreactivity of iba-1 in the microglia was dramatically increased. The microglia displayed enlarged nuclei and remarkably thick and short processes. With marked increase in the number of processes, their short processes displayed overlapping. Concomitantly, fully activated microglia were found in the nerve fiber layer and retinal ganglion cell layer corresponding to the area of retinal injury in animals with ocular hypertension. RGC loss was significantly increased from 17.4% in PB control OH retina to 28.3% in LPS group (# $p=0.007$). The increased RGC death should not be due to direct neurotoxic effect of LPS as it has been shown that LPS did not exert direct neurotoxicity (Bronstein et al., 1995). Dysregulated responses or over-activation of microglia is considered to be destructive and dangerous for neighboring neurons because of the harmful effects of free-radicals produced by fully activated microglia (Ladeby et al., 2005; Block et al., 2007).

3.2 Restricted activation of microglia is neuroprotective to RGC under COH

In contrast to conventional stimulation, activation of microglia/macrophages can be modulated by the cytokines secreted by infiltrated T-lymphocytes, or the local CNS environment, which is named as restricted (appropriate) stimulation. Immune suppressive cytokines that released from CD4+/CD25+ regulatory T cells or Th2 cells, such as IL-4, IL-10 or TGF-β can markedly modulate the activation state of microglia/macrophages (Kipnis et al., 2004). The macrophages are at an "alternative activated" M2 phenotype. These M2 macrophages promote angiogenesis, matrix remodeling and suppress destructive immunity (Sica et al., 2006).

MCP-1/CCL2 is a β-chemokine involved in the activation and recruitment of monocytic cells to injury sites (Zhang and Koninck, 2006). MCP-1/CCL2 can either induce neuroprotection or neurodestruction depending on the experimental model (Galasso et al., 2000; Eugenin et al., 2003; Kalehua et al., 2004). Using MCP-1/CCL2, the activation states of microglia can be manipulated, they can exert divergent effects on RGC survival under COH. Our results demonstrated different morphologies of microglia, which are correlated to the severity of neuronal loss in an experimental rat glaucoma model. Compared to fully activated state of microglia in the retina (1000 ng MCP-1), a unique semi-activated phenotype of microglia was found in the 10/100 ng MCP-1 group(s) (Chiu et al., 2010). The nuclei were slightly enlarged and processes of microglia were significantly shortened with moderate thickening, and there was no overlapping of processes. Concomitant to the changes in microglial morphology, RGC loss appeared to be correlated with the activation status of microglia. Two weeks after the first laser, OH with intravitreous injection of PB resulted in 17.4% RGC loss. Injection of 10 ng of MCP-1 decreased the RGC loss to 10.3%, and 100 ng of MCP-1 significantly reduced RGC loss to 3.4% (** $p<0.001$, MCP-1 100 ng vs. PB). Further increase of MCP-1 to 1000 ng did not decrease but significantly increased RGC loss to 21.2%. At one month after the first laser treatment, compared to the PB control, MCP-1 100 ng significantly reduced RGC loss from 19.1% to 5.1% (* $p<0.001$).

The protective effects of microglia can be accomplished by producing neurotrophic molecules such as IGF-1 (Streit, 2005; Butovsky, et al., 2006a). Previous brain ischemia studies have shown that activated microglia can produce neurotrophic molecules such as IGF-1 (O'Donnell et al., 2002; Butovsky et al., 2006a; Lalancette-Hebert et al., 2007). Our study showed that after four weeks under COH, IGF-1 immunoreactivity was markedly reduced in the retinas with PB. In the 100 ng MCP-1-treated group, the immunoreactivity of IGF-1 was up-regulated and restored to normal level.

Similar phenomenon is also observed in oral feeding of herbal medicine, wolfberry polysaccharides, in this model (Chiu et al., 2009). One to 100 mg/kg LBP exerted the best neuroprotection and elicited moderately activated microglia in the inner retina with ramified appearance but thicker and focally enlarged processes. When activation of microglia was attenuated by intravitreous injection of macrophage/microglia inhibitory factor (MIF), protective effect of 10 mg/kg LBP was attenuated. Therefore, restricted activation of microglia under ocular hypertension is neuroprotective to the survival of RGCs.

4. Conclusion

Taken together, it is the time for us to reconsider how to categorize the activation state of microglia (Chang et al., 2009). First, the resting state with lots of processes and small size of cell body in morphology; second, the semi-activated state (police state or M2 phenotype) with thick and short processes and large size of cell body; third, the fully activated state (army state or M1 phenotype) with very thick processes and very large size of cell body with sometimes amoeboid shape. The army state of microglia can produce free-radicals including nitric oxide, superoxide and different pro-inflammatory cytokines. In contrast, the police state of microglia can produce trophic factor without releasing free-radicals. While resting microglia can be considered to be a security guard for immune surveillance, semi-activated (M2 activated) microglia can be regarded as a police officer to prevent any bad situation for further neuroinflammation and to protect citizen neurons without miss-firing by-stander neurons, and fully activated (M1 activated) microglia can function as army responsible to fight in a battle. Nevertheless, the by-stander neurons will be damaged unavoidably.

Our findings using the COH model, demonstrate a distinct morphology of microglia in response to neuroprotective dose of MCP-1/CCL2, and wolfberry. Definition of this distinct morphology will help future studies to understand the biological mechanisms of neuroprotective microglia, opening up a new avenue of manipulating microglia to elicit neuroprotective effects in neurodegeneration.

5. Acknowledgment

The work done by this laboratory has been or is currently supported by The Glaucoma Foundation, USA; American Health Assistant Foundation, USA; HKU Alzheimer's Disease Research Network under Strategic Theme Research on Healthy Aging; University Strategic Research Theme on Drug Discovery; Research Fund for the Control of Infectious Diseases (09080822) from Food and Health Bureau of Hong Kong SAR Government; General Research Fund (761609M) from Research Grant Council; Azalea (1972) Endowment Fund, HKU Seed Funding for Basic Research (201011159058), and HKU Small Project Funding (200907176185).

6. References

Benoit M, Desnues B, Mege J-L. 2008. Macrophage Polarization in Bacterial Infections. The Journal of Immunology 181:3733-3739.

Block ML, Zecca L, Hong JS. 2007. Microglia-mediated neurotoxicity: uncovering the molecular mechanisms. Nature Reviews Neuroscience 8:57-69.

Bronstein DM, Perez-Otano I, Sun V, Mullis Sawin SB, Chan J, Wu GC, Hudson PM, Kong LY, Hong JS, McMillian MK. 1995. Glia-dependent neurotoxicity and neuroprotection in mesencephalic cultures. Brain Res 704:112-116.

Butovsky O, Koronyo-Hamaoui M, Kunis G, Ophir E, Landa G, Cohen H, Schwartz M. 2006a. From the Cover: Glatiramer acetate fights against Alzheimer's disease by inducing dendritic-like microglia expressing insulin-like growth factor 1. Proc Natl Acad Sci U S A 103:11784-11789.

Butovsky O, Kunis G, Koronyo-Hamaoui M, Schwartz M. 2007. Selective ablation of bone marrow-derived dendritic cells increases amyloid plaques in a mouse Alzheimer's disease model. Eur J Neurosci 26:413-416.

Butovsky O, Landa G, Kunis G, Ziv Y, Avidan H, Greenberg N, Schwartz A, Smirnov I, Pollack A, Jung S, Schwartz M. 2006b. Induction and blockage of oligodendrogenesis by differently activated microglia in an animal model of multiple sclerosis. J Clin Invest 116:905-915.

Chan HC, Chang RCC, Ip AKC, Chiu K, Yuen WH, Zee SY, So KF. 2007. Neuroprotective effects of Lycium barbarum Lynn on protecting retinal ganglion cells in an ocular hypertension model of glaucoma. Exp Neurol 203:269-273.

Chang RCC, Chiu K, Ho YS, So KF. 2009. Modulation of Neuroimmune Responses on Glia in the Central Nervous System: Implication in Therapeutic Intervention against Neuroinflammation. Cellular & Molecular Immunology 6:317-326.

Chiu K, Chan HC, Yeung SC, Yuen WH, Zee SY, Chang RCC, So KF. 2009. Modulation of microglia by Wolfberry on the survival of retinal ganglion cells in a rat ocular hypertension model J Ocul Biol Dis Inform 2:127-136.

Chiu K, Chang RCC, So KF. 2007. Laser induced rat chronic ocular hypertension model. Journal of Visualized Experiments 10: http://www.jove.com/index/ Details.stps?ID=549.

Chiu K, Yeung SC, So KF, Chang RCC. 2010a. Modulation of morphological changes of microglia and neuroprotection by monocyte chemoattractant protein-1 in experimental glaucoma. Cellular & Molecular Immunology 7:61-68.

Chiu K, Zhou Y, Yeung SC, Lok CKM, Chan OOC, Chang RCC, So KF, Chiu JF. 2010b. Up-Regulation of Crystallins is Involved in the Neuroprotective Effect of Wolfberry on Survival of Retinal Ganglion Cells in Rat Ocular Hypertension Model. J Cell Biochem 110:311-320.

Davalos D, Grutzendler J, Yang G, Kim JV, Zuo Y, Jung S, Littman DR, Dustin ML, Gan WB. 2005. ATP mediates rapid microglial response to local brain injury in vivo. Nat Neurosci 8:752-758.

Eugenin EA, D'Aversa TG, Lopez L, Calderon TM, Berman JW. 2003. MCP-1 (CCL2) protects human neurons and astrocytes from NMDA or HIV-tat-induced apoptosis. J Neurochem 85:1299-1311.

Forrester JV. 2009. Privilege revisited: an evaluation of the eye's defence mechanisms. Eye 23:756-766.

Galasso JM, Liu Y, Szaflarski J, Warren JS, Silverstein FS. 2000. Monocyte chemoattractant protein-1 is a mediator of acute excitotoxic injury in neonatal rat brain. Neuroscience 101:737-744.

Geissmann F, Auffray C, Palframan R, Wirrig C, Ciocca A, Campisi L, Narni-Mancinelli E, Lauvau G. 2008. Blood monocytes: distinct subsets, how they relate to dendritic cells, and their possible roles in the regulation of T-cell responses. Immunol Cell Biol 86:398-408.

Huang P, Qi Y, Xu YS, Liu JH, Liao DP, Zhang SSM, Zhang C. 2010. Serum Cytokine Alteration is Associated With Optic Neuropathy in Human Primary Open Angle Glaucoma. J Glaucoma 19:324-330.

Kalehua AN, Nagel JE, Whelchel LM, Gides JJ, Pyle RS, Smith RJ, Kusiak JW, Taub DD. 2004. Monocyte chemoattractant protein-1 and macrophage inflammatory protein-2 are involved in both excitotoxin-induced neurodegeneration and regeneration. Exp Cell Res 297:197-211.

Kigerl KA, Gensel JC, Ankeny DP, Alexander JK, Donnelly DJ, Popovich PG. 2009. Identification of Two Distinct Macrophage Subsets with Divergent Effects Causing either Neurotoxicity or Regeneration in the Injured Mouse Spinal Cord. The Journal of Neuroscience 29:13435-13444.

Kipnis J, Avidan H, Caspi RR, Schwartz M. 2004. Dual effect of CD4(+)CD25(+) regulatory T cells in neurodegeneration: A dialogue with microglia. Proc Natl Acad Sci U S A 101:14663-14669.

Kipnis J, Schwartz M. 2002. Dual action of glatiramer acetate (Cop-1) in the treatment of CNS autoimmune and neurodegenerative disorders. Trends in Molecular Medicine 8:319-323.

Kremmer S, Kreuzfelder E, Klein R, Bontke N, Henneberg-Quester KB, Steuhl KP, Grosse-Wilde H. 2001. Antiphosphatidylserine antibodies are elevated in normal tension glaucoma. Clin Exp Immunol 125:211-215.

Ladeby R, Wirenfeldt M, Garcia-Ovejero D, Fenger C, Dissing-Olesen L, Dahnau I, Finsen B. 2005. Microglial cell population dynamics in the injured adult central nervous system. Brain Research Reviews 48:196-206.

Lalancette-Hebert M, Gowing G, Simard A, Weng YC, Kriz J. 2007. Selective ablation of proliferating microglial cells exacerbates ischemic injury in the brain. J Neurosci 27:2596-2605.

Lam TT, Kwong JMK, Tso MOM. 2003. Early glial responses after acute elevated intraocular pressure in rats. Invest Ophthalmol Vis Sci 44:638-645.

Luo XG, Chiu K, Lau FHS, Lee VWH, Yung KKL, So KF. 2009. The Selective Vulnerability of Retinal Ganglion Cells in Rat Chronic Ocular Hypertension Model at Early Phase. Cell Mol Neurobiol 29:1143-1151.

Maruyama I, Ohguro H, Ikeda Y. 2000. Retinal ganglion cells recognised by serum autoantibody against gamma-enolase found in glaucoma patients. Invest Ophthalmol Vis Sci 41:1657-1665.

Naskar R, Wissing M, Thanos S. 2002. Detection of early neuron degeneration and accompanying microglial responses in the retina of a rat model of glaucoma. Invest Ophthalmol Vis Sci 43:2962-2968.

Neufeld AH. 1999. Microglia in the optic nerve head and the region of parapapillary chorioretinal atrophy in glaucoma. Arch Ophthalmol 117:1050-1056.

Nimmerjahn A, Kirchhoff F, Helmchen F. 2005. Resting microglial cells are highly dynamic surveillants of brain parenchyma in vivo. Science 308:1314-1318.

O'Donnell SL, Frederick TJ, Krady JK, Vannucci SJ, Wood TL. 2002. IGF-I and microglia/macrophage proliferation in the ischemic mouse brain. Glia 39:85-97.

Polazzi E, Altamira LEP, Eleuteri S, Barbaro R, Casadio C, Contestabile A, Monti B. 2009. Neuroprotection of microglial conditioned medium on 6-hydroxydopamine-induced neuronal death: Role of transforming growth factor beta-2. J Neurochem 110:545-556.

Polazzi E, Gianni T, Contestabile A. 2001. Microglial cells protect cerebellar granule neurons from apoptosis: Evidence for reciprocal signaling. Glia 36:271-280.

Polazzi E, Monti B. 2010. Microglia and neuroprotection: From in vitro studies to therapeutic applications. Prog Neurobiol 92:293-315.

Quigley HA. 1996. Number of people with glaucoma worldwide. Br J Ophthalmol 80:389-393.

Resnikoff S, Pascolini D, Etya'ale D, Kocur I, Pararajasegaram R, Pokharel GP, Mariotti SP. 2004. Global data on visual impairment in the year 2002. . Bull World Health Organ 82:844-851.

Romano C, Barrett DA, Li ZZ, Pestronk A, Wax MB. 1995. Anti-rhodopsin antibodies in sera from patients with normal-pressure glaucoma. Invest Ophthalmol Vis Sci 36:1968-1975.

Romano C, Li ZZ, Arendt A, Hargrave PA, Wax MB. 1999. Epitope mapping of anti-rhodopsin antibodies from patients with normal pressure glaucoma. Invest Ophthalmol Vis Sci 40:1275-1280.

Schori H, Kipnis J, Yoles E, WoldeMussie E, Ruiz G, Wheeler LA, Schwartz M. 2001. Vaccination for protection of retinal ganglion cells against death from glutamate cytotoxicity and ocular hypertension: Implications for glaucoma. Proc Natl Acad Sci U S A 98:3398-3403.

Schwartz M. 2007. Modulating the immune system: a vaccine for glaucoma? Can J Ophthalmol 42:439-441.

Schwartz M, Butovsky O, Bruck W, Hanisch UK. 2006. Microglial phenotype: is the commitment reversible? Trends Neurosci 29:68-74.

Schwartz M, Ziv Y. 2008. Immunity to self and self-maintenance: a unified theory of brain pathologies. Trends in Immunology 29:211-219.

Sica A, Schioppa T, Mantovani A, Allavena P. 2006. Tumour-associated macrophages are a distinct M2 polarised population promoting tumour progression: Potential targets of anti-cancer therapy. Eur J Cancer 42:717-727.

Tezel G. *2010,* doi:10.1016/j.exer.2010.07.009. The immune response in glaucoma: A perspective on the roles of oxidative stress. Exp Eye Res In Press, Corrected Proof.

Tezel G, Edward DP, Wax MB. 1999. Serum autoantibodies to optic nerve head glycosaminoglycans in patients with glaucoma. Arch Ophthalmol 117:917-924.

Tezel G, Seigel GM, Wax MB. 1998. Autoantibodies to small heat shock proteins in glaucoma. Invest Ophthalmol Vis Sci 39:2277-2287.

Tezel G, Wax MB. 1999. Inhibition of caspase activity in retinal cell apoptosis induced by various stimuli in vitro. Invest Ophthalmol Vis Sci 40:2660-2667.

Tezel G, Wax MB. 2000. The mechanisms of hsp27 antibody-mediated apoptosis in retinal neuronal cells. J Neurosci 20:3552-3562.

Tezel G, Yang JJ, Wax MB. 2004. Heat shock proteins, immunity and glaucoma. Brain Res Bull 62:473-480.

Wang X, Tay SSW, Ng YK. 2000. An immunohistochemical study of neuronal and glial cell reactions in retinae of rats with experimental glaucoma. Exp Brain Res 132:476-484.

Wax MB, Barrett DA, Pestronk A. 1994. Increased incidence of paraproteinemia and autoantibodies in patients with normal-pressure glaucoma. Am J Ophthalmol 117:561-568.

Wax MB, Tezel G. 2009. Immunoregulation of retinal ganglion cell fate in glaucoma. Exp Eye Res 88:825-830.

Wax MB, Tezel G, Edward PD. 1998a. Clinical and ocular histopathological findings in a patient with normal-pressure glaucoma. Arch Ophthalmol 116:993-1001.

Wax MB, Tezel G, Kawase K, Kitazawa Y. 2001. Serum autoantibodies to heat shock proteins in glaucoma patients from Japan and the United States. Ophthalmology 108:296-302.

Wax MB, Tezel G, Saito I, Gupta RS, Harley JB, Li ZZ, Romano C. 1998b. Anti-Ro/SS-A positivity and heat shock protein antibodies in patients with normal-pressure glaucoma. Am J Ophthalmol 125:145-157.

Yang JJ, Patil RV, Yu H, Gordon M, Wax MB. 2001a. T cell subsets and sIL-2R/IL-2 levels in patients with glaucoma. Am J Ophthalmol 131:421-426.

Yang JJ, Tezel G, Patil RV, Romano C, Wax MB. 2001b. Serum autoantibody against glutathione S-transferase in patients with glaucoma. Invest Ophthalmol Vis Sci 42:1273-1276.

Zhang J, Koninck Y. 2006. Spatial and temporal relationship between monocyte chemoattractant protein-1 expression and spinal glial activation following peripheral nerve injury. J Neurochem 97:772-783.

15

Stem Cell Based Therapies for Glaucoma

Hari Jayaram, Silke Becker and G. Astrid Limb
UCL Institute of Ophthalmology & Moorfields Eye Hospital
United Kingdom

1. Introduction

Glaucoma remains one of the leading causes of blindness worldwide. In England and Wales glaucoma is a major or contributory factor for 12-14% of all registrations for blindness and partial sight, second only to macular degeneration (Bunce et al., 2010). The worldwide burden is more significant, with glaucoma being the second leading cause of global blindness after cataract (Resnikoff et al., 2004). It has been estimated that 60.5 million people worldwide would be affected by glaucoma by 2010, with the figure expected to rise to 80 million by 2020 (Quigley and Broman, 2006).

Current treatments for glaucoma comprise the lowering of intraocular pressure by eye drops, laser procedures or drainage surgery. However, as implied by the statistics above, many patients experience significant visual loss due to degeneration of retinal ganglion cells (RGCs) despite the advances in the treatments currently available. The need for novel therapies exists for such patients, in particular those with end stage glaucoma, where the maintenance of a small number of surviving RGCs may yet permit a reasonable quality of life (Much et al., 2008). Stem cell therapies developed in the laboratory and translated to clinical practice provide an exciting and realistic hope for those affected by degenerative retinal diseases including glaucoma. This chapter will discuss three mechanisms by which stem cell therapies may potentially offer hope to patients with end stage glaucoma, namely local RGC replacement, optic nerve regeneration and stem cell mediated neuroprotection.

2. Sources of stem cells

Stem cells are characterised by their capacity for unlimited self-renewal and ability to differentiate into different cell types. The term progenitor cell is often applied to multipotent cells with a capacity for self-renewal, however this chapter will use the term stem cell to encompass all progenitor and precursor cell types.

An ideal candidate for developing stem cell based therapies would be readily available, easy to expand in culture, possess an acceptable long term safety profile and be autologous in nature, in order to avoid the need to modulate the host immune response and prevent rejection. Unfortunately a cell type that fulfils all these criteria remains elusive, however current research is directed towards a limited number of cell types which themselves exhibit certain advantages or disadvantages. Such cell populations may be sourced from three broad categories - embryonic or foetal tissue, adult tissue and reprogrammed cells (Figure 1).

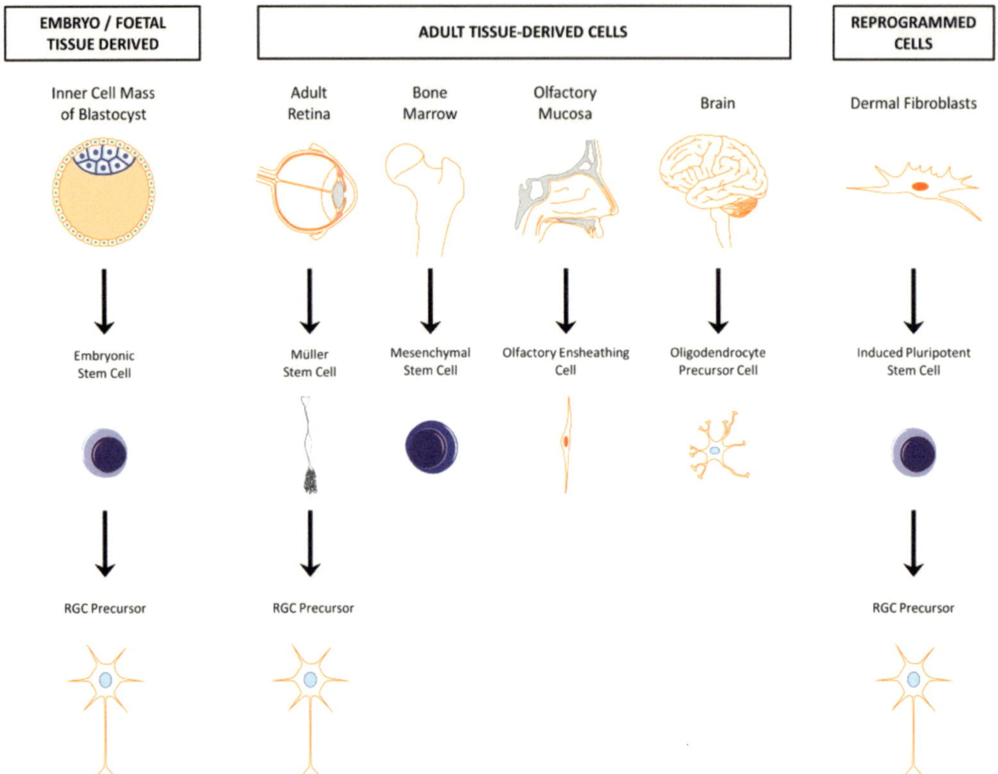

Fig. 1. Summary of the sources of cells that may be potentially used for cell based therapies in glaucoma. (Figure composed using Motifolio Inc. diagrams)

2.1 Embryonic stem cells

Embryonic stem cells (ESCs) arise from the inner cell mass of the blastocyst, which is formed at about five days after fertilisation in humans. Such cells are often sourced from excess tissue obtained from embryo donations and fertility treatments and have been associated with ethical objections due to controversies regarding the use of such tissue for research. However they possess an unlimited capacity for self-renewal with an ability to differentiate into any of the cell types within the human body (Evans and Kaufman, 1981). ESCs have been proposed as ideal candidates for cell based therapies to treat human retinal diseases, due their capacity to migrate and differentiate into different cell types. ESCs have been differentiated *in vitro* into neurons (Bibel et al., 2004) as well as retinal pigmented epithelium (RPE) (Hirano et al., 2003), but controlling their differentiation has proved challenging. In the absence of appropriate intracellular signals, ESCs appear to differentiate towards a neuronal fate by default (Hemmati-Brivanlou and Melton, 1997), although differentiation into retina specific precursors often involves complex laboratory protocols (Osakada et al., 2009). A drawback of a pluripotent cell type is the risk of teratoma formation by uncontrolled growth of transplanted ESCs (Hentze et al., 2007) which remains a major concern. In addition, safety concerns derived from the observed chromosomal instability of cultured ESCs (Moon et al., 2011) require further investigation.

2.2 Adult tissue-derived stem cells

Adult tissue-derived stem cells offer an alternative for the development of cell based therapies which circumvents the ethical controversies surrounding foetal and embryonic tissue. Up to date, various sources of adult stem cells have been investigated for their potential ability to regenerate or replace retinal neurons which are described below.

2.2.1 Müller stem cells

The concept of central nervous system (CNS) regeneration from glial cells has become more accepted in recent years. Radial glia within the brain have been shown to act as neural stem cells within the developing mammalian nervous system, with the ability to generate both new neurons and glia (Merkle et al., 2004). Müller glia are the radial glia of the retina and have been shown to share a common lineage with retinal neurons and to derive from a common multipotent progenitor (Turner and Cepko, 1987). Studies in zebrafish have demonstrated that the ability of this species to regenerate retina is due to the presence of Müller glia with stem cell characteristics (Bernardos et al., 2007). Pharmacological depletion of the ganglion cell layer has been shown to induce a regenerative response in this species, which is characterised by Müller glial cells re-entering the cell cycle and producing neuronal progenitor cells that repopulate the ganglion cell layer (Fimbel et al., 2007).

Although a capacity for regeneration similar to that seen in the zebrafish has not been observed in higher species, a population of Müller glia with stem cell characteristics has been identified in the adult human retina (Lawrence et al., 2007). These cells express markers of neural progenitors *in vitro* and a proportion of them are able to express markers of mature retinal neurons in response to various culture conditions (Lawrence et al., 2007). Data from our laboratory exploring transplantation of these cells in a rodent model of ganglion cell depletion shows that pre-differentiated cells are able to integrate within the host RGC layer and cause partial restoration of the scotopic threshold response, which is a marker of RGC function in the rat electroretinogram (Singhal et al., 2009).

Such cell lines are easily obtained from cadaveric donor retinae (Limb et al., 2002) and further studies may reveal whether it is possible to obtain patient specific cell lines from peripheral retinal biopsies, leading to the possibility of developing an autologous grafting strategy.

2.2.2 Mesenchymal stem cells

Mesenchymal stem cells are most commonly obtained from bone marrow biopsies and umbilical cord blood and have been considered as candidates for autologous cell transplantation. Pharmacological methods have been used to mobilise haematopoetic stem cells from the bone marrow into the bloodstream to facilitate their harvesting for transplantation (Uy et al., 2008) rather than employing more invasive bone marrow trephine techniques. The mobilisation of mesenchymal stem cells is more difficult than that of haematopoietic stem cells, with several strategies showing promise in animal models (Pitchford et al., 2009). During development mesenchymal stem cells differentiate into bone, cartilage and muscle. However they have been reported to de-differentiate *in vitro* into other cell types including neurons and glia, although at present there is much controversy surrounding this ability (Krabbe et al., 2005). As will be discussed later, this cell type is likely to have a more significant role in neuroprotective strategies rather than neuronal replacement, due to their ability to secrete cytokines.

2.2.3 Oligodendrocyte precursor cells

Oligodendrocyte precursor cells (OPCs) are a type of neural stem cells responsible for the generation of oligodendrocytes during normal development, and for re-myelination of the white matter in the adult CNS (Watanabe et al., 2002). They are the commonest proliferative cell type in the adult CNS (Dawson et al., 2003). OPCs have been reported to exhibit some stem cell characteristics (Nunes et al., 2003) and neuroprotective potential *in vitro* (Wilkins et al., 2001), which have led to investigations into their potential use for stem cell based therapies to treat neurodegenerative conditions including glaucoma.

2.2.4 Olfactory ensheathing cells

Olfactory tissue is unique within the CNS, in that continuous removal and regeneration of tissue occurs throughout life. The sensory axons that project to the olfactory bulb are closely associated with specialised cells known as olfactory ensheathing cells (OECs). OECs are glial cells which lie within the nasal mucosa and olfactory bulb and characteristically ensheathe axons of the olfactory nerve. Transplantation of these cells has been used to support regenerating axons in animal models of spinal cord injury and to restore function (Li et al., 2008). Due to the relative ease by which nasal mucosal biopsies may be obtained, these cells may potentially constitute a source of cells through which autologous transplantation strategies may be developed in the future. There is considerable molecular heterogeneity and functional diversity of OECs with much work still taking place in animal models (Su and He, 2010). Further investigation into the gene expression and cell fate determination of these cells will facilitate the development of more robust protocols to isolate and expand the OEC progenitor/stem cell population within this complex tissue.

2.3 Induced pluripotent stem cells

The characterisation of induced pluripotent stem cells (iPS) cells has created an alternative potential cell source for transplantation in regenerative medicine. Takahashi & Yamanaka (Takahashi and Yamanaka, 2006) demonstrated that by retroviral induction of Oct3/4, Sox2, c-Myc and Klf4, pluripotent stem cell lines could be derived from fibroblast cultures. Further study of these "reprogrammed" iPS cells showed that their biological behaviour was indistinguishable from that of ESCs (Wernig et al., 2007). Subsequent modifications to the original protocol have enabled iPS cell lines to be created without the use of viral vectors (Okita et al., 2008) and without induction of the oncogene c-Myc (Nakagawa et al., 2008) which may be associated with an increase in tumorigenesis. However before such cells can be used in human therapies, safety concerns regarding the effect of the reactivation of pluripotency, alterations in target cells and characterisation of these cells need to be addressed (Jalving and Shepers, 2009).

3. Potential of stem cells for retinal ganglion cell replacement

One of the strategies to restore vision in glaucoma patients after RGCs have been lost or irreversibly damaged is their functional replacement by autologous or heterologous transplantation.

It is generally accepted that damage to the neural retina during glaucoma is restricted to the impairment of function and subsequently degeneration of RGCs (Kerrigan-Baumrind et al., 2000; Quigley and Green, 1979), making these cells ideal candidates for early cell replacement strategies. Recent evidence indicates, however, that in addition to damage to

the optic nerve, prolonged elevation of intraocular pressure may also induce degeneration or loss of function of other retinal neural cell types, most notably of amacrine cells (Hernandez et al., 2009). Similar observations have been made in other retinal degenerative diseases such as retinitis pigmentosa, which is characterized not only by the loss of rod, but also of cone photoreceptors and by major morphological changes of other surviving retinal neurons (Fariss et al., 2000). Therefore early intervention may be preferable, if cell replacement strategies are to succeed, in order to restrict the number of cells types which need to be transplanted. In addition, the correct establishment of synaptic connections between transplanted RGC and native cells may be facilitated, providing that the stratified structure of the retina with its circuitry and at least some of the connections of the RGCs through the optic nerve and the optic chiasm to the lateral geniculate nucleus are preserved.
At present, research has mostly focused on the identification of suitable cells, which can be differentiated towards RGCs and their precursors, as well as the experimental conditions required for the optimal expression of their molecular markers. Furthermore, a small number of studies have investigated the electrophysiological properties of the RGC precursors generated *in vitro* and their transplantation into *in vivo* models. Although research has been conducted into the functional replacement of RGCs, and potential candidate stem cells have been identified, there are currently no cell-based therapeutic options that are either available to patients or tested in clinical trials. Establishment of cell based therapies to replace or regenerate RGCs, as with any other cell based therapy, would require validation protocols for safety, efficacy and long term survival of the transplanted cells. In the following sections we will review the potential of human ES cells, iPS cells and adult human Müller stem cells for the generation and transplantation of RGCs and their precursors.

3.1 Human embryonic stem cells as a prospective source of RGCs

Most evidence for the differentiation of ESCs into retinal progenitors and their potential for retinal transplantation has been provided by animal studies. Murine ESCs have been shown to generate RGC-like cells *in vitro* by differentiation protocols using various growth and differentiating factors. This has resulted in the expression of markers such as Ath5, Brn3b, RPF-1, Thy-1 and Isl-1 (Jagatha et al., 2009), which are characteristically expressed by RGCs. Rx/rax-expressing murine ESCs, which were treated with retinoic acid to induce neural commitment, expressed markers of RGCs and horizontal cells, displayed electrophysiological properties consistent with RGCs and were able to integrate *ex vivo* into mouse retinae (Tabata et al., 2004). Importantly, when mouse ESCs, which had been differentiated into eye-like structures, were co-cultured with retinal explants following damage to the inner retinal cells, migration into the RGC layer as well as expression of the RGC markers HuD and Brn3b were observed (Aoki et al., 2007).
Proof of concept that human ESCs can successfully differentiate into retinal neurons has been provided by xenologous transplantation. Following intravitreal injection into the adult mouse eye, human ESCs formed structures reminiscent of the developing optic cup and expressed markers of a wide range of retinal progenitors and neurons (Aoki et al., 2009).
In addition transplanted murine ESCs have been shown to integrate into the inner and outer nuclear as well as the inner plexiform layers of the retinae of host mice with retinal degeneration. Transplanted cells adopted a morphology consistent with and displayed molecular markers of a wide range of retinal neurons, such as βIII-tubulin and NeuN, calretinin, PKC-α and rhodopsin (Meyer et al., 2006).

In addition, Lamba et al. have recently provided evidence that human ESCs can generate retinal progenitors with high efficiency, expressing a number of molecular markers usually observed in the developing retina. These cells have shown exceptional correlation between their levels of expression of genes specific for differentiating neurons and the developmental stage of the retina, including markers of RGC and amacrine cells, which constitute the inner retina, i.e. HuD/C, Pax6, neurofilament-M and Tuj1 (Lamba et al., 2006).

Transplantation of human ESC-derived neural and retinal progenitors into animal models of retinal degeneration has been extensively studied by several groups. Neural precursors derived from human ESCs have been transplanted subretinally and intravitreally into mice, where they have been shown to be able to integrate into the retina and survive for long periods of time after grafting. Although these cells mostly displayed photoreceptors markers (Banin et al., 2006), such findings have provided evidence that human ESCs have the potential to form retinal neurons following engraftment. These results have been further supported by additional evidence that human ESCs can adopt a neural morphology and express neural retinal markers following transplantation and differentiating treatment in an *in vivo* murine model of RGC depletion, without giving rise to teratomas (Hara et al., 2010).

Although human ESCs have shown potential for use in RGC replacement therapies for glaucoma, major disadvantages associated with the use of human ESCs still remain. Ethical constraints relating to the use of these cells, their limited availability and safety issues regarding teratoma formation are likely to curtail the translation of ESCs for human RGC replacement to the clinical setting. Further work should therefore be aimed towards identifying alternative sources of cells that may safely and efficiently replace these cells in the glaucomatous eye without these ethical and practical constraints.

3.2 RGC differentiation of induced pluripotent stem cells

Some of the disadvantages of human ESCs have been addressed by the development of iPS cells, which have been proposed as a viable source of cells for autologous transplantation. The generation of iPS cells does not require the destruction of embryonic tissue and therefore does not have the same ethical implications as work with ESCs, which have been a limitation in a large number of developed countries. In addition, iPS cells can be derived from and tailored to the patient, making cells more widely available and rendering immunosuppressive therapy following transplantation redundant. To date, few studies have investigated the potential for iPS cells in stem cell treatment of retinal degenerative diseases, although recently some progress has been made to generate iPS cell-derived RGC-like cells.

Parameswaran et al. have recently provided evidence that iPS cells, which originated from reprogrammed mouse embryonic fibroblasts by transfection with Oct3/4, Sox2, Klf4 and c-Myc, can give rise to both RGCs and photoreceptors *in vitro*. They reported that neural induction and exposure to conditioned media from E14 rat retinal cells augmented the expression of Ath1, Brn3b, RPF1 and Irx2, which regulate RGC differentiation, while the retinal progenitor markers Sox2, Rx and Chx10 were reduced. Importantly, the same study reported that the generated RGC-like cells displayed tetrodotoxin-sensitive voltage-dependent sodium currents, which is a hallmark of functional neurons (Parameswaran et al., 2010).

Chen et al. have used a similar approach by creating iPS cells from reprogrammed murine fibroblasts, which had been transduced with Oct3/4, Sox2, c-Myc and Klf4, to generate RGC-like cells. These cells expressed markers of retinal progenitor cells, i.e. Pax6, Rx, Otx2,

Lhx2 and nestin, the levels of which were attenuated after differentiation towards a RGC fate. Differentiation was accompanied by expression of markers of RGC progenitors such as Brn3b and Isl-1, as well as Thy-1.2, a marker of mature RGCs. However, transplanted cells did not engraft into murine retina following intravitreal injection and they retained their pluripotency as demonstrated by their ability to form intraocular teratomas (Chen et al., 2010).

These studies illustrate major problems associated with the transplantation of cells derived from iPS cells, which need to be addressed. In particular, as described by Chen et al., the ability of iPS to form teratomas and therefore their potential to form cancerous growths may prove problematic. These findings suggest that preparation of iPS cell derived RGC progenitors for individual patients may need to undergo extensive validation for safety and efficacy, making them likely to be impractical and expensive for autologous therapies.

3.3 Müller stem cells as a source of RGCs for glaucoma therapies

The lack of regenerative potential of the human retina *in vivo* may be due to presently unknown inhibitory factors within the fully developed retina, since human Müller glia cells with stem cell characteristics have been reported to retain the ability to divide indefinitely *in vitro* (Limb et al., 2002). Until further research can elucidate the nature of these inhibitory factors, it is however unlikely that treatment options involving re-activation of endogenous Müller stem cells in the adult human retina can be developed. Cell replacement by transplantation of Müller stem cell-derived retinal neural progenitors may therefore currently offer a more promising strategy to restore visual function after irreversible damage or substantial loss of RGCs in glaucoma.

Müller glia with stem cell characteristics have been demonstrated to be predominantly located in the peripheral sections of the adult human retina (Bhatia et al., 2009). Human Müller stem cells can be easily isolated from cadaveric donor retina, and these cells can be grown and expanded indefinitely *in vitro,* and express markers of neural progenitor cells, such as Sox2, Notch1, Pax6, Shh and Chx10, as well as markers of Müller glia cells and retinal neurons e.g. CRALBP, HuD, PKC, and peripherin (Lawrence et al., 2007). When cultured under differentiating conditions in the presence of extracellular matrix and growth factors, enriched populations of cells expressing markers of specific retinal neurons can be obtained (Bhatia et al., 2011; Lawrence et al., 2007; Singhal et al., manuscript submitted).

This is illustrated by the fact that Müller stem cells cultured under various conditions develop a neuronal morphology and upregulate their expression of retinal neural and RGC precursor markers such as βIII-tubulin, Brn3b, Isl-1 and rhodopsin. Simultaneously expression levels of the neural progenitor marker Pax6 and the glial cell marker vimentin are also attenuated (Bhatia et al., 2011), indicating that existing Müller stem cell lines may have the potential to form RGC precursors.

However at present, intraocular transplantation studies using Müller stem cells have been conducted using mostly undifferentiated cells. Initially Lawence et al. reported integration of subretinally transplantated Müller stem cells into neonatal Lister Hooded rats and adult dystrophic RCS rats. Engrafted cells were shown to express the photoreceptor markers recoverin and rhodopsin, the RGC marker HuD as well as calretinin, which identifies RGCs and amacrine cells (Lawrence et al., 2007). Although integration of undifferentiated Müller stem cells has been observed after subretinal transplantation into adult dystrophic RCS rats, these cells were located in all retinal layers and did not selectively locate to the ganglion cell layer or adopt RGC-like morphology (Singhal et al., 2008).

Undifferentiated Müller stem cells have also been used for intravitreal and subretinal transplantation in a rat model of glaucoma. Although only few of the transplanted cells expressed the Müller glia and astrocyte marker GFAP, expression of βIII-tubulin indicates that at least some of the transplanted cells were able to adopt a neural phenotype. Interestingly, many of the grafted cells showed a migratory phenotype and aligned towards the host retina, in particular the optic nerve head, although they did not migrate and disseminate within the retina (Bull et al., 2008).

Recently it has been reported that Müller stem cells can be differentiated into RGC precursors, which integrate into the retina after intravitreal injection and can partly restore function in RGC-depleted retina as measured by electroretinography (Singhal et al., 2009). Although at present understanding of Müller stem cell differentiation towards RGC precursors is limited, previous work with this cell type has shown that they may have the potential for therapeutic regeneration of RGC function in glaucoma. In particular the maturity of Müller stem cells may potentially decrease the risk of teratoma formation. In addition, their ontogenetic proximity to retinal neurons may likely facilitate the development of protocols not only to successfully derive and transplant RGC precursors, but also to induce endogenous retinal regeneration without the need for transplantation.

3.4 Barriers to successful stem cell transplantation

Although some progress has been made regarding the successful production, delivery, integration and survival of RGC progenitors, major obstacles for successful engraftment and functional restoration remain and will be discussed below. These include the host immune response and extracellular matrix, which form a barrier for cell integration into the healthy host retina. During retinal degenerative processes, there is abnormal deposition of extracellular matrix, mainly chondroitin sulphate proteoglycans, which are responsible for the formation of glial scarring (gliosis). In addition, accumulation of microglia occurs, which has been shown to surround transplanted cells, inhibit their migration and induce their death (Singhal et al., 2008). Additionally, effective migration and integration of the transplanted cells has been suggested to be dependent upon their ontogenetic stage (MacLaren et al., 2006). These requirements will be discussed in more detail below.

3.4.1 Modulation of the host extracellular matrix

Various transplantation studies using a wide range of cells derived from ESCs as well as Müller stem cells have concluded that successful engraftment into the healthy adult retina is impeded by extracellular matrix components and the physical barrier of the inner limiting membrane (Chacko et al., 2003; Johnson et al., 2010b). This is unlikely to be influenced by the route of cell delivery, since transplantation by either intravitreal or subretinal injection did not yield integration of transplanted cells into the healthy host retina in the adult rat (Bull et al., 2008). In addition dissemination of the transplanted cells within the retina has been reported to be highly restricted (Banin et al., 2006). Conversely, integration of transplanted cells has been demonstrated in neonates (Chacko et al., 2003) or in the adult retina following injury (Chacko et al., 2003), indicating that these environments may be more permissive for successful engraftment.

Glaucomatous changes of the retina are generally accompanied by reactive gliosis as well as remodelling and deposition of extracellular matrix components (Guo et al., 2005). Increased production of chondroitin sulphate proteoglycans (CSPGs), which have been shown to

inhibit rat optic nerve regeneration after crush injury (Selles-Navarro et al., 2001) and reduce axonal and dendritic growth (Zuo et al., 1998), has been demonstrated following CNS and spinal cord damage (Bradbury et al., 2002). CSPGs have also been reported to form a barrier to cell migration following transplantation in animal models (Singhal et al., 2008) (Figure 2). Furthermore, degradation of CSPGs has been shown to enhance dendritic and axonal regeneration following brain and spinal cord injury (Bradbury et al., 2002; Zuo et al., 1998).
As a result of these findings, the effects of modulation of extracellular matrix components have recently been explored in conjunction with retinal progenitor transplantation. Evidence has been provided to show that co-administration of chondroitinase ABC or erythropoietin, which has been reported to upregulate MMP-2 (Wang et al., 2006), greatly increases the number of cells, which successfully integrate into the host retina (Singhal et al., 2008; Suzuki et al., 2007). Similarly, the integration of murine neonatal retinal cells into the adult rat host retina by *ex vivo* transplantation has been shown to be augmented by the induction of MMP-2 (Suzuki et al., 2006).

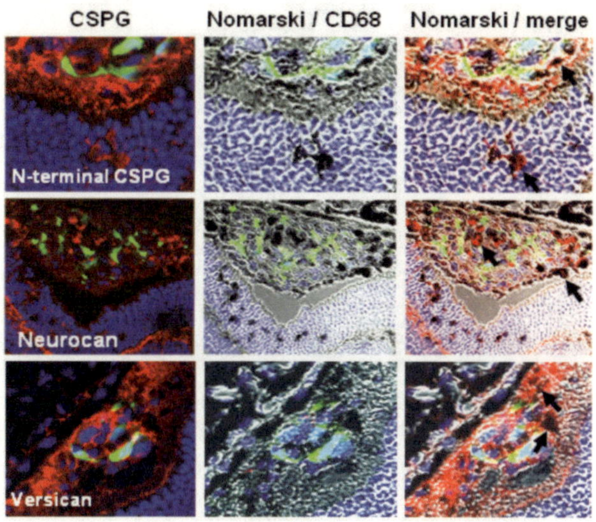

Fig. 2. Confocal imaging of rodent retina 2 weeks after subretinal transplantation of Müller stem cells. Sections on the left column shows the transplanted cells (green) surrounded by N-terminal CSPG, neurocan and versican (red). The middle column shows the same sections under Nomarski illumination to illustrate the accumulation of CD68 positive microglia (black). The column on the right shows the merged images under Nomarski illumination illustrating co-localization (arrows) of CD68 positive cells and CSPGs (red) surrounding the transplanted cells (green) (from Singhal et al., 2008).

3.4.2 Modulation of the host immune response

A successful transplantation scheme requires long term survival of the grafted cells. Allogeneic grafts induce a host immune response, leading to rejection and failure of the transplant. However cell survival is greatly increased by systemic immunosuppression of the recipient following allogeneic cell transplantation into the eye (West et al., 2010). Triple therapy with oral immunosuppressives has recently been used to increase survival of xenografted Müller stem cells to 2 to 3 weeks, although microglia and macrophage activation was observed and transplants were destroyed after 4 weeks (Bull et al., 2008). Activation of phagocytic microglia, the resident immune cells of the CNS, which may promote axonal degeneration of RGCs and of the optic nerve, is frequently observed during glaucoma (Ebneter et al., 2010; Yuan and Neufeld, 2001). In transplantation models, microglia prevent the migration of transplanted cells into the retina (Singhal et al., 2008) (Figure 3). Suppression of the intraocular immune response and inhibition of microglial activation by intravitreal injection of triamcinolone acetonide may therefore promote the integration and the survival of RGC precursors into retinae with glaucomatous changes. Intravitreal injection of triamcinolone acetonide in combination with oral immunosuppression and anti-inflammatory medication has previously been shown to greatly reduce microglial activation against the xenograft (Singhal et al., 2008; Singhal et al., 2010).

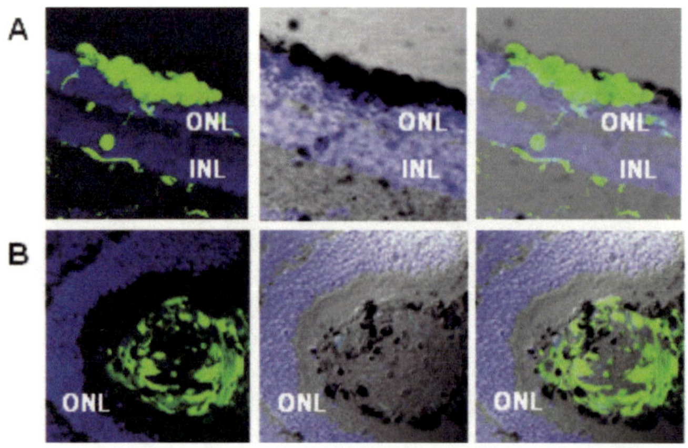

Fig. 3. **A**. Müller stem cells (green) accumulate in the subretinal space and do not migrate into the retina. Middle image shows Nomarski illumination identifying CD68 positive cells (black) in the same retinal section. Right figure shows Nomarski illumination identifying co-localization of transplanted cells with microglial cells expressing CD68 (black).
B. Transplanted cells can be seen forming a large cluster in the subretinal space 2 weeks after transplantation. Middle image shows localization of microglia (black) around the transplanted cells (green). Right figure shows microglia (black) surrounding the transplanted cells (green) and resembling a granuloma-type structure (From Singhal et al., 2008).

In experimental animal models, immune-tolerization of embryos or neonates by intraperitoneal injection of grafted cells may be used to further reduce the host immune response (Billingham et al., 1953).

3.4.3 Ontogenetic stage of transplanted cells

Currently the role played by the ontogenetic stage of transplanted RGC precursors upon their integration into host retina, as well as on functionality of the engrafted cells, has not been investigated. Previous transplantation studies have demonstrated that stem cells isolated from adult individuals rarely migrated into the healthy adult retina (Johnson et al., 2010a; Lawrence et al., 2007; Singhal et al., 2008), while embryonic and neonatal retinal progenitors and other stem cells have been shown to successfully integrate into the host retina (Warfvinge et al., 2001; Wojciechowski et al., 2004), suggesting that the developmental stage of the transplant may be crucial for successful migration and functional integration.

Several studies have investigated the role of the developmental stage of grafted retinal neurons for successful incorporation into the host retina. Based on this work, it has been concluded at least in the case of photoreceptor transplantation that early postnatal post-mitotic precursors or cells of a similar ontogenetic stage are the most promising candidates for transplantation in terms of their ability to migrate and disseminate into the retina and differentiate towards a functional phenotype (MacLaren et al., 2006).

However, more recent studies have suggested that there may be no need for transplantation of photoreceptor progenitors for these cells to integrate, as fully mature photoreceptors retain the ability to integrate into the mature retina upon transplantation (Gust and Reh, 2011). Moreover, integration of photoreceptors derived from human Müller glia into the degenerated rat retina has shown to be independent from NRL expression by these cells (Jayaram et al., unpublished observations).

In addition the developmental phase of transplanted cells will likely have major implications on treatment safety, with less differentiated cells posing a greater risk of tumorigenesis. In fact, a number of studies using cells derived from embryonic stem or iPS cells have reported the occurrence of teratomas (Arnhold et al., 2004; Chen et al., 2010), whereas no formation of cancerous growths was reported after transplantation of adult-derived stem cells.

In summary, future research will be needed to elucidate the effects of the ontogenetic stage of transplanted RGC precursors on graft integration, function and safety.

3.5 Strategies to measure functional outcome

With the development of methods for the transplantation of RGC in glaucoma, the measurement of functional outcomes will become increasingly important. It can be anticipated, however, that these will encompass techniques currently available for the monitoring of disease progression. Electrophysiological measurements are widely used to assess glaucomatous damage both in patients and in experimental animal models and will likely continue to play a major role in evaluating treatment success. Some of these protocols have been standardized by the International Society for Clinical Electrophysiology of Vision (ISCEV) guidelines (Holder et al., 2007; Marmor et al., 2009), although they may be complemented by other methods established for laboratory use.

The pattern ERG is currently one of the most useful techniques to assess glaucomatous damage in patients. It generally utilizes a black and white checkerboard stimulus with pattern reversal as prescribed by the ISCEV standards (Holder et al., 2007). The pattern ERG has been shown to be reduced in patients with glaucoma and correlates with visual field defects (Wanger and Persson, 1983). In addition the use of variable check sizes may be advisable to assess the extent of glaucomatous change (Bach et al., 1988). Recently multifocal pattern electroretinograms have been demonstrated to be reduced in glaucoma patients (Monteiro et al., 2011; Stiefelmeyer et al., 2004), although other studies have reported that localized reductions of the signal amplitude could not be correlated with visual field defects (Klistorner et al., 2000). Since this method requires good accommodation and fixation (Holder et al., 2007), it is widely used in human subjects, while its applicability to animal models is limited.

Preclinical studies will likely favour methods employing Ganzfeld stimulation, which are relatively easy to apply to a laboratory setting. The most commonly used of these is the scotopic threshold response, a low intensity light response with stimulation below the psychophysical threshold, which has be ascribed to RGC function, although it may species-dependently contain contributions from amacrine cells (Frishman et al., 1996; Korth et al., 1994; Sieving, 1991). More recently the photopic negative response has been established as a measure of RGC function (Viswanathan et al., 1999), although other cellular origins, such as glia and amacrine cells, have been suggested (Machida et al., 2008). However, at present this has not been assimilated into ISCEV guidelines.

Pattern reversal, pattern onset/offset or flash visual evoked potentials can be used to assess RGC and optic nerve function. Although they are usually employed in a clinical setting (Odom et al., 2010), especially the flash, the pattern onset/offset visual evoked potentials may potentially be used for experimental applications in animals (Huang et al., 2011; Ver Hoeve et al., 1999). Recently multifocal mapping of visual evoked potentials has been developed (Hasegawa and Abe, 2001), but has not been widely applied to practice. However, for clinical purposes perimetry will remain important, as gains in the visual field of patients may indicate whether potential RGC cell therapies are successful.

4. Optic nerve regeneration

It has been considered critical for the functional success of RGC replacement therapies in glaucoma that transplanted cells form axons, restore the optic nerve and establish new connections with their physiological targets. The optic nerve has traditionally been thought to be incapable of renewal, with axonal damage invariably leading to the degeneration of RGC somata and resulting in the irreparable loss of vision.

A range of studies has investigated the effects of peripheral nerve transplantation on RGC survival as well as axonal sprouting and re-growth. Extensive evidence has been presented that autologous grafts of peripheral nerves can protect axotomized RGCs from cell death and in addition can promote the regeneration and re-growth of axons. Some studies have even shown that after transplantation of peripheral nerves, RGCs regenerated long axons, which extended into the superior colliculus, where they formed synapses in their physiological target region (Aguayo et al., 1991; Vidal-Sanz et al., 1991).

Other cell types such as OECs and macrophages have been suggested to augment axon formation. The promoting effect of OECs on neurite formation may likely be contact-mediated (Leaver et al., 2006). In addition, macrophages have been reported to promote axonal growth, probable through the release of oncomodulin and activation of the protein kinase Mst3b and Ca^{2+}/calmodulin kinases as downstream effectors (Lorber et al., 2009 ; Yin et al., 2006).

Distinct growth factors have been identified which may affect optic nerve regeneration. A combination of fibroblast growth factor 2 (FGF2), neurotrophin 3 (NT3) and brain derived neurotrophic factor (BDNF) (Logan et al., 2006) has been reported to stimulate axonal outgrowth of RGCs. Furthermore a range of molecules have been identified, which can reduce dendrite formation, e.g. Nogo-A, myelin-associated glycoprotein and components of the extracellular matrix such as proteoglycans (Koprivica et al., 2005; Su et al., 2009; Wong et al., 2003). Many of these inhibitory factors converge on the small G-protein RhoA, inhibition of which has been shown to result in stimulation of axon formation (Bertrand et al., 2005).

Interestingly, the length of new axons grown from cultured RGCs has been reported to be reduced after the developmental age at which synaptic connections in the superior colliculus are formed, although the proportion of cells generating axons was not altered (Goldberg et al., 2002).

The formation and guidance of axons from RGCs to their targets during development have been intensively investigated. Netrins, semaphorins, laminin, erythropoietin-producing hepatocellular receptor/Eph receptor-interacting protein, Wnt and slits have been shown to act as chemo-attractants and repellants during optic nerve development in the embryo (Erskine and Herrera, 2007; McLaughlin and O'Leary, 2005). Interestingly, some of these guiding signals have been reported to be retained or restored following injury in the adult brain (Bahr and Wizenmann, 1996), which may help to guide axons formed by transplanted RGCs to the right targets. Additionally it has been shown that following transplantation of embryonic retinal tissue, connections to the superior colliculus are successfully established (Seiler et al., 2010).

5. Stem cell mediated neuroprotection in glaucoma

The pathophysiological mechanisms implicated in RGC loss seen in glaucoma have led to the development of neuroprotective strategies becoming a major focus of current glaucoma research (Danesh-Meyer, 2011). Contemporary research in stem cell mediated neuroprotection for glaucoma has been developed on the backdrop of promising work performed in models of neurodegenerative disease affecting other parts of the CNS.

Glaucomatous RGC loss and neuronal degeneration in other neurodegenerative conditions share mechanisms such as oxidative stress, impairment of axonal transport, excitotoxicity and inflammation (Baltmr et al., 2010) making neuroprotective strategies relevant to patients affected by both conditions.

Stem cell derived strategies for neuroprotection, if successful, offer several theoretical advantages over conventional pharmacological approaches. Should transplanted cells integrate within the host retina, it is possible that a single treatment may provide long term neuroprotection offering support to surviving neurons. The observation that endogenous neural stem cells are able to migrate to the site of injury in ischaemic stroke and differentiate into mature neurons (Felling and Levison, 2003), gives rise to the possibility of a similar phenomenon occurring with transplanted cells in the context of glaucoma, with such cells potentially responsible for the provision of local support.

Stem cells are able to facilitate local neuronal survival by the production of several neurotrophic factors. This multifactorial effect has been demonstrated in animal models of CNS disease (Corti et al., 2007) and work in a rodent model of Parkinson's Disease showed that neural stem cell transplantation conferred a more significant neuroprotective benefit than both a single injection of neurotrophins or prolonged delivery via local infusion (Yasuhara et al., 2006). Transplantation of neural progenitors in animal models of neurodegenerative disease has been shown to confer neuroprotection via an immunomodulatory mechanism (Pluchino et al., 2005). Alteration of the microenvironment surrounding damaged RGCs, perhaps through immune mediated actions of transplanted cells, may help promote local neuronal survival.

A major beacon of hope in stem cell research is the concept of autologous transplantation. Such a strategy would minimise the risk of graft rejection and prevent a lifetime of potentially toxic immunosuppressive therapy for patients. Neuroprotective strategies involving Müller stem cells, bone marrow derived mesenchymal stem cells and OECs offer realistic potential for autologous transplantation. However, more work is still necessary to design practical approaches to obtain suitable tissue for this purpose, as well as to derive functional cells that can be used for transplantation. Should current concerns regarding the safety of iPS cells for therapeutic use be overcome (Jalving and Shepers, 2009), these reprogrammed adult somatic cells offer an exciting avenue for the development of autologous therapies in the future.

Mesenchymal stem cell mediated neuroprotection has been demonstrated following transplantation in various models of retinal degeneration (Arnhold et al., 2007; Inoue et al., 2007; Lu et al., 2010; Zhang and Wang, 2010). This phenomenon is likely to be secondary to the secretion of neurotrophic factors such as BDNF, ciliary neurotrophic factor (CNTF), nerve growth factor (NGF), insulin like growth factor 1 (IGF1) and FGF2 (Cho et al., 2005; Labouyrie et al., 1999) which are known to offer protection to damaged retina. These observations, coupled with promising results showing neuroprotection in models of CNS degenerative disease (Andrews et al., 2008; Karussis et al., 2008; Parr et al., 2007; Torrente and Polli, 2008), have led to this category of stem cells becoming a focus for the development of cell-based neuroprotective strategies to treat glaucoma.

Disruption of the retrograde axonal transport of BDNF has been shown to be involved in the pathophysiology of glaucoma (Pease et al., 2000) and attempts to upregulate expression of BDNF (Martin et al., 2003) and CNTF (Pease et al., 2009) using gene therapy have been shown to attenuate RGC loss in experimental models. A reduction in RGC loss has been observed in rodents with raised intraocular pressure following intravitreal transplantation of mesenchymal stem cells (Johnson et al., 2010a; Yu et al., 2006). The latter reported increased levels of CNTF, BDNF and FGF within the retinae of treated eyes, which were hypothesised to be responsible for this neuroprotective effect. Survival of the cells was observed at up to five weeks, but currently there is a lack of data describing long term graft survival and a prolonged neuroprotective effect, both of which will be essential for such a therapy to be translated to the clinic.

Despite suggestions that mesenchymal stem cells may possess a capacity to migrate from the systemic circulation into diseased tissue, migration into chronically damaged neural tissue is regarded as being limited, and hence strategies for cell delivery would be best served by direct injection into affected tissue. In the context of glaucoma models, cells administered via an intravenous approach were unable to be detected in the eye and had no effect in attenuating RGC loss (Johnson et al., 2010a).

The neuroprotective effect of transplanted cells may be optimised further by enhancing the neurotrophin secreting ability of cells through either cytokine driven protocols or gene therapy techniques. Proof of concept for this idea was demonstrated in a model of cerebral ischaemia where intravenous infusion of mesenchymal stem cells genetically modified to deliver BDNF to the cerebral circulation provided a greater neuroprotective effect than untreated cells (Nomura et al., 2005). This principle has been successfully applied to a rodent model of RGC damage induced by optic nerve transection (Levkovitch-Verbin et al., 2010). Mesenchymal stem cells were induced to secrete high levels of BDNF, VEGF and Glial Derived Neurotrophic Factor by using a cytokine driven protocol *in vitro*. Intravitreal transplantation of both modified and untreated mesenchymal stem cells produced similar neuroprotective effects when compared to sham injection. One interpretation of these findings would be that even small amounts of trophic factor release, as seen with untreated cells, may confer neuroprotection. However a more realistic argument may be that the severity of optic nerve transection is such that even the higher levels of trophic factors delivered by the modified cells would be unlikely to prevent RGC death. Further research into the role of cell populations that have enhanced neurotrophin secreting capability in models of glaucoma may provide further insight into the therapeutic potential of such an approach.

Inflammation has frequently been associated with neurodegenerative disease. It is commonly observed as a consequence of acute injuries including trauma and stroke, but is also a characteristic feature of demyelinating disease where autoimmune processes are central to the pathophysiology. Mesenchymal stem cells derived from the bone marrow are known to have the ability to modulate the inflammatory response. There is much hope and optimism in the field of multiple sclerosis that these cells may provide *in situ* immunomodulation and neuroprotection (Payne et al., 2011) with the results of clinical trials eagerly awaited. It is quite feasible that this mechanism may be applicable to glaucomatous RGC loss, however further studies are required to investigate this possibility.

The observation that OPCs exhibit neuroprotective properties *in vitro* (Wilkins et al., 2001) has led to some interest in their role as a potential candidate for cell-based therapies in a model of glaucoma. Interestingly OPCs were only able to demonstrate a neuroprotective effect following concomitant activation of pro-inflammatory cells using zymozan (Bull et al., 2009). The neuroprotective effect was not contact-mediated and was attributed to the release of diffusible trophic factors from the activated OPCs. A potential risk of transplanting such cells into glaucomatous eyes is the potential of excessive myelination, which carries the theoretical risk of blocking the transmission of light within the eye and reducing the electrical conduction of RGCs. However further studies into the nature of the trophic factors released by these cells may aid the design of further novel neuroprotective strategies to treat glaucoma.

OEC transplantation has been observed to increase axonal regeneration in models of spinal cord injury (Ramon-Cueto and Valverde, 1995). These initial observations led to the development of further studies into the potential of these cells to develop novel treatments for optic nerve disorders and glaucoma. *In vitro* work has demonstrated that OECs cause ensheathment of RGCs without the process of myelination occurring (Plant et al., 2010). Transplantation of OECs into the distal stump of transected optic nerves provided further evidence of regeneration of several axons (Li et al., 2003; Wu et al., 2010) that were supported by the transplanted cells. Following transretinal delivery into normal rodent eyes, OECs migrate along the RGC layer into the optic nervehead demonstrating ensheathment of RGC axons by the cytoplasm of transplanted cells (Li et al., 2008). It is possible that this process may provide some mechanical support to compromised axons, which may subsequently be able to maintain sufficient functional vision if therapies can be developed for patients with end stage glaucoma.

Evidence from models of spinal cord transection suggests that OEC transplantation is associated with an increased secretion of neurotrophins such as BDNF which appears to correlate with the neuroprotective effect (Sasaki et al., 2006). However it was not clear whether the BDNF was secreted by the transplanted cells or by activation of endogenous cells. Attempts to combine OEC transplantation with concomitant neurotrophin administration have shown promising results to date. Combination therapy in a model of optic nerve crush resulted in restoration of the latency of the visual evoked potential to almost 90% of normal levels with retrograde RGC labelling suggesting of axonal regeneration (Liu et al., 2010).

Future studies using these cells directed towards attenuating glaucomatous RGC loss may focus upon the potential of external support of RGC axons exiting via the lamina cribrosa as well as internal neuroprotection mediated by the provision of trophic factors. In addition further study into the functional characteristics of OECs is required as well as investigation of the effects of OEC in models of experimental glaucoma.

The perfect stem cell-based therapy to treat glaucoma would involve the activation of endogenous stem cells to repair damaged RGCs and thus restore function. The damaged CNS lacks plasticity and neuronal regeneration is notoriously difficult due to a lack of trophic cues (Hou et al., 2008) and the inhibitory nature of the microenvironment (Asher et al., 2001). Nevertheless there is growing evidence that endogenous neural stem cells may proliferate in response to brain injury such as stroke (Felling and Levison, 2003). Although only a proportion of new cells differentiate into new neurons and survive in the long term (Naylor et al., 2005), methods have been established to enhance the proliferation of endogenous neural stem cells following ischaemic injury (Ninomiya et al., 2006).

With respect to damaged neurons within the retina, it may be the Müller glia that hold the key for endogenous reactivation. Their well-documented capacity to regenerate retinal neurons in the teleost retina (Bernardos et al., 2007; Fimbel et al., 2007) and the known presence of similar cells in adult human retina (Lawrence et al., 2007) would make these cells a promising target around which studies of endogenous stem cell repair could be developed.

6. Conclusion

The rapidly evolving field of stem cell research offers exciting potential in the long term for innovative therapies moving from bench to bedside in patients who are affected by advanced glaucoma. Although regeneration of the optic nerve itself may be unrealistic with current scientific knowledge, further studies into local retinal ganglion replacement and neuroprotective mechanisms using transplanted stem cells may offer hope that such treatments may be translated to patients in years to come.

7. Acknowledgements

Supported by The Medical Research Council (MRC), UK (Grants G0900002 and G0701341). HJ holds a Fellowship from the MRC and the Royal College of Surgeons of Edinburgh.
Also supported by Fight for Sight and the NIHR Biomedical Research Centre for Ophthalmology Moorfields Eye Hospital NHS Foundation Trust and UCL Institute of Ophthalmology, UK

8. References

Aguayo, A.J., Rasminsky, M., Bray, G.M., Carbonetto, S., McKerracher, L., Villegas-Perez, M.P., Vidal-Sanz, M., Carter, D.A., 1991. Degenerative and regenerative responses of injured neurons in the central nervous system of adult mammals. Philos Trans R Soc Lond B Biol Sci 331, 337-343.

Andrews, E.M., Tsai, S.Y., Johnson, S.C., Farrer, J.R., Wagner, J.P., Kopen, G.C., Kartje, G.L., 2008. Human adult bone marrow-derived somatic cell therapy results in functional recovery and axonal plasticity following stroke in the rat. Exp Neurol 211, 588-592.

Aoki, H., Hara, A., Niwa, M., Motohashi, T., Suzuki, T., Kunisada, T., 2007. An in vitro mouse model for retinal ganglion cell replacement therapy using eye-like structures differentiated from ES cells. Exp Eye Res 84, 868-875.
Aoki, H., Hara, A., Niwa, M., Yamada, Y., Kunisada, T., 2009. In vitro and in vivo differentiation of human embryonic stem cells into retina-like organs and comparison with that from mouse pluripotent epiblast stem cells. Dev Dyn 238, 2266-2279.
Arnhold, S., Absenger, Y., Klein, H., Addicks, K., Schraermeyer, U., 2007. Transplantation of bone marrow-derived mesenchymal stem cells rescue photoreceptor cells in the dystrophic retina of the rhodopsin knockout mouse. Graefes Arch Clin Exp Ophthalmol 245, 414-422.
Arnhold, S., Klein, H., Semkova, I., Addicks, K., Schraermeyer, U., 2004. Neurally selected embryonic stem cells induce tumor formation after long-term survival following engraftment into the subretinal space. Invest Ophthalmol Vis Sci 45, 4251-4255.
Asher, R.A., Morgenstern, D.A., Moon, L.D., Fawcett, J.W., 2001. Chondroitin sulphate proteoglycans: inhibitory components of the glial scar. Prog Brain Res 132, 611-619.
Bach, M., Hiss, P., Rover, J., 1988. Check-size specific changes of pattern electroretinogram in patients with early open-angle glaucoma. Doc Ophthalmol 69, 315-322.
Bahr, M., Wizenmann, A., 1996. Retinal ganglion cell axons recognize specific guidance cues present in the deafferented adult rat superior colliculus. J Neurosci 16, 5106-5116.
Baltmr, A., Duggan, J., Nizari, S., Salt, T.E., Cordeiro, M.F., 2010. Neuroprotection in glaucoma - Is there a future role? Exp Eye Res 91, 554-566.
Banin, E., Obolensky, A., Idelson, M., Hemo, I., Reinhardtz, E., Pikarsky, E., Ben-Hur, T., Reubinoff, B., 2006. Retinal incorporation and differentiation of neural precursors derived from human embryonic stem cells. Stem Cells 24, 246-257.
Bernardos, R.L., Barthel, L.K., Meyers, J.R., Raymond, P.A., 2007. Late-stage neuronal progenitors in the retina are radial Muller glia that function as retinal stem cells. J Neurosci 27, 7028-7040.
Bertrand, J., Winton, M.J., Rodriguez-Hernandez, N., Campenot, R.B., McKerracher, L., 2005. Application of Rho antagonist to neuronal cell bodies promotes neurite growth in compartmented cultures and regeneration of retinal ganglion cell axons in the optic nerve of adult rats. J Neurosci 25, 1113-1121.
Bhatia, B., Singhal, S., Lawrence, J.M., Khaw, P.T., Limb, G.A., 2009. Distribution of Muller stem cells within the neural retina: evidence for the existence of a ciliary margin-like zone in the adult human eye. Exp Eye Res 89, 373-382.
Bhatia, B., Singhal, S., Tadman, D.N., Khaw, P.T., Limb, G.A., 2011. SOX2 is required for adult human muller stem cell survival and maintenance of progenicity in vitro. Invest Ophthalmol Vis Sci 52, 136-145.
Bibel, M., Richter, J., Schrenk, K., Tucker, K.L., Staiger, V., Korte, M., Goetz, M., Barde, Y.A., 2004. Differentiation of mouse embryonic stem cells into a defined neuronal lineage. Nat Neurosci 7, 1003-1009.
Billingham, R.E., Brent, L., Medawar, P.B., 1953. Actively acquired tolerance of foreign cells. Nature 172, 603-606.
Bradbury, E.J., Moon, L.D., Popat, R.J., King, V.R., Bennett, G.S., Patel, P.N., Fawcett, J.W., McMahon, S.B., 2002. Chondroitinase ABC promotes functional recovery after spinal cord injury. Nature 416, 636-640.

Bull, N.D., Irvine, K.A., Franklin, R.J., Martin, K.R., 2009. Transplanted oligodendrocyte precursor cells reduce neurodegeneration in a model of glaucoma. Invest Ophthalmol Vis Sci 50, 4244-4253.

Bull, N.D., Limb, G.A., Martin, K.R., 2008. Human Muller stem cell (MIO-M1) transplantation in a rat model of glaucoma: survival, differentiation, and integration. Invest Ophthalmol Vis Sci 49, 3449-3456.

Bunce, C., Xing, W., Wormald, R., 2010. Causes of blind and partial sight certifications in England and Wales: April 2007-March 2008. Eye (Lond) 24, 1692-1699.

Chacko, D.M., Das, A.V., Zhao, X., James, J., Bhattacharya, S., Ahmad, I., 2003. Transplantation of ocular stem cells: the role of injury in incorporation and differentiation of grafted cells in the retina. Vision Res 43, 937-946.

Chen, M., Chen, Q., Sun, X., Shen, W., Liu, B., Zhong, X., Leng, Y., Li, C., Zhang, W., Chai, F., Huang, B., Gao, Q., Xiang, A.P., Zhuo, Y., Ge, J., 2010. Generation of retinal ganglion-like cells from reprogrammed mouse fibroblasts. Invest Ophthalmol Vis Sci 51, 5970-5978.

Cho, K.J., Trzaska, K.A., Greco, S.J., McArdle, J., Wang, F.S., Ye, J.H., Rameshwar, P., 2005. Neurons derived from human mesenchymal stem cells show synaptic transmission and can be induced to produce the neurotransmitter substance P by interleukin-1 alpha. Stem Cells 23, 383-391.

Corti, S., Locatelli, F., Papadimitriou, D., Del Bo, R., Nizzardo, M., Nardini, M., Donadoni, C., Salani, S., Fortunato, F., Strazzer, S., Bresolin, N., Comi, G.P., 2007. Neural stem cells LewisX+ CXCR4+ modify disease progression in an amyotrophic lateral sclerosis model. Brain 130, 1289-1305.

Danesh-Meyer, H.V., 2011. Neuroprotection in glaucoma: recent and future directions. Curr Opin Ophthalmol 22, 78-86.

Dawson, M.R., Polito, A., Levine, J.M., Reynolds, R., 2003. NG2-expressing glial progenitor cells: an abundant and widespread population of cycling cells in the adult rat CNS. Mol Cell Neurosci 24, 476-488.

Ebneter, A., Casson, R.J., Wood, J.P., Chidlow, G., 2010. Microglial activation in the visual pathway in experimental glaucoma: spatiotemporal characterization and correlation with axonal injury. Invest Ophthalmol Vis Sci 51, 6448-6460.

Erskine, L., Herrera, E., 2007. The retinal ganglion cell axon's journey: insights into molecular mechanisms of axon guidance. Dev Biol 308, 1-14.

Evans, M.J., Kaufman, M.H., 1981. Establishment in culture of pluripotential cells from mouse embryos. Nature 292, 154-156.

Fariss, R.N., Li, Z.Y., Milam, A.H., 2000. Abnormalities in rod photoreceptors, amacrine cells, and horizontal cells in human retinas with retinitis pigmentosa. Am J Ophthalmol 129, 215-223.

Felling, R.J., Levison, S.W., 2003. Enhanced neurogenesis following stroke. J Neurosci Res 73, 277-283.

Fimbel, S.M., Montgomery, J.E., Burket, C.T., Hyde, D.R., 2007. Regeneration of inner retinal neurons after intravitreal injection of ouabain in zebrafish. J Neurosci 27, 1712-1724.

Frishman, L.J., Shen, F.F., Du, L., Robson, J.G., Harwerth, R.S., Smith, E.L., 3rd, Carter-Dawson, L., Crawford, M.L., 1996. The scotopic electroretinogram of macaque after retinal ganglion cell loss from experimental glaucoma. Invest Ophthalmol Vis Sci 37, 125-141.

Goldberg, J.L., Klassen, M.P., Hua, Y., Barres, B.A., 2002. Amacrine-signaled loss of intrinsic axon growth ability by retinal ganglion cells. Science 296, 1860-1864.

Guo, L., Moss, S.E., Alexander, R.A., Ali, R.R., Fitzke, F.W., Cordeiro, M.F., 2005. Retinal ganglion cell apoptosis in glaucoma is related to intraocular pressure and IOP-induced effects on extracellular matrix. Invest Ophthalmol Vis Sci 46, 175-182.

Gust, J., Reh, T.A., 2011. Adult donor rod photoreceptors integrate into the mature mouse retina. Invest Ophthalmol Vis Sci.

Hara, A., Taguchi, A., Aoki, H., Hatano, Y., Niwa, M., Yamada, Y., Kunisada, T., 2010. Folate antagonist, methotrexate induces neuronal differentiation of human embryonic stem cells transplanted into nude mouse retina. Neurosci Lett 477, 138-143.

Hasegawa, S., Abe, H., 2001. Mapping of glaucomatous visual field defects by multifocal VEPs. Invest Ophthalmol Vis Sci 42, 3341-3348.

Hemmati-Brivanlou, A., Melton, D., 1997. Vertebrate embryonic cells will become nerve cells unless told otherwise. Cell 88, 13-17.

Hentze, H., Graichen, R., Colman, A., 2007. Cell therapy and the safety of embryonic stem cell-derived grafts. Trends Biotechnol 25, 24-32.

Hernandez, M., Rodriguez, F.D., Sharma, S.C., Vecino, E., 2009. Immunohistochemical changes in rat retinas at various time periods of elevated intraocular pressure. Mol Vis 15, 2696-2709.

Hirano, M., Yamamoto, A., Yoshimura, N., Tokunaga, T., Motohashi, T., Ishizaki, K., Yoshida, H., Okazaki, K., Yamazaki, H., Hayashi, S., Kunisada, T., 2003. Generation of structures formed by lens and retinal cells differentiating from embryonic stem cells. Dev Dyn 228, 664-671.

Holder, G.E., Brigell, M.G., Hawlina, M., Meigen, T., Vaegan, Bach, M., 2007. ISCEV standard for clinical pattern electroretinography--2007 update. Doc Ophthalmol 114, 111-116.

Hou, S.T., Jiang, S.X., Smith, R.A., 2008. Permissive and repulsive cues and signalling pathways of axonal outgrowth and regeneration. Int Rev Cell Mol Biol 267, 125-181.

Huang, T.L., Chang, C.H., Lin, K.H., Sheu, M.M., Tsai, R.K., 2011. Lack of protective effect of local administration of triamcinolone or systemic treatment with methylprednisolone against damages caused by optic nerve crush in rats. Exp Eye Res 92, 112-119.

Inoue, Y., Iriyama, A., Ueno, S., Takahashi, H., Kondo, M., Tamaki, Y., Araie, M., Yanagi, Y., 2007. Subretinal transplantation of bone marrow mesenchymal stem cells delays retinal degeneration in the RCS rat model of retinal degeneration. Exp Eye Res 85, 234-241.

Jagatha, B., Divya, M.S., Sanalkumar, R., Indulekha, C.L., Vidyanand, S., Divya, T.S., Das, A.V., James, J., 2009. In vitro differentiation of retinal ganglion-like cells from embryonic stem cell derived neural progenitors. Biochem Biophys Res Commun 380, 230-235.

Jalving, M., Shepers, H., 2009. Induced pluripotent stem cells: will they be safe? Curr Opin Mol Ther 11, 383-393.

Johnson, T.V., Bull, N.D., Hunt, D.P., Marina, N., Tomarev, S.I., Martin, K.R., 2010a. Neuroprotective effects of intravitreal mesenchymal stem cell transplantation in experimental glaucoma. Invest Ophthalmol Vis Sci 51, 2051-2059.

Johnson, T.V., Bull, N.D., Martin, K.R., 2010b. Identification of barriers to retinal engraftment of transplanted stem cells. Invest Ophthalmol Vis Sci 51, 960-970.

Karussis, D., Kassis, I., Kurkalli, B.G., Slavin, S., 2008. Immunomodulation and neuroprotection with mesenchymal bone marrow stem cells (MSCs): a proposed

treatment for multiple sclerosis and other neuroimmunological/neurodegenerative diseases. J Neurol Sci 265, 131-135.
Kerrigan-Baumrind, L.A., Quigley, H.A., Pease, M.E., Kerrigan, D.F., Mitchell, R.S., 2000. Number of ganglion cells in glaucoma eyes compared with threshold visual field tests in the same persons. Invest Ophthalmol Vis Sci 41, 741-748.
Klistorner, A.I., Graham, S.L., Martins, A., 2000. Multifocal pattern electroretinogram does not demonstrate localised field defects in glaucoma. Doc Ophthalmol 100, 155-165.
Koprivica, V., Cho, K.S., Park, J.B., Yiu, G., Atwal, J., Gore, B., Kim, J.A., Lin, E., Tessier-Lavigne, M., Chen, D.F., He, Z., 2005. EGFR activation mediates inhibition of axon regeneration by myelin and chondroitin sulfate proteoglycans. Science 310, 106-110.
Korth, M., Nguyen, N.X., Horn, F., Martus, P., 1994. Scotopic threshold response and scotopic PII in glaucoma. Invest Ophthalmol Vis Sci 35, 619-625.
Krabbe, C., Zimmer, J., Meyer, M., 2005. Neural transdifferentiation of mesenchymal stem cells--a critical review. APMIS 113, 831-844.
Labouyrie, E., Dubus, P., Groppi, A., Mahon, F.X., Ferrer, J., Parrens, M., Reiffers, J., de Mascarel, A., Merlio, J.P., 1999. Expression of neurotrophins and their receptors in human bone marrow. Am J Pathol 154, 405-415.
Lamba, D.A., Karl, M.O., Ware, C.B., Reh, T.A., 2006. Efficient generation of retinal progenitor cells from human embryonic stem cells. Proc Natl Acad Sci U S A 103, 12769-12774.
Lawrence, J.M., Singhal, S., Bhatia, B., Keegan, D.J., Reh, T.A., Luthert, P.J., Khaw, P.T., Limb, G.A., 2007. MIO-M1 cells and similar muller glial cell lines derived from adult human retina exhibit neural stem cell characteristics. Stem Cells 25, 2033-2043.
Leaver, S.G., Harvey, A.R., Plant, G.W., 2006. Adult olfactory ensheathing glia promote the long-distance growth of adult retinal ganglion cell neurites in vitro. Glia 53, 467-476.
Levkovitch-Verbin, H., Sadan, O., Vander, S., Rosner, M., Barhum, Y., Melamed, E., Offen, D., Melamed, S., 2010. Intravitreal injections of neurotrophic factors secreting mesenchymal stem cells are neuroprotective in rat eyes following optic nerve transection. Invest Ophthalmol Vis Sci 51, 6394-6400.
Li, Y., Li, D., Khaw, P.T., Raisman, G., 2008. Transplanted olfactory ensheathing cells incorporated into the optic nerve head ensheathe retinal ganglion cell axons: possible relevance to glaucoma. Neurosci Lett 440, 251-254.
Li, Y., Sauve, Y., Li, D., Lund, R.D., Raisman, G., 2003. Transplanted olfactory ensheathing cells promote regeneration of cut adult rat optic nerve axons. J Neurosci 23, 7783-7788.
Limb, G.A., Salt, T.E., Munro, P.M., Moss, S.E., Khaw, P.T., 2002. In vitro characterization of a spontaneously immortalized human Muller cell line (MIO-M1). Invest Ophthalmol Vis Sci 43, 864-869.
Liu, Y., Gong, Z., Liu, L., Sun, H., 2010. Combined effect of olfactory ensheathing cell (OEC) transplantation and glial cell line-derived neurotrophic factor (GDNF) intravitreal injection on optic nerve injury in rats. Mol Vis 16, 2903-2910.
Logan, A., Ahmed, Z., Baird, A., Gonzalez, A.M., Berry, M., 2006. Neurotrophic factor synergy is required for neuronal survival and disinhibited axon regeneration after CNS injury. Brain 129, 490-502.
Lorber, B., Howe, M.L., Benowitz, L.I., Irwin, N., 2009. Mst3b, an Ste20-like kinase, regulates axon regeneration in mature CNS and PNS pathways. Nat Neurosci 12, 1407-1414.

Lu, B., Wang, S., Girman, S., McGill, T., Ragaglia, V., Lund, R., 2010. Human adult bone marrow-derived somatic cells rescue vision in a rodent model of retinal degeneration. Exp Eye Res 91, 449-455.

Machida, S., Raz-Prag, D., Fariss, R.N., Sieving, P.A., Bush, R.A., 2008. Photopic ERG negative response from amacrine cell signaling in RCS rat retinal degeneration. Invest Ophthalmol Vis Sci 49, 442-452.

MacLaren, R.E., Pearson, R.A., MacNeil, A., Douglas, R.H., Salt, T.E., Akimoto, M., Swaroop, A., Sowden, J.C., Ali, R.R., 2006. Retinal repair by transplantation of photoreceptor precursors. Nature 444, 203-207.

Marmor, M.F., Fulton, A.B., Holder, G.E., Miyake, Y., Brigell, M., Bach, M., 2009. ISCEV Standard for full-field clinical electroretinography (2008 update). Doc Ophthalmol 118, 69-77.

Martin, K.R., Quigley, H.A., Zack, D.J., Levkovitch-Verbin, H., Kielczewski, J., Valenta, D., Baumrind, L., Pease, M.E., Klein, R.L., Hauswirth, W.W., 2003. Gene therapy with brain-derived neurotrophic factor as a protection: retinal ganglion cells in a rat glaucoma model. Invest Ophthalmol Vis Sci 44, 4357-4365.

McLaughlin, T., O'Leary, D.D., 2005. Molecular gradients and development of retinotopic maps. Annu Rev Neurosci 28, 327-355.

Merkle, F.T., Tramontin, A.D., Garcia-Verdugo, J.M., Alvarez-Buylla, A., 2004. Radial glia give rise to adult neural stem cells in the subventricular zone. Proc Natl Acad Sci U S A 101, 17528-17532.

Meyer, J.S., Katz, M.L., Maruniak, J.A., Kirk, M.D., 2006. Embryonic stem cell-derived neural progenitors incorporate into degenerating retina and enhance survival of host photoreceptors. Stem Cells 24, 274-283.

Monteiro, M.L., Hokazono, K., Cunha, L.P., Oyamada, M.K., 2011. Multifocal pattern electroretinography for the detection of neural loss in eyes with permanent temporal hemianopia or quadrantanopia from chiasmal compression. Br J Ophthalmol.

Moon, S.H., Kim, J.S., Park, S.J., Lim, J.J., Lee, H.J., Lee, S.M., Chung, H.M., 2011. Effect of chromosome instability on the maintenance and differentiation of human embryonic stem cells in vitro and in vivo. Stem Cell Res 6, 50-59.

Much, J.W., Liu, C., Piltz-Seymour, J.R., 2008. Long-term Survival of Central Visual Field in End-Stage Glaucoma. Ophthalmology 115, 1162-1166.

Nakagawa, M., Koyanagi, M., Tanabe, K., Takahashi, K., Ichisaka, T., Aoi, T., Okita, K., Mochiduki, Y., Takizawa, N., Yamanaka, S., 2008. Generation of induced pluripotent stem cells without Myc from mouse and human fibroblasts. Nat Biotechnol 26, 101-106.

Naylor, M., Bowen, K.K., Sailor, K.A., Dempsey, R.J., Vemuganti, R., 2005. Preconditioning-induced ischemic tolerance stimulates growth factor expression and neurogenesis in adult rat hippocampus. Neurochem Int 47, 565-572.

Ninomiya, M., Yamashita, T., Araki, N., Okano, H., Sawamoto, K., 2006. Enhanced neurogenesis in the ischemic striatum following EGF-induced expansion of transit-amplifying cells in the subventricular zone. Neurosci Lett 403, 63-67.

Nomura, T., Honmou, O., Harada, K., Houkin, K., Hamada, H., Kocsis, J.D., 2005. I.V. infusion of brain-derived neurotrophic factor gene-modified human mesenchymal stem cells protects against injury in a cerebral ischemia model in adult rat. Neuroscience 136, 161-169.

Nunes, M.C., Roy, N.S., Keyoung, H.M., Goodman, R.R., McKhann, G., 2nd, Jiang, L., Kang, J., Nedergaard, M., Goldman, S.A., 2003. Identification and isolation of multipotential neural progenitor cells from the subcortical white matter of the adult human brain. Nat Med 9, 439-447.

Odom, J.V., Bach, M., Brigell, M., Holder, G.E., McCulloch, D.L., Tormene, A.P., Vaegan, 2010. ISCEV standard for clinical visual evoked potentials (2009 update). Doc Ophthalmol 120, 111-119.

Okita, K., Nakagawa, M., Hyenjong, H., Ichisaka, T., Yamanaka, S., 2008. Generation of mouse induced pluripotent stem cells without viral vectors. Science 322, 949-953.

Osakada, F., Ikeda, H., Sasai, Y., Takahashi, M., 2009. Stepwise differentiation of pluripotent stem cells into retinal cells. Nat Protoc 4, 811-824.

Parameswaran, S., Balasubramanian, S., Babai, N., Qiu, F., Eudy, J.D., Thoreson, W.B., Ahmad, I., 2010. Induced pluripotent stem cells generate both retinal ganglion cells and photoreceptors: therapeutic implications in degenerative changes in glaucoma and age-related macular degeneration. Stem Cells 28, 695-703.

Parr, A.M., Tator, C.H., Keating, A., 2007. Bone marrow-derived mesenchymal stromal cells for the repair of central nervous system injury. Bone Marrow Transplant 40, 609-619.

Payne, N., Siatskas, C., Barnard, A., Bernard, C.C., 2011. The prospect of stem cells as multi-faceted purveyors of immune modulation, repair and regeneration in multiple sclerosis. Curr Stem Cell Res Ther 6, 50-62.

Pease, M.E., McKinnon, S.J., Quigley, H.A., Kerrigan-Baumrind, L.A., Zack, D.J., 2000. Obstructed axonal transport of BDNF and its receptor TrkB in experimental glaucoma. Invest Ophthalmol Vis Sci 41, 764-774.

Pease, M.E., Zack, D.J., Berlinicke, C., Bloom, K., Cone, F., Wang, Y., Klein, R.L., Hauswirth, W.W., Quigley, H.A., 2009. Effect of CNTF on retinal ganglion cell survival in experimental glaucoma. Invest Ophthalmol Vis Sci 50, 2194-2200.

Pitchford, S.C., Furze, R.C., Jones, C.P., Wengner, A.M., Rankin, S.M., 2009. Differential mobilization of subsets of progenitor cells from the bone marrow. Cell Stem Cell 4, 62-72.

Plant, G.W., Harvey, A.R., Leaver, S.G., Lee, S.V., 2010. Olfactory ensheathing glia: Repairing injury to the mammalian visual system. Exp Neurol.

Pluchino, S., Zanotti, L., Rossi, B., Brambilla, E., Ottoboni, L., Salani, G., Martinello, M., Cattalini, A., Bergami, A., Furlan, R., Comi, G., Constantin, G., Martino, G., 2005. Neurosphere-derived multipotent precursors promote neuroprotection by an immunomodulatory mechanism. Nature 436, 266-271.

Quigley, H.A., Broman, A.T., 2006. The number of people with glaucoma worldwide in 2010 and 2020. Br J Ophthalmol 90, 262-267.

Quigley, H.A., Green, W.R., 1979. The histology of human glaucoma cupping and optic nerve damage: clinicopathologic correlation in 21 eyes. Ophthalmology 86, 1803-1830.

Ramon-Cueto, A., Valverde, F., 1995. Olfactory bulb ensheathing glia: a unique cell type with axonal growth-promoting properties. Glia 14, 163-173.

Resnikoff, S., Pascolini, D., Etya'ale, D., Kocur, I., Pararajasegaram, R., Pokharel, G.P., Mariotti, S.P., 2004. Global data on visual impairment in the year 2002. Bull World Health Organ 82, 844-851.

Sasaki, M., Hains, B.C., Lankford, K.L., Waxman, S.G., Kocsis, J.D., 2006. Protection of corticospinal tract neurons after dorsal spinal cord transection and engraftment of olfactory ensheathing cells. Glia 53, 352-359.

Seiler, M.J., Aramant, R.B., Thomas, B.B., Peng, Q., Sadda, S.R., Keirstead, H.S., 2010. Visual restoration and transplant connectivity in degenerate rats implanted with retinal progenitor sheets. Eur J Neurosci 31, 508-520.

Selles-Navarro, I., Ellezam, B., Fajardo, R., Latour, M., McKerracher, L., 2001. Retinal ganglion cell and nonneuronal cell responses to a microcrush lesion of adult rat optic nerve. Exp Neurol 167, 282-289.

Sieving, P.A., 1991. Retinal Ganglion-Cell Loss Does Not Abolish the Scotopic Threshold Response (STR) of the Cat and Human ERG. Clinical Vision Sciences 6, 149-158.

Singhal, S., Jayaram, H., Bhatia, B., Salt, T.E., Khaw, P.T., Limb, G.A., 2009. Retinal Ganglion Cell (RGC) Precursors Derived From Adult Human Muller Stem Cells Exhibit Neural Function in vitro and Partially Restore RGC Function in vivo. Invest. Ophthalmol. Vis. Sci. 50, 5138-.

Singhal, S., Lawrence, J.M., Bhatia, B., Ellis, J.S., Kwan, A.S., Macneil, A., Luthert, P.J., Fawcett, J.W., Perez, M.T., Khaw, P.T., Limb, G.A., 2008. Chondroitin sulfate proteoglycans and microglia prevent migration and integration of grafted Muller stem cells into degenerating retina. Stem Cells 26, 1074-1082.

Singhal, S., Lawrence, J.M., Salt, T.E., Khaw, P.T., Limb, G.A., 2010. Triamcinolone attenuates macrophage/microglia accumulation associated with NMDA-induced RGC death and facilitates survival of Muller stem cell grafts. Exp Eye Res 90, 308-315.

Stiefelmeyer, S., Neubauer, A.S., Berninger, T., Arden, G.B., Rudolph, G., 2004. The multifocal pattern electroretinogram in glaucoma. Vision Res 44, 103-112.

Su, Y., Wang, F., Teng, Y., Zhao, S.G., Cui, H., Pan, S.H., 2009. Axonal regeneration of optic nerve after crush in Nogo66 receptor knockout mice. Neurosci Lett 460, 223-226.

Su, Z., He, C., 2010. Olfactory ensheathing cells: biology in neural development and regeneration. Prog Neurobiol 92, 517-532.

Suzuki, T., Akimoto, M., Imai, H., Ueda, Y., Mandai, M., Yoshimura, N., Swaroop, A., Takahashi, M., 2007. Chondroitinase ABC treatment enhances synaptogenesis between transplant and host neurons in model of retinal degeneration. Cell Transplant 16, 493-503.

Suzuki, T., Mandai, M., Akimoto, M., Yoshimura, N., Takahashi, M., 2006. The simultaneous treatment of MMP-2 stimulants in retinal transplantation enhances grafted cell migration into the host retina. Stem Cells 24, 2406-2411.

Tabata, Y., Ouchi, Y., Kamiya, H., Manabe, T., Arai, K., Watanabe, S., 2004. Specification of the retinal fate of mouse embryonic stem cells by ectopic expression of Rx/rax, a homeobox gene. Mol Cell Biol 24, 4513-4521.

Takahashi, K., Yamanaka, S., 2006. Induction of pluripotent stem cells from mouse embryonic and adult fibroblast cultures by defined factors. Cell 126, 663-676.

Torrente, Y., Polli, E., 2008. Mesenchymal stem cell transplantation for neurodegenerative diseases. Cell Transplant 17, 1103-1113.

Turner, D.L., Cepko, C.L., 1987. A common progenitor for neurons and glia persists in rat retina late in development. Nature 328, 131-136.

Uy, G.L., Rettig, M.P., Cashen, A.F., 2008. Plerixafor, a CXCR4 antagonist for the mobilization of hematopoietic stem cells. Expert Opin Biol Ther 8, 1797-1804.

Ver Hoeve, J.N., Danilov, Y.P., Kim, C.B., Spear, P.D., 1999. VEP and PERG acuity in anesthetized young adult rhesus monkeys. Vis Neurosci 16, 607-617.

Vidal-Sanz, M., Bray, G.M., Aguayo, A.J., 1991. Regenerated synapses persist in the superior colliculus after the regrowth of retinal ganglion cell axons. J Neurocytol 20, 940-952.

Viswanathan, S., Frishman, L.J., Robson, J.G., Harwerth, R.S., Smith, E.L., 3rd, 1999. The photopic negative response of the macaque electroretinogram: reduction by experimental glaucoma. Invest Ophthalmol Vis Sci 40, 1124-1136.

Wang, L., Zhang, Z.G., Zhang, R.L., Gregg, S.R., Hozeska-Solgot, A., LeTourneau, Y., Wang, Y., Chopp, M., 2006. Matrix metalloproteinase 2 (MMP2) and MMP9 secreted by erythropoietin-activated endothelial cells promote neural progenitor cell migration. J Neurosci 26, 5996-6003.

Wanger, P., Persson, H.E., 1983. Pattern-reversal electroretinograms in unilateral glaucoma. Invest Ophthalmol Vis Sci 24, 749-753.

Warfvinge, K., Kamme, C., Englund, U., Wictorin, K., 2001. Retinal integration of grafts of brain-derived precursor cell lines implanted subretinally into adult, normal rats. Exp Neurol 169, 1-12.

Watanabe, M., Toyama, Y., Nishiyama, A., 2002. Differentiation of proliferated NG2-positive glial progenitor cells in a remyelinating lesion. J Neurosci Res 69, 826-836.

Wernig, M., Meissner, A., Foreman, R., Brambrink, T., Ku, M., Hochedlinger, K., Bernstein, B.E., Jaenisch, R., 2007. In vitro reprogramming of fibroblasts into a pluripotent ES-cell-like state. Nature 448, 318-324.

West, E.L., Pearson, R.A., Barker, S.E., Luhmann, U.F., Maclaren, R.E., Barber, A.C., Duran, Y., Smith, A.J., Sowden, J.C., Ali, R.R., 2010. Long-term survival of photoreceptors transplanted into the adult murine neural retina requires immune modulation. Stem Cells 28, 1997-2007.

Wilkins, A., Chandran, S., Compston, A., 2001. A role for oligodendrocyte-derived IGF-1 in trophic support of cortical neurons. Glia 36, 48-57.

Wojciechowski, A.B., Englund, U., Lundberg, C., Warfvinge, K., 2004. Survival and long distance migration of brain-derived precursor cells transplanted to adult rat retina. Stem Cells 22, 27-38.

Wong, E.V., David, S., Jacob, M.H., Jay, D.G., 2003. Inactivation of myelin-associated glycoprotein enhances optic nerve regeneration. J Neurosci 23, 3112-3117.

Wu, M.M., Fan, D.G., Tadmori, I., Yang, H., Furman, M., Jiao, X.Y., Young, W., Sun, D., You, S.W., 2010. Death of axotomized retinal ganglion cells delayed after intraoptic nerve transplantation of olfactory ensheathing cells in adult rats. Cell Transplant 19, 159-166.

Yasuhara, T., Matsukawa, N., Hara, K., Yu, G., Xu, L., Maki, M., Kim, S.U., Borlongan, C.V., 2006. Transplantation of human neural stem cells exerts neuroprotection in a rat model of Parkinson's disease. J Neurosci 26, 12497-12511.

Yin, Y., Henzl, M.T., Lorber, B., Nakazawa, T., Thomas, T.T., Jiang, F., Langer, R., Benowitz, L.I., 2006. Oncomodulin is a macrophage-derived signal for axon regeneration in retinal ganglion cells. Nat Neurosci 9, 843-852.

Yu, S., Tanabe, T., Dezawa, M., Ishikawa, H., Yoshimura, N., 2006. Effects of bone marrow stromal cell injection in an experimental glaucoma model. Biochem Biophys Res Commun 344, 1071-1079.

Yuan, L., Neufeld, A.H., 2001. Activated microglia in the human glaucomatous optic nerve head. J Neurosci Res 64, 523-532.

Zhang, Y., Wang, W., 2010. Effects of bone marrow mesenchymal stem cell transplantation on light-damaged retina. Invest Ophthalmol Vis Sci 51, 3742-3748.

Zuo, J., Neubauer, D., Dyess, K., Ferguson, T.A., Muir, D., 1998. Degradation of chondroitin sulfate proteoglycan enhances the neurite-promoting potential of spinal cord tissue. Exp Neurol 154, 654-662.

16

Functional and Structural Evaluation of Retrobulbar Glaucomateus Damage

Kaya N Engin
Bagcilar Education and Research Hospital,
Department of Ophthalmology Istanbul
Turkey

1. Introduction

Glaucoma represents a group of neurodegenerative diseases characterized by structural damage to the optic nerve and the slow, progressive death of retinal ganglion cells (RGCs). Elevated intraocular pressure (IOP) is traditionally considered to be the most important risk factor for glaucoma, and treatment options for the disease have hitherto been limited to its reduction. However, visual field loss and RGC death continue to occur in patients with well controlled IOPs (Chidlow et al, 2007). Currently, increased IOP has been excluded from the definition of glaucoma, considered a major risk factor, and glaucoma has been defined as an optic neuropathy. Though we have effective medical and surgical therapies at hand, progressive visual loss is still a prevalent symptom in glaucoma cases. Evidence today proves that glaucomatous damage proceeds from RGCs to the brain (Weinreb, 2007).

The ophthalmologist is fully aware that he/she is dealing with the whole visual system -not just the globe, in many neuro-ophthalmic disorders, knowing a defect in the visual field can be due to much pathology from the globe to cortex. Today, we should take areas beyond the retina and optic nerve into consideration in glaucoma follow ups as well. If we recall the anatomy, it is as follows: the retina, optic nerves, optic chiasm, optic tracts, lateral geniculate nuclei (LGN), other brainstem primary visual nuclei (superior colliculus, pretectum), hypothalamic nuclei, pulvinar and accessory optic system, geniculostriate (optic) radiations, striate cortex, visual association areas, and related interhemispheric connections constitute the primary visual sensory system in humans. The optic nerve consists of four segments: intraocular (1 mm in length), intraorbital (about 25 to 30 mm), intracanalicular (about 9 to 10 mm), and intracranial (about 16 mm). Thus, the entire length of the optic nerve from the globe to the optic chiasm is about 5 to 6 cm.

Behind the laminar cribrosa, the optic nerve abruptly increases in diameter from 3 mm to 4 mm in midorbit and to 5 mm intracranially. The optic chiasm derives from the merging of the two optic nerves and sits 10.7 ± 2.4 mm above the dorsum of the sella turcica. Occasionally, the intracranial optic nerves are shorter, and the chiasm may lie directly above the sella in a position that is called "prefixed." More commonly, the optic chiasm is positioned 10 to 12 mm above the insertion of the diaphragma sellae onto the dorsum. The significance of this region arises from the fact that lateral fibers originating from the temporal side of the globe directly pass it, while medial fibers originating from the nasal side cross over to the opposite hemisphere (Figure 1). As the retinofugal fibers pass through the chiasm, they form the optic tracts immediately posterior to the optic chiasm. Each tract begins at the posterior notch of the chiasm and is separated from the other optic tract by the pituitary stalk inferiorly and the third ventricle more superiorly. Most of the fibers in the optic tract terminate in the ipsilateral LGN. With the accessory fibers from other nuclei they form the optic radiation (geniculocalcarine fiber tract) and constitute the "posterior" visual pathway that projects to the primary visual cortex. The primary visual cortex goes by many names, such as striate cortex, area 17, or as used in experimental research, V1. These visual fibers then turn medially above and below the occipital horn to terminate in the mesial surface of the occipital lobe, the striate (calcarine) cortex. The visual cortex extends anteriorly toward the splenium of the corpus callosum and is separated into a superior and an inferior portion by the calcarine fissure, which runs horizontally (Sadun, 2007).

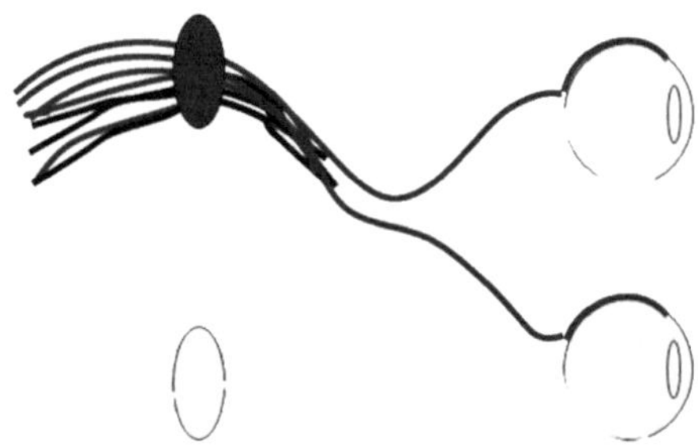

Fig. 1. Cross-over of nasal and temporal fibers in optic chiasm.

2. Glaucoma as a brain disease

2.1 Histopathological studies

Gupta and Yücel have provided primary evidence that glaucomatous damage extends from RGCs to vision centers in the brain. They have observed degenerative and/or neurochemical changes in the LGN, magno-, parvo-, and koniocellular pathways, and changes in metabolic activity in both the LGN and visual cortex in glaucoma (Gupta & Yücel, 2003). The same group elicited many subsequent studies in this area thereafter. In an experimental primate model of unilateral glaucoma, they observed degenerative changes in magnocellular, parvocellular, and koniocellular pathways in the LGN, and these changes are presented in relation to IOP and the severity of optic nerve damage. Neuropathological findings were also present in LGN layers driven by the unaffected fellow eye. Finally, there was information on changes in the visual cortex in relation to varying degrees of RGC loss (Yucel et al, 2003).

The first clinicopathological case of human glaucoma, demonstrating degenerative changes in the brain involving the intracranial optic nerves, LGN, and visual cortex have been reported by the same group. Postmortem specimens of a 79 year old, healthy white male - with a large cup to disc ratio of 0.9, deep excavation and loss of the inferotemporal rim, was compared with 4 controls in the same age group. Optic nerve atrophy in glaucoma compared to control optic nerves was pronounced. Marked axonal loss was also evident inferiorly in the right and left glaucoma optic nerves. Compared to the control, there was striking overall LGN shrinkage in glaucoma. Nissl stained sections showed magnocellular parvocellular neurons with smaller, more globoid cytoplasm and smaller nucleus in glaucoma compared to stellate neurons seen in the controls. Lipofuscin pigment deposits occupied more of the cytoplasm in glaucoma compared to the controls. In the visual cortex

representing the visual field defect, cortical ribbon thickness reduction was easily discernible compared to the controls (Gupta et al, 2006).
They also put forward that numerous similarities exist between glaucoma and neurodegenerative diseases, such as Alzheimer's and Parkinson's disease. Similarities include the selective loss of neuron populations, transsynaptic degeneration in which disease spreads from injured neurons to connected neurons, and common mechanisms of cell injury and death. Mechanisms involved in central visual system damage in glaucoma included oxidative injury and glutamate toxicity, as seen in neurodegenerative diseases. Similar to many neurodegenerative diseases, those changes have been histopathologically proven to be prevented by the use of Memantine (Gupta & Yücel, 2007).
In the light of these studies, the importance of IOP-independent strategies in the treatment of glaucoma increases, while studies for in vivo demonstration of brain damage in patients with glaucoma accelerate. For this purpose, the most commonly used technology is magnetic resonance imaging (MRI).
The first key findings have been obtained with Functional MRI (fMRI). Increases in neuronal activity are accompanied by changes in blood oxygenation that give rise to changes in the MR signal. First, local concentrations of deoxyhemoglobin generate magnetic field gradients along the blood vessels reduce the MR signal. Second, increases in neuronal activity result in decreases in the local oxygen extraction fraction in the blood that, in turn, causes a corresponding drop in the local concentration of deoxyhemoglobin. The net reduction of deoxyhemoglobin during brain activity manifests in an increase in MR signal known as blood oxygenation level dependent (BOLD) signals. Mapping BOLD signals is called "Retinotopic Organisation" (Duncan et al, 2007).
Another important MRI technique for imaging visual pathways is Diffusion-Tensor MRI (DTI). It is based on the movement principle of fluids in a plane connected to the nerve. Water diffusion in biological tissues, such as white matter occurs preferentially parallel to the orientation of axons. Such diffusion is known as anisotropic diffusion which depends on the structural environment of white matter. DTI provides a complete description of water diffusion in three dimensions. Radial ($\lambda 1$) and axial diffusivities ($\lambda 2$, $\lambda 3$) form anisotropy and it is estimated as fractional anisotropy (FA). Axial diffusivities can be expressed as a single value, $\lambda//$. A nerve can be traced with anisotropy maps, a process referred to as "Tractography" (Nucifora et al, 2007) (Figure 2).

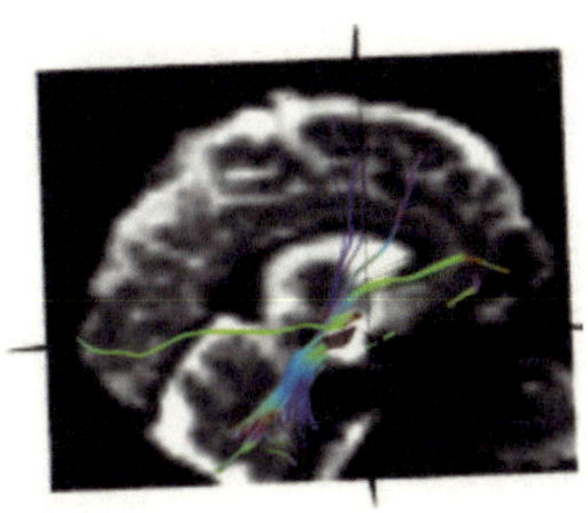

Fig. 2. Imaging nerve fibers with "Tractography" method.

2.2 Animal studies

Retrobulbar neuro-degeneration could be demonstrated in experimental glaucoma models with different MRI techniques. In a rat model of chronic glaucoma, choline reduction in the visual cortex was revealed with proton magnetic resonance spectroscopy. Relative to the creatine level, the choline level was found to be significantly lower in the left glaucomatous visual cortex than the right control visual cortex in all animals. In addition, a marginally significant increase in the glutamate level was observed in the glaucomatous visual cortex. Authors concluded that, measurement of the Cho:Cr reduction in the visual cortex may be a noninvasive biomarker for this disease (Chan et al, 2009).

In a DTI study with 7T MRI, experimental glaucoma was performed on seven rats by substantial photocoagulation of the episcleral and limbal veins of the right eyes with Argon laser, whereas the left eye served as the control. It was shown for the first time that *in vivo* DTI can be successfully applied to detect axonal density changes occurring in the rat model of glaucoma. As much as 10% decrease in axonal density of the glaucomatous ON was detected in enlarged B_0 coronal plane images by an approximately 30% increase in $\lambda 1$ and 5% decrease in FA with no significant change in that of $\lambda//$. In the same study, those findings are also histopathologically confirmed (Hui et al, 2007).

2.3 Retrobulber imaging in humans

The optical nerve is of specific importance since it is among structures heavily influenced by glaucomatous neuro-degeneration and it provides information on the ipsilateral eye. In a study conducted with conventional MRI in patients with glaucoma, it was reported that the diameter of the optic nerve was significantly lower, and that the optic chiasm was shorter in comparison with that of the controls and those findings correlated with deterioration in MD values rather than c/d ratios (Kashiwagi et al, 2004).

In a more recent study, as a biomarker for axonal loss in glaucomatous optic atrophy, the retrobulbar optic nerve was diameter measured by ultrafast high-resolution MRI at 3T. Included in the study was one eye each from 47 subjects, of whom 9 had no eye disease, 16 had preperimetric glaucoma, 11 had a glaucomatous mean visual field defect of <10 dB and 11 of >10 dB. OND was found to be correlated best with the retinal nerve fiber layer thickness measured by an optic coherence tomography (Lagrèze et al, 2009).

Another study was conducted in 26 patients with primary open-angle glaucoma (POAG), and 26 control subjects. In the patient group, the presence of white matter hyperintensities (WMH) was evaluated more on fluid-attenuated inversion recovery images of the brain. Both the area of the optic nerves and the magnetisation transfer ratio (MTR) measured in the chiasm and in the grey and white matter of the calcarine fissure were lower. Authors used Conventional MRI and magnetisation transfer imaging of the brain and optic pathway and concluded that, POAG leads to optic nerve atrophy and degeneration of the optic pathway. The finding of the increase in the number of WMH implies that cerebrovascular disease may play a role in the pathogenesis of POAG (Kitsos et al, 2009).

One of most important techniques in the structural evaluation of nervous tissue is DTI. The optical tract in humans could be imaged from CGL to calcarine sulcus using this method (Sherbondy et al, 2008). Garaci et al. examined glaucomatous damage in humans over 16 patients with POAG and 10 control subjects. Sixteen patients with POAG were examined. Glaucoma severity was clinically assessed with the use of a six-stage system based on static threshold visual field parameters. DTI was performed with a 3-T MR unit. Mean diffusivity (MD) and fractional anisotropy (FA) maps were automatically created. Regions of interest were positioned in three spots for each evaluation. They found that, the optic radiations and optic nerves of patients with glaucoma, compared to the control subjects, had significantly

higher MD and significantly lower FA. A negative correlation between the mean FA for the optic nerves and glaucoma stage was reported (Garaci et al, 2009). Optic radiations were evaluated in another DTI study conducted with a 3T high-field magnetic resonance scanner in 50 glaucoma patients and 50 healthy age-matched controls in which anterograde and retrograde transneuronal rarefaction of the optic radiation were reported (Engelhorn et al, 2011)
The study emphasizing the importance of functionally examining the optical pathways in terms of glaucoma was conducted by Duncan et al. This study, which was first to in vivo confirm of interconnection between glaucoma and the brain, also used the 3T MRI and fMRI technique. Six asymmetric POAG patients with one glaucomatous eye and a less affected "fellow" eye were included. Patients' fellow eyes had markedly fewer visual field abnormalities relative to the glaucomatous eye. A long and complicated stimulus was given to the patients in three sessions to produce neuronal activity. The template fitting technique was used to project patterns of visual field loss onto the cortex. A comparison was made between the BOLD responses to the scotoma-mapping stimulus and the PSD from visual field testing for each patient yielding PSDDIF scores. A "pointwise" comparison of thresholds throughout the visual field to fMRI responses in corresponding locations of V1 was also conducted. They demonstrated that the pattern of VF loss observed using SAP is reflected by the pattern of BOLD activity in V1, and fMRI responses correlate with visual function thresholds (Duncan et al, 2007).
With a similar methodology, decreased cortical activity in the primary visual cortex of cases with POAG have been reported once again. The resultant cortical depression is stated to be unrelated to interocular differences in results of polarimetry, OCT, and ophthalmoscopy, but is negatively correlated with PSD of visual field analysis (Qing et al, 2010).
Imaging of CGL constitutes a great challenge. Arterial Spin Labeling fMRI -which provides direct measures of functional cerebral blood flow (CBF) changes, was used by Lu et al. in five healthy subjects. In this study, the baseline CBF in each LGN was estimated by averaging the signal measured during the off period (e.g. lack of hemispheric stimulus) for that LGN (Lu et al, 2008).
The Occipital Proton MR Spectroscopy technique, which detects low levels of N-Acetylaspartate in cortex areas receiving poor stimulation, was tried in patients with glaucoma and age-dependent macula degeneration. However, on the contrary to the above mentioned animal study, a reduction in metabolite levels in areas matching the progressive visual field in those patients could not be observed (Boucard et al, 2007).

3. Clinical evaluation of glaucomatous neuro-degeneration

3.1 Introduction

Above, we mentioned the possibilities provided by recent medicine via retrobulbar glaucomatous damage and the compatibility of resultant structural and functional findings with each other and histopathological and animal studies. In recent practice, we most frequently use Optical Coherence Tomography (OCT) and Visual Fields (VF), in decreasing order, in order to structurally and functionally examine glaucomatous damage in the eye. We have current knowledge regarding either advantages and disadvanteges of these two techniques or congruity of the data obtained. Although VF have been known to be a subjective method in glaucoma follow-ups, studies in large series revealed that OCT also possesses its own individual variability. Three factors that contribute to Retinal Nerve Fiber Layer (RNFL) variability in this range were identified. First, diseases of the inner retina can contribute to artifactual thickening in some patients. Second, the individual variation in the visual field to disc mapping plays a role. Finally, the location of blood vessels, as well as the degree to which they are included by the RNFL algorithm, affects variability. Therefore, there is a considerable variability in the relationship between structure and function in glaucoma, even when care is taken to ensure that the data are of the highest quality (Hood et al, 2009). In addition, myopia (Rauscher et al, 2009) and the OCT technology used (Knight et al, 2009) are included in other variables. RNFL thickness, on the other hand, consists of two parts: RGC axons and nonaxon portion. Hood et al. assumes that the loss in the thickness of the axon portion is proportional to local field sensitivity loss, when field loss is expressed on a linear scale. That is, a 3-dB loss is associated, on average, with a loss of one half of the axon portion of the RNFL thickness, whereas the nonaxon portion is assumed to remain constant with RGC loss (Hood et al, 2007). However, the recently recognized approach is that glaucomatous damage affects both structure and function in linear proportion (Hood et al, 2009; Knight et al, 2009).

In our study, we examined the glaucoma - brain relation using a 1.5 T MRI device, which was in clinical use, and with DTI-MRI in terms of structure and with fMRI in terms of function; moreover, we examined those techniques with OCT and VF, respectively. In this manner, we aimed to non-invasively and comprehensively demonstrate eye - brain connection in glaucoma in humans, develop a method convenient for clinical use in order to use both in the diagnosis and follow-up of glaucoma and in studies with large case series, and finally to establish a strong reference for studies on the pathogenesis, follow-up and treatment of glaucoma.

3.2 Material and method

The eyes of an asymmetrical glaucoma patient and a healthy subject are included in this study. Care was taken that the control subject and patient did not have any known additional ocular, neurological or systemic diseases. Flow analysis was performed with color Doppler ultrasonography in the carotid, ophthalmic, posterior ciliar and central retinal arteries in order to eliminate ischemic pathology. While the central VF and MD and PSD values of the patient were recorded for functional analysis, retrobulbar assessment was performed with fMRI. Structural analyzes were completed by comparing c/d ratios with OCT and mean RNFL and ganglion cell (GCC) values with DTI. While the bilateral eyes of the patient were compared with each other and with the control, compatibility between structural and functional analyzes of globe and optic pathways was also evaluated.

DTI imaging

Imaging was performed with a 1.5 T Avanto Siemens (Erlangen, Germany) MRI device in Bakırköy Dr. Sadi Konuk Training and Research Hospital. Imaging protocol consisted of obtaining a high resolution T1 weighed (1x1x1mm) MPRAGE sequence, and fMRI time series images and diffusion weighed images, which are necessary for diffusion tensor imaging (DTI). For DTI, diffusion weighed images in 30 different directions and with 2 different b values (b=0,1000) were obtained. Imaging parameters were determined as TR=8200ms, TE=90ms, 2 mean, 3x3x3 isotropic voxel dimensions, a total of 60 slices and imaging duration of approximately 8 minutes. Diffusion weighed images were first separated from non-brain sections using FSL software. Using MedINRIA software on those images, diffusion tensor maps and fiber tractographs were created. Moreover, magnification was applied on b0 coronal plane images obtained from the same region and optic nerve morphologies were also evaluated on this plane (Figure 3).

DTI data analysis

A ROI (region on interest) 3 mm distance from the optic nerve was selected (Figure 4) and DTI parametric characteristic values (λ1, λ2, λ3) of the optic nerve were calculated. Using those measurements, FA and MD values were also estimated using formulas.

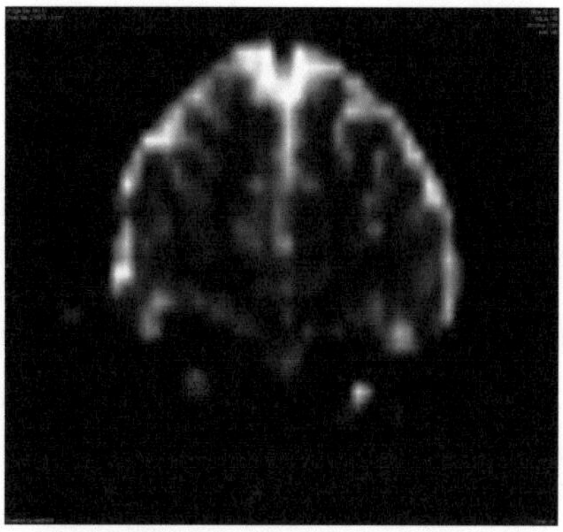

Fig. 3. Imaging optic nerve on b0 coronal plane images.

$$FA = \frac{\sqrt{3\left[(\lambda_1 - \langle\lambda\rangle)^2 + (\lambda_2 - \langle\lambda\rangle)^2 + (\lambda_3 - \langle\lambda\rangle)^2\right]}}{\sqrt{2(\lambda_1^2 + \lambda_2^2 + \lambda_3^2)}}, \langle\lambda\rangle = \frac{\lambda_1 + \lambda_2 + \lambda_3}{3}$$

Tracts have been drawn according to the ROIs, fiber count (SL), mean fiber length (d) and fiber volume (V) were recorded. Approximate slice areas were calculated with formula (A=V/d). Moreover, morphologies of the optic nerve were evaluated using b0 coronal plane images obtained from the same region.

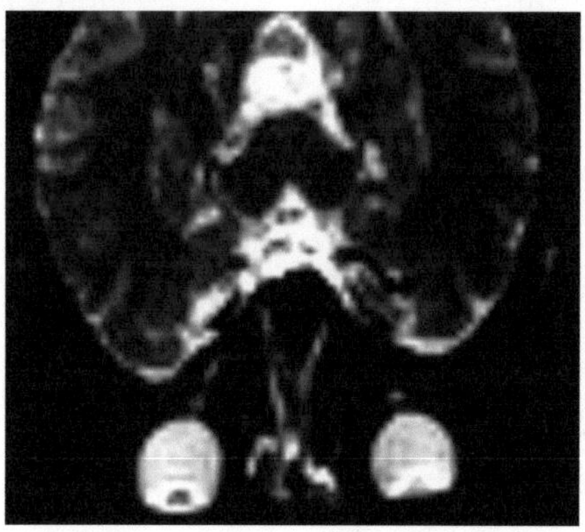

Fig. 4. ROI determination for diffusion analysis with DTI.

fMRI imaging

All fMRI imaging procedures were performed at Bakırköy Dr. Sadi Konuk Research Hospital using a 1.5 T Siemens MRI device. An anatomic image was obtained in 128 fractions in 1x1x1 cm resolution with a high resolution T1 weighed 3D GRE sequence. Functional MRI images were obtained with a GE-EPI sequence. In a 64x64 data collection matrix, 29 fractions covering visual cortex were obtained in resolutions of 3x3x3 mm voxel dimensions. TR was 2900ms, TE

30 was ms and the flip angle was 90 degrees. Sequential two imaging procedures were performed for the left and right eye of the patient with glaucoma. Thus, 544 volumes including 272 volumes for each eye were obtained from each individual.

Stimulation

Visual stimulation was prepared using OpenGL library and it was displayed by reflecting onto a mirror inside the MRI via an LCD projector and transparent curtain during the experiment. The visual field angle was measured as 40^0 on a horizontal plane and 25^0 on a vertical plane. The visual field was divided into five rings, each consisting of 12 sectors, and small spaces were left in order to differentiate each sector from the other. During the experiment, test subjects were asked to focus on the center point of the stimulation. Half of the selected 60 regions in the visual field along 67 blocks were flashed at a frequency of 8 Hz in the form of 4x4 chess boards. 68. No stimulation left in the block and the subject looked at blank screen.

fMRI data analyses

All functional analyzes were performed with SPM5 (by the Wellcome Department of Imaging Neuroscience, London, England). Following standard movement correction and fraction time correction procedures, all functional images were blurred using a Gausian spatial filter with FWHM of 5mm for modeling fMRI data, each of the 60 regions in the visual field were taken as a regressor and those regressors were used in the general linear model in SPM5. To model fMRI data, each regressor was convolved with standard hemodynamic response function.
For each of the 60 regions divided on the visual field, SPM(t) maps giving statistics of activation in relevant regions were created. Those maps were masked in the form of ($t > 3.12$, $p < 0.001$).
In order to compare activations occurring in the visual cortex, the visual field regions most heavily influenced by glaucoma were determined in each patient and activations occurring in the stimulation of those regions were calculated. For this purpose, voxel clusters exceeding the cut-off value in SPM(t) maps of each region were found and the percent change in BOLD was measured using fMRI corresponding to those clusters (Figure 5).

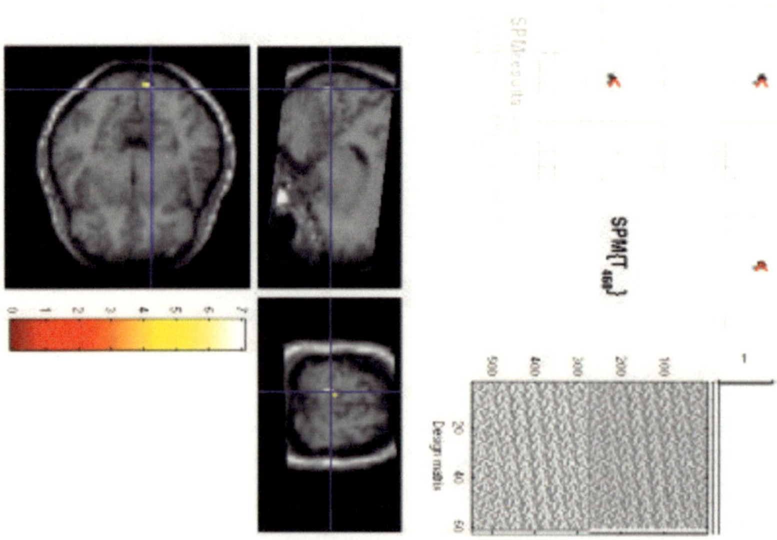

Fig. 5. Determination of BOLD signal in particular voxels

3.3 Results

In examinations performed with a Color Doppler ultrasonography, vascular anomaly was not observed in subjects. When the OCT findings of subjects (Table 1) were compared with the DTI diffusion analyzes (Table 2), reduction in all diffusion parameters in the eye with severe glaucoma relative to the other eye was observed for AC with asymmetrical involvement. In the comparison with the control, a reduction in MD and SL values was observed. High values in both mildly and severely glaucomatous eyes of AC were obtained relative to control.

		c/d	RNFL	GCC	PSD	MD
Control	Right	0.02	102.90	94,30	1,66	0,04
	Left	0	102.94	97,09	1,82	0,02
AC	Right	0,18	102,80	109,25	2,18	-2,75
	Left	0,45	71,04	82,16	11,13	-22,15

Table 1. OCT and VF findings of the control and the patient. RNFL: Retinal nerve fiber layer analysis, GCC: Ganglion cell counting, PSD: Pattern Standard Deviation, MD: Mean Deviation.

		FA	λ1	λ2	λ3	MD	SL	V	d	A
Control	Right	0,17	3,21	2,63	2,08	2,64	4	185,083	20.05	9,23
	Left	0,15	3,41	2,96	2,57	2,98	4	158.64	20,78	7,63
AC	Right	0,37	2,54	1,69	1,19	1,806	4	350,967	13,50	26
	Left	0,325	2,08	1,43	1,07	1,526	2	134,987	12	11,25

Table 2. Diffusion analysis findings of the control and the patient. FA: Fractional anisotropy, λ1: Radial diffusivity, λ2, λ3: Axial diffusivities, MD: Mean diffusivity, SL: Nerve fiber count, V: Volume, d: Maximum length, a: approximate cross-sectional area.

In b0 coronal plane images, when the control eyes (Figure 6A) and eyes with symmetrical involvement were compared, deterioration in the optic nerve diffusion of severely glaucomatous eyes of the patient with asymmetrical involvement was observed (Figure 6B)

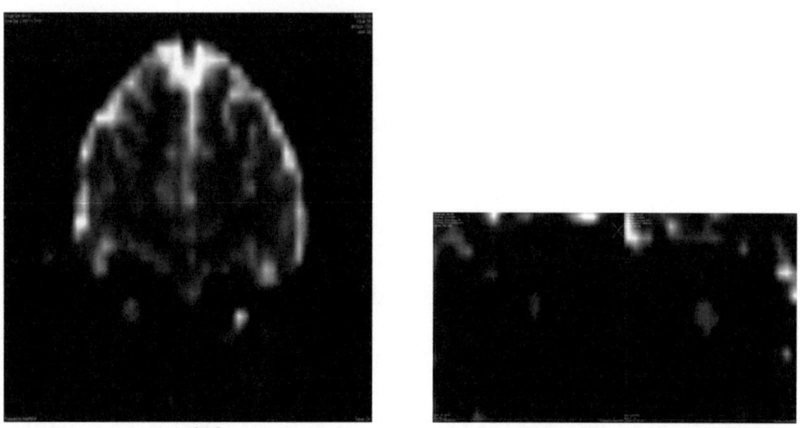

(A) (B)

Fig. 6. b0 coronal plane images of control (A) and AC with severe glaucoma in left eye (B).

In comparison with the control (Figure 7B) and opposite eye, a decrease in the thickness of the optic nerve on the severely glaucomatous side in the patient with asymmetrical involvement (Figure 7A) was clearly observed in optic nerve tractographies.

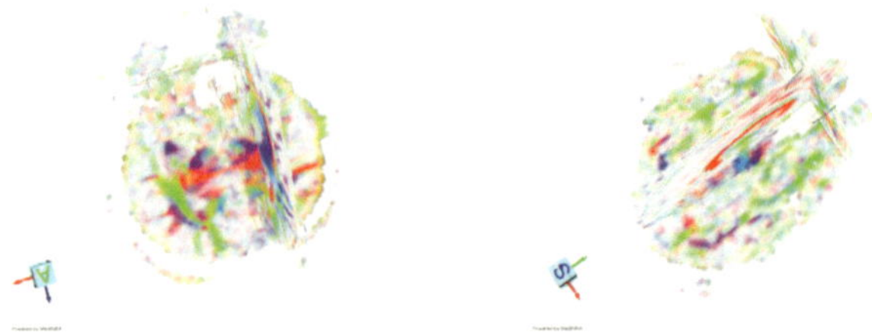

(A) (B)

Fig. 7. Color FA map optic nerve tractography of control (A) and AC with severe glaucoma in left eye (B).

In fMRI analyzes, data analyzes were performed with reference to VF obtained in subjects. BOLD signals obtained from each quadrant were recorded (Table 3). In the sensitive field analysis, success could not be gained since BOLD could not be obtained in all voxels.

	Upper Right		Upper Left		Lower Left		Lower Right	
	Left	Right	Left	Right	Left	Right	Left	Right
Control	2.68	2.34	2.81	2.44	2.8	2.57	2.75	2.4
AC	1.72*	1.25	1.26	1.73	1.31	1.76	1.29	1.75

Table 3. Recorded BOLD signals from each quadrant of the control and the patient with severe glaucoma in left eye. *Enhanced BOLD values in the severely effected eye.

In comparative analyzes on quadrants with VF defect, in the patient with asymmetrical involvement, BOLD values in the eye with heavier defect were lower than that of the other eye (Figures 8A and B).

3.4 Discussion

Glaucoma is a group of ocular diseases characterized with progressive optic nerve damage and loss of vision. Despite recent treatments efficiently reducing IOP, they reserve the above mentioned characteristics. This condition made neuro-protection a high-priority issue in glaucoma (Weinreb, 2007). However, studies focused on the glaucoma - brain relation, which have increased in number in recent years, have shown us that the posterior aspect of the retina and the head of the optic nerve should be considered when IOP-independent treatment is developed, and moreover, diffusion of neurodegeneration in the brain should be taken into consideration in the diagnosis and follow-up of glaucoma. More importantly, it is obvious that the damage is sustained (Yücel et al, 2003). Therefore, in this study, we aimed to create bulbar-retrobulbar, structural-functional integrity in the evaluation of glaucomatous neurodegeneration.

The DTI examination, the structural examination arm of our study, was performed in two stages. In DTI diffusion analyzes, the observation of reduction in all parameters in the severely glaucomatous eye in comparison with the other eye in the patient with

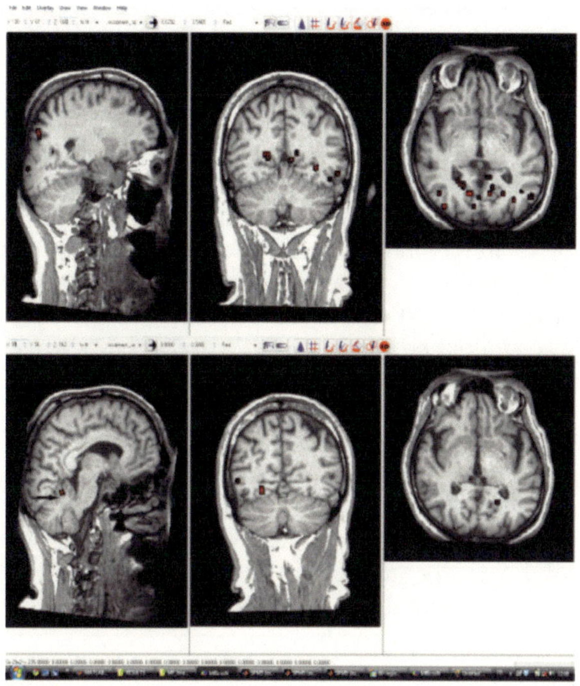

Fig. 8. For AC, BOLD signals of right eye inferior temporal quadrant (A) and left eye inferior temporal quadrant. Arrow: BOLD signal obtained in cerebellum due to movement of the patient

asymmetrical involvement is partially compatible with the literature. In the experimental glaucoma study conducted by Hui et al. on a mouse model, a decrease in FA values and an increase in $\lambda 1$ values were observed in the optic nerve in glaucomatous eye and an increase in $\lambda 1$ between Day 8 and Day 21 was found to be statistically significant (Hui et al, 2007). On the contrary, in the single study conducted on humans, an increase in MD values in addition to a decrease in FA values, which were parallel to findings of Hui et al., were reported (Garaci et al, 2009). Direct correlation of diffusion analyzes with findings of eye is not yet present in the literature.

Morphological findings obtained in the second stage of DTI outcomes are compatible with the literature. Degeneration in the glaucomatous optic nerve could be histologically demonstrated in mice (Hui et al, 2007), monkeys and humans (Gupta et al, 2006). Moreover, the degeneration could be demonstrated, as we imaged in humans using 1.5T and in the optic nerve on the coronal plane of small mice with 7T DTI, but it was reported as reduction rather than a temporal loss (Hui et al, 2007). Those findings match the above studies conducted on glaucoma patients with conventional MRI (Kashiwagi et al, 2004). On the contrary, lower volume in the control relative to the patient values can be explained on the basis that the diameter of optic nerve may have significant (in the range of 4-9 mm) inter-individual variation (Stark & Bradley, 1996).

In our study, functional evaluation was performed with VF and fMRI. However, it was observed that VF defects were also correlating with DTI findings. In fact, a defect in the visual field may originate from a pathology in any location ranging from the retina to the cortex (Landers et al, 2004). It was reported that in normo-tensive glaucoma, deeper depressions were observed in the VF of the patient with ischemia in the brain MRI (Suzuki et al, 2004). In our study, in the comparative analysis of quadrants with VF defect, it was found that in the patient with asymmetrical involvement, BOLD values of the eye with serious defect were lower than that of the other eye.

The outstanding study of Duncan et al. (Duncan et al, 2007) is the only study in the literature where functional analysis with VF and MRI was conducted in glaucoma. In the study, the imaging of a defect of VF in the brain with 3T MRI using a long and complex stimulation was achieved. It is also possible to perform those precise analyzes using our multifocal mapping method; however, 3T MRI was used in the original method (Vanni et al, 2005). In the study, since BOLD could not be obtained in all voxels in sensitive area analysis with 1.5 T MRI, success could not be gained; however, an occipital cortex BOLD activity difference could be demonstrated in the highly asymmetrical patient.

In our study, an important aim, in our opinion, was to develop a method compatible with MRI devices routinely used in clinics, because we believe that large case series can only be obtained with this approach. Studies existing in the literature were performed with 3T MRI devices, which were generally used for experimental purposes, and with 6-7T MRI devices, which were solely used for experimental purposes. Moreover, there is no study in the literature which examines structural and functional ophthalmological diagnosis methods and DTI-MRI and fMRI techniques in combination.

In this pro-study, the glaucoma-brain connection has been demonstrated in humans. Visual pathways from the retina to the cerebral cortex have been evaluated both structurally and functionally with routine clinical instruments. Furthermore, results obtained were concordant with OCT and VF, in structural and functional analysis.

5. Conclusions

After many years of subsequent precious studies on glaucoma-brain connection, Gupta and Yucel conclude "Glaucoma as a neurodegenerative disease is a valid working hypothesis to understand neural injury in the visual system. Observations suggest that mechanisms independent of IOP are also implicated in glaucomatous degeneration. This paradigm may stimulate the discovery of innovative IOP-independent strategies to help prevent loss of vision in glaucoma patients".

Strategies independent from IOP, concerning the area beyond the optic nerve head, are needed in the evaluation and treatment of glaucoma. Currently, it is possible to image visual pathways from the optic nerve to the cerebral cortex both structurally and functionally. As our pro-study showed, routine clinical instruments are also adequate for clinical trials to reveal the glaucoma-brain connection; however, more sophisticated techniques are being developed to illuminate that relation further. Better understanding of retrobulbar glaucomatous damage will enable us to determine more efficient diagnosis, follow-up and treatment strategies and facilitate the answering of some questions which remain unknown about this disease.

6. Acknowledgments

The author wish to thank to other members of "3B Study group" Bulent Yemişci MD (Bağcılar Education and Research Hospital, Dept Ophthalmology), Sibel Bayramoğlu MD,

Nurten Turan MD (Bakırköy ŞK Education and Research Hospital, Dept of Radiology), Cengizhan Öztürk MD PhD Prof, Onur Özyurt Msc, Esin Karahan Msc (Bosphorus University, Dept of Biomedical Engineering) for their ongoing efforts in imaging glaucomatous neurodegeneration, and to Gülgün Engin MD Prof (Istanbul University, Istanbul Faculty of Medicine, Dept of Radiology) for employing her drawing skills for the artwork in this chapter.

7. References

Boucard CC, Hoogduin JM, van der Grond J, Cornelissen FW. (2007). Occipital proton magnetic resonance spectroscopy (1H-MRS) reveals normal metabolite concentrations in retinal visual field defects. *PLoS ONE* 2(2): e222.

Chan KC, So KF, Wu EX. (2009). Proton magnetic resonance spectroscopy revealed choline reduction in the visual cortex in an experimental model of chronic glaucoma. *Exp Eye Res* 88(1):65-70.

Chidlow G, Wood JP, Casson RJ. (2007). Pharmacological neuroprotection for glaucoma. *Drugs* 67(5):725-759.

Duncan RO, Sample PA, Weinreb RN, Bowd C, Zangwill LM. (2007). Retinotopic organization of primary visual cortex in glaucoma: Comparing fMRI measurements of cortical function with visual field loss. *Prog Retin Eye Res* 26(1):38-56.

Engelhorn T, Michelson G, Waerntges S, Struffert T, Haider S, Doerfler A. (2011). Diffusion Tensor Imaging Detects Rarefaction of Optic Radiation in Glaucoma Patients. *Acad Radiol* Mar 4. [Epub ahead of print]

Garaci FG, Bolacchi F, Cerulli A, Melis M, Spanò A, Cedrone C, Floris R, Simonetti G, Nucci C. (2009). Optic nerve and optic radiation neurodegeneration in patients with glaucoma: in vivo analysis with 3-T diffusion-tensor MR imaging. *Radiology* 252(2):496-501.

Gupta N, Yücel YH. (2003). Brain changes in glaucoma. *Eur J Ophthalmol* 13 Suppl 3:S32-535.

Gupta N, Ang LC, de Tilly LN, Bidaisee L, Yucel YH. (2006). Human glaucoma and neural degeneration in intracranial optic nerve, LGN, and visual cortex. *Br J Ophthalmol* 90:674–678.

Gupta N, Yücel YH. (2007). Glaucoma as a neurodegenerative disease. *Curr Opin Ophthalmol* 18(2):110-114.

Hui ES, Fu QL, So KF, Wu EX. (2007). Diffusion tensor MR study of optic nerve degeneration in glaucoma. *Conf Proc IEEE Eng Med Biol Soc 2007* 2007:4312-4315.

Hood DC, Anderson SC, Wall M, Kardon RH. (2007). Structure versus function in glaucoma: an application of a linear model. *Invest Ophthalmol Vis Sci* 48:3662–3668.

Hood DC, Anderson SC, Wall M, Raza AS, Kardon RH. (2009). A Test of a Linear Model of Glaucomatous Structure–Function Loss Reveals Sources of Variability in Retinal Nerve Fiber and Visual Field Measurements *Invest Ophthalmol Vis Sci* 50:4254–4266

Kashiwagi K, Okubo T, Tsukahara S. (2004). Association of magnetic resonance imaging of anterior optic pathway with glaucomatous visual field damage and optic disc cupping. *J Glaucoma* 13(3):189-195.

Kitsos G, Zikou AK, Bagli E, Kosta P, Argyropoulou MI. (2009). Conventional MRI and magnetisation transfer imaging of the brain and optic pathway in primary open-angle glaucoma. *Br J Radiol* 82(983):896-900.

Knight OJ, Chang RT, Feuer WJ, Budenz DL. (2009). Comparison of retinal nerve fiber layer measurements using time domain and spectral domain optical coherent tomography. *Ophthalmology* 116(7): 1271–1277.

Landers J, Tang KC, Hing S. (2004). A visual field abnormality: ocular or cerebral cause? *Clin Experiment Ophthalmol* 32(2):219-222.

Lagrèze WA, Gaggl M, Weigel M, Schulte-Mönting J, Bühler A, Bach M, Munk RD, Bley TA. (2009). Retrobulbar optic nerve diameter measured by high-speed magnetic resonance imaging as a biomarker for axonal loss in glaucomatous optic atrophy. *Invest Ophthalmol Vis Sci* 50(9):4223-4228.

Lu K, Perthen JE, Duncan RO, Zangwill LM, Liu TT. (2008). Noninvasive measurement of the cerebral blood flow response in human lateral geniculate nucleus with arterial spin labeling fMRI. *Hum Brain Mapp* 29(10):1207-14.

Nucifora PGP, Verma R, Lee S, Melhem ER. (2007). Diffusion-Tensor MR Imaging and Tractography: Exploring Brain Microstructure and Connectivity. *Radiology* 245:367-384.

Qing G, Zhang S, Wang B, Wang N. (2010). Functional MRI signal changes in primary visual cortex corresponding to the central normal visual field of patients with primary open-angle glaucoma. *Invest Ophthalmol Vis Sci* 51(9):4627-4634.

Rauscher FM, Sekhon N, Feuer WJ, Budenz DL. (2009). Myopia affects retinal nerve fiber layer measurements as determined by optical coherence tomography. *J Glaucoma* 18(7): 501–505.

Sadun AA, Glaser JS, Bose S. (2007). Anatomy of the Visual Sensory System, In: *Duane's Ophthalmology*, Tasman W, Jaeger EA, (Eds.), Chapter 34, Lippincott Williams & Wilkins, ISBN 978-0-7817-6855-9, Philadelphia, PA, USA.

Sherbondy AJ, Dougherty RF, Napel S, Wandell BA. (2008). Identifying the human optic radiation using diffusion imaging and fiber tractography. *J Vis* 8(10):1-11.

Smith SM. (2002). Fast robust automated brain extraction. *Human Brain Mapping* 17(3):143-155

Stark DD, Bradley WG. (1996). Magnetic Resonance Imaging In: *Orbit*, Scott W. Pp 988-1028. Mosby, Missouri,USA.

Suzuki J, Tomidokoro A, Araie M, Tomita G, Yamagami J, Okubo T, Masumoto T. (2004). Visual field damage in normal-tension glaucoma patients with or without ischemic changes in cerebral magnetic resonance imaging. *Jpn J Ophthalmol* 48(4):340-344.

Vanni S, Henriksson L, James AC. (2005). Multifocal fMRI mapping of visual cortical areas. *Neuroimage* 27(1):95-105.

Weinreb RN. (2007). Glaucoma neuroprotection: What is it? Why is it needed? *Can J Ophthalmol* 42(3):396-398.

Yücel YH, Zhang Q, Weinreb RN, Kaufman PL, Gupta N. (2003). Effects of retinal ganglion cell loss on magno-, parvo-, koniocellular pathways in the LGN and visual cortex in glaucoma. *Prog Retin Eye Res* 22(4):465-481.

17

Central Changes in Glaucoma: Neuroscientific Study Using Animal Models

Kazuyuki Imamura et al.*
Dept. Systems Life Engineering, Maebashi Institute of Technology, Maebashi-shi, Japan

1. Introduction

The relatively high incidence of glaucoma has become a serious health problem in the rapidly aging society (Elolia and Stokes, 1998; Klein et al., 1992; Leske, 1983; Salive et al., 1992). Adequate animal models are thus urgently needed to develop an effective remedy(s) of glaucoma or even to prevent its occurence. Death of retinal ganglion cells (RGC) death is the major pathological feature of glaucoma, and has been studied extensively at the level of the retina focused on the optic nerve head. Visual field deficit caused by the loss of RGCs in glaucoma must be accompanied by morphological and physiological changes in the higher visual centers. However, limited knowledge is available concerning the trans-synaptic changes, in morphology and physiology, induced in the central visual system by glaucoma.

Our basic premise is that the centripetal changes in glaucoma may precede those in the eye, because compensation processes for the deteriorating function are, in general, much fast or strongly expressed in the central system than peripheral system due to the increased level of complexity in the former. Provided that this is the case, the detection of central changes is critical for establishing the early diagnosis of glaucoma in its initial stage.

The number of photoreceptors in the retina is about one billion, while that of optic nerve fibers is about one hundred and twenty million. By a simple calculation, therefore, it is likely that there is substantial afferent convergence or integration within neural network of the retina before visual output sent out along the centripetal pathway. Thus, abnormal retinal outputs in glaucoma to the lateral geniculate nucleus (LGN) are thought to induce compensatory responses in thalamic and visuocortical neurons. We would like to examine such changes in morphology and physiology as a harbinger of glaucomatous changes in visual function.

---

*Masamitsu Shimazawa[1], Hirotaka Onoe[2], Yasuyoshi Watanabe[2], Kiyoshi Ishii[3], Chihiro Mayama[3], Takafumi Akasaki[4], Satoshi Shimegi[5], Hiromichi Sato[5], Kazuhiko Nakadate[6], Hideaki Hara[1] and Makoto Araie[4]
[1]*Molecular Pharmacology, Dept. Biofunctional Evaluation, Gifu Pharmaceutical Univ., Gifu-shi, Gifu 501-1196, Japan*
[2]*RIKEN Center for Molecular Imaging Science, Japan*
[3]*Dept. Ophthalmology, Graduate School of Medicine and Faculty of Medicine, Univ. of Tokyo, Japan*
[4]*Dept. Intelligent System, Faculty of Computer Science and Engineering, Kyoto Sangyo University, Kyoto-shi, Japan*
[5]*Lab. Cognitive and Behavioral Neuroscience, Graduate School of Medicine, Osaka University, Toyonaka-shi, Japan*
[6]*Dept. Histology and Neurobiology, Graduate School of Medicine, Dokkyo Medical University, Japan*

A monkey model of unilateral hypertension glaucoma has been successfully created by laser irradiation to the trabecular meshwork: experimental monkeys exhibited, when ophthalmologically examined, sustained and reproducible increase in intraocular pressure (IOP) for a relatively long period (Shimazawa et al., 2006a, b). Lately, experimentally induced changes in the primary visual pathway were reported findings by ophthalmological examinations of monkeys studied by using PET in monkeys with unilateral hepertension glaucoma. In addition, the time course of changes in appearance of the optic disk and thickness of the retinal nerve fiber layer (RNFL) measured by scanning laser ophthalmoscopy (HRT) and scanning laser polarimetry (GDx), exhibited corresponding changes in hypertension glaucoma of human. The latter measurement was in good correlations with RNFL thickness determined histologically (Shimazawa et al., 2006b). Visual field loss in glaucomatous monkeys was also studied by a behavioral method (Sasaoka et al., 2005).

In this chapter, we describe a set of new findings we obtained for the centripetal changes in hypertension glaucoma, which is experimentally induced by unilateral laser coagulation of the trabeclar meshwork of monkeys. Data-analysis methods employed here include: imaging with positoron emission tomography (PET), neuroanatomical tracing, immunohistochemical staining, and electrophysiological single-unit recording.

2. Two new findings in glaucomatous monkeys obtained by PET

PET is a powerful, noninvasive imaging technology widely used in examination of brain function (Giovacchini et al., 2011). As reported previously (Imamura et al., 2009), we found in a PET study with 2-[^{18}F]fluoro-2-deoxy-glucose on glaucomatous monkeys that monocular visual stimulation of the affected eye yielded significantly reduced neural responses in the occipital areas of visual cortices. Intriguingly, the reduction in response was limited to the cortex ipsilateral to the affected eye, indicating the unique vulnerability of ipsilateral visual cortex in glaucomatous monkeys (Imamura et al., 2009).

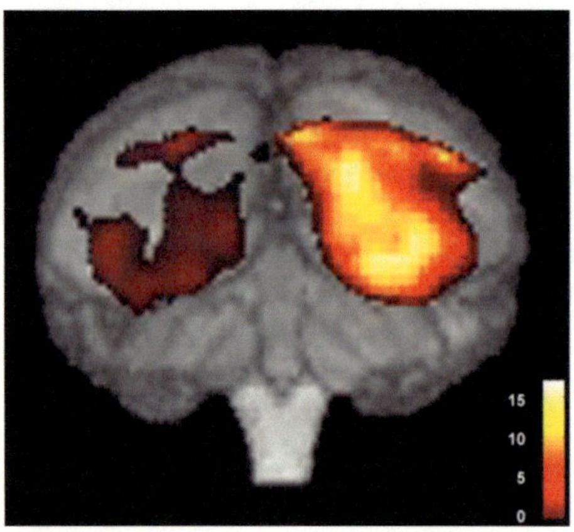

Fig. 1. A symmetric activation of occipital cortex in glaucomatous monkey. Modified from NeuroReport, (Imamura et al., 2009)

Characteristic pattern of ^{18}FDG uptake during monocular activation is shown as a back view of monkey brain. Statistical parametric mapping (SPM) analysis was performed using six images obtained form two model monkeys. The results of SPM analysis (t-values), with data from six

PET images for each eye of two monkeys, are superimposed on the T1 image of one monkey. The color scale indicated the t-value, the level of significance ($P<0.05$, red to $P<0.00001$, white). Note that left visual cortex ipsilateral to the affected eye exhibited significantly lower activity, suggesting deterioration of function in the ipisilateral visual pathway.

Next, using [^{11}C]PK11195, a PET tracer for peripheral benzodiazepine receptors, we found selective binding in the LGN of glaucomatous monkeys, while no binding was found in other brain regions. In the central nervous system, the expression of peripheral benzodiazepine receptors are limited to the activated microglia, which in turn exhibits neurotoxic, neurotrophic and neuroprotective activities by releasing several types of cytokines, including NO, TNF-α, and IL-1ß. The binding of [^{11}C]PK11195 was earlier reported only in the diseased brain, for example, in multiple sclerosis (Vowinckel et al., 1997), herpes encephalitis (Cagnin, et al., 2001b), and Alzheimer disease (Cagnin, et al., 2001a). In short, the present finding indicates that, in our model monkeys, hypertension glaucoma induces the activation of the microglia in the LGN suggestive of some functional changes in the LGN.

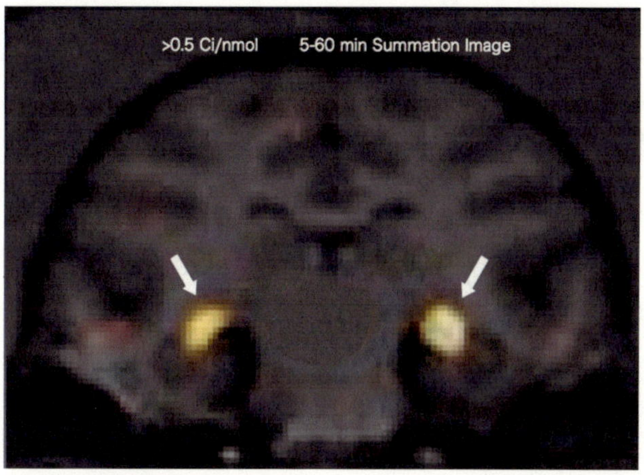

Fig. 2. Accumulation of [^{11}C]PK11195 activity in the LGN. A PET summation image is superimposed on an MRI T1 image. The PET image in the frontal plane shows selective accumulation of activity in the LGN of both hemispheres (arrows). Modified from NeuroReport, (Imamura et al., 2009)

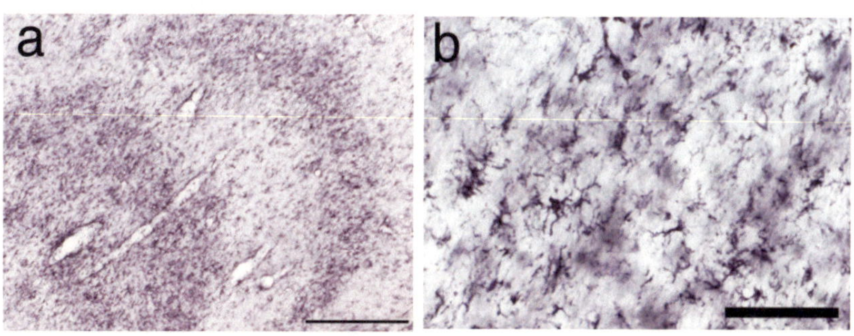

Fig. 3. Immunohistochemical staining of activated microglia in the LGN of glaucomatous monkey. Higher power view of a stained layer is shown (b). Scale bars show 500 μm (a) and 200 μm (b), respectively.

To clarify the above point, we further performed an immunohistochemical study using specific antibody against activated microglia (Graeber et al., 1994). Results indicated that the immunoreactivity was confined indeed to the LGN layers that normally receive afferent inputs from the glaucoma-affected eye. The termination pattern of retinal axons in the LGN is known to eye-selective, with one layer receiving input only from one eye. Accordingly, the staining pattern we found was complimentary between the left and right and left LGNs. Immunohistochemical staining was performed using CR3/43 antibody, which selectively recognizes activated microglia. Laminar selective staining (a) was found. The stained layers were found to receive inputs from the glaucomatous eye.

3. Selective damage of centripetal visual pathway ipsilateral to affected eye

Next we asked why the activity in the visual cortex was selectively reduced in the hemisphere ipsilateral to the affected eye. We performed neuroanatomical tracing experiments using wheat germ agglutinin (WGA) as an anterograde tracer. WGA was injected into normal eye of naive monkeys and both normal and affected eyes of the glaucomatous monkeys. After a survival period of 3 days for anterograde transport of the tracer, the animals were perfused with 4 % paraformaldehyde, the brain was removed and immunohistochemical staining of thin LGN section was performed using an anti-WGA antibody (Gong & LeDoux, 2003).

First, in the case of the normal eye of a naive monkey, individual layers of the LGN that receive input from the injected eye were stained (Fig. 4). At higher magnification (Fig. 5), it was clearly seen that postsynaptic neurons were transsynaptically labeled with some granular staining pattern that reflected endings of the afferent nerve fibers (Fig. 5).

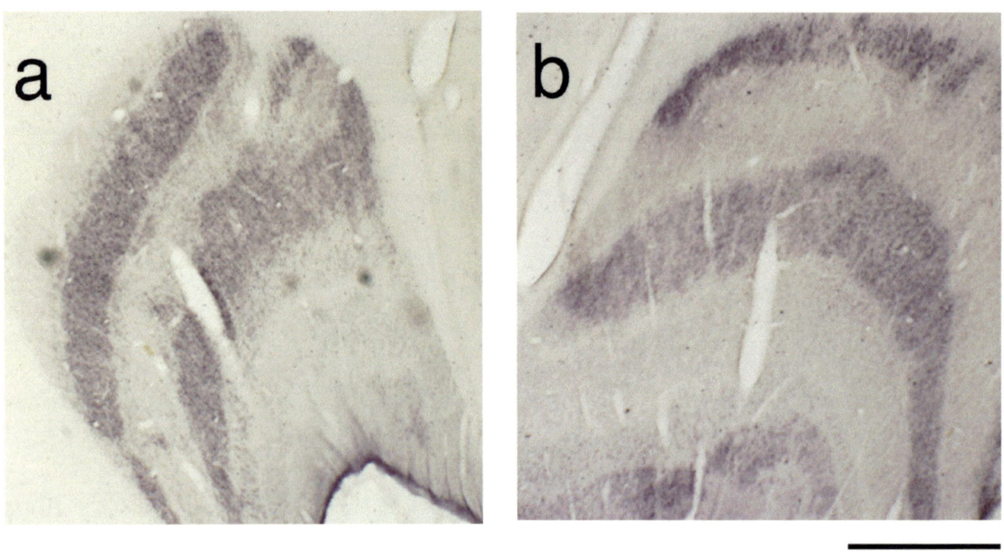

Fig. 4. Immunohistochemical staining of normal LGN, using anti-WGA antibody after monocular injection of WGA In the case of naive animal, the left (a) and right (b) LGN exhibit complementary staining pattern of layers that receive afferents from the injected eye. Scale, 1 mm.

Fig. 5. Transsynaptic transport of WGA in the LGN. Labeling of postsynaptic neurons was found in the form of granular, presumably presynaptic, staining in a layer of the LGN. Scale, 50 μm.

Figure 6 shows the results of a case, in which the tracer was injected into the normal eye of glaucomatous monkey. A complementary staining pattern similar to that found with the aforementioned case was obtained. In addition, discordant staining was sometimes found invading into neighboring layers that should be free of the input from the injected eye.
Finally, a tracer injection was performed into the affected eye of the glaucomatous monkey. In one of the two monkeys examined, no transport of WGA was found in the LGN, while in the other animal selective staining was found only in the input-receiving layers of the LGN contralateral to the injected eye. No staining was found in the ipsilateral LGN (Fig. 7).

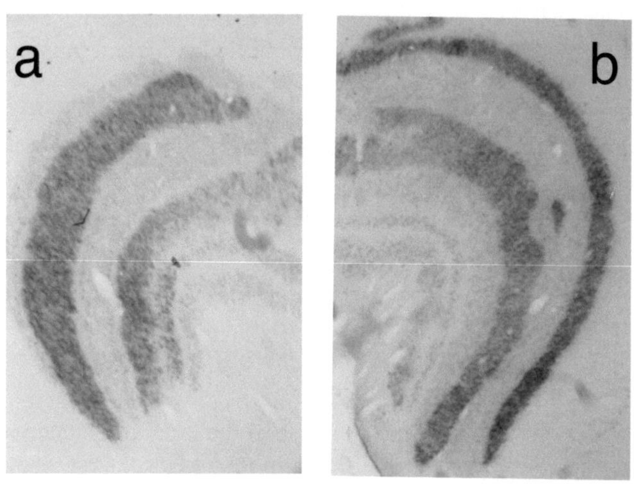

Fig. 6. Staining pattern of the left (a) and right (b) LGN of glaucomatous monkey when WGA was injected into the fellow eye. Scale, 1 mm.

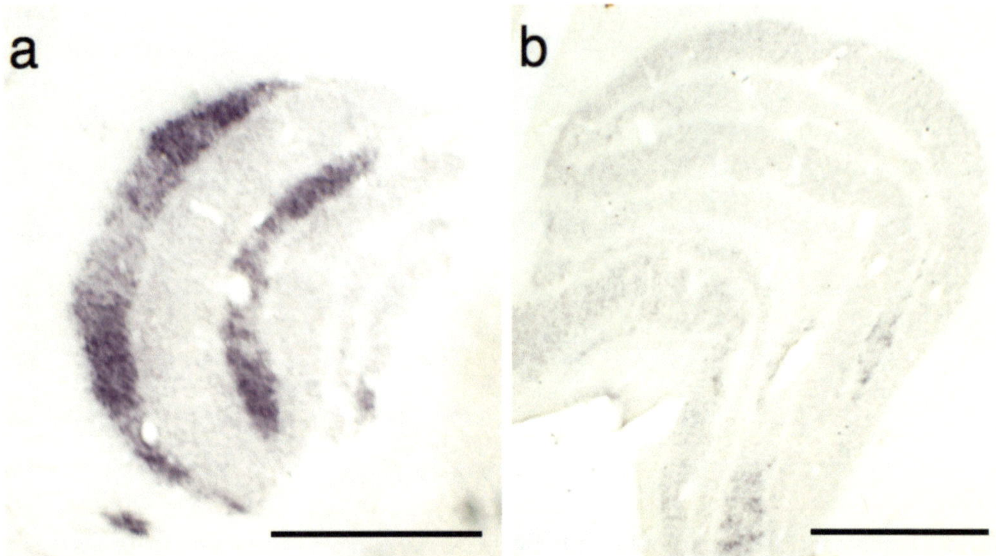

Fig. 7. Staining pattern of the left (a) and right (b) LGN of glacomatous monkey when WGA was injected into the affected eye. Scale, 1 mm.

In the right LGN, the staining was found in layers 6 and 4 and a part of 1, all of which usually receive input from the injected eye. In the left LGN ipsilateral to the glaucomatous eye, some faint staining was seen in the ventrolateral parts of layers 5 and 3. These results indicate that the normal retinal projection to the LGN was reserved only for in the contralatral pathway, strongly suggesting that the ipsilateral pathway was vulnerable to the elevation of IOP. This asymmetry indicated that injury of retinal ganglion cells in the temporal retina was more severe than that in the nasal retina. Interestingly, reduction of nasal-temporal asymmetry was reported in normal-tension glaucoma (Asano et al., 2007). Likewise, in strabismic amblyopes, reduced monocular activation was selectively detected only in visual cortex ipsilateral to the deprived eye (Imamura et al., 1997). Taken together, the present result suggest the high vulnerability of the ipsilateral projection in these pathophysiological conditions.

Electronmicroscopic examinations revealed that the optic nerve fibers derived from the glaucomatous eye were shrunken and damaged. In particular, the outer part was damaged more severely than the central part of the nerve trunk (Fig. 8). It was reported that in humans, optic nerve axons are not instructed to establish a retinotopic order within the initial portion of the visual pathway (Fitzgibbon and Taylor, 1996). However, in our model monkeys, vulnerability of the outer part of the optic nerve is frequently found.

4. Mechanisms of the induction of activated microglia in the LGN of glaucomatous animals

To obtain clues for the activation of the microglia in the LGN of glaucomatous monkeys, the following experiments were performed in the mouse LGN. First, we suspected that the microglia in the LGN was activated as a consequence of the substantial reduction of neural activity in the retina of the glaucomatous monkeys. Then, under isoflurane anesthesia, one eye of the mouse was injected with either tetrodotoxin (TTX), a sodium channel blocker, or

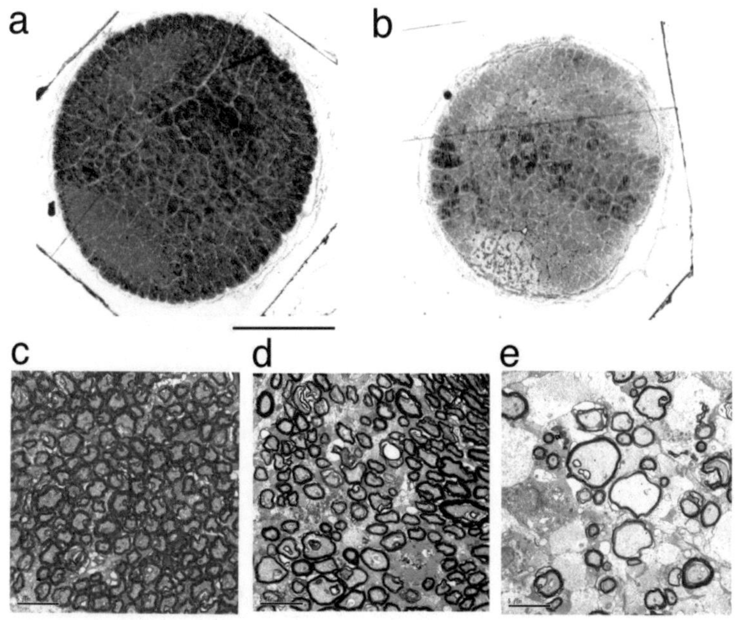

Fig. 8. Electronmicroscopic view of the optic nerve.
In lower-power view, it is clear that the optic nerve derived from the glaucomatous eye (b) is profoundly damaged when compared with that from the fellow eye (a). Scale, 1mm. In the high-power view, severe demyelination was observed in the outer part of the optic nerve (e), while the central dark portion exhibit a trace of myelinated fibers (d). However, the density of myelinated fibers was reduced in (d) and (e) compared with the optic nerve from the fellow eye (c).

N-methyl-D aspartate (NMDA), an agonist of NMDA-type glutamatergic receptors to suppress neuronal electrical activity or enhance excitability of retinal cells, respectively. One week after the respective eye injection, animals were perfused and immunohistochemical analysis was performed using antibodies to zif268 protein, a neuronal activity marker, and ionized calcium binding adaptor molecules 1 (Iba 1), a marker of microglia. In mice, the superior colliculus (SC) is the major recipient site of the retinal afferents. As expected, an asymmetrical staining pattern of Zif268 was seen in the SC of the mice monocularly injected with TTX (Fig. 9), while little difference was found in the SC of NMDA-injected mice (not shown). Rather, a slight enhancement was found in the SC contralateral to the NMDA-injected eye.

These results showed that each of the two chemical injected into one eye affected retinal neuronal activities in an expected manner. In the LGN of these mice, for sure, the activated microglias were induced following the TTX injection, although their number was small when compared with that following monocular enucleation, a measure that is much stronger than the former (Fig. 10). Taken together, these findings suggested that when the retinal activity was substantially outside of a certain range, activated microglia were induced in the LGN.

In our monkey model, the retinal activity was clearly suppressed in the IOP-elevated (laser-irradiated) eye, because immunostaining of visual cortical sections with an anti-Zif268

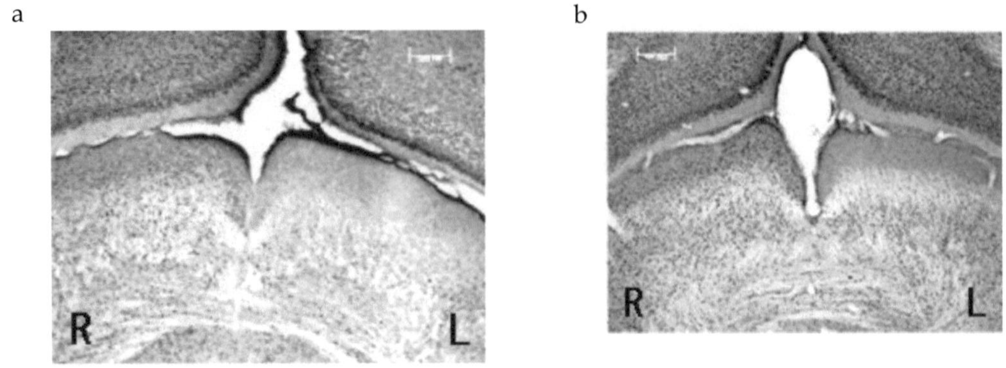

Fig. 9. Immunohistochemical staining of the superior colliculus (SC) of the TTX-injected mouse (a) and enucleated mouse (b) with an anti-zif268 antibody.
The left SC was free of zif268-positive nuclear staining, indicating neuronal activity of the right eye was suppressed by the injection of TTX or the enucleation of eyeball.

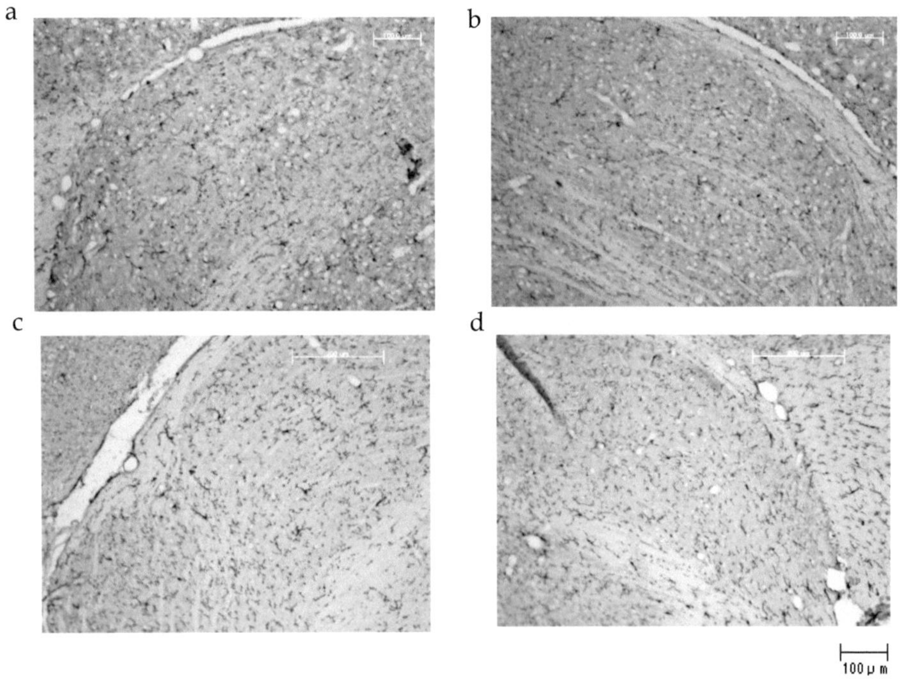

Fig. 10. Iba1 immunostaining of the mouse LGN. Right (a, c) and left (b, d) LGN of the mice, in which their right eye was injected with TTX (a, b) or enucleated (c, d), respectively.

antibody clearly exhibited ocular dominance patches indicating that neuronal activity was suppressed in columns corresponding to the glaucomatous eye (Fig. 11). Under this situation, the microglia are activated in the LGN. This means that maintenance of an adequate level of the retinal activity is critical in keeping the extent of microglia activation low in the central visual pathway.

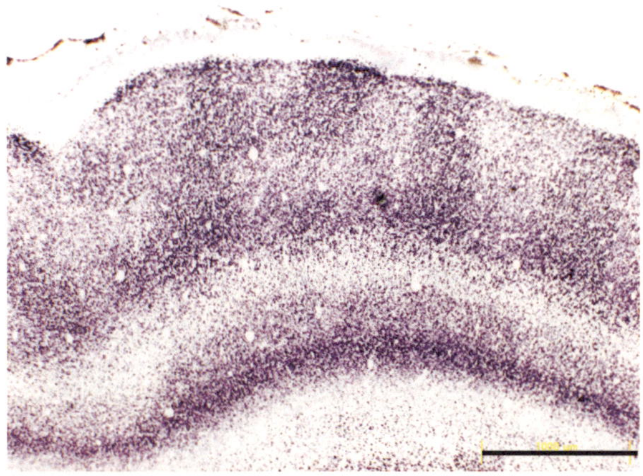

Fig. 11. Ocular dominance patches revealed by zif268 immunohistochemistry of the visual cortex of glaucomatous monkey. Scale, 1.0 mm.

A recent in vivo two-photon imaging study (Wake et al., 2009) reported that resting microglia contact with synapses once an hour and that this contact is neuronal activity-dependent. Intriguingly, transient ischemia prolonged the contact for one hour and presynaptic buttons disappeared after that. These finding is consistent with our findings in the LGN of glaucomatous monkeys.

5. Electrophysiological recordings of LGN neurons in monkey with experimentally-induced glaucoma

5.1 Background

Single-neuron recording from the primate LGN is useful for studying abnormalities in visual responses in experimental glaucoma (Smith et al., 1993). The primate LGN was selected as a primary site for investigation because of its striking similarities to the human LGN (Spear et al., 1994; O'Keefe et al., 1998) and the response properties of LGN neurons in normal monkeys have been extensively studied (Lee et al., 1979; McClurkin and Marrocco, 1984; Wilson and Forestner, 1995; Usrey and Reid, 2000; Levitt et al., 2001).

Yücel et al. (2000) obtained the following findings for the parvo (P) and magnocelular (M) laminas that receive inputs from the glaucomatous eye: i) there was a significant loss of LGN relay neurons, ii) the loss increased with increase in extent of the RGC loss, iii) neuronal atrophy occurred as measured with decrease in the cross-sectional area of neurons stained with parvalbumin, and iv) the degree of atrophy in the M and P pathways was linearly related to the extent of RGC loss. These are the first findings in the central nervous system that when transsynaptic degeneration occurs, and the extent of target neuron loss in the brain center linearly increases with increasing loss of afferent fibers (Yücel et al., 2001).

More specifically, one recent report has engaged our interest by reporting the expansion of visual receptive fields in the SC after the experimental elevation of IOP in one eye (King et al., 2006). They authors suggested that the expansion was induced by enlargement of dendritic field diameter of the retinal ganglion cells due to the elevation of IOP (Ahmed et al., 2001). Thus, along the same line or reasoning, we investigated electrophysiologically the following matters: i) characterization of the neural changes in the LGN of glaucomatous

monkeys, particularly focusing on size changes in minimum response field (MRF) of neurons, ii) to determine whether the extent of such changes differ between the P- and M pathways, and iii) to compare the changes in response properties of LGN neurons between stimulation of glaucomatous and normal eyes.
Three adult male cynomologus monkeys (Macaca fascicularis, GM1-3, Table 1) were used.

Subject I.D.	Eye	initial IOP mmHg	Age at the 1st LI (postnatal months)	Age at the 2nd LI (postnatal months)	Final IOP mmHg	C/D ratio (HRT)	Age at the start of Physiological Recordings (postnatal months)
GM1	R	-			22.3	0.149	90
	L	-	62	62	46.7	0.720	
GM2	R	20.5			14.0	0.063	61
	L	18.0	54	55	29.7	0.526	
GM3	R	16.5			17.2	0.271	59
	L	15.0	51	51	38.7	0.740	

Table 1. Experimental subjects
IOP, intraocular pressure; LI, laser irradiation; HRT, ophthalmological examination by Heidelberg Retina Tomography; -, no measurement. Data in GM2 and GM3 were cited from 2 monkeys out of 11 previously described in (Shimazawa et al., 2006).

5.2 Changes in IOP and funduscopic images of the glaucomatous monkeys

The experimental manipulation and IOP changes that follow over time are summarized for each of the three experimental monkeys in Table 1. In the present study, experimental glaucoma was induced in the left eye. All the three with glaucoma survived for 6 months or longer.
Figure 12 shows the time course of changes in IOP of monkeys GM2 and GM3. Within one month after laser irradiation, the IOP of the treated left eye was significantly elevated and remained high over the following three months. For GM1, however, IOP was measured twice a day (~12 hr apart) only at four different timings. At postnatal month 63, IOPs were 53.3 ± 2.22 and 21.0 in glaucomatous and normal eye, respectively. At postnatal month 66, IOPs were still significantly elevated for glaucomatous eye as compared to the normal (52.6 ± 2.51 vs 19.8 ± 1.28, $p < 0.0001$, student t-test). There was little variation in IOP measurements within a day.
Figure 13 shows representative funduscopic images obtained from GM2 using HRT. The results of optic disk examinations are summarized in Table 2. The reference plane of HRT was 50 μm deep from the temporal edge of the papilla. The "cup" area and "cup volume are defined, respectively, as a 2D and 3D space deeper below the reference plane. The cup/disk area ratio of the optic disk (C/D ratio) is defined as the average diameter of the cup area divided by that of the disk or the optic nerve head in the retina. The C/D ratio, cup area, volume, and depth were substantially higher in the left eye, which consistently exhibited high IOPs (Table 2). The rim area and rim volume (green and blue areas in Figs. 13 **c** and **d**) reflecting the mean thickness of the nerve fiber lamina, appeared to be smaller in the glaucomatous eye (Fig. 13d). Cupping of the optic papilla was clearly observable in the left eye of the three experimental animals. Albeit the three showed a similar C/D ratios at the time of physiological recording, ophthalmological examinations estimated the severity of their glaucomatous changes as GM1 > 3 > 2 in a decreasing order.

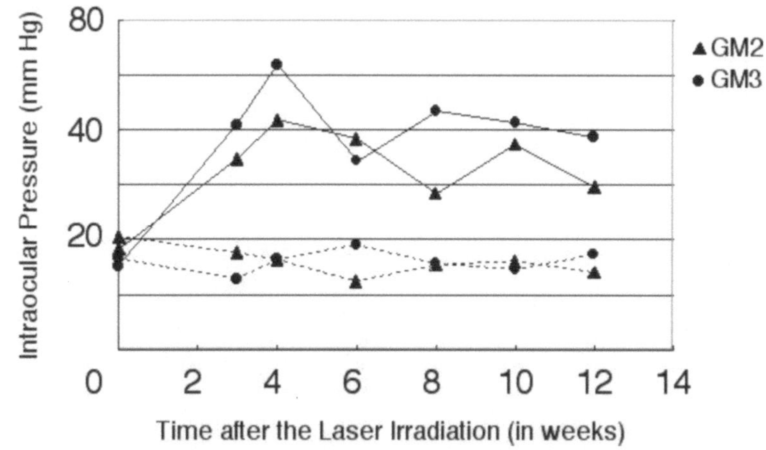

Fig. 12. Time course of changes in IOP (monkey GM2, triangles and GM3, circles) following laser irradiation. Solid lines and dotted lines indicate IOPs of the treated and untreated eyes, respectively. Each data point shows the mean of three measurements. Two measurements were taken within a day (~12 hr apart) on the four different days of examinations to determine the short-term fluctuation in IOP measurements (monkey GM1). Irradiation was performed about one month before the first measurement (i.e. postnatal month 62). At postnatal month 63, IOPs of glaucomatous and normal eyes were 53.3 ± 2.22 (mean ± standard deviation) and 21.0 mmHg, respectively. At postnatal month 66, IOPs were still significantly different (52.6 ± 2.51 vs 19.8 ± 1.28, $p < 0.0001$, Student t-test). IOPs of GM2 and GM3 were cited from 2 monkeys out of 11 previously described in (Shimazawa et al., 2006).

5.3 Impairment of electrophysiological responses

Referencing a brain map of the macaque monkey, lacquer-coated stainless steel electrodes with relatively low impedance (0.5 MΩ at 50 Hz) were initially used to locate the position of the LGN, based on the standard stereotaxic procedure. Then, a glass-coated, high-impedance (>2.0 MΩ at 50 Hz) tungsten microelectrode (Levick, 1972) was introduced into the LGN through a guide cannula vertically placed in the agar-sealed chamber. Action potentials of single neurons were conventionally amplified and monitored on a storage oscilloscope. Minimum response fields (MRFs) (Hubel and Wiesel, 1961; Barlow et al., 1967; Cleland et al., 1983) were routinely mapped with a moving, high contrast light slit and a small spot of flashing light. The border of response fields was repeatedly examined before a circle with an appropriate diameter was respectively assigned to them as authentic MRFs.

The LGN in each cerebral hemisphere represents the nasal hemifield of the contralateral eye, and the temporal hemifield of the ipsilateral eye. The LGN is a thalamic relay structure in the centripetal; projection pathway of the visual system composed of 6 principal laminae of neurons, each of which receives eye-specific inputs: laminae 1, 4, and 6 receive inputs from the contralateral eye, while laminae 2, 3, and 5, input from the ipsilateral eye (Perry et al., 1984). By electrode penetrations that pass vertically through the entire extent of the LGN, it is possible to record from relay neurons of two main types, P- and M neurons, which have receptive fields in approximately corresponding regions of the visual field for the two eyes. Upon the completion of single-neuron recording, we histologically confirmed our assignment of the laminar location to each of many recorded neurons along a given track, using micromanipulator reading during recording.

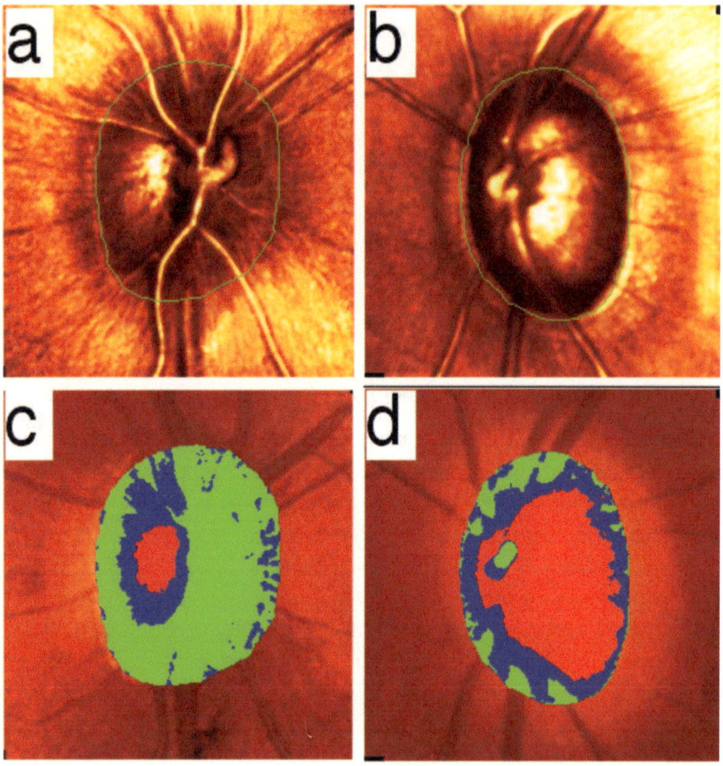

Fig. 13. Representative confocal images (**a** and **b**) of the optic disc and topographic images of HRT (**c** and **d**) in normal (**a** and **c**) and glaucomatous (**b** and **d**) eyes of monkey GM2. Red areas in the optic discs (**c** and **d**) indicate "cupping". Green and Blue areas in **c** and **d** indicate the so-called "rim area", reflecting change in nerve fiber layers (NFL). In the left eye with high IOP, mean NFL thickness was less than in the right eye (0.157 vs. 0.315 mm).

	GM1		GM2		GM3	
	Right	Left	Right	Left	Right	Left
Disk Area (mm2)	1.322	1.647	1.643	1.676	1.807	1.754
Cup Area (mm2)	0.198	1.182	0.103	0.882	0.49	1.297
Cup/Disk Area Ratio	0.149	0.72	0.063	0.526	0.271	0.74
Rim Area (mm2)	1.123	0.465	1.54	0.793	1.317	0.457
Height Variation Contour (mm)	0.315	0.367	0.487	0.216	0.347	0.154
Cup Volume (mm3)	0.017	0.327	0.008	0.154	0.079	0.668
Rim Volumn (mm3)	0.234	0.082	0.574	0.112	0.305	0.055
Mean Cup Depth (mm)	0.117	0.347	0.127	0.226	0.175	0.538
Maxmum Cup Depth (mm)	0.374	0.699	0.419	0.559	0.534	0.953
Cup Shape Measure	-0.22	0.003	-0.271	-0.109	-0.21	0.067
Mean RNFL Thickness	0.21	0.13	0.315	0.157	0.231	0.126
RNFL Cross Section Area (mm2)	0.868	0.597	1.432	0.724	1.015	0.594
Intraocular Pressure (mmHg)	22.3	46.7	14	29.7	17.2	38.7

Table 2. Ophthalmological examination by HRT. Data in GM2 and GM3 were cited from 2 monkeys out of 11 previously described in (Shimazawa et al., 2006).

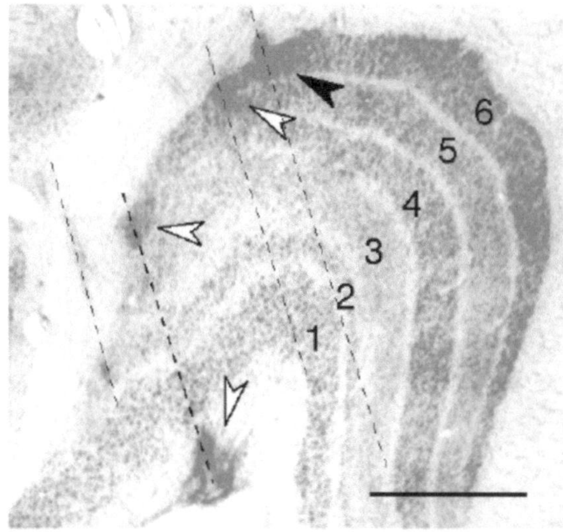

Fig. 14. Histological reconstruction of the recording tracks on Nissl-stained coronal sections obtained from a monkey.
Four arrowheads indicate electrolytic lesions on the recording tracks (dotted lines). The solid arrowhead indicates the location of a neuron whose responses are shown in Fig. 16. Note that the most medial penetration directly entered the magnocellular layers. The numbers indicate the 6 main laminas of the monkey lateral geniculate nucleus. Scale bar 1 mm.

Figure 14 shows an example of a photomicrograph of a Nissl-stained coronal section at the middle level of the LGN in the left hemisphere ipsilateral to the glaucomatous eye. No gross abnormality is noted in Nissl morphology. We first determined the lamina location of each recorded neuron from the stereotypical shift in eye preference of the receptive fields as our recording electrode was advanced vertically through the different LGN laminas.
Previous studies showed that, up to an eccentricity of 30 degrees, the MRF of LGN neurons in monkey was smaller than three degrees (Schiller et al., 1976; Lee et al., 1979; Bauer et al., 1999; McClurkin et al., 1991; White et al., 2001; Solomon et al., 2002). Solomon et al. (2002) reported that the classical center radius (r_c) of parvo- and magnocellular cells could be estimated by the following equations, respectively:

Parvo: $r_c = \exp(0.11x-3.4)$
Magno: $r_c = \exp(0.07x-2.4)$
x, eccentricity (in degree)

Figure 15 shows plots of the MRF of LGN neurons obtained from monkeys GM1 (Fig. 15**a**), GM2 (Fig. 15**c**), and GM3 (Fig. 15**e**) with respective scores for injury found in the head of the optic nerve (Figs. 15**b**, **d**, and **f**). Using more than 10 microelectrode penetrations, we covered the visual field out to ~40 degrees eccentricity in the peripheral visual field.
On stimulation of the normal eye, many small MRFs (each about 1 visual degree across) were found in the peri-foveal region (left plots with a cluster of black circles in Figs. 15**a**, **c**, and **e**). However, no corresponding cluster of small MRFs was found in the central visual field upon stimulation of the glaucomatous eye (right plots with red circles in Fig. 15**a**, **c**, and **e**). This was particularly clear in monkeys GM1 and GM3, because of the relative lack of spatial overlap of plotted MRFs.

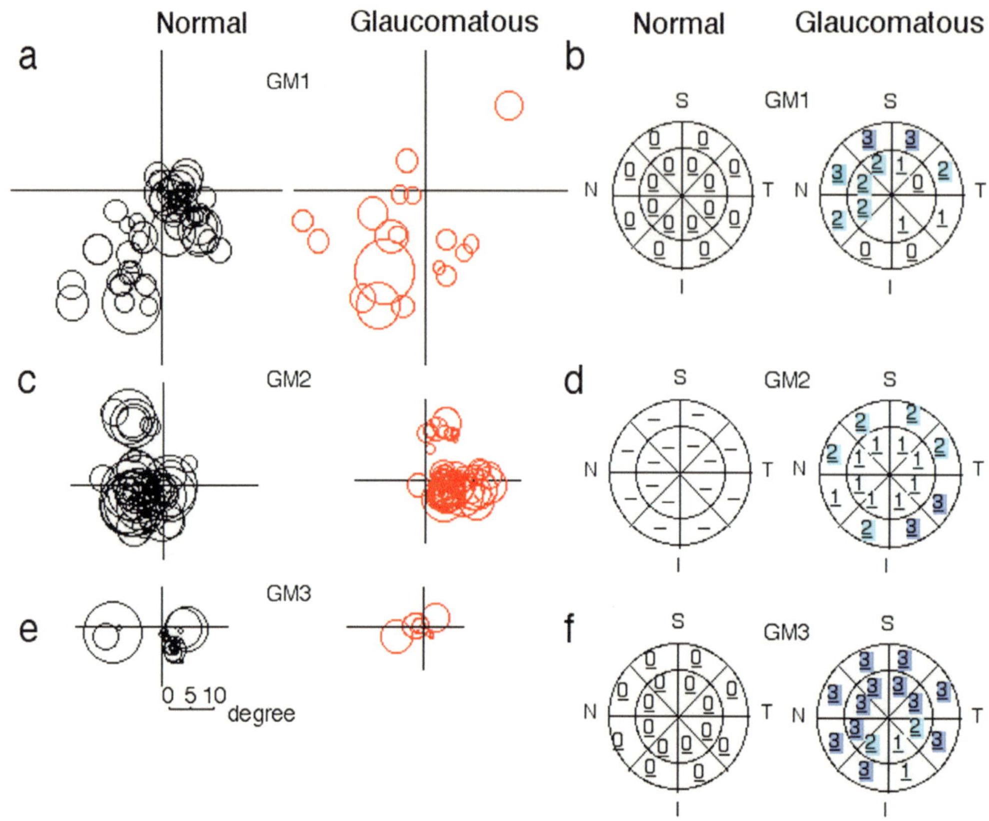

Fig. 15. Plots of the minimum response field (MRF) and diagrams that show injury to the optic nerves in three monkeys (**a** and **b**, monkey GM1; **c** and **d**, monkey GM2; **e** and **f**, monkey GM3).
The MRF of each LGN neurons is rendered as a circle and its boundary indicated by black (normal eye responses, left plots) or red (glaucomatous eye responses, right plots) circles. The horizontal meridian is drawn as a line connecting the two foveas, and the vertical meridian as a line midway between two optic disks. The scale bar shown under the plots for the normal eye of GM3 is common to all MRF plots. Based on the protocol of Sanches et al. (1986), injury to the optic nerve was evaluated histologically (Perry and Cowey, 1985; Wassle et al., 1990; Harwerth et al., 1999). Cross-sections were divided into 16 sectors (8 equal-sized pies, each further halved by an intersecting ring) and the degree of injury in each sector was evaluated microscopically at x 100 with an increasing order of severity: 0, normal; 1, mild (partial atrophy found without hypertrophy of connective tissue); 2, moderate (atrophy of axons with hypertrophy of connective tissue); 3, severe (complete lack of normal axons). S, I, N, and T indicate orientation of the optic nerve head as superior, inferior, nasal, and temporal, respectively.

The pattern and degree of injury to the optic nerve head varied among the three monkeys. Monkeys GM1 and GM3 exhibited more severe injury in the nasal-superior than other sectors, while mild injury was found uniformly in the central sectors of monkey GM3 (Figs. 15**b**, **d**, and **f**). Consistent with this finding, MRFs for the glaucomatous eye were mostly missing from the temporal-inferior visual field of GM1 and GM3.

Intriguingly, we found many extremely large MRFs (>10 degree) in all three monkeys (Figs. 15**a**, **c**, and **e**), suggesting an abnormality in the neural mechanism controlling the size of MRFs in the LGN of glaucomatous monkeys.

5.4 Stimulation of glaucomatous and normal eyes

The enlargement of the MRF size of single LGN neurons was observed for both stimulation of normal and glaucomatous eyes (Fig. 15**a**, **c**, and **e**). In the overwhelming majority of 252 recorded neurons, irrespective of which eye was stimulated, the size of MRFs was much larger than one degree across. In GM1, the median MRF size was 4-5 degrees across, while it was 2-3 and 1-2 degrees in GM2 and GM3, respectively (Fig. 16**a-c**). The Wiscoxon signed

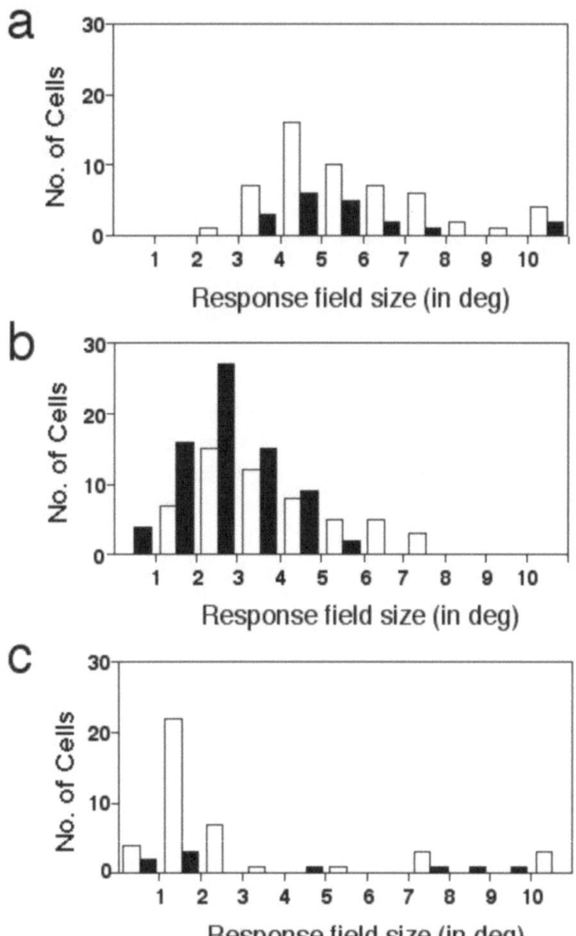

Fig. 16. Frequency histograms of neurons with different MRF sizes in three monkeys (**a**: monkey GM1, **b**: monkey GM2, **c**: monkey GM3).
Filled columns indicate neurons that responded to stimulation of the glaucomatous eye, while open columns indicate those that responded to stimulation of the normal eye. Numbers 2 to 10 on the abscissa indicate size of minimum response field between (n-1) < x ≤ n degrees. Neurons with response field larger than 10 degrees were grouped together as >10.

rank test (using Prism 4, GraphPad Software Inc., CA U.S.A.) showed that the median derived from the three monkeys was significantly larger in the normal eyes than those in glaucomatous eyes ($P<0.037$).
Responses to stimulation of the normal eye were more common than to that of the glaucomatous eye in all three monkeys, although the distribution pattern of neurons in the histogram was similar for the two eyes in GM1 and GM2.
Since susceptibility to elevated IOP may differ between different types of RGCs, we suspected the presence of comparable differences in the LGN. However, we found no marked difference in overall MRF size increase between P and M neurons in the glaucomatous LGN laminas. This conclusion was based on examination of 170 neurons in P laminas and 73 neurons in M laminas, both of which were included in Fig. 16. We concluded that effects of elevated IOP on MRF size could be obtained in both M- and P-neurons.

5.5 Size-tuning curve of LGN neurons

To gain insight into the cellular mechanism underlying the enlargement of LGN receptive fields in glaucomatous monkeys, we investigated their size-tuning properties objectively by stimulating them with a drifting sinusoidal grating patches whose size varied randomly (Akasaki et al., 2002). For the sake of efficiency of the experiments, the application of the objective method was limited to only a part of neurons recorded (N=34) in the above-cited study. Activities of the thus-isolated single neurons were continuously fed to an audio monitor during receptive-field mapping and quantitative data were acquired using a time-stamping board (Lisberger Tech., San Francisco) at a sampling rate of 1 MHz.
Results shown in Figure 17 were obtained from a lamina-6 P neuron whose recording site is shown in Fig. 14 (solid arrow head). Raster plots and PSTHs of the responses to stimuli given to the right normal eye with three different sizes of grating patches are shown in Figs. 17**a**, **b**, and **c**. The resultant stimulus size-tuning curve is shown in Fig. 17**d**. This neuron had a MRF of 12.5 degrees. The response of this neuron was suppressed one time with a patch size of about 21 degrees across (Figs. 17**b** and **d**), but became strong again with increase in patch sizes beyond 28 degrees (Figs. 17**c** and **d**).
Three types of size-tuning behavior were recognized. Two representative size-tuning curves are shown in Figure 18 (**b** and **c**). First, a neuron with a small MRF exhibited the maximum response at 1.4 degrees, and the response remained strongly suppressed (down to ~ 40% of the maximum) when the patch size was increased beyond this size (Fig. 18**b**). However, having a large MRF of 7.0 degrees, another neuron exemplified in Fig. 18**c** exhibited relatively weak suppression (~73%) with increases in the stimulus patch size beyond 2.1 degrees, which elicited the peak response. With further increase in stimulus size, the response of this type of cells often became stronger to make a second peak. The third type exhibited no measurable suppression.
A population of 39 neurons, including 5 not assessed quantitatively, from 7 recording tracks was classified into the three types groups, with about three-quarters of neurons (30 of 39) exhibiting either weak or no suppression at all.
Next, in 34 neurons quantitatively assessed neurons out of the 39 mentioned above, we directly compared the two kinds of size estimates: one derived from manually plotted MRFs and the other, the receptive field size indices derived from size-tuning curves. The correlation coefficient (r) was 0.76 and the slope of the fitted line was 1.04, indicating a good correlation between the two measures (Fig. 18**a**, $p<0.001$). Most of the points were located

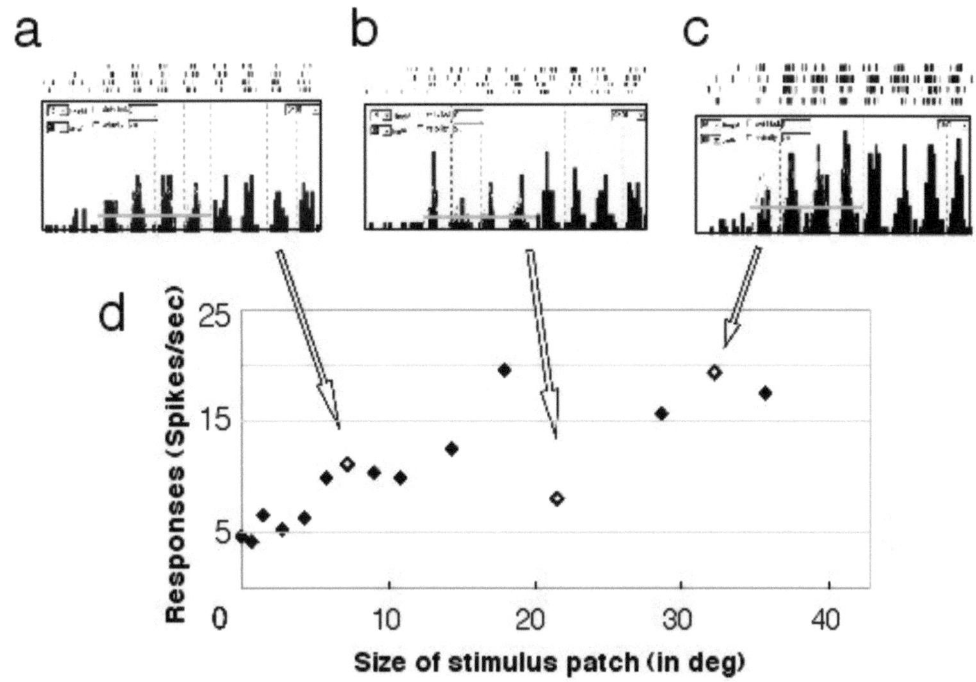

Fig. 17. An example of size-tuning tests.
Three representative peristimulus time histograms (PSTHs) and raster plots (**a**, **b**, **c**) are shown for stimulus sizes indicated by the three open diamonds in **d**. The number of repetition was 6 and bin size was 50 ms for each PSTH. The scale bar under PSTH **c** indicates one sec and is common to **a** and **b**. Mean firing rate (spikes/s) for the first 2 sec after the start of stimulus drift (gray lines in PSTHs) was plotted (filled diamonds) against grating patch size in degrees. The recording site of this neuron is shown in Fig. 14.

above the diagonal dotted line, indicating that the size of MRFs was mostly smaller than the size indices derived from the objective measurements.
In short, the present findings indicate: i) the MRF is usually smaller than the size of the grating patch that evoked the maximum response, while there is a significant correlation between these two measures, and ii) the enlargement of receptive fields of LGN neurons in glaucomatous monkeys was often accompanied by the lack of strong surround suppression.
Increase in the cell receptive field size was recently shown in the rat superior colliculus following increase in IOP in one eye (King et al., 2006). The authors suggested that the increase in receptive-field size was related to increase in the size of the dendritic arbors of surviving ganglion cells in the retina. Thus, by the same token, the morphological changes in surviving ganglion cells at the affected eye likely contribute to the emergence of the enlarged receptive fields in the LGN found in the present study.
However, unlike the above-noted findings for rat collicular cells, here in LGN neurons of experimentally induced hypertension glaucomatous monkeys, we found that receptive fields were enlarged with visual stimulation of not only the glaucomatous eye but also the normal eye, which exhibited normal IOP. We suspect that, in the case of LGN neurons, receptive-field enlargement was due to modification of the balance between excitation and

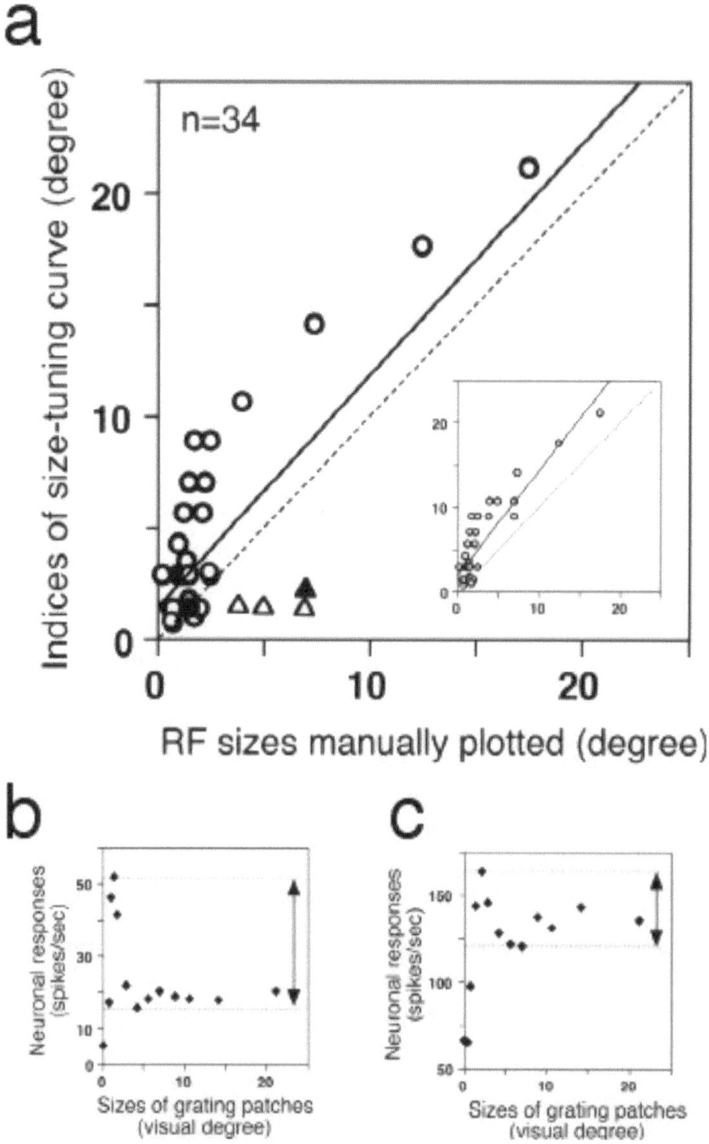

Fig. 18. Correlation between the size of manually plotted MRF and that based on size-tuning curves.

In **a**, the minimum size of the grating patch that evoked the maximum response (peak value or first inflection) was used as a size index for the size-tuning curve. All triangles indicate a group of cells which exhibited a dissociation of these two measures. Size-tuning curves of two representative neurons are shown in **b** (filled square in **a**) and **c** (filled triangle in **a**). In **b** and **c**, the dotted lines with double-headed arrows indicate maximum and minimal responses (i.e. extent of suppression). The solid lines in **a** are fitted by (y=1.04x+1.53) and (y=1.25x+1.87) for the ***inset*** (triangles excluded), respectively. The dotted lines in **a** are diagonal lines. Data points plotted in **a** appear less than 34 (n=34) because of overlap involving several points.

inhibition. It has been shown that experimental scotoma induces functional reorganization of the primary visual cortex, with enlargement of the receptive fields of neurons representing the region surrounding scotoma into the regions corresponding to scotoma representation (Chino et al., 1992; Gilbert and Wiesel, 1992; Darian-Smith and Gilbert, 1995). When visual stimulation with a discrete patch activates a cluster of thalamic neurons that relay their out put to the cortex, the corresponding feedback projections from the cortex appear to reinforce the core of the thalamic activity by densely focusing on the most active relay neurons while indirectly inhibiting neighboring thalamic neurons in the fringe (Marrocco et al., 1982). This feedback projection narrows the thalamic responsive zone, restricts receptive field sizes, and alters neuronal response properties (Webb et al., 2002).
Cortico-thalamic feedback was excitatory when the receptive fields of cortical and thalamic neurons overlapped, but inhibitory when they did not (Tsumoto et al., 1978). Corticofugal feedback also affects the generation of length tuning in the visual pathway: length tuning of LGN neurons was released from cortical control when the visual cortex was cooled (Murphy and Sillito, 1987). In short, the robust effects of corticofugal feedback on geniculate neuron activity suggest that this feedback contributes to the emergence of extremely large MRFs in the LGN in the abnormal conditions.

6. Functional implications

The onset of clinical signs is commonly much delayed in glaucomatous patients. Visual abnormality is first noted when injury to the retina has already significantly progressed. In parallel, behavioral measurements in glaucomatous monkeys showed that abnormality in the detection threshold of visual targets was mild despite the severity of injury to the retina (Sasaoka et al., 2005). This suggests the presence of a high level of neural plasticity in the adult brain that compensates for the loss of function due to retinal injury. We found the abnormal enlargement of receptive fields not only with stimulation of the glaucomatous eye but also of the normal eye, suggesting that the mechanism triggering this type of adult plasticity does not reside locally in the retina or even the LGN, but outside of them, probably in visual cortex. This line of reasoning further urges us to study the visual cortex to detect early sign of hypertension glaucoma.
An apparent analogy may be drawn here to the well-known somatosensory field compensation observed in the case of "phantom limbs" (Ramachandran and Rogers-Ramachandran, 2000). In general, the central nervous system readily undergoes reorganization when normal afferents are removed, to compensate for lost function (Wall et al., 1986). Although the basic phenomenology seems to be real in the somatosensory system, in the visual system likelihood of a similar long-term cortical reorganization after retinal lesions is far from settled (Smirmakis et al., 2005). Unlike the acute sensory disturbance induced by cutting or crushing of the optic nerve, in hypertensive glaucoma apoptotic cell death of retinal ganglion cells evolves slowly over a long period of time. The unilateral hypertension model of glaucoma in monkeys thus provides a unique opportunity for not only pathophysiological study on glaucoma ethiology but also study on adult plasticity in the central visual pathways.

7. Conclusion

A relatively high incidence of glaucoma has become a serious problem in the modern aging society. In our investigation, we focused on the neural changes along the central visual pathway in experimentally induced, hypertension glaucoma. First, we used PET in monkeys with unilateral hypertension glaucoma. In 2-[^{18}F]fluoro-2-deoxy-glucose studies, monocular visual stimulation of the affected eye yielded significantly reduced neural responses in the occipital areas. The reduction in response was limited to the visual cortex ipsilateral to the affected eye, indicating the unique vulnerability of ipsilateral visual cortex in experimental unilateral glaucoma. Next, in anatomical tracing experiments with WGA, we found in the glaucomatous eye that the retinal projection was selectively damaged in the ipsilateral pathway to the LGN, whereas the contralateral projection was relatively-well preserved. Third, in [^{11}C]PK11195 positron emission tomography and immunohistochemical studies, selective accumulation of activated microglia, a sign of neural degeneration, was found bilaterally in the LGN. The accumulation of activated microglia in the LGN is induced plausibly due to the abnormal, either suppressed or enhanced retinal electrical activity. Fourth, in the electrophysiological study on unilateral hypertension glaucomatous monkeys, we found that: i) the existence of "blind" regions in the visual field, in which no receptive field could be found despite multiple penetrations throughout each LGN, ii) the mean size of receptive fields was increased in both glaucomatous-eye-recipient and normal-eye-recipient LGN laminae, iii) the size was significantly larger for the normal-eye than those for glaucomatous eye. In glaucomatous monkeys, receptive field properties of responsive LGN neurons often exhibited little modification except in the receptive-field size. This form of adult plasticity may play a role in neuronal compensation in the central visual pathway of retinal input due to glaucoma. In addition to reduce the ganglion cell death, it is suggested that the enhancement of neural plasticity in the central visual pathway is also important for the remedy of glaucoma. In short, the current findings in experimental hypertension glaucoma seem to support our basic premise that the neural changes along the central visual pathway in glaucoma may precede those in the eye, against the backgroung of the former's high degree of compensation for the deteriorating function.

8. Acknowledgements

We are grateful to Dr. T. Kasamatsu for his invaluable suggestions. We also thank Dr. M. Connolly for critical reading of the manuscript. This work was supported in part by a grant (GONI & II) from Santen Pharmaceutical Co., Ltd. and a consignment expense from the Molecular Imaging Program on 'Research Basis for Exploring New Drugs' from the Ministry of Education, Culture, Sports, Science, and Technology (MEXT) of Japan. We also thank to our previous coworkers involved in some of the experiments appearing in the present paper.

9. References

Ahmed F.A.K.M., Chaudhary, P., & Sharma, S.C. (2001). Effects of increased intraocular pressure on rat retinal ganglion cells. *Int. J. Devl. Neurosci.*, 19, pp. (209-218)

Akasaki, T., Sato, H., Yoshimura, Y., Ozeki, H., & Shimegi, S. (2002). Suppressive effects of receptive field surround on neuronal activity in the cat primary visual cortex. *Neurosci. Res.*, 43, pp. (207-220)

Asano, E., Mochizuki, K., Sawada, A., Nagasaka, E., Kondo, Y., & Yamamoto T. (2007). Decreased nasal-temporal asymmetry of the second-order kernel response of

mulitifocal electroretinograms in eyes with normal-tension glaucoma. *Jpn. J. Ophthalmol.*, 51, 5, pp. (379-389)
Barlow, H.B., Blakemore, C., & Pettigrew, J.D. (1967). The neural mechanism of binocular depth discrimination. *J. Physiol.*, 193 pp. (327-342)
Bauer, U., Scholz, M., Levitt, J.B., Obermayer, K., & Lund, J.S. (1999). A model for the depth-dependence of receptive field size and contrast sensitivity of cells in layer 4C of macaque striate cortex. *Vision Res.*, 39, pp. (613-629)
Cagnin, A, Brooks D.J., Kennedy A.M., Gunn R.N., Myers, R., Turkheimer F.E., Jones, T., & Banati, R.B. (2001a). In-vivo measurement of activated microglia in dementia. *Lancet*, 358, pp. (9280)
Cagnin, A., Myers, R., Gunn, R.N., Lawrence, A.D., Stevens, T., Kreutzberg, G.W., Jones, T., Banati, R.B. (2001b). In vivo visualization of activated glia by [^{11}C] (R)-PK11195-PET following herpes encephalitis reveals projected neuronal damage beyond the primary focal lesion. *Brain*, 124, 10, pp. (2014-2017)
Chino, Y.M., Kaas, J.H., Smith, E.L., 3rd, Langston, A.L., & Cheng, H. (1992). Rapid reorganization of cortical maps in adult cats following restricted deafferentation in retina. *Vision Res.*, 32, pp. (789-796)
Cleland, B.G., Lee, B.B., & Vidyasagar, T.R. (1983). Response of neurons in the cat's lateral geniculate nucleus to moving bars of different length. *J. Neurosci.*, 3, pp. (108-116)
Darian-Smith, C., & Gilbert, C.D. (1995). Topographic reorganization in the striate cortex of the adult cat and monkey is cortically mediated. *J. Neurosci.*, 15 pp. (1631-1647)
Elolia, R., & Stokes, J. (1998). Monograph series on aging-related diseases: XI. Glaucoma. *Chronic Dis. Can.*, 19, pp. (157-169)
Fischer, B., & Kruger, J. (1974). The shift-effect in the cat's lateral geniculate neurons. *Exp.* Brain Res., 21, pp. (225-227)
Fitzgibbon, T., & Taylor, S.F. (1996). Retinotopy of the human retinal nerve fibre layer and optic nerve head. *J. Comp. neurol.*, 375, 2, pp. (238-251)
Gilbert, C.D., & Wiesel, T.N. (1992). Receptive field dynamics in adult primary visual cortex. *Nature*, 356, pp. (150-152)
Giovacchini, G., Squitieri, F., Esmaelizadeh, M, Milano, A., Mansi, L., & Clarmiello A. (2011). PET translates neurophysiology into images: A review to stimulate a network between neuroimaging and basic research. *J. Cell Physiol.*, 226 4, pp. (948-961)
Gong, S, & LeDoux, M.S. (2003). Immunohistochemical detection of wheat germ agglutinin-horseradish peroxisase (WGA-HRP). *J. Neurosci. Methods*, 26, 1, pp. (25-34)
Graeber, M.B., Bise, K., & Mehraein, P. (1994). CR3/43, a merker for activated human microglia: application to diagnostic neuropathology. *Neurophathol. Appl. Neurobiol.*, 20, 4, pp. (406-408)
Harwerth, R.S., Carter-Dawson, L., Shen, F., Smith, E.L., 3rd, & Crawford, M.L. (1999). Ganglion cell losses underlying visual field defects from experimental glaucoma. *Invest. Ophthalmol. Vis. Sci.*, 40, pp. (2242-2250)
Hubel, D.H., & Wiesel, T.N. (1961). Integrative action in the cat's lateral geniculate body. *J. Physiol.*, 155, pp. (385-398)
Imamura, K., Richter, H., Fischer, H. Lennerstrand, G., Franzén, Rydberg, A., Andersson, J., Schneider, H., Onoe, H., Watanabe, Y., & Långström, B. (1997). Reduced activity in the extrastriate visual cortex of individuals with strabismic amblyopia. *Neuroscience Lett.*, 225, pp. (173-176)

Imamura, K., Onoe, H., Shimazawaa, M., Nozaki, S., Wada, Y., Kato, K., Nakajima, H., Mizuma, H., Onoe, K., Taniguchi, T., Sasaoka, M., Hara, H., Tanaka, S, Araie, M., & Watanabe, W. (2009). Molecular imaging reveals unique degenerative changes in experimental glaucoma. *NeuroReport*, 20, pp. (139-144)

King, W.M., Sarup, V., Sauve, Y., Moreland, C.M., Carpenter, D.O., & Sharma, S.C. (2006). Expansion of visual receptive fields in experimental glaucoma. *Vis. Neurosci.*, 23, pp. (137-142)

Klein, B.E., Klein, R., & Linton, K.L. (1992). Intraocular pressure in an American community. The Beaver Dam Eye Study. *Invest. Ophthalmol. Vis. Sci.*, 33, pp. (2224-2228)

Lee, B.B., Creutzfeldt, O.D., & Elepfandt, A. (1979). The responses of magno- and parvocellular cells of the monkey's lateral geniculate body to moving stimuli. *Exp. Brain Res.*, 35, pp. (547-557)

Leske, M.C. (1983). The epidemiology of open-angle glaucoma: a review. *Am. J. Epidemiol.*, 118, pp. (166-191)

Levick, W.R. (1972). Another tungsten micro-electrode. *Med. Biol. Eng.*, 10, pp. (510-515)

Levitt, J.B., Schumer, R.A., Sherman, S.M., Spear, P.D., & Movshon, J.A. (2001). Visual response properties of neurons in the LGN of normally reared and visually deprived macaque monkeys. *J. Neurophysiol.*, 85, pp. (2111-2129)

Marrocco, R.T., McClurkin, J.W., & Young, R.A. (1982). Modulation of lateral geniculate nucleus cell responsiveness by visual activation of the corticogeniculate pathway. *J. Neurosci.*, 2, pp. (256-263)

McClurkin, J.W., & Marrocco, R.T. (1984). Visual cortical input alters spatial tuning in monkey lateral geniculate nucleus cells. *J. Physiol.*, 348, pp. (135-152)

McClurkin, J.W., Gawne, T.J., Richmond, B.J., Optican, L.M., & Robinson, D.L. (1991) Lateral geniculate neurons in behaving primates. I. Responses to two-dimensional stimuli. *J. Neurophysiol.*, 66, pp. (777-793)

Murphy, P.C., & Sillito, A.M. (1987). Corticofugal feedback influences the generation of length tuning in the visual pathway. *Nature*, 329, pp. (727-729)

O'Keefe, L.P., Levitt, J.B., Kiper, D.C., Shapley, R.M., & Movshon, J.A. (1998). Functional organization of owl monkey lateral geniculate nucleus and visual cortex. *J. Neurophysiol.*, 80, pp. (594-609)

Perry, V.H., & Cowey, A. (1985). The ganglion cell and cone distributions in the monkey's retina: implications for central magnification factors. *Vision Res.*, 25, pp. (1795-1810)

Perry, V.H., Oehler, R., & Cowey, A. (1984). Retinal ganglion cells that project to the dorsal lateral geniculate nucleus in the macaque monkey. *Neurosci.*, 12, pp. (1101-1123)

Ramachandran, V.S., & Rogers-Ramachandran, D. (2000). Phantom limbs and neural plasticity. *Arch. Neurol.*, 57, pp. (317-320)

Salive, M.E., Guralnik, J., Christen, W., Glynn, R.J., Colsher, P., & Ostfeld, A.M. (1992). Functional blindness and visual impairment in older adults from three communities. *Ophthalmology*, 99, pp. (1840-1847)

Sanchez, R.M., Dunkelberger, G.R., & Quigley, H.A. (1986). The number and diameter distribution of axons in the monkey optic nerve. *Invest. Ophthalmol. Vis. Sci.*, 27, pp. (1342-1350)

Sasaoka, M., Hara, H., & Nakamura, K. (2005). Comparison between monkey and human visual fields using a personal computer system. *Behav. Brain Res.*, 161, pp. (18-30)

Schiller, P.H., Finlay, B.L., & Volman, S.F. (1976). Quantitative studies of single-cell properties in monkey striate cortex. I. Spatiotemporal organization of receptive fields. *J. Neurophysiol.*, 39, pp. (1288-1319)

Shimazawa, M., Taniguchi, T., Sasaoka, M., & Hara, H. (2006a). Nerve fiber layer measurement using scanning laser polarimetry with fixed corneal compensator in normal cynomolgus monkey eyes. *Ophthalmic Res.*, 38, pp. (1-7)

Shimazawa, M., Tomita, G., Taniguchi, T., Sasaoka, M., Hara, H., Kitazawa, Y., & Araie, M. (2006b). Morphometric evaluation of changes with time in optic disc structure and thickness of retinal nerve fibre layer in chronic ocular hypertensive monkeys. *Exp. Eye Res.*, 82, pp. (427-440)

Smith, E.L,, 3rd, Chino, Y. M., Harwerth, R. S., Ridder, W. H., 3rd, Crawford, M.L.J., & DeSantis, L. (1993). Retinal inputs to the monkey's lateral geniculate nucleus in experimental glaucoma. *Clinical Vision Sci.*, 8, pp. (113-139)

Smirnakis, S.M., Brewer, A.A., Schmid, M.C., Tolias, A.S., Schuz, A., Augath, M., Inhoffen, W., Wandell, B.A., & Logothetis, N.K. (2005). Lack of long-term cortical reorganization after macaque retinal lesions. *Nature*, 435, pp. (300-307)

Solomon, S.G., White, A.J., & Martin, P.R. (2002). Extraclassical receptive field properties of parvocellular, magnocellular, and koniocellular cells in the primate lateral geniculate nucleus. *J. Neurosci.*, 22, pp. (338-349)

Spear, P.D., Moore, R.J., Kim, C.B., Xue, J.T., & Tumosa, N. (1994). Effects of aging on the primate visual system: spatial and temporal processing by lateral geniculate neurons in young adult and old rhesus monkeys. *J. Neurophysiol.*, 72, pp. (402-420)

Tsumoto, T., Creutzfeldt, O.D., & Legendy, C.R. (1978). Functional organization of the corticofugal system from visual cortex to lateral geniculate nucleus in the cat (with an appendix on geniculo-cortical mono-synaptic connections). *Exp. Brain Res.*, 32, pp. (345-364)

Usrey, W.M., & Reid, R.C. (2000). Visual physiology of the lateral geniculate nucleus in two species of new world monkey: Saimiri sciureus and Aotus trivirgatis. *J. Physiol.*, 523, 3, pp. (755-769)

Vowinckel, E., Reutens, D., Becher B., Evans, A., Owens, T., & Antel J.P. (1997). PK11195 binding to the peripheral benzodiazepine receptor as a marker of microglia activation in multiple sclerosis and experimental autoimmune encephalomyelitis. *J. Neurosci. Res.*, 50, 2, pp. (345-353)

Wake, H., Moorhouse, A.J., Jinno, S., Kohsaka S., & Nabekura, J. (2009). Resting microglia directly monitor the functional state of synapses in vivo and determine the fate of ischemic terminals. *J. Neurosci.*, 29, 13, pp. (3974-3980)

Wall, J.T., Kaas, J.H., Sur, M., Nelson, R.J., Felleman, D.J., & Merzenich, M.M. (1986). Functional reorganization in somatosensory cortical areas 3b and 1 of adult monkeys after median nerve repair: possible relationships to sensory recovery in humans. *J. Neurosci.*, 6, pp. (218-233)

Wassle, H., Grunert, U., Rohrenbeck, J., & Boycott, B.B. (1990). Retinal ganglion cell density and cortical magnification factor in the primate. *Vision Res.*, 30, pp. (1897-1911)

Webb, B.S., Tinsley, C.J., Barraclough, N.E., Easton, A., Parker, A., & Derrington, A.M. (2002). Feedback from V1 and inhibition from beyond the classical receptive field modulates the responses of neurons in the primate lateral geniculate nucleus. *Vis. Neurosci.*, 19, pp. (583-592)

White, A.J., Solomon, S.G., & Martin, P.R. (2001). Spatial properties of koniocellular cells in the lateral geniculate nucleus of the marmoset Callithrix jacchus. *J. Physiol.*, 533, pp. (519-535)

Wilson, J.R., & Forestner, D.M. (1995). Synaptic inputs to single neurons in the lateral geniculate nuclei of normal and monocularly deprived squirrel monkeys. *J. Comp. Neurol.*, 362, pp. (468-488)

Yücel, Y.H., Zhang, Q., Gupta, N., Kaufman, P.L., & Weinreb, R.N. (2000). Loss of neurons in magnocellular and parvocellular layers of the lateral geniculate nucleus in glaucoma. *Arch. Ophthalmol.*, 118, pp. (378-384)

Yücel, Y.H., Zhang, Q., Weinreb, R.N., Kaufman, P.L., & Gupta, N. (2001). Atrophy of relay neurons in magno- and parvocellular layers in the lateral geniculate nucleus in experimental glaucoma. *Invest. Ophthalmol. Vis. Sci.*, 42, pp. (3216-3222)

18

Using Artificial Neural Networks to Identify Glaucoma Stages

Gustavo Santos-García and Emiliano Hernández Galilea
Department of Surgery. Faculty of Medicine, Universidad de Salamanca
Spain

1. Introduction

Glaucoma is one of the principal causes of blindness in the world[1]. It is an illness which has an asymptomatic form until advanced stages, thus early diagnosis represents an important objective to achieve with the aim that people who present Glaucoma maintain the best visual acuity throughout life, thereby improving their quality of life.
An Artificial Neural Network (ANN) is proposed for the diagnosis of Glaucoma. Automated combination and analysis of information from structural and functional diagnostic techniques were performed to improve Glaucoma detection in the clinic.
In our work we contribute the inclusion of Artificial Intelligence and neuronal networks in the diverse systems of clinical exploration and autoperimetry and laser polarimetry, with the objective of facilitating the adequate staging in a rapid and automatic way and thus to be able to act in the most adequate manner possible.
Data from clinical examination, standard perimetry and analysis of the nerve fibers of the retina with scanning laser polarimetry (NFAII;GDx) were integrated in a system of Artificial Intelligence. Different tools in the diagnosis of Glaucoma by an automatic classification system were explained based on ANN. In the present work an analysis of 106 eyes, in accordance with the stage of glaucomatous illness was used to develop an ANN. Multilayer perceptron was provided with the Levenberg-Marquardt method. The learning was carried out with half of the data and with the training function of gradient descent w/momentum backpropagation and was checked by the diagnosis of a Glaucoma expert ophthalmologist. A correct classification of each eye in the corresponding stage of Glaucoma has been achieved. Specificity and sensitivity are 100%. This method provides an efficient and accurate tool for the diagnosis of Glaucoma in the stages of glaucomatous illness by means of AI techniques.

2. Clinical, structural and functional examination in Glaucoma

Glaucoma is one of the principal causes of blindness in the world. Glaucoma is an ocular disease and it is the second leading cause of blindness worldwide and responsible for 20% of blindness in Europe. Glaucoma is also an age related disease and has age-adjusted prevalence of 1.55%, therefore the increase in elderly population in the world will increase the number of patients with Glaucoma in the coming decades. This increase in patients with Glaucoma will enlarge the socioeconomic cost associated to visual deficient diseases. Therefore efforts should

[1] Research supported by Spanish project DESAFIOS10 TIN2009-14599-C03-01.

be made to improve the diagnosis and treatment of this disease (European Glaucoma Society, 2008; Gordon et al., 2002; Huang & Chen, 2005; Quigley, 1985).

Glaucoma is an optic neuropathy characterized by progressive loss of retinal ganglion cells, changes in the optic nerve head and associated visual field loss (Fig. 1). There are a variety of risk factors for Glaucoma, the most important of which is intraocular pressure, IOP (Quigley et al., 1994). Primary open angle Glaucoma has an adult onset, is usually bilateral, and has no symptoms until late in the disease when patients lose their central vision. An understanding of the etiology and anatomical changes associated with Glaucoma is critical for early diagnosis of the disease and preserving sight (Song et al., 2005). Different studies have shown that structural and functional techniques for detecting Glaucoma often identify different Glaucoma patients when Glaucoma severity is not too advanced (Bowd et al., 2001; Zangwill et al., 2001), and that combining structural and functional techniques can improve Glaucoma detection (Caprioli, 1992; Mardin et al., 2006; Shah et al., 2006).

A variety of risk factors may predispose an individual to either the development of Glaucoma or disease progression. The Ocular Hypertension Treatment Study (Gordon et al., 2002) suggested that several factors predisposed patients who had ocular hypertension without ophthalmoscopic or perimetric evidence of Glaucoma to develop Glaucoma. Patients who were older, had a larger cup-disc ratio at the start of the trial, greater elevation of IOP, or thinner corneas appeared to be more likely to develop Glaucoma. Pressure-independent factors that may predict the onset of Glaucoma or ocular hypertension may include genetic predisposition, altered optic-nerve microcirculation, systemic hypotension, race, or myopia (Gordon et al., 2002).

Quigley and collaborators observed histological evidence that there is a substantial loss of axons of the optic nerve before the first defects in the visual field appear (Quigley, 1985). Other studies have found clinical evidence of this same fact (Quigley et al., 1989; Sommer et al., 1991).

The functional studies performed today in clinical practice, fundamentally the conventional computerized perimetry (static, threshold, white stimulus on white background), do not appear to be optimal nor sufficiently sensitive to detect early functional damage in many individuals (Fig. 2). A high number of ocular hyper tense subjects and suspect of Glaucoma with normal standard visual fields present alterations of the visual function in other tests (Johnson et al., 1993; Sample et al., 1993).

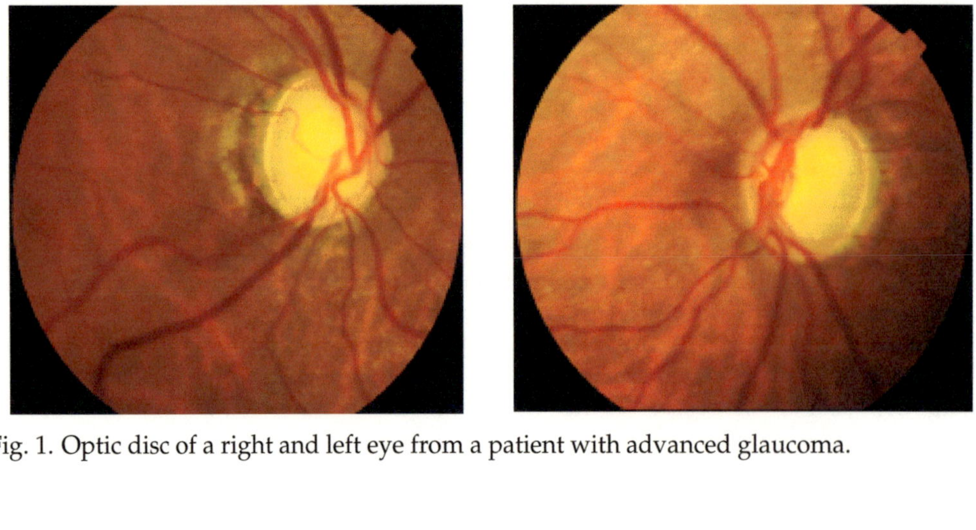

Fig. 1. Optic disc of a right and left eye from a patient with advanced glaucoma.

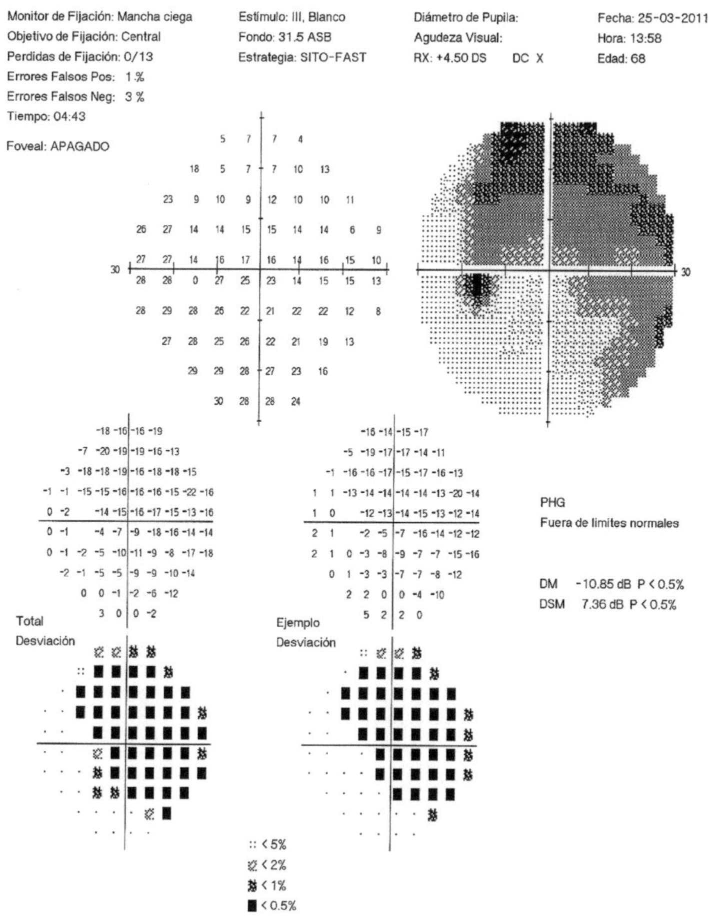

Fig. 2. Example for standard automated perimetry: Humphrey field analyzer test.

The single most effective method of diagnosing Glaucoma, therefore, is evaluating the optic nerve to determine if any injury has occurred. Direct examination of the optic nerve fibers at the optic nerve is essential in the diagnosis of Glaucoma, but is another non sensitive technique, in addition, normal eyes may have an optic nerve indistinguishable from those of incipient stages of Glaucoma. Other exploratory techniques are objective and reliable to detect Glaucoma before visual field loss, where search includes the technical photographic study of the layer of the retinal nerve fiber.

Today there is almost total unanimity in that the structural changes in the fiber layer of the retina and the neuro-retinal ring of the optic papilla precede the development of losses of visual field and it is admitted that the demonstration of specific alterations in the nerve fiber layer of the retina or in the papilla of the optic nerve allows the identification of a simple chronic Glaucoma in the most incipient phase of its clinical evolution independently of the ocular pressure and still in the absence of loss of visual field (Sharma et al., 2008; Tjon-Fo-Sang et al., 1996; Uchida et al., 1996; Weinreb et al., 1995).

Until now, the most universally accepted finding to establish a definitive diagnosis of Glaucoma was loss of visual field, but it is now considered that, even with more sophisticated techniques, it requires a significant loss of optic nerve fibers to document the visual field loss (Sample et al., 1993). In Glaucoma optic neuropathy a progressive loss of retinal ganglion cells occurs and consequently a decrease in thickness of retinal nerve fibers layer. It is known that the decrease of these fibers begins up to five years before it functional damage established with perimetry can be detected. Functional and structural injury in Glaucoma is present and the measurements of changes in the optic nerve could be correlated with damage observed in the visual field. The availability of devices to allow the analysis of the thickness of the fibers layer is very important (Bowd et al., 2001; Shah et al., 2006).

As glaucomatous structural injury progresses, changes develop in the contour of the optic nerve. These features of glaucomatous optic neuropathy include diffuse or focal thinning of the neuroretinal rim, enlargement of the cup, notching, and/or excavation. Different methods have been used to document the status of the optic nerve and retinal nerve fiber layer, RNFL (Lin et al., 2007). The evaluation of the nerve fiber layer of the retina with photographic techniques has shown to have technical limitations and the possibility of high frequencies of false positives (Peli et al., 1986).

The direct exploration of the fibers by digital videoophthalmolgraphy of the peripapillar area described by Caprioli (Caprioli, 1990; Caprioli & Miller, 1988; 1989; Caprioli et al., 1989) was one of the first attempts to achieve an objective measure based on the digitalized images of the Rodenstock analyser. From the images of the retina surface and of a plane of reference in the retina surface itself the thickness of the RNFL is inferred. With this procedure Caprioli himself described, for the first time, the typical pattern of "camelÕs hump". Among the inconveniences the necessity of the reference plane is outstanding, which supposes the exigence that this be constant so that the measures of monitoring are valid since they originated a great variability of the measures obtained. This variability, nonetheless, is less than that of the measurements of the papilla structures performed in the comparative study of Miller & Caprioli (1991), which though it limits its clinical applications, demonstrates its utility.

Currently there are commercially available versions of optical imaging techniques (Figures 3 and 4): scanning laser polarimetry with variable corneal compensation (GDx VCC), confocal scanning laser ophthalmoscopy (HRT II, Heidelberg Retina Tomograph), and optical coherence tomography (Stratus OCT) to discriminate between healthy eyes and eyes with glaucomatous visual field loss. The sensitivities at high specificities were similar among the best parameters from each instrument (Medeiros et al., 2004).

Scanning laser polarimetry (SLP) is a technology used to assess the RNFL in order to detect early glaucomatous damage. This technology has several potential advantages. Because less biological variability is expected in the region of the RNFL than the optic-nerve head, clinicians have the ability to define a narrower range of normal RNFL measurements. SLP has another advantage, that of being independent of a reference plane. Therefore, the retardation value that is measured by SLP refers to the RNFL and is not dependent upon measurements of any other ocular region when considering change over a period of time (Medeiros et al., 2004; Weinreb et al., 1995).

Laser polarimetry is a technology that uses a polarized laser diode as light source (780 nm). It is a confocal ellipsometric laser measuring a total delay of light reflected from the retina and from these data determines the thickness of the RNFL (microns) point by point in the peripapillary region. Currently apparatus is being presented as a novelty compared to previous versions that can compensate corneal birefringence on an individual basis for each patient (Zhou, 2006).

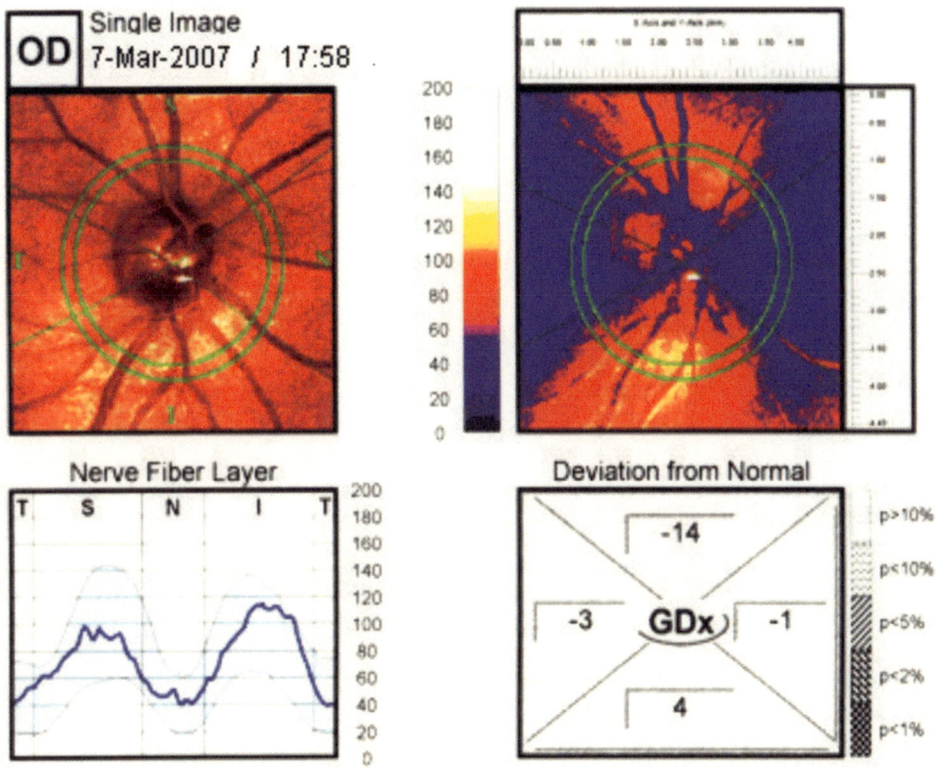

Fig. 3. Analysis with laser polarimetry for the measurement of the thickness of the layer of retinal nerve fibres using the NFA-II, GDX fibres analyser for a normal patient.

Scanning laser ophthalmoscopy. which is embodied in the Heidelberg Retinal Tomograph (Heidelberg Instruments, Inc., Heidelberg, Germany), is a highly reproducible technology that provides a means of obtaining objective measurements of optic-nerve topography. However, this technology was not fundamentally designed to generate RNFL assessments and there are limitations in relying on topography to detect glaucomatous progression (Bowd et al., 2002; Zangwill et al., 2001).

Another technology that has recently been utilized for Glaucoma detection is optical coherence tomocraphy, OCT (Fig. 5). OCT is a high resolution technology that generates direct measurements of the retina and RNFL thickness with a high degree of test-retest variability. However, few normative data for this technology exist at this time. OCT generates a single optical slice through the peripapillary RNFL, which may provide less information than a broad sampling of the entire RNFL profile provided by Scanning laser polarimetry (Burgansky-Eliash et al., 2005; Ferreras et al., 2008; Huang & Chen, 2005; Lu et al., 2008; Medeiros et al., 2005; 2004; Zangwill et al., 2001).

Glaucoma diagnosis is based on a range of normal measurements with the objective of finding eyes that are outside what is considered normal. There are two challenges for physicians when using structural testing. The first is diagnosis of the disease and the second is monitoring the known disease for progression.

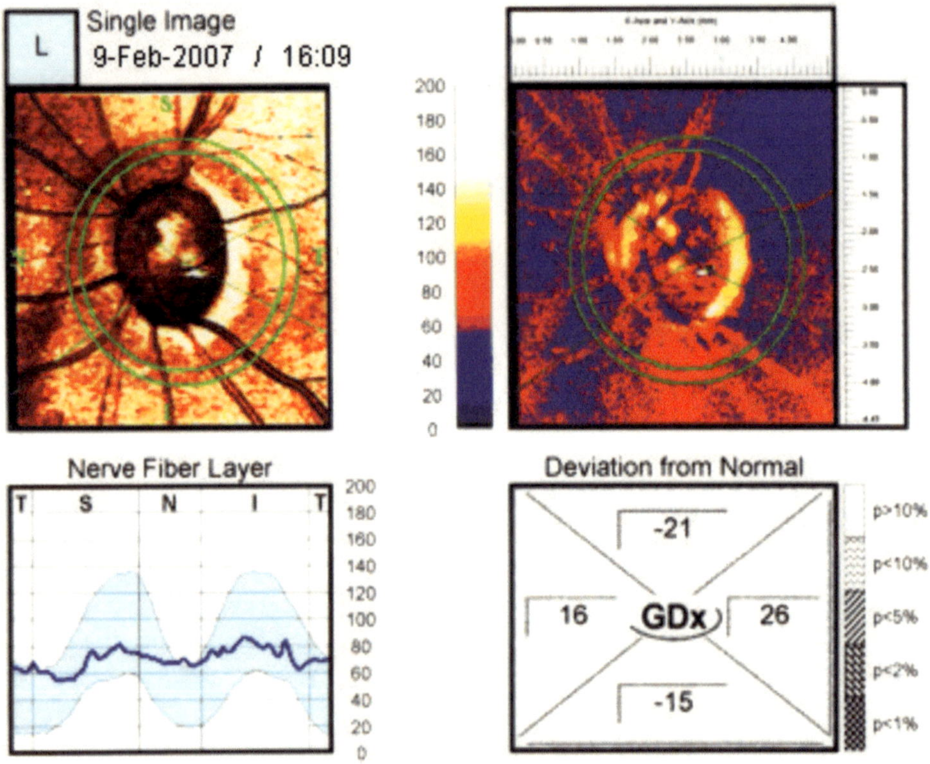

Fig. 4. Analysis with laser polarimetry for the measurement of the thickness of the layer of retinal nerve fibres using the NFA-II, GDX fibres analyser for a glaucomatous patient with stage 5 Glaucoma.

3. Diagnosis of Glaucoma by automatic systems

In ophthalmology applications of ANN have been used for the interpretation of the visual field for recognition and evaluation of the cell population of corneal endothelium (Ruggeri & Pajaro, 2002) and recognition of retinographs and angiofluorescent graphs in diabetic retinopathy (Gardner et al., 1996; Sivakumar et al., 2005).

Goldbaum et al. (1994) used the models of neuronal networks of multi-layer perceptron trained by retropropagation in the interpretation and classification of visual fields.

The methods of perimetric examination have contributed indices to analyze the visual field, but in no case was a clinical diagnosis included. The expert systems were the following step and were formed by programs specially designed to solve problems and to give diagnoses, taking into account the human experience accumulated. Based on the curve of accumulated defect, the indices and the influence of the false positives and negatives on the indices, they have been able to carry out classifications of the normal, doubtful or pathological visual fields in different degrees (Antón et al., 1995).

Other more complete programs integrated the analysis of the family and personal antecedents, the intraocular pressure, the papilla excavation indice and the state of the visual field, to similarly emit a clinical judgment.

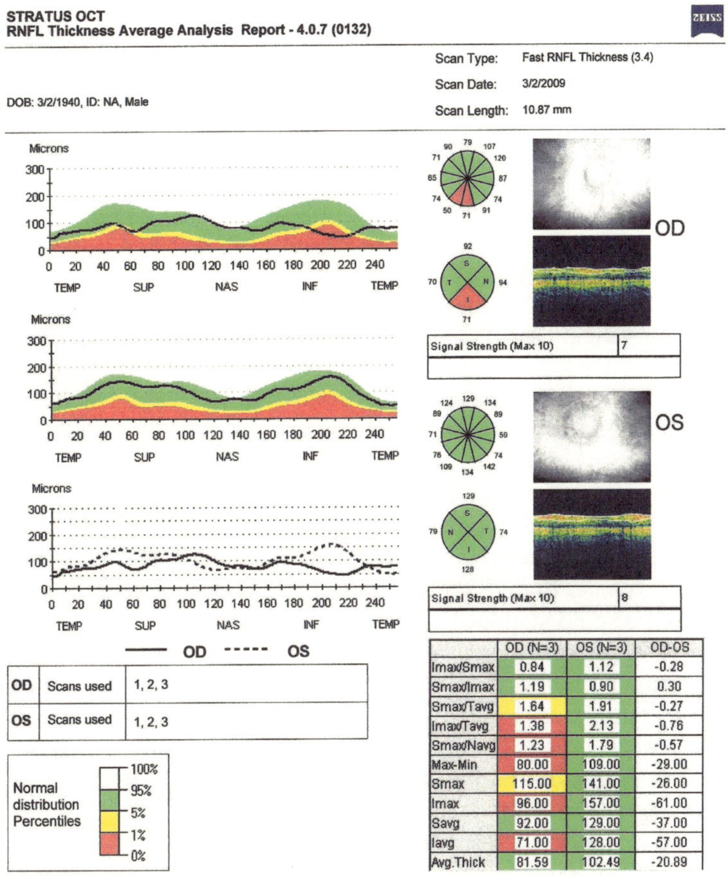

Fig. 5. Optical coherence tomography (OCT).

For the classification and diagnosis of the defects in the visual field a problem of discrimination into diagnostic categories has been proposed in accordance with the distribution and profundity of the lesions and, therefore, it is necessary to know the characteristics or patterns that allow the classification of each case. Moreover, the method chosen must be capable of treating qualitative and quantitative variables and perform with asymmetric variables of distribution or that are very distanced from a normal distribution. With these premises the list of usable procedures have been discriminant with logistic regression and the neuronal networks.

Antón et al. (1997) used the ANN for the interpretation of the incipient perimetric lesions produced in glaucoma and conclude that both the networks and the logistic regression are capable of differentiating between the incipient perimetric lesions produced by the glaucoma and those produced by other illnesses with important precision. They add that if these methods were applied to the PALOC, or another perimetric test, more sensitive to glaucomatous functional lesions than conventional perimetry, it would be a great aid for the identification and interpretation of the defects produced by this neuropathy.

Brigatti et al. (1996) also use the ANN to classify patients into normal or glaucomatous. They include automated data of the visual field, such as average defects, variances of corrected losses and fluctuation in the short term, and structural data such as radius of excavation, volume of disc and thickness of the nerve fiber layer. On including the data for the visual field and the structural data the results are better than when the data are used separately. The sensitivity with the data together was 90% and the specificity 84%. Only with the structural data a sensitivity of 87% and specificity of 56% were achieved and the results were 84% and 86% respectively if only the functional data were trained.

Recently, the Ocular Hypertension Treatment Study has shown that approximately 50% of individuals who convert to glaucomatous optic neuropathy do not have detectable changes in standard automated perimetry. The results suggest that structural change precedes functional change. Therefore, a significant application of a different type of technology would provide a means of establishing a diagnosis of glaucoma prior to any detectable functional abnormalities in vision.

Artificial neural networks were reported to be able to differentiate between glaucoma and normal visual field status at least as well as trained readers (Bengtsson et al., 2005; Goldbaum et al., 1994; Lietman et al., 1999).

Artificial neural networks have been trained on different optic nerve head imaging analyzer parameters to classify eyes as glaucomatous or healthy in accordance with confocal scanning laser ophthalmoscopy (Brigatti et al., 1996; Uchida et al., 1996). Using this method, the neural network classifier is trained to detect a relationship between input (parameters of structural study) and a predefined gold-standard diagnosis by comparing its prediction with the labeled diagnosis and by learning from its mistakes.

Neural network techniques differ from basic statistical techniques such as linear discriminant function because they can adapt to the distribution of the data rather than assume a predefined distribution. The success of statistical or neural network classification methods is most often measured by reporting areas under the receiver operating characteristic curve or by reporting sensitivity at different specificities.

It was also reported that machine learning classifiers discriminate better between normal and glaucomatous fields than do global visual field indices (Goldbaum et al., 2002; Lietman et al., 1999). Global visual field indices are far from ideal as diagnostic tools, however, because they condense all threshold data into one number, resulting in loss of valuable spatial information, and visual field indices are not particularly sensitive to early localized glaucomatous visual field loss (Asman et al., 1992; Chauhan et al., 1989).

Disc topography data have also been added to visual field data to improve the diagnostic ability of ANNs (Brigatti et al., 1996).

Lietman et al. (1999) has determined a feed-forward neural network with a single hidden layer and was trained to recognize visual field defects previously collected in a longitudinal follow-up glaucoma study, and then tested on fields taken from the same study but not used in the training. The receiver operating characteristics of the network were then compared with the previously determined performance of other algorithms on the same data set.

ANNs have been suggested as tools for interpretation of automated visual field test results in patients with glaucoma (Goldbaum et al., 1994; Lietman et al., 1999). Other types of machine learning classifiers, such as support vector machines or committee machines, have also been reported to interpret visual fields adequately (Gordon et al., 2002).

Using the optic disc topography parameters of the Heidelberg Retina Tomograph neural network techniques can improve differentiation between glaucomatous and non-glaucomatous eyes. Trained neural networks, with global and regional Heidelberg Retina Tomograph parameters used as input, improve on previously proposed parameters for discriminating between glaucomatous and nonglaucomatous eyes (AIGS, 2004; Bowd et al., 2002; 2001; 2004).

Neural networks and other machine classifiers seem to have a great potential to become a useful clinical tool in the diagnosis of glaucomatous visual field loss, and may be of value in the study of the performance of a range of types of data inputs with different machine classifiers.

4. Developing an artificial neural network

4.1 Neural networks

Rumelhart & McClelland (1986) presented the *backpropagation learning algorithm* in a year that can be considered the cornerstone of the ANNs recent history. ANN models have been extensively studied and applied in recent years in the hope of reaching human performance in different fields, including, for instance, automatic speech recognition, image processing, and biomedical applications (Arbib, 1995; Azuaje et al., 1999; Chan et al., 2002; Hernández Galilea et al., 2007; Lippmann & Kukolich, 1995; Lippmann & Shahian, 1997; Papalolukas et al., 2002; Peña Reyes & Sipper, 2000; Santos-García, 1990; Santos-García et al., 2004; Tu et al., 1998; Villar-Gómez & Santos-García, 1994; Widrow & Lehr, 1990). Actually, neurocomputing is blossoming almost daily in both theoretical and practical approaches. ANNs are generally more robust and outperform other computational tools in solving problems such as: classification, clustering, modeling, forecasting, optimization and association.

There are several models of neural nets according to their relevant features: topology, type of learning algorithm, degree of learning supervision, and so on. Classical ANN models are: Hopfield networks, Carpenter-Grossberg networks (Adaptative resonance theory), Kohonen networks (self-organizing feature maps), and backpropagation multilayer perceptron networks (Lippmann, 1987).

ANNs are empirical models in nature, however they obtain accurate and robust solutions for more or less precisely formulated problems and for complex phenomena that are only understood through experimental data.

4.2 Multilayer perceptron networks

A *neural network* is defined in mathematical terms as a graph with the following properties: (1) each node i, called *neuron* (Fig. 6), is associated with a state variable x_i storing its current output; (2) each junction between two neurons i and k, called *synapse* or *link*, is associated with a real weight ω_{ik}; (3) a real threshold θ_i, called *activation threshold*, is associated with each neuron i; (4) a *transfer function* $f_i[n_k, \omega_{ik}, \theta_i, (k \neq i)]$ is defined for each neuron, and determines the activation degree of the neuron as a function of its threshold, the weights of the input junctions and the outputs n_k of the neurons connected to its input synapses. In our case, the transfer function has the form $f(\sum_k \omega_{ik} n_k - \theta_i)$, where $f(x)$ is a sigmoidal function, defined by $f(x) = 1/(1 + e^{(\nu - x)})$, which corresponds to the continuous and derivable generalization of the step function (Hecht-Nielsen, 1990; Lippmann, 1987; Santos-García et al., 2008).

Multilayer perceptrons are networks with one or more layers of nodes between the layer of input units and the layer of output nodes; Fig. 7 shows a three-layer perceptron. These layers contain hidden units or nodes which obtain their input from the previous layer and output their results to the next layer, to both of which they are fully-connected. Nodes within each layer are not connected and have the same transfer function.

The strength of the multilayer perceptron originates from the use of non-linear sigmoidal functions in the nodes. If the nodes were linear elements, then monolayer networks with

appropriately selected weights could repeat the calculations carried out by a multilayer network (Widrow & Sterns, 1985). A multilayer perceptron with a non-linear step function and a hidden layer can solve problems in which the decision regions are open or closed convex regions. In the case of perceptrons with one hidden layer, problems with arbitrary decision regions can be solved, but more complex regions will need a greater number of nodes in the network (Hornik et al., 1995; Ilachinski, 2001).
Fundamental characteristics of a multilayer perceptron network are: (*i*) it is an adaptative method which permits the carrying out of non-linear statistics; (*ii*) fitting is made by a gradient method using the training data; (*iii*) a multilayer perceptron with three layers with step transference functions can solve any problem with arbitrary decision regions; (*iv*) noise in the patterns, the same as in the statistical fitting, does not impede their classification; (*v*) training of the connection weights must be very great; (*vi*) backpropagation algorithm usually finds the global minimum of the error function.

4.3 The backpropagation algorithm

The accuracy of the multilayer perceptron depends basically on the correct weights between nodes. The backpropagation training algorithm is an algorithm for adjusting those weights which uses a gradient descent method to minimize the mean quadratic error between the actual outputs of the perceptron and the desired outputs (Lippmann, 1987).
Let x^k_{ij} and y^k_{ij} be the input and output, respectively, for the i pattern of node j of layer k. Let ω^k_{ij} be the weight of the connection of neuron j of layer k with neuron i of the previous layer. By definition of the perceptron by layers, the following relationships are fulfilled

$$x^k_{ij} = \sum_l \omega^k_{lj} y^{k-1}_{il}; \quad y^k_{ij} = f(x^k_{ij})$$

The mean quadratic error function between the real output of the perceptron and the desired output, for a particular pattern i, is defined as $E_i = \frac{1}{2}\sum_{j,k}(y^k_{ij} - d^k_{ij})^2$, where d^k_{ij} is the desired output for pattern i of node j of layer k. In order to minimize the error function we use the descending gradient function, considering the error function E_p and the weight sequence $\omega^k_{ij}(t)$, started randomly at time $t = 0$, and adapted to successive discrete time intervals. We then have $\omega^k_{ij}(t+1) = \omega^k_{ij}(t) - \eta\, \partial E_l / \partial \omega^k_{ij}(t)$, where η is the so-called *learning rate constant*.
We can conclude that $w_{ij}(t+1) = w_{ij}(t) + \eta \delta_j x'_i$, where x'_i is the output of neuron i, and δ_j is an error term for node j. For output neurons, it must be $\delta_j = y_j(1-y_j)(d_j - y_j)$. For a hidden node j, $\delta_j = x'_j(1-x'_j)\sum_k \delta_k w_{jk}$, where k ranges over all neurons in the layers above neuron j. Internal node thresholds are adapted in a similar manner.

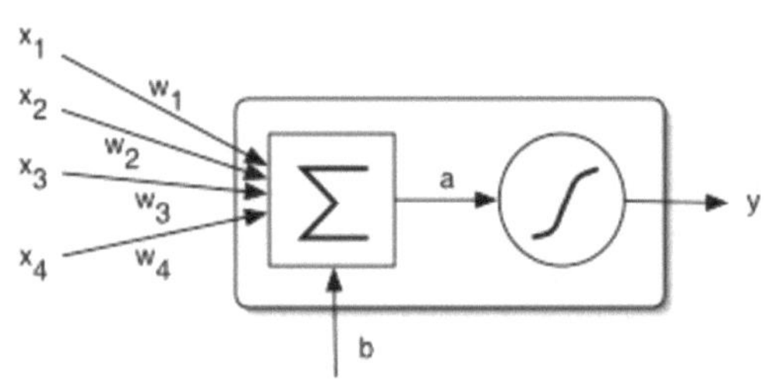

Fig. 6. Behaviour of an artificial neuron.

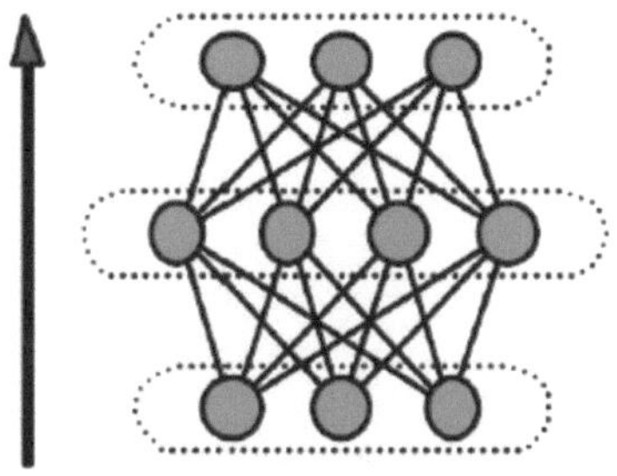

Fig. 7. A fully-connected, three-layer feed-forward perceptron neural network.

The high performance usually achieved with this backpropagation algorithm is rather surprising if we take into account the fact that the gradient method, of which the backpropagation training algorithm is a generalization, can find a local minimum of the error function instead of the desired global minimum. Some ideas for improving performance and reducing the appearance of local minimums are, for example, the addition of new nodes in the hidden layers, the lowering of the gain term used for the adaptation of weights and, above all, the initial training with a different set of random weights.

4.4 Matlab and Toolbox Neural Networks

Matlab (The MathWorks Inc, Natick, MA) is a high-level technical computing language and interactive environment for algorithm development, data visualization, data analysis, and numeric computation. It can be used in a wide range of applications, including signal and image processing, and computational biology. In an easily used environment Matlab integrates numerical analysis, the computation of matrices, the processing of signals and graphics, where the problems and solutions are expressed in a similar way to how they are expressed mathematically, avoiding the traditional programming. Matlab is an interactive system whose basic element of data is the matrix, which does not require to be dimensioned. The Matlab language is a high-level matrix/array language with control flow statements, functions, data structures, input/output, and object-oriented programming features. It allows both *programming in the small* to rapidly create quick programs you do not intend to reuse. You can also do *programming in the large* to create complex application programs intended for reuse. Neural Network Toolbox provides tools for designing, implementing, visualizing, and simulating neural networks. Neural Network Toolbox supports feedforward networks, radial basis networks, dynamic networks, self-organizing maps, and other proven network paradigms.

There are other work environments with neuronal networks. Some of them are Neural Works Professional II (Neural-Ware Inc., Pittsburgh, PA), SAS Enterprise Miner Software (SAS Institute Inc., Cary, NC), and Neural Connection (SPSS Inc., Chicago, IL).

5. ANN as a tool to identifier Glaucoma stages

For the diagnosis of Glaucoma, we propose a system of *Artificial Intelligence* that employs ANNs and integrates, jointly, the analysis of the nerve fibers of the retina from the study with scanning laser polarimetry (NFAII;GDx), perimetry and clinical data.

The present work shows an analysis of 106 eyes of 53 patients, in accordance with the stage of glaucomatous illness in which each eye was found. The groups defined include stage 0,

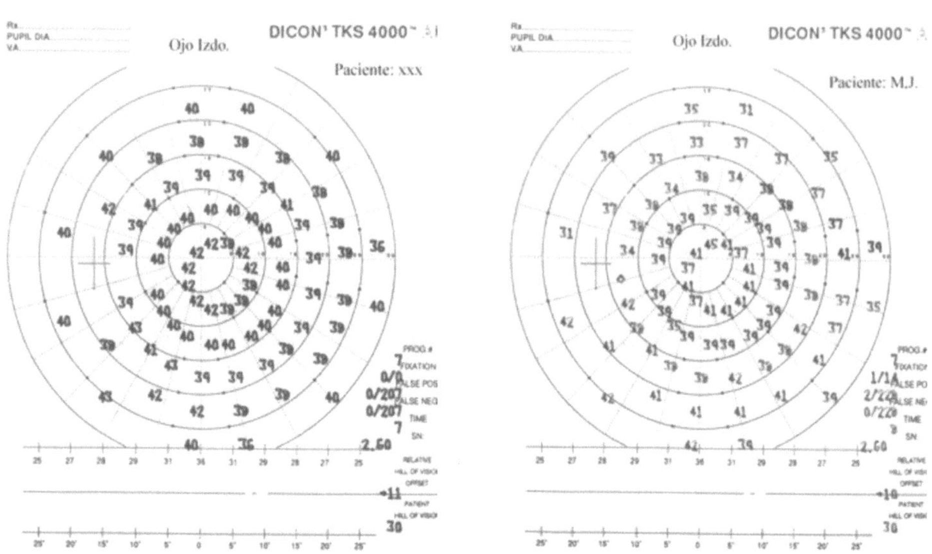

Fig. 8. Perimetry of a left eye of a normal patient (left image). Perimetry of a left eye of a patient (right image).

which corresponds to normal eyes; stage 1, for ocular hypertension; 2, for early Glaucoma; 3, for established Glaucoma; 4, for advanced Glaucoma and 5, for terminal Glaucoma. The developed ANN is a 16–30–1 multilayer perceptron provided with the Levenberg-Marquardt method (Franco Suárez-Bárcena et al., 2000; Lippmann, 1987; Widrow & Lehr, 1990).

5.1 Stages to classify

To classify the eyes in groups, besides studying IOP (Goldmann tonometry) and the ophthalmoscopic study of the optic disc by means of biometry using Volk aspheric lens (Quigley et al., 1994) Dicon TKS 4000 autoperimetry (Fig. 8) has been used for the analysis of the visual field and laser polarimetry for the measurement of the thickness of the layer of retinal nerve fibers using the NFA-II, GDX fiber analyser (Figures 3 and 4).
A classification into different groups was performed taking into account each eye of each patient separately. Thus, and taking into account the classification proposed by Caprioli (1992):

- Stage 0 (normal eye): Within this group were included patients whose IOP was lower than 21 mmHg and there was no effect on papilla nor the visual field nor of the parameters of the analyzer of the RNFL.
- Stage 1 (ocular hypertension): Formed by all the eyes that only presented an IOP equal to or greater than 21mmHg and both the exploration and the functional tests and the analysis of the RNFL were within normality.
- Stage 2 (early Glaucoma): They were eyes that presented an altered IOP and some of the following diagnostic data: effect on the papilla, incipient alteration of the visual field, decrease in the number of retinal nerve fibers.

- Stage 3 (established Glaucoma): Those eyes had IOP equal to or greater than 21 mmHg with involvement of the papilla, from moderate to significant alteration of the visual field as well as alteration of the RNFL analyzer parameters.
- Stage 4 (advanced Glaucoma): Those eyes that presented an IOP superior to 21 mmHg and an important effect, ophthalmoscopically demonstrable, on the papilla, an important alteration of the visual field and a significant alteration of the parameters of the analyser of RNFL.
- Stage 5 (terminal Glaucoma): If as well as the alterations in the IOP (equal to or greater than 21mmHg) there was papilla excavation with atrophy, the visual field with alterations proper to the terminal stage and alteration of the parameters of the analysis of the RNFL.

Table 1 shows a basic descriptive statistic by stage of the illness for the variables of study: Chamber, IOP, Papilla and Mean. These qualitative and quantitative variables are taken from the history and from the visual field of the individual. The intervals of confidence of the mean have been considered with a coefficient of confidence of 95%.

5.2 ANN variables

The input neurons receive the values of 16 input variables and the output neuron obtains the value of the output variable that corresponds with the stage of the Glaucoma for each eye. The definition of the 16 variables of input of the neuronal network consists of:

- **AGE**. Age of the patient.
- **CHAMBER**. Depth of the anterior chamber of the ocular globe.
- **IOP**. Intraocular pressure—expressed in millimetres of mercury.
- **OPTIC DISC**. Cup-to-disc ratio. If the result was less than 0.4, 0 was assigned; if between 0.4–0.5, 1 was assigned; if between 0.5–0.6, 2 was assigned and if between 0.7–0.9, 3 was assigned.

	CHAMBER *Depth of the chamber* (category)	**IOP** *Intraocular pressure* (mmHg)	**PAPILA** *Evaluation of the papilla (E/P)* (category)	**MEDIA** *Total mean of isopters of* 15°, 20°, 25°, 30°
STAGE 0 (normal eye)	$2,00 \pm 0,00$	$20,00 \pm 0,00$	$0,00 \pm 0,00$	$42,61 \pm 0,83$
STAGE 1 (ocular hypertension)	$2,00 \pm 0,36$	$22,29 \pm 0,70$	$0,00 \pm 0,00$	$41,70 \pm 1,85$
STAGE 2 (early Glaucoma)	$2,22 \pm 0,51$	$22,55 \pm 1,34$	$0,11 \pm 0,25$	$41,61 \pm 1,28$
STAGE 3 (established Glaucoma)	$2,13 \pm 0,25$	$23,96 \pm 0,89$	$0,93 \pm 0,10$	$40,39 \pm 1,32$
STAGE 4 (advanced Glaucoma)	$1,92 \pm 0,39$	$22,76 \pm 2,62$	$1,61 \pm 0,31$	$41,17 \pm 0,99$
STAGE 5 (terminal Glaucoma)	$1,93 \pm 0,21$	$25,21 \pm 2,61$	$1,54 \pm 0,31$	$39,07 \pm 2,80$
UNIVERSE	$2,02 \pm 0,12$	$23,63 \pm 0,89$	$0,94 \pm 0,16$	$40,49 \pm 1,00$

Table 1. Basic descriptive statistics by stage of illness for the variables of study: Chamber, IOP, Papilla and Mean. The intervals of confidence of the mean with coefficient of confidence of 95%.

- **FIXATION**. Fixation losses by the patient from all those performed during the autoperimetry testing of visual field examination.
- **NS, TS, NI, TI**. Average of the values of the visual field in the superior nasal, superior temporal, inferior nasal and inferior temporal quadrant, respectively.
- **MEAN**. Mean of all the values of the visual field.
- **NORMAL DEVIATION SUPERIOR, INFERIOR, TEMPORAL, NASAL**. Difference of the thickness of the nerve fibre layer employing the GDX program in the superior, inferior, temporal and nasal quadrant, respectively, for our patient compared with the normal patient of the same race and age.
- **NUMBER**. Experimental number extracted from all the values on acquiring an image employing NFA-II, GDX.
- **MEAN THICKNESS**. Mean of the thickness of all the pixels of the image; utilising the 65,536 points in an image considered valid.

The unaffected patients present a constant value in the variable of depth of the anterior chamber. The Mann-Whitney test establishes that there are no significant differences between the stage of illness groups for this variable. The graph of error for the variable chamber reveals that the different trustworthiness intervals of the affected patients overlap.

5.3 ANN results

The used ANN is a multilayer perceptron with backpropagation with a hidden layer provided with the Levenberg-Marquardt method. The input layer consists of 16 neurons, the hidden layer has 30 neurons and the output layer is a single neuron. The single neuron output layer with a logistic transfer function provided the network output: glaucomatous stage of the eye. The implementation of the ANN model has been carried out by means of the scientific computation platform R2010 *M*atlab, using the toolbox of *N*eural Networks (The MathWorks Inc, Natick, MA). Once the model had been defined, half the data were randomly employed to train the ANN. The learning was carried out with half of the data and with the training function of gradient descent w/momentum backpropagation and was checked by the diagnosis of an ophthalmologist, expert in glaucoma. The evolution of the process of learning is shown in Figure 9.

The model of neuronal network has been evaluated from the other half of the data. A 100% correct classification of each eye in the corresponding stage of glaucoma has been achieved. Therefore, the specificity and sensitivity are 100%.

With regard to the variable IOP, the unaffected patients take a constant value. There is a significant difference between the group of patients without illness and those affected regarding the variable IOP (p=0,001), according to the Mann-Whitney test. The graph of error for the variable IOP (Fig. 10) shows that the different intervals of confidence of the affected patients are overlapped among themselves.

The unaffected and ocular hypertense patients, which is to say, belonging to groups 0 and 1 do not present variation in the variable of relation excavation/papilla. There is a significant difference between the groups of subjects without illness and those affected with regard to the variable PAPILLA (p=0,004) according to the Mann-Whitney test.

Regarding the variable of mean, which represents the perimetric functional capacity and corresponds to the mean of all the values obtained from the visual field by autoperimetry there is a significant difference between the group of subjects without illness and the affected patients with respect to the mean variable (p=0,022), according to the Mann-Whitney test.

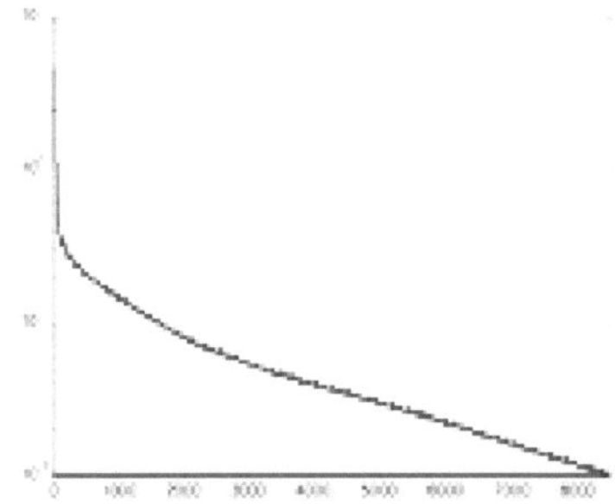

Fig. 9. Training evolution of our proposed ANN model.

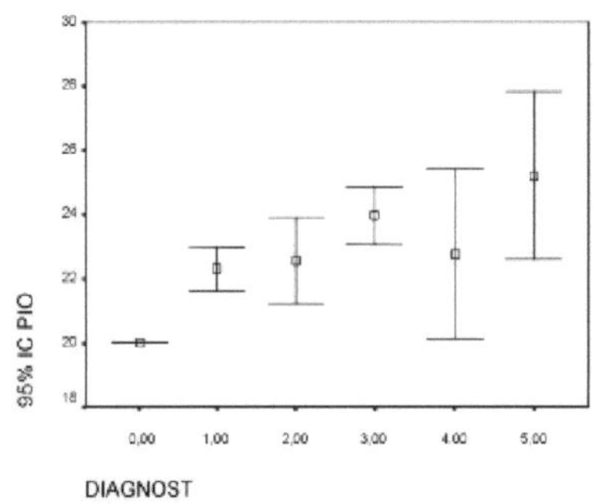

Fig. 10. Graph of error of the variable IOP referring to the Intraocular Pressure in mmHg for each of the groups (0,00 Stage 0 (normal eye): IOP was inferior to 21 mmHg; 1,00 Stage1 (ocular hypertension $\geq$ 21 mmHg; 2,00 Stage 2 (early Glaucoma); 3,00 Stage 3 (established Glaucoma); 4,00 Stage 4 (advanced Glaucoma); 5,00 Stage 5 (terminal Glaucoma)) of illness. The confidence intervals of the mean of coefficient of confidence of 95%.

6. Discussion

Glaucoma constitutes a pathology of multifactorial etiology, thus establishing an objective alteration in the different diagnostic tests represents the principal element for the performance of a certain diagnosis of glaucoma. This fact is especially transcendent in those situations in which the possible precocious diagnosis entails a therapeutic action which in a fundamental way affects the prognosis of the illness.

At present no diagnostic test can be considered alone and constitute in itself a diagnostic criterion. It is accepted that IOP is a risk factor, without being considered a specific and discriminatory element of glaucoma, in addition, when the term of normotensional or low pressure glaucoma has been established to define a variant in which the glaucomatous neuropathy takes place without the participation of an elevated pressure. Nonetheless, it continues to represent an objective clinical parameter and highly reproducible, clearly correlated with the development of the illness, being, moreover, one of the factors of risk which can be medically and surgically acted upon.

It is evident that in spite of the increase of specificity and sensitivity of the diagnostic tests which are applied to glaucoma, such as computerised perimetry or the analysis of the nerve fibers of the retina, clinical judgment persists as the primordial element, based on the phenotypic characteristics of the patient, the clinical signs and monitoring, all performed by an expert evaluator in glaucoma.

With regard to the clinical significance, the most relevant datum of the exploration in glaucoma is the ophthalmoscopic evaluation of the papilla (Sommer et al., 1991). It is simple for an ophthalmologist to recognize a glaucomatous alteration of the papilla in the case of terminal (G4) or advanced (G5) glaucoma and even, in its case, to discriminate the papilla alteration for the group of established glaucoma (G3). Nevertheless, incipient alterations entail a greater difficulty in discrimination.

The cup-to-disc ratio has been considered a valid parameter to discriminate between normal and glaucomatous subjects as well as to quantify the progress of the disease. At present, however, another series of findings are included that complete the clinical evaluation, as are the disc haemorrhages in splinter, the presence of optic head notch, more frequent on the temporal side. This last has been considered as a relatively specific parameter of incipient glaucomatous damage (Fingeret et al., 2005).

The structural alterations produced in glaucoma can be determined through the study of clinical signs and the ophthalmic examination of the papilla. Nonetheless, the functional alterations are more precocious. These alterations are demonstrated in the study of the visual field which contributes the translation of the damage of ganglion cells of the retina in the context of glaucomatous illness.

We therefore consider that even when the mean functional capacity is not the only parameter to be evaluated it results, in our study to be a relatively non-specific datum as it is unable to differentiate between the different groups in accordance with the stages of the glaucomatous illness. Nevertheless, and even when the criteria of selection were sufficient to not include defects of refraction, opacities of lens or artefacts, due to other pathologies, this fact has not influenced, in a fundamental manner, the results of the autoperimetry.

The variability of the perimetry as an exploratory method, as well as the lack of reproducibility, is one of its principal inconveniences. Perhaps the most important is that it is a subjective test that, moreover, depends on the training and collaboration of the patient. This fact is even more important in the present forms of perimetry whose test is of greater complexity than that of the conventional one (Racette et al., 2008; Sakata et al., 2007).

Autoperimetry is a very simplified method regarding training of the patient and monitoring of the test, allowing its management by unqualified personnel. Moreover, it is performed in a short period of time. The interpretation of the field is relatively simple and comparable with conventional perimetries, using a more simple series of algorithms, they cannot be compared with the more diffused standards of the computerized perimeters, nonetheless permit a rapid interpretation.

The evaluation of the campimetric defects, however, are not exclusively based on the quantitative results, but also on the qualitative characteristics, such as the location, shape and extension of the scotomas. The diagnostic efficiency is greater when the indexes that incorporate these characteristics are considered (Sommer et al., 1991).

The incipient lesions do not present a high specificity, thus the interpretation of a visual field lacks objectivity and is based both on the clinical experience from which the results are analysed and from the evaluation of the contralateral eye and the performance of the test on more occasions.

For all these reasons the use of a system of Artificial Intelligence has been proposed so that analysing the parameters obtained in the perimetry such as the indexes and spatial considerations it will be possible to produce a diagnosis (Burgansky-Eliash et al., 2005; Henson et al., 1997; Huang & Chen, 2005).

Diverse authors have developed neuronal networks and confirmed their utility in the differentiation and spatial classification of the perimetric defects, after training the neuronal network and an index of specificity and sensitivity of over 80% has been established in the different studies (Antón et al., 1997; Henson et al., 1997).

In our study, and commencing from the efficacy of the systems of neuronal networks applied to the recognition of the visual fields in glaucomatous pathology we have performed the design of a neuronal network with the objective of, employing the great quantity of indexes, parameters, variables and algorithms derived from the autoperimetry and the analysis of the CNFR by laser polarimetry, being able to carry out an assignation of patients in the diverse subgroups of evolution of the primary glaucoma of open angle.

At present the clinical exploration does not contribute sufficient data to produce a diagnosis or establish the adequate stage of evolution. Equally it is not possible to differentiate among the group of ocular hypertension Those who should be treated, since later they develop a glaucoma. This possibility of discrimination at present settles in an essential manner, in functional tests like perimetry or in the objective quantification of the structural damage of the optic nerve. Similarly, none of these tests can be considered in an isolated fashion, as we have mentioned previously. Even when both possess a high index of correlation it is not possible to forego the data from clinical exploration to perform a certain diagnosis. In addition, in the interpretation of the clinical and quantitative data it is necessary in all cases that an expert participates which in many cases is found in the context of the exploration (Bowd et al., 2002; 2005; Goldbaum et al., 2005; Shah et al., 2006; Zhu et al., 2010).

In the neuronal network designed for our study a total of 16 variables of work were used which formed the inputs for the neuronal network, establishing the diagnosis as the only variable of output of the model. The layer of neurons of input was composed by indices of polarimetry together with parameters from the autoperimetry and those derived from the clinical exploration. The occult/hidden layer was composed by thirty nodes or neurons and a single output to constitute a neuronal network of multilayer perceptron with retropropagation.

For the function of training the data of 50% of the patients of our data base were used including normal and glaucomatous patients in diverse stages at random, achieving with a total of 8000 cycles an adequate model to achieve the threshold of mean error of the neuronal network. The performance of classification of the designed network was validated with the remainder of the data of the other 50% of the patients of the database.

We have been able to prove that the assignation to each of the subgroups of evolution of glaucoma was 100% achieving a specificity and sensitivity of 100%. Mutlukan & Keating (1994) achieves similar percentages with a neuronal network of retropropagation designed for the identification of visual fields with three layers with a hidden layer of 40 nodes.

The updating and improvement of technological tools of systems like Bayesian machine learning (Boden et al., 2007; Bowd et al., 2008) or the neuronal networks where the interpretation of structural methods such as optical coherence tomography or GDx polarimetry and functional ones such as standard automated perimetry can be combined will increase the yield in the detection of glaucoma and its progression.

7. References

AIGS (2004). Glaucoma diagnosis structure and function reports and consensus statements, *1st Global AIGS Consensus Meeting on Structure and Function in the Management of Glaucoma*, Kugler Publications, Amsterdam.

Antón, A., Jordano, J. & Maquet, J. (1995). Sistema experto de diagnóstico de glaucoma: "glaucom easy", *Archivos de la Sociedad Española de Oftalmología* **69**: 23–28.

Antón, A., Zangwill, L., Emdadi, A. & Weinreb, R. N. (1997). Nerve fiber layer measurements with scanning laser polarimetry in ocular hypertension, *Arch Ophthalmol* **115**(3): 331–4.

Arbib, M. (1995). *Handbook of brain theory and neural netwoks*, MIT Press, Cambridge, MA.

Asman, P., Heijl, A., Olsson, J. & Rootzen, H. (1992). Spatial analyses of glaucomatous visual fields; a comparison with traditional visual field indices, *Acta Ophthalmol (Copenh)* **70**(5): 679–86.

Azuaje, F., Dubitzky, W., Lopes, P., Black, N., Adamson, K., Wu, X. & White, J. A. (1999). Predicting coronary disease risk based on short-term rr interval measurements: a neural network approach, *Artif Intell Med* **15**(3): 275–97.

Bengtsson, B., Bizios, D. & Heijl, A. (2005). Effects of input data on the performance of a neural network in distinguishing normal and glaucomatous visual fields, *Invest Ophthalmol Vis Sci* **46**(10): 3730–6.

Boden, C., Chan, K., Sample, P. A., Hao, J., Lee, T. W., Zangwill, L. M., Weinreb, R. N. & Goldbaum, M. H. (2007). Assessing visual field clustering schemes using machine learning classifiers in standard perimetry, *Invest Ophthalmol Vis Sci* **48**(12): 5582–90.

Bowd, C., Chan, K., Zangwill, L. M., Goldbaum, M. H., Lee, T. W., Sejnowski, T. J. & Weinreb, R. N. (2002). Comparing neural networks and linear discriminant functions for glaucoma detection using confocal scanning laser ophthalmoscopy of the optic disc, *Invest Ophthalmol Vis Sci* **43**(11): 3444–54.

Bowd, C., Hao, J., Tavares, I. M., Medeiros, F. A., Zangwill, L. M., Lee, T. W., Sample, P. A., Weinreb, R. N. & Goldbaum, M. H. (2008). Bayesian machine learning classifiers for combining structural and functional measurements to classify healthy and glaucomatous eyes, *Invest Ophthalmol Vis Sci* **49**(3): 945–53.

Bowd, C., Medeiros, F. A., Zhang, Z., Zangwill, L. M., Hao, J., Lee, T. W., Sejnowski, T. J., Weinreb, R. N. & Goldbaum, M. H. (2005). Relevance vector machine and support vector machine classifier analysis of scanning laser polarimetry retinal nerve fiber layer measurements, *Invest Ophthalmol Vis Sci* **46**(4): 1322–9.

Bowd, C., Zangwill, L. M., Berry, C. C., Blumenthal, E. Z., Vasile, C., Sanchez-Galeana, C., Bosworth, C. F., Sample, P. A. & Weinreb, R. N. (2001). Detecting early glaucoma by assessment of retinal nerve fiber layer thickness and visual function, *Invest Ophthalmol Vis Sci* **42**(9): 1993–2003.

Bowd, C., Zangwill, L. M., Medeiros, F. A., Hao, J., Chan, K., Lee, T. W., Sejnowski, T. J., Goldbaum, M. H., Sample, P. A., Crowston, J. G. & Weinreb, R. N. (2004). Confocal scanning laser ophthalmoscopy classifiers and stereophotograph evaluation for prediction of visual field abnormalities in glaucoma-suspect eyes, *Invest Ophthalmol Vis Sci* **45**(7): 2255–62.

Brigatti, L., Hoffman, D. & Caprioli, J. (1996). Neural networks to identify glaucoma with structural and functional measurements, *Am J Ophthalmol* **121**(5): 511–21.

Burgansky-Eliash, Z., Wollstein, G., Chu, T., Ramsey, J. D., Glymour, C., Noecker, R. J., Ishikawa, H. & Schuman, J. S. (2005). Optical coherence tomography machine learning classifiers for glaucoma detection: a preliminary study, *Invest Ophthalmol Vis Sci* **46**(11): 4147–52.

Caprioli, J. (1990). The contour of the juxtapapillary nerve fiber layer in glaucoma, *Ophthalmology* **97**(3): 358–65; discussion 365–6.

Caprioli, J. (1992). Discrimination between normal and glaucomatous eyes, *Invest Ophthalmol Vis Sci* **33**(1): 153–9.

Caprioli, J. & Miller, J. M. (1988). Videographic measurements of optic nerve topography in glaucoma, *Invest Ophthalmol Vis Sci* **29**(8): 1294–8.

Caprioli, J. & Miller, J. M. (1989). Measurement of relative nerve fiber layer surface height in glaucoma, *Ophthalmology* **96**(5): 633–39; discussion 639–41.

Caprioli, J., Ortiz-Colberg, R., Miller, J. M. & Tressler, C. (1989). Measurements of peripapillary nerve fiber layer contour in glaucoma, *Am J Ophthalmol* **108**(4): 404–13.

Chan, K., Lee, T. W., Sample, P. A., Goldbaum, M. H., Weinreb, R. N. & Sejnowski, T. J. (2002). Comparison of machine learning and traditional classifiers in glaucoma diagnosis, *IEEE Trans Biomed Eng* **49**(9): 963–74.

Chauhan, B. C., Drance, S. M. & Lai, C. (1989). A cluster analysis for threshold perimetry, *Graefes Arch Clin Exp Ophthalmol* **227**(3): 216–20.

European Glaucoma Society, E. (2008). *Terminology and Guidelines for Glaucoma*, Ed. Dogma, Savona, Italy.

Ferreras, A., Pablo, L. E., Pajarin, A. B., Larrosa, J. M., Polo, V. & Honrubia, F. M. (2008). Logistic regression analysis for early glaucoma diagnosis using optical coherence tomography, *Arch Ophthalmol* **126**(4): 465–70.

Fingeret, M., Medeiros, F. A., Susanna, R., J. & Weinreb, R. N. (2005). Five rules to evaluate the optic disc and retinal nerve fiber layer for glaucoma, *Optometry* **76**(11): 661–8.

Franco Suárez-Bárcena, I., Santos-García, G., E., H. G. & A., F. S. (2000). Aplicación de redes neuronales a la clasificación clínica en estadíos de glaucoma, *76 Congreso de la Sociedad Española de Oftalmología*, Madrid.

Gardner, G. G., Keating, D., Williamson, T. H. & Elliott, A. T. (1996). Automatic detection of diabetic retinopathy using an artificial neural network: a screening tool, *Br J Ophthalmol* **80**(11): 940–4.

Goldbaum, M. H., Sample, P. A., Chan, K., Williams, J., Lee, T. W., Blumenthal, E., Girkin, C. A., Zangwill, L. M., Bowd, C., Sejnowski, T. & Weinreb, R. N. (2002). Comparing machine learning classifiers for diagnosing glaucoma from standard automated perimetry, *Invest Ophthalmol Vis Sci* **43**(1): 162–9.

Goldbaum, M. H., Sample, P. A., White, H., Colt, B., Raphaelian, P., Fechtner, R. D. & Weinreb, R. N. (1994). Interpretation of automated perimetry for glaucoma by neural network, *Invest Ophthalmol Vis Sci* **35**(9): 3362–73.

Goldbaum, M. H., Sample, P. A., Zhang, Z., Chan, K., Hao, J., Lee, T. W., Boden, C., Bowd, C., Bourne, R., Zangwill, L., Sejnowski, T., Spinak, D. & Weinreb, R. N. (2005). Using unsupervised learning with independent component analysis to identify patterns of glaucomatous visual field defects, *Invest Ophthalmol Vis Sci* **46**(10): 3676–83.

Gordon, M. O., Beiser, J. A., Brandt, J. D., Heuer, D. K., Higginbotham, E. J., Johnson, C. A., Keltner, J. L., Miller, J. P., Parrish, R. K., n., Wilson, M. R. & Kass, M. A. (2002). The ocular hypertension treatment study: baseline factors that predict the onset of primary open-angle glaucoma, *Arch Ophthalmol* **120**(6): 714–20; discussion 829–30.

Hecht-Nielsen, R. (1990). *Neurocomputing*, Addison-Wesley, Reading, MA.

Henson, D. B., Spenceley, S. E. & Bull, D. R. (1997). Artificial neural network analysis of noisy visual field data in glaucoma, *Artif Intell Med* **10**(2): 99–113.

Hernández Galilea, E., Santos-García, G. & Suárez-Bárcena, I. (2007). Identification of glaucoma stages with artificial neural networks using retinal nerve fibre layer analysis and visual field parameters, *in* E. Corchado, J. Corchado & A. Abraham (eds), *Innovations in Hybrid Intelligent Systems*, Vol. 44 of *Advances in Intelligent and Soft Computing*, Springer Berlin / Heidelberg, pp. 418–424.

Hornik, K., Stinchcombe, M., White, H. & Auer, P. (1995). Degree of approximation results for feedforward networks approximating unknown mappings and their derivatives, *Neural Computation* **6**(6): 1262–1275.

Huang, M. L. & Chen, H. Y. (2005). Development and comparison of automated classifiers for glaucoma diagnosis using stratus optical coherence tomography, *Invest Ophthalmol Vis Sci* **46**(11): 4121–9.

Ilachinski, A. (2001). *Cellular automata*, World Scientific Publishing Company.

Johnson, C. A., Adams, A. J., Casson, E. J. & Brandt, J. D. (1993). Blue-on-yellow perimetry can predict the development of glaucomatous visual field loss, *Arch Ophthalmol* **111**(5): 645–50.

Lietman, T., Eng, J., Katz, J. & Quigley, H. A. (1999). Neural networks for visual field analysis: how do they compare with other algorithms?, *J Glaucoma* **8**(1): 77–80.

Lin, S. C., Singh, K., Jampel, H. D., Hodapp, E. A., Smith, S. D., Francis, B. A., Dueker, D. K., Fechtner, R. D., Samples, J. S., Schuman, J. S. & Minckler, D. S. (2007). Optic nerve head and retinal nerve fiber layer analysis: a report by the american academy of ophthalmology, *Ophthalmology* **114**(10): 1937–49.

Lippmann, R. (1987). An introduction to computing with neural nets, *IEEE ASSP Magazine* **4**: 4–22.

Lippmann, R. & Kukolich, L. (1995). Using neural networks to predict the risk of cardiac bypass operations, *in* S. Rogers & D. Ruck (eds), *Applications and science of artificial neural networks*, SPIE, pp. 650–660.

Lippmann, R. P. & Shahian, D. M. (1997). Coronary artery bypass risk prediction using neural networks, *Ann Thorac Surg* **63**(6): 1635–43.

Lu, A. T., Wang, M., Varma, R., Schuman, J. S., Greenfield, D. S., Smith, S. D. & Huang, D. (2008). Combining nerve fiber layer parameters to optimize glaucoma diagnosis with optical coherence tomography, *Ophthalmology* **115**(8): 1352–7, 1357 e1–2.

Mardin, C. Y., Peters, A., Horn, F., Junemann, A. G. & Lausen, B. (2006). Improving glaucoma diagnosis by the combination of perimetry and hrt measurements, *J Glaucoma* **15**(4): 299–305.

Medeiros, F. A., Zangwill, L. M., Bowd, C., Vessani, R. M., Susanna, R., J. & Weinreb, R. N. (2005). Evaluation of retinal nerve fiber layer, optic nerve head, and macular thickness measurements for glaucoma detection using optical coherence tomography, *Am J Ophthalmol* **139**(1): 44–55.

Medeiros, F. A., Zangwill, L. M., Bowd, C. & Weinreb, R. N. (2004). Comparison of the gdx vcc scanning laser polarimeter, hrt ii confocal scanning laser ophthalmoscope, and stratus oct optical coherence tomograph for the detection of glaucoma, *Arch Ophthalmol* **122**(6): 827–37.

Miller, E. & Caprioli, J. (1991). Regional and long-term variability of fundus measurements made with computer-image analysis, *Am J Ophthalmol* **112**(2): 171–6.

Mutlukan, E. & Keating, D. (1994). Visual field interpretation with a personal computer based neural network, *Eye (Lond)* **8 (Pt 3)**: 321–3.

Papalolukas, C., Fotiadis, D. I., Likas, A. & Michalis, L. K. (2002). An ischemia detection method based on artificial neural networks, *Artif Intell Med* **24**: 167–178.

Peña Reyes, C. A. & Sipper, M. (2000). Evolutionary computation in medicine: an overview, *Artif Intell Med* **19**: 1–23.

Peli, E., Hedges, T. R. & Schwartz, B. (1986). Computerized enhancement of retinal nerve fiber layer, *Acta Ophthalmol (Copenh)* **64**(2): 113–22.

Quigley, H. A. (1985). Better methods in glaucoma diagnosis, *Arch Ophthalmol* **103**(2): 186–9.

Quigley, H. A., Dunkelberger, G. R. & Green, W. R. (1989). Retinal ganglion cell atrophy correlated with automated perimetry in human eyes with glaucoma, *Am J Ophthalmol* **107**(5): 453–64.

Quigley, H. A., Enger, C., Katz, J., Sommer, A., Scott, R. & Gilbert, D. (1994). Risk factors for the development of glaucomatous visual field loss in ocular hypertension, *Arch Ophthalmol* **112**(5): 644–9.

Racette, L., Medeiros, F. A., Zangwill, L. M., Ng, D., Weinreb, R. N. & Sample, P. A. (2008). Diagnostic accuracy of the matrix 24-2 and original n-30 frequency-doubling technology tests compared with standard automated perimetry, *Invest Ophthalmol Vis Sci* **49**(3): 954–60.

Ruggeri, A. & Pajaro, S. (2002). Automatic recognition of cell layers in corneal confocal microscopy images, *Comput Methods Programs Biomed* **68**(1): 25–35.

Rumelhart, D. & McClelland, J. (1986). *Parallel distributed processing*, MIT Press, Cambridge, MA.

Sakata, L. M., Deleon-Ortega, J., Arthur, S. N., Monheit, B. E. & Girkin, C. A. (2007). Detecting visual function abnormalities using the swedish interactive threshold algorithm and matrix perimetry in eyes with glaucomatous appearance of the optic disc, *Arch Ophthalmol* **125**(3): 340–5.

Sample, P. A., Taylor, J. D., Martinez, G. A., Lusky, M. & Weinreb, R. N. (1993). Short-wavelength color visual fields in glaucoma suspects at risk, *Am J Ophthalmol* **115**(2): 225–33.

Santos-García, G. (ed.) (1990). *The Hopfield and Hamming networks applied to the automatic speech recognition of the five Spanish vowels*, Artificial Neural Nets and Genetic Algorithms, Springer-Verlag, Wien.

Santos-García, G., Palomino, M. & Verdejo, A. (2008). Rewriting logic using strategies for neural networks: an implementation in maude, *in* J. M. Corchado, S. Rodríguez, J. Llinas & J. M. Molina (eds), *International Symposium on Distributed Computing and Artificial Intelligence (DCAI 2008)*, Vol. 50 of *Advances in Soft Computing*, Springer, Salamanca, pp. 424–433.

Santos-García, G., Varela, G., Novoa, N. & Jiménez, M. F. (2004). Prediction of postoperative morbidity after lung resection using an artificial neural network ensemble, *Artificial Intelligence in Medicine* **30**(1): 61–69.

Shah, N. N., Bowd, C., Medeiros, F. A., Weinreb, R. N., Sample, P. A., Hoffmann, E. M. & Zangwill, L. M. (2006). Combining structural and functional testing for detection of glaucoma, *Ophthalmology* **113**(9): 1593–602.

Sharma, P., Sample, P. A., Zangwill, L. M. & Schuman, J. S. (2008). Diagnostic tools for glaucoma detection and management, *Surv Ophthalmol* **53 Suppl1**: S17–32.

Shields, M. B. (1992). *Textbook of glaucoma*, 3rd ed edn, : Williams & Wilkins, Baltimore [etc.].

Sivakumar, R., Ravindran, G., Muthayya, M., Lakshminarayanan, S. & Velmurughendran, C. U. (2005). Diabetic retinopathy analysis, *J Biomed Biotechnol* **2005**(1): 20–27.

Sommer, A., Katz, J., Quigley, H. A., Miller, N. R., Robin, A. L., Richter, R. C. & Witt, K. A. (1991). Clinically detectable nerve fiber atrophy precedes the onset of glaucomatous field loss, *Arch Ophthalmol* **109**(1): 77–83.

Song, X., Song, K. & Chen, Y. (2005). A computer-based diagnosis system for early glaucoma screening, *Conf Proc IEEE Eng Med Biol Soc* **6**: 6608–11.

Tjon-Fo-Sang, M. J., de Vries, J. & Lemij, H. G. (1996). Measurement by nerve fiber analyzer of retinal nerve fiber layer thickness in normal subjects and patients with ocular hypertension, *Am J Ophthalmol* **122**(2): 220–7.

Tu, J. V., Weinstein, M. C., McNeil, B. J. & Naylor, C. D. (1998). Predicting mortality after coronary artery bypass surgery: what do artificial neural networks learn? the steering committee of the cardiac care network of ontario, *Med Decis Making* **18**(2): 229–35.

Uchida, H., Brigatti, L. & Caprioli, J. (1996). Detection of structural damage from glaucoma with confocal laser image analysis, *Invest Ophthalmol Vis Sci* **37**(12): 2393–401.

Villar-Gómez, R. & Santos-García, G. (1994). Multilayer perceptron applied to the automatic speech recognition of the spanish vowels, *Sci Bull, Ser A: Appl Math Phys* **56**.

Weinreb, R. N., Shakiba, S. & Zangwill, L. (1995). Scanning laser polarimetry to measure the nerve fiber layer of normal and glaucomatous eyes, *Am J Ophthalmol* **119**(5): 627–36.

Widrow, B. & Lehr, M. (1990). 30 years of adaptative neural networks: Perceptron, madaline, and backpropagation, *Proceedings of the IEEE*, Vol. 78, pp. 1415–1442.

Widrow, B. & Sterns, S. (1985). *Adaptive signal processing*, Prentice Hall.

Zangwill, L. M., Bowd, C., Berry, C. C., Williams, J., Blumenthal, E. Z., Sanchez-Galeana, C. A., Vasile, C. & Weinreb, R. N. (2001). Discriminating between normal and glaucomatous eyes using the heidelberg retina tomograph, gdx nerve fiber analyzer, and optical coherence tomograph, *Arch Ophthalmol* **119**(7): 985–93.

Zhou, Q. (2006). Retinal scanning laser polarimetry and methods to compensate for corneal birefringence, *Bull Soc Belge Ophtalmol* **302**: 89–106.

Zhu, H., Crabb, D. P., Schlottmann, P. G., Lemij, H. G., Reus, N. J., Healey, P. R., Mitchell, P., Ho, T. & Garway-Heath, D. F. (2010). Predicting visual function from the measurements of retinal nerve fiber layer structure, *Invest Ophthalmol Vis Sci* **51**(11): 5657–66.